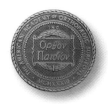

American Academy of Orthopaedic Surgeons

OKU

Orthopaedic Knowledge Update:

Trauma

3

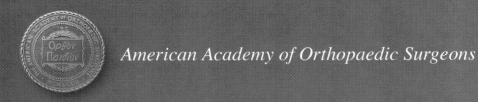

American Academy of Orthopaedic Surgeons

OKU

Orthopaedic Knowledge Update:

Trauma

3

Edited by
Michael R. Baumgaertner, MD
Paul Tornetta III, MD

Developed by
Orthopaedic Trauma Association

Published 2005
by the American Academy of Orthopaedic Surgeons
6300 North River Road
Rosemont, IL 60018
1-800-626-6726

Third Edition
Copyright ©2005 by the
American Academy of Orthopaedic Surgeons

ISBN

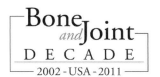

Bone *and* Joint
DECADE
— 2002 - USA - 2011 —

Acknowledgments

Editorial Board, OKU: Trauma 3

Jeffrey O. Anglen, MD, FACS
Department of Orthopaedics
Indiana University and Purdue University
Indianapolis, Indiana

Michael R. Baumgaertner, MD
Department of Orthopaedics
Yale University
New Haven, Connecticut

Jens R. Chapman, MD
Department of Orthopaedics
University of Washington Harborview Medical Center
Seattle, Washington

Kenneth J. Koval, MD
Dartmouth Hitchcock Medical Center
Lebanon, New Hampshire

Mark C. Reilly, MD
Department of Orthopaedics
New Jersey Medical School
Newark, New Jersey

Emil H. Schemitsch, MD
Chief of the Orthopedic Division
St. Michael's Hospital
University of Toronto
Toronto, Ontario, Canada

Andrew H. Schmidt, MD
Department of Orthopaedics
Hennepin County Medical Center
Minneapolis, Minnesota

Michael D. Stover, MD
Department of Orthopaedics
Loyola University Medical Center
Maywood, Illinois

David C. Teague, MD
Health Science-Department of Orthopaedics
University of Oklahoma
Oklahoma City, Oklahoma

Paul Tornetta III, MD
Department of Orthopaedics
Boston Medical Center
Boston, Massachusetts

Orthopaedic Trauma Association Board of Directors, 2005-2006

Paul Tornetta III, MD
President
Michael J. Bosse, MD
President-Elect
Robert A. Probe, MD
Secretary
Alan L. Jones, MD
Chief Financial Officer
Roy Sanders, MD
Immediate Past President
James P. Stannard, MD
Member at Large
Richard E. Buckley
Member at Large
Melvin P. Rosenwasser, MD
Member at Large
Ross K. Leighton, MD
Annual Program Chair

American Academy of Orthopaedic Surgeons Board of Directors, 2005

Stuart L. Weinstein, MD
President
Richard F. Kyle, MD
First Vice President
James H. Beaty, MD
Second Vice President
Edward A. Toriello, MD
Treasurer
Robert W. Bucholz, MD
James H. Herndon, MD
Gordon M. Aamoth, MD
Oheneba Boachie-Adjei, MD
Frances A. Farley, MD
Kristy Weber, MD
Frank B. Kelly, MD
Dwight W. Burney III, MD
Matthew S. Shapiro, MD
Mark C. Gebhardt, MD
Andrew N. Pollak, MD
Joseph C. McCarthy, MD
Leslie L. Altick
William L. Healy, MD
Karen L. Hackett (*Ex-Officio*), FACHE, CAE

Staff

Mark Wieting, *Chief Education Officer*
Marilyn L. Fox, PhD, *Director, Department of Publications*
Lisa Moore, *Managing Editor*
Keith Huff, *Senior Editor*
Kathleen Anderson, *Medical Editor*
Mary Steermann, *Manager, Production and Archives*
Sophie Tosta, *Assistant Production Manager*
Susan Morritz Baim, *Production Coordinator*
Michael Bujewski, *Database Coordinator*
Courtney Astle, *Production Database Associate*
Karen Danca, *Production Assistant*

Contributors

Samuel G. Agnew, MD, FACS
Pee Dee Orthopaedic Associates
Florence, South Carolina

Daniel T. Altman, MD
Director, Orthopaedic Spine Trauma
Department of Orthopaedic Surgery
Allegheny General Hospital
Pittsburgh, Pennsylvania

Marisa P. Andrews, CPC, CST
Coding Quality Assessment and Education
  Supervisor
Anesthesia Department
Scott and White Hospital
Temple, Texas

Jeffrey O. Anglen, MD, FACS
Department of Orthopaedics
Indiana University and Purdue University
Indianapolis, Indiana

Carlo Bellabarba, MD
Department of Orthopaedics
University of Washington Harborview
  Medical Center
Seattle, Washington

Michael J. Bellino, MD
Assistant Professor
Orthopaedic Surgery Department
Stanford University Medical Center
Stanford, California

Mohit Bhandari, MD, MSc, FRCSC
Clinical Epidemiology and Biostatistics
  Department
McMaster University
Hamilton, Ontario, Canada

Christopher M. Bono, MD
Assistant Professor of Orthopaedic Surgery
Department of Orthopaedic Surgery
Boston University Medical Center
Boston, Massachusetts

Michael J. Bosse, MD
Orthopaedic Trauma Surgeon
Department of Orthopaedic Surgery
Carolinas Medical Center
Charlotte, North Carolina

Michael E. Brage, MD
Assistant Professor of Clinical Orthopaedic
  Surgery
Department of Orthopaedics
University of California
San Diego, California

Greg A. Brown, MD, PhD
Assistant Professor
Department of Orthopaedic Surgery
University of Minnesota
Minneapolis, Minnesota
Regions Hospital
Saint Paul, Minnesota

Lisa K. Cannada, MD
Assistant Professor
Assistant Chief of Orthopaedics/Trauma
Department of Orthopaedics
Grady Memorial Hospital
Atlanta, Georgia

DuWayne A. Carlson, MD
Orthopaedic Traumatologist
Department of Orthopaedics Indianapolis
Methodist Hospital
Indianapolis, Indiana

Jens R. Chapman, MD
Department of Orthopaedics
University of Washington Harborview
  Medical Center
Seattle, Washington

Peter A. Cole, MD
Associate Professor
University of Minnesota
Chief
Department of Orthopaedic Surgery
Regions Hospital
Saint Paul, Minnesota

Cory A. Collinge, MD
Orthopaedic Specialty Associates
Fort Worth, Texas

Carol Copeland, MD
Shock Trauma Orthopaedics
Baltimore, Maryland

Charles N. Cornell, MD
Professor of Clinical Orthopedic Surgery
Weill Medical College of Cornell University
Department of Orthopedics
Hospital for Special Surgery
New York, New York

Kyle F. Dickson, MD
Associate Professor of Orthopaedic Surgery
Tulane University School of Medicine
New Orleans, Louisiana

Douglas R. Dirschl, MD
Department of Orthopaedics
University of North Carolina at Chapel Hill
Chapel Hill, North Carolina

Paul J. Dougherty, MD
Chief, Orthopaedic Trauma Division
Orthopaedic Surgery Residency
  Program Director
Henry Ford Hospital
Detroit, Michigan

Kenneth A. Egol, MD
Chief Trauma Service
Department of Orthopaedic Surgery
New York University Hospital for Joint
  Diseases
New York, New York

Jonathan S. Erulkar, MD
Department of Orthopaedics and
  Rehabilitation
Yale University School of Medicine
New Haven, Connecticut

John M. Flynn, MD
Attending Surgeon
Department of Orthopaedics
The Children's Hospital of Philadelphia
Assistant Professor
Department of Orthopaedics
University of Pennsylvania School of
  Medicine
Philadelphia, Pennsylvania

Robert A. Gallo, MD
Department of Orthopaedics
Allegheny General Hospital
Pittsburgh, Pennsylvania

John T. Gorczyca, MD
Department of Orthopaedics
University of Rochester Medical Center
Rochester, New York

Andrew Green, MD
Associate Professor
Chief Shoulder and Elbow Surgery
Department of Orthopaedic Surgery
Brown Medical School
Providence, Rhode Island

Gary S. Gruen, MD
Professor
Vice Chairman
Orthopaedic Surgery
University of Pittsburgh
Pittsburgh, Pennsylvania

Zbigniew Gugala, MD, PhD
The Joseph Barnhart Department of
  Orthopaedic Surgery
Baylor College of Medicine
Houston, Texas

George J. Haidukewych, MD
Assistant Professor
Director, Orthopedic Trauma Service
Mayo Clinic
Rochester, Minnesota

Langdon Hartsock, MD, FACS
Department of Orthopaedic Surgery
Medical University of South Carolina
Charleston, South Carolina

Thomas Higgins, MD
Department of Orthopaedics
University of Utah
Salt Lake City, Utah

Clifford B. Jones, MD
Associate Clinical Professor
Department of Orthopaedics
Michigan State University
Orthopaedic Associates of Grand Rapids
Spectrum Health Medical Center
Michigan State University
Grand Rapids, Michigan

David M. Kahler, MD
Associate Professor
Director of Orthopaedic Trauma
Department of Orthopaedic Surgery
University of Virginia
Charlottesville, Virginia

Philip James Kregor, MD
Associate Professor and Director
Division of Orthopaedic Trauma
Vanderbilt Orthopaedic Institute
Nashville, Tennessee

Christian Krettek, MD
Professor and Chairman
Trauma Department
Hannover Medical School
Hannover, Germany

Brian K. Kwon, MD, PhD, FRCSC
Assistant Professor
Department of Orthopaedics
Combined Neurosurgical and Orthopaedic
  Spine Program
University of British Colombia
Vancouver, British Columbia, Canada

Loren Latta, PE, PhD
Professor and Director of Research
Department of Orthopaedics and
  Rehabilitation
University of Miami, School of Medicine
Miami, Florida

Richard T. Laughlin, MD
Associate Professor and Program Director
Department of Orthopaedic Surgery
Wright State University, School of Medicine
Dayton, Ohio

Mark A. Lee, MD
Assistant Professor
Department of Orthopaedic Surgery
University of California, Davis Medical
  Center
Sacramento, California

Ross K. Leighton, MD, FRCSC, FACS
Associate Professor
Department of Surgery
Halifax, Nova Scotia, Canada

Ronald W. Lindsey, MD
Professor of Orthopaedic Surgery
The Joseph Barnhart Department of
  Orthopaedic Surgery
Baylor College of Medicine
Houston, Texas

Ellen J. MacKenzie, PhD
Center for Injury Research and Health
  Policy
Bloomberg School of Hygiene and Public
  Health
Johns Hopkins University
Baltimore, Maryland

J. L. Marsh, MD
Professor of Orthopedics
University of Iowa Hospitals and Clinics
Iowa City, Iowa

Timothy P. McHenry, MD
Department of Orthopaedics and
  Rehabilitation
Brooke Army Medical Center
Fort Sam Houston, Texas

Michael D. McKee, MD, FRCSC
Associate Professor
Division of Orthopaedic Surgery
Department of Surgery
St. Michael's Hospital and the University of
  Toronto
Toronto, Canada

Wolfgang A. Menth-Chiari, MD
Staff Trauma Surgeon
Department of Traumatology
University of Vienna Medical School
Vienna, Austria

Theodore Miclau, MD
Professor and Vice Chairman
Department of Orthopaedic Surgery
University of California
San Francisco General Hospital
San Francisco, California

William J. Mills, MD
Assistant Professor
Department of Orthopaedic Surgery
University of Washington Harborview
  Medical Center
Seattle, Washington

Michael A. Miranda, MD
Director of Orthopedic Trauma
Department of Orthopedic Surgery
Orthopedic Associates
Hartford Hospital
Hartford, Connecticut

Sohail K. Mirza, MD
Department of Orthopaedics
University of Washington Harborview
  Medical Center
Seattle, Washington

Berton R. Moed, MD
Professor and Chairman
Department of Orthopaedic Surgery
Saint Louis University School of Medicine
Saint Louis, Missouri

Steven J. Morgan, MD
Associate Professor
Department of Orthopaedics
University of Colorado
Denver, Colorado

Sean E. Nork, MD
Associate Professor
Department of Orthopaedic Surgery
University of Washington Harborview
  Medical Center
Seattle, Washington

Brent Norris, MD
Associate Professor
Director Orthopaedic Trauma Fellowship
Department of Orthopaedic Surgery
University of Tennessee
Chattanooga, Tennessee

William T. Obremskey, MD, MPH
Department of Orthopedics
Vanderbilt University
Nashville, Tennessee

Peter J. O'Brien, MD, FRCSC
Associate Professor
Head, Division of Orthopaedic Trauma
Department of Orthopaedics
University of British Colombia
Vancouver, British Columbia, Canada

Robert F. Ostrum, MD
Director of Orthopaedic Trauma
Department of Orthopaedic Surgery
Cooper Hospital/University Medical Center
Camden, New Jersey

James Powell, MD
Clinical Associate Professor
Department of Surgery
University of Calgary
Calgary, Alberta, Canada

Robert A. Probe, MD
Chairman, Division of Orthopaedic Surgery
Department of Surgery
Scott and White Memorial Hospital and
  Clinic
Temple, Texas

Kevin J. Pugh, MD
Director, Division of Trauma
Department of Orthopaedics
The Ohio State University
Columbus, Ohio

Thomas J. Puschak, MD
Orthopaedic Spine Surgeon
Department of Orthopaedics
Panorama Orthopedics
Golden, Colorado

Gregory Rafijah, MD
Director of Hand Surgery
Department of Orthopaedic Surgery
Harbor-UCLA Medical Center
Torrance, California

Nalini Rao, MD
Department of Orthopaedics
Associates in Infectious Disease
Pittsburgh, Pennsylvania

J. Spence Reid, MD
Department of Orthopaedics
Penn State University
Hershey, Pennsylvania

William M. Ricci, MD
Assistant Professor
Department of Orthopaedic Surgery
Washington University School of Medicine
  at Barnes-Jewish Hospital
Saint Louis, Missouri

Charles M. Richart, MD
Associate Director of Trauma and Surgical
  Critical Care
Saint Luke's Hospital of Kansas City
Saint Luke's Surgical Specialists
Saint Luke's Hospital
Kansas City, Missouri

Marie D. Rinaldi, BA
Department of Surgery
New Jersey Medical School
Newark, New Jersey

David Ring, MD
Department of Orthopaedics
Massachusetts General Hospital
Boston, Massachusetts

Craig S. Roberts, MD
Associate Professor
Residency Director
Department of Orthopaedic Surgery
University of Louisville
Louisville, Kentucky

M.L. Routt Jr, MD
Professor
University of Washington Orthopaedics and
   Sports Medicine Department
Harborview Medical Center
Seattle, Washington

S. Robert Rozbruch, MD
Director, Institute for Limb Lengthening
   and Reconstruction
Department of Orthopedic Surgery
Hospital for Special Surgery
New York, New York

David A. Sanders, MD
Department of Orthopaedics
London Health Sciences Center
London, Ontario, Canada

Rick C. Sasso, MD
Assistant Professor
Clinical Orthopaedic Surgery
Indiana University School of Medicine
Indiana Spine Group
Indianapolis, Indiana

David M. Scher, MD
Assistant Professor of Orthopaedic Surgery
Department of Orthopaedic Surgery
New York University Hospital for Joint
   Diseases
New York, New York

Susan A. Scherl, MD
Assistant Professor
Department of Orthopaedic Surgery and
   Rehabilitation
The University of Nebraska
Omaha, Nebraska

Gregory J. Schmeling, MD
Associate Professor
Director, Division of Orthopaedic Trauma
Department of Orthopaedic Surgery
Medical College of Wisconsin
Milwaukee, Wisconsin

Andrew H. Schmidt, MD
Department of Orthopaedics
Hennepin County Medical Center
Minneapolis, Minnesota

Alexandra K. Schwartz, MD
Assistant Clinical Professor
Department of Orthopaedic Surgery
University of California, San Diego
San Diego, California

Michael Sirkin, MD
Chief, Orthopaedic Trauma Service
University of Medicine and Dentistry, New
   Jersey Medical School
Newark, New Jersey

Joseph F. Slade III, MD
Associate Professor of Yale Orthopaedics
   and Director of Yale Hand and Upper
   Extremity
Yale University
New Haven, Connecticut

Douglas G. Smith, MD
Department of Orthopaedics
University of Washington Harborview
   Medical Center
Seattle, Washington

Adam Starr, MD
Department of Orthopaedic Surgery
University of Texas Southwestern Medical
   Center
Dallas, Texas

David Stephen, MD, FRCSC
Director of Orthopedic Trauma
Assistant Professor, University of Toronto
Department of Orthopedics
Sunnybrook and Women's College Health
   Sciences Centre
Toronto, Ontario, Canada

David Templeman, MD
Department of Orthopaedic Surgery
University of Minnesota
Minneapolis, Minnesota

Roger Torga-Spak, MD
The Joseph Barnhart Department of
   Orthopaedic Surgery
Baylor College of Medicine
Houston, Texas

Pat Torres, RHIT, CCS, CPC
Compliance Manager, Coding and Billing
Corporate Compliance
Scott and White Memorial Hospital
Temple, Texas

Bruce Trahan, MHA, CHE
Director
Department of Orthopaedic Surgery
Scott and White Memorial Hospital and
   Clinic
Temple, Texas

Roman Ullrich, MD
Associate Professor of Anesthesia and
   General Intensive Care
Department of Anesthesia and General
   Intensive Care
University of Vienna
Vienna, Austria

Alexander R. Vaccaro, MD
Professor
Department of Orthopaedic Surgery
Thomas Jefferson University Hospital and
   the Rothman Institute
Philadelphia, Pennsylvania

David A. Volgas, MD
Assistant Professor
Division of Orthopaedic Surgery
University of Alabama at Birmingham
Birmingham, Alabama

David S. Weisman, MD
Clinical Assistant Professor
Department of Orthopaedics
UMDNS Robert Wood Johnson Medical
   School
New Brunswick, New Jersey

Philip R. Wolinsky, MD
Associate Professor
Department of Orthopaedic Surgery
University of California, Davis Medical
   Center
Sacramento, California

James J. Yue, MD
Assistant Professor
Department of Orthopaedics and
   Rehabilitation
Yale University School of Medicine
New Haven, Connecticut

Boris A. Zelle, MD
Department of Orthopaedics
University of Pittsburgh
Pittsburgh, Pennsylvania

Daniel Zinar, MD
Chair, Department of Orthopaedic Surgery
Harbor-UCLA Medical Center
Torrance, California

Bruce H. Ziran, MD
Associate Professor of Orthopaedic Surgery
Saint Elizabeth Health Center Orthopaedics
Northeast Ohio Universities College of
   Medicine
Youngstown, Ohio

Preface

The American Academy of Orthopaedic Surgeons launched the *Orthopaedic Knowledge Update* series in 1984, and specialty OKU volumes in 1994, to promote "learner-centered education" and to provide a useful, comprehensive, and accessible synthesis of the information available from the latest peer-reviewed orthopaedic literature. Those goals have consistently been met in the subsequent editions of OKU and in the specialty-oriented volumes, including the first two editions of OKU Trauma, published in 1996 and 2000.

Dramatic advances in acute fracture care, as well as contemporary issues involving the delivery, reimbursement, and evaluation of trauma care make the publication of this third edition of OKU Trauma especially timely and necessary. We have chosen to enhance the exclusively anatomic organization of previous editions (divided into upper and lower extremity, spine and pelvis fractures) by creating three entirely new sections that address special trauma considerations, the delivery and assessment of fracture care, and managing the sequelae of acute injury. Thus, the text begins with an up-to-date assessment of new outcome measurements, new practice models, and new technologies. Next, an entire section is devoted to the management of multiple trauma, fracture healing problems, and fracture sequelae. A final section on special problems and considerations in the management of pediatric and geriatric fractures has been added. As in previous editions,

each fully referenced chapter provides annotations to the most current, peer-reviewed literature discussed by authors.

OKU Trauma 3 has been written by more than 90 volunteer authors from the Orthopaedic Trauma Association. To coordinate and publish such a volume, great teamwork is required, and we are particularly fortunate and grateful for the skill and effort provided by our section editors: Jeffrey O. Anglen, MD; Jens R. Chapman, MD; Kenneth J. Koval, MD; Mark C. Reilly, MD; Emil H. Schemitsch, MD; Andrew H. Schmidt, MD; Michael D. Stover, MD; and David C. Teague, MD, as well as the contributions of the Academy staff. We are confident that this third edition of OKU Trauma is the best yet, will provide you with immediate valuable "pearls" in your approach to the care of trauma patients, and will subsequently serve as your primary fracture management reference. If you scan the table of contents and peruse any chapter, we think that you will quickly agree.

Michael R. Baumgaertner, MD
Paul Tornetta III, MD
Editors

Table of Contents

Section 2: The Polytrauma Patient and Fracture Healing

Section Editor: Emil H. Schemitsch, MD

Section 3: Upper Extremity

Section Editor: Andrew H. Schmidt, MD

Section 4: Axial Skeleton—Including Spine and Pelvis

Section Editors: Jens R. Chapman, MD
Michael D. Stover, MD

Section 5: Lower Extremity

Section Editors: Mark C. Reilly, MD
David C. Teague, MD

American Academy of Orthopaedic Surgeons

Section 6: Geriatric and Pediatric Trauma

Section Editor: Kenneth J. Koval, MD

Section 1

New Measurements and New Technology

Section Editor:
Jeffrey O. Anglen, MD, FACS

Chapter 1

Guide for Orthopaedic Outcome Instruments

William T. Obremskey, MD, MPH

Outcomes Assessment

Outcomes research has become the buzzword of clinical researchers, insurance companies, and health care delivery corporations. Outcome can be defined as the patient's end result from treatment of a disease. The term "end result" was coined by Codman in 1914.[1] He proposed that knowledge of the end result for patients should be the parameter by which medical/surgical treatment be judged. His concept that hospitals use outcome assessment to measure and improve quality was not well accepted in his time. Weinstein and Deyo[2] proposed complete outcome assessment to include patient well-being or health status, costs, expectations, and biologic status. This chapter will define outcome instruments, describe common outcome instruments, and explain their use in research and practice.

The types of outcomes that are important for patients include not only clinical outcomes, but also health-related outcomes and functional outcomes. Clinical outcomes (such as range of motion, radiographic union, implant loosening, and infection) have been the focus of clinical research in orthopaedic surgery. Significant literature supports the observation that good clinical outcomes (range of motion or a healed fracture) do not necessarily translate into good functional outcomes. Health-related quality of life (HRQOL) involves patients' perceptions of how they are functioning as affected by their overall health. Functional outcomes assess patient function at the most complete level as an individual in society. The areas of patient function include mental health, social function, role function (such as worker, spouse, and parent), physical function, and activities of daily living.

Why Assess Outcomes?

A better understanding of the factors that are important to patients in their recovery will enable physicians to improve the quality of health care and patient satisfaction. In addition, new medical and surgical treatments are increasingly questioned by patients' insurance companies and government payors. As health care decision making becomes more centralized, it is necessary for physicians and health organizations to produce evidence that a treatment improves a patient's overall physical function and quality of life. Physicians and/or health care institutions that gather data showing clinical effectiveness will be strongly positioned for health care contracting. HRQOL outcomes and classic clinical outcomes can help physicians provide patients and payors with high-quality information that they may use to make decisions regarding health care.

Types of Outcome Instruments

Outcome patient-based instruments can be categorized as generic, disease-specific, region-specific, joint- and injury-specific, and patient-specific measures. Clinicians and health service researchers use the HRQOL and functional outcome instruments that are appropriate for their needs. The use of patient-based measures in orthopaedic literature has increased significantly in the past 10 years. A recent review of the major orthopaedic journals indicated that from 1991 to 2001 the use of patient-based measures increased from 8% overall to 18%.[3] Common patient outcome instruments include the Medical Outcomes Study Short Form 36-Item Health Survey (SF-36), Quality of Well-Being scale (QWB), Sickness Impact Profile (SIP), and the EuroQuol (EQ-5D). These generic instruments measure general health status that includes physical symptoms and function as well as emotional dimensions of health. These instruments are broad in scope and are useful in comparing the health status of individuals with different diseases or patients from different populations and different cultures. The disadvantage of generic instruments is that they may not be able to detect subtle differences among patients with the same disease process or changes in individual patients over time. The Musculoskeletal Functional Assessment (MFA) and the Short Musculoskeletal Functional Assessment (SMFA) questionnaires are generic outcome instruments that were designed to assess musculoskeletal conditions of overuse and arthritis as well as provide quality of life data. The use of generic patient-specific outcomes has become so commonplace that some granting institutions require that a generic outcome instrument be included in the design of a clinical project.

The most commonly used disease-specific outcome instrument in orthopaedics is the Western Ontario and McMaster University Arthritis Index (WOMAC), designed to assess osteoarthritis of the upper and lower extremities. Disease-specific instruments have been developed for patients with cardiovascular disease, closed head injuries, colorectal cancer, and chronic obstructive pulmonary disease as well as other disease processes.

Region-specific instruments are available for upper and lower extremities. The upper extremity measures include the Disabilities of the Arm, Shoulder, and Hand (DASH) outcome measure and the Upper Extremity Function Scale. Lower extremity instruments include the Toronto Extremity Salvage Score and the American Academy of Orthopaedic Surgeons' (AAOS) Musculoskeletal Outcomes Data Collection and Management System (MODEMS) lower extremity instruments. These region-specific and disease-specific measures may not be sensitive enough to detect small changes in musculoskeletal conditions of differing severity or over time. The disease-specific and region-specific measures are designed to gather some HRQOL information as well.

Numerous patient-based outcome instruments that are joint- and injury-specific have been developed and have been used in orthopaedic studies in the past 10 years. Some are in common use, such as the Harris Hip Score or Iowa Ankle and Knee Scores. Other questionnaires are quite specific, such as the Wheelchair Users Shoulder Pain Index Score. Other instruments that have been described are the Western Ontario Shoulder Instability questionnaire, the Shoulder Pain Disability Index, the Simple Shoulder Test, the Shoulder Disability Questionnaire, the Lysholm knee score, a carpal tunnel syndrome functional instrument, and the Roland-Morris low back pain score. Many of these scales, such as the Wheelchair Users Shoulder Pain Index Score, are quite specific for disease processes in patient populations and are not applicable to a large number of patients or conditions. The advantage to using these instruments is that they may be quite sensitive in identifying subtle changes in a patient's specific condition. For example, the Western Ontario Shoulder Instability questionnaire asks specific questions about shoulder position and sensations of instability that may not be asked on more generalized scales. Individual patient scores on these questionnaires are also not generalizeable or comparable to general populations. None of the joint- and injury-specific instruments have been scientifically developed or validated, except the carpal tunnel syndrome functional instrument. Scientific development and validation of an outcome instrument is time-consuming and costly. It is not cost effective unless an instrument is developed for a common problem or can be used for a variety of problems.

Patient-specific measures are individualized questionnaires in which patients are able to choose items from a customized questionnaire based on Item Response Theory (see http://www.edres.org/irt/ for additional information).[4] The different patient-specific measures that are available are useful for individual patients with the same disorders, but it is difficult to extrapolate such data to a more general population. The instruments take significant time to complete and are probably not appropriate for assessing patients with musculoskeletal conditions.

Additional outcome measures that may be useful are the Visual Analog Scale (VAS) and work disability questionnaires. The pain VAS is a commonly used and accepted alternative measure of pain severity. Patients mark their level of pain on a 10-cm line (0 equals no pain and 10 equals severe pain). The VAS is a validated tool for quantitatively assessing a patient's pain. The DASH questionnaire has a separate work module that determines in which areas a patient has difficulties at work.[5]

Which Outcome Measure to Use?

Because multiple patient-based outcome questionnaires are available, it can be difficult for clinicians and researchers to decide which outcome measures are best for their purposes. Any HRQOL or functional outcome questionnaire must be psychometrically sound (psychometrics is the science of making a questionnaire reliable and reproducible). This requires adequate reliability, validity, and responsiveness. Validity includes face validity, context validity, and construct validity with convergent and discriminative validity, the discussion of which is beyond the scope of this chapter. Which type of outcome measurement is to be used is based on the needs of each researcher or clinician. Researchers studying a specific joint and injury disease process may choose a specific outcome measure. Clinicians who want to use one instrument for all patients to assess outcomes will select a generic-, disease-, or region-specific outcome instrument. The generally recommended approach would be to select a generic- or disease-specific instrument in addition to a region-specific or joint-specific outcome measure. Although the ability of disease-specific or region-specific instruments to judge generic HRQOL issues has not been well studied, the MFA, SMFA and DASH questionnaires may have some advantages for judging specific and generic outcome measures. A recent review of six orthopaedic journals found that the SF-36 was the most common patient-specific health questionnaire used. This instrument, along with the Roland-Morris questionnaire for back pain and the WOMAC questionnaire for osteoarthritis, were the most commonly used outcome instruments.[3]

Outcome Instrument Details

Generic Instruments

The four most widely used and evaluated patient-based instruments that are appropriate for use in the assessment of musculoskeletal disease and/or injury are the SF-36, SIP, EQ-5D, and QWB, which forms the backbone of the Quality Adjusted Life Years (QALYs) methodology. These scales share the common characteristic of assessing all areas of human activity, including physical, psychologic, social, and role functioning. They also share the characteristic of assessing the patient as a whole (from the patient's perspective) and not as an organ system, disease, or limb. They are internally consistent, reproducible, and discriminative between clinical conditions of different severity. They are also sensitive to change in health status over time and are not physician administered.

The SF-36 is the most widely applied general health status instrument.[6] Its 36 scaled questions (0 = poor to 100 = best) relate to the following eight functional subscales: bodily pain, role function (physical), role function (emotional), social function, physical function, energy/ fatigue, mental health, and general health and vitality perceptions. There is no single aggregate scale; the subscales can be combined into a Physical Component Score and a Mental Component Score. The SF-36 has been validated to be reliable and reproducible. It can be administered by the patient or interviewer as well as by telephone or mail and takes only 10 minutes to complete. These features make it appealing and practical for use in a busy office or clinic setting. This instrument may have a ceiling effect (scores are concentrated at best function) for patients with musculoskeletal conditions. This means that clinically important functional problems may not be adequately characterized using this scale because the disability is too minimal to be assessed. Patients with mild to moderate dysfunction (such as overuse injuries or minor fractures) may score near the highest possible scores, and further improvement cannot be measured. The SF-36 has a particular weakness in assessing upper extremity function.

The SIP, a 136-item endorsable statement questionnaire (if a statement of function applies to their current situation, patients respond with either "yes" or "no"), requires trained interviewers to administer and takes 30 minutes to complete.[7] Twelve different domains are assessed, scored independently, and aggregated into a physical and a psychosocial subscale as well as into one aggregate score. The scale is 0 to 100 points; the higher the score, the worse the disability. Patients with scores above 30 have seriously diminished quality of life. The SIP has also been used to assess patients with multiple health conditions and makes comparisons of the impact of disease on health possible. It has been used to assess patients with musculoskeletal trauma with good success. Because of the difficulty and length of its administration, the SIP may be most useful for well-funded outcome studies or controlled trials. It is likely that it also has a ceiling effect, in which lesser degrees of musculoskeletal dysfunction are not identified.

The EQ-5D assesses health status in five dimensions (mobility, self-care, usual activities, pain/discomfort, and anxiety/depression). The first three dimensions are dependent on physical functioning. Patients are asked to choose between three responses for level of pain (no pain or discomfort, moderate pain or discomfort, or extreme pain or discomfort). If chronic pain is well controlled, it may be mild, but there is no option for this response in the EQ-5D. The different possible states are then weighted and used to calculate the final score. The weight of each health state is based on a study population that develops preferences from 0 to 1 and correlate to worst health versus best health. The scores can be used in economic analyses such as a cost utility analysis.

The QWB is an interviewer-administered, 78-item questionnaire and one of the most useful scales for cost-effectiveness studies.[8] It also is considered to be more sensitive to small changes in functional status than other similar scales. Multiplying data from large populations by the number of years of life expectancy and cost per intervention gives the QALY and cost per year of well life expectancy. QALYs provide a methodology for making difficult decisions regarding resource allocation. When orthopaedic interventions such as hip arthroplasty and hip fracture fixation have been studied using this methodology, they have fared well. The QWB physical function scale also likely has ceiling effects.

These are examples of general health status instruments that have broad acceptance and the ability to compare the functional impact of various diseases. Disease-specific or condition-specific instruments offer increased sensitivity and limit the floor and ceiling effects. The general health status instruments and their attributes are listed in Table 1.

All of the HRQOL scores derived from using these instruments are significantly affected by a patient's comorbidities, age, and sex. This factor has been best described with the SF-36. One study showed that the comorbidities of arthritis back pain and depression have the greatest effect on altering a HRQOL score.[6] Understanding this effect is important in the interpretation of HRQOL scores. The SF-36 has been published with normative values for the US population and also for patients with multiple comorbidities. These comorbidities impact the mean scores of the SF-36 subscales of physical function, role function (physical), bodily pain, general health, and vitality.[6]

Normative values of the SF-36 also vary with age and sex. This is most evident when comparing physical function scores across age groups. Specific subscales of the SF-36 have also been analyzed and stratified for age and sex. Investigators need to be aware of these variances when using a HRQOL survey to assess a patient's functional recovery, and patients' scores may need to be compared with those of their appropriate age group to

TABLE 1 | HRQOL Instruments and Scoring Resources

Instrument	Method	Training Required	Time to Complete	Target Population	Conditions	Source
SF-36	Self or interviewer	2 hours	5 to 10 minutes	All	General HRQOL measures	Medical Outcomes Trust 20 Park Plaza Suite 1014 Boston, MA 02116-4313
SIP	Self or interviewer	1 week	30 minutes	All	General HRQOL measures	Ann Skinner 624 N. Broadway Room 647 Baltimore, MD 21205
WOMAC	Self	1 week	10 minutes	Patients with arthritis	Arthritis	Jane Campbell London Health Science Center, Suite 303 South Campus 375 South St. London, Ontario N6A 4G5 Canada
Nottingham Health Profile	Self	1 week	10 minutes	All	General HRQOL measures	Jim McEwan Dept. of Public Health University of Glasgow Glasgow G128QQ Scotland
QWB	Trained interviewer	2 weeks	12 minutes	All	General HRQOL measures	Holly Teetzel Dept. of Family and Preventive Medicine Box 0622 University of California San Diego 9500 Gilman Drive La Jolla, CA 92093
AAOS Upper extremity, lower extremity, spine and pediatrics	Self or interviewer	1 week	Variable depending on modules used; 10 to 40 minutes	Patients with specific regions of disease/injury or specific age	HRQOL applied to regional or specific age groups in the musculoskeletal population	Director Research and Scientific Affairs American Academy of Orthopaedics 6300 N. River Road Rosemont, IL 60018
MFA	Self or interviewer	2 hours	20 minutes	Patients with musculoskeletal disease	HRQOL measure applied to patients with musculoskeletal disease	http://www.AAOS.org/ outcomes
SMFA	Self or interviewer	1 hour	10 minutes	Patients with musculoskeletal disease	HRQOL measure applied to patients with musculoskeletal disease	http://www.AAOS.org/ outcomes

(Reproduced with permission from Obremskey WT, Swiontkowski MF: Evaluation of outcomes for musculoskeletal injury, in *Skeletal Trauma*. Philadelphia, PA, WB Saunders, 1998, pp 731-741.)

obtain a more accurate assessment of functional capacity.

The MFA instrument, a 101-item questionnaire, was developed and validated as a generic health questionnaire with a large emphasis on the impact of musculoskeletal injuries/conditions.[9,10] It was developed as a tool for outcome research projects and randomized controlled trials. It has been tested for responsiveness, validity, and reliability. The MFA may provide the community clinician with more detail, but administering the MFA may be more demanding on staff and patients than is necessary for routine use. The MFA has also been published with reference values to population norms.[11]

The SMFA was developed for clinicians who are trying to routinely and quantitatively compare patient progress over time as well as with that of patients from other settings. The SMFA is a 46-item, self-administered instrument that takes 10 to 15 minutes to complete.[12] The SMFA has two parts. Part 1 (the dysfunction index) has four categories: daily activities, emotional status, arm/hand function, and mobility. Each question has a Likert five-point response format, ranging from one point for good function to five points for poor function. The scores in Part 1 categories can be totaled to create the dysfunction index, which scores 34 items that assess a patient's perception of functional performance. Part 2 (the bother index) has 12 items that assess the degree that patients are bothered in recreation and leisure, sleep and rest, work, and family. The five-point response ranges from one point (no problems) to five points (extremely bothered). Each category of the dysfunction index is normalized to a total score (range, 0 to 100). The scores of the dysfunction and bother index are also normalized on a scale from 0 to 100, so that the high scores indicate poor function.

It has been shown to be feasible to administer the SMFA in community and university clinic settings without disrupting the daily flow of the office and with good patient compliance and acceptance. If a busy clinic desires to use only a single instrument for all conditions being studied, the MFA or SMFA questionnaire provides general health and area-specific information with fewer floor and ceiling effects than the SF-36 or WOMAC.[13]

Disease-Specific Instruments

The WOMAC is a 24-question scale that is divided into three dimensions (pain, stiffness, and physical function). The WOMAC is self-administered, available in 65 languages, and has been validated. It is widely used in the evaluation of patients with knee and hip osteoarthritis.[14] It is a reliable and responsive measure of outcome and has been used in diverse clinical and interventional studies. It is the most widely used instrument for measuring outcomes in patients with osteoarthritis, and it is the most commonly used outcome instrument for assessing patients who have undergone hip and knee arthroplasty.

Region-Specific Instruments

In 1993, the AAOS and members of the Council of Musculoskeletal Specialty Societies began to pool resources to develop questionnaires that could be used for musculoskeletal injuries and conditions in an office setting and allow local, regional, and national collection of patient-specific outcome data. The database, MODEMS, incorporated the SF-36, demographic and comorbidity information, and included questionnaires specific for the upper extremity (DASH), lower extremity, and pediatric patients and patients with spinal injuries. The AAOS established a research institute to oversee the MODEMS project. The instrument was validated and takes 10 to 30 minutes to

complete. The AAOS conducted a trial project to make national data available and collected data on more than 30,000 patients in 3 months.[15] The AAOS sponsored a national database for MODEMS collection, but discontinued it in April 2000 (decreased data were accrued because physicians were concerned about central data registry). The MODEMS questionnaires, however, are still available for use. These questionnaires provide HRQOL data with the SF-36 as well as area-specific and disease-specific information; therefore, it is a good instrument for comprehensive evaluation.

The Upper Extremity Function Scale is an eight-item, self-administered questionnaire that was designed to measure the impact of upper extremity dysfunction on overall patient function. This instrument was tested in patients with work injuries and carpal tunnel syndrome.[16] The Upper Extremity Function Scale demonstrated good internal consistency, few floor effects, and excellent convergent and discriminant validity. Convergent validity is confirmed if patient, injury, or treatment factors produce outcome results that are expected (for example, anatomic joint reductions have improved range of motion or higher function scores), and discriminate validity is confirmed if patient, injury, or treatment factors have divergent outcome results as expected (for example, open comminuted articular fractures have worse outcomes than closed simple shaft fractures).

Joint- and Injury-Specific Instruments

The Toronto Extremity Salvage Score is a 30-question instrument that measures physical function after tumor resection.[17] This instrument is used to assess patients who have undergone musculoskeletal oncology salvage surgery and has been shown to have high validity and responsiveness in this population.

The Simple Shoulder Test was developed as a joint-specific measure of shoulder function status.[18] It was based on patients' functional ability to perform extremes of motion. This instrument includes 12 functional questions with endorsable ("yes" or "no") responses. It has been used in studies of shoulder degenerative joint disease as well as rotator cuff tears.

The Roland-Morris questionnaire, a 24-item instrument that assesses low back pain, is derived from the SIP.[19] Although this questionnaire has undergone several revisions, it is commonly used for assessing patients with low back pain.

The Harris Hip Score is a commonly used instrument for the preoperative and postoperative assessment of patients who have undergone joint arthroplasty. It incorporates pain assessment, walking distances, physical function, and range of motion into an overall score. It has been used commonly in published studies, but it has never been scientifically developed or validated.

The Iowa Ankle and Knee Scores is an instrument that was developed for the long-term assessment of patients with tibial fractures.[20] Iowa Ankle and Knee Scores are based on a 100-point scale that incorporates the patient's self-assessment of pain and function as well as data from the physical examination (range of motion, gait, and deformity). This instrument provides a joint-specific measure of outcome, but it has never been scientifically developed or validated.

Recommendations for Clinical Outcomes Research and Assessment

Outcomes assessment involves the routine collection of HRQOL data to evaluate the effectiveness of patient care. Outcomes assessment instruments are often administered at the clinician's office and typically provide the type of data in which health care payors are interested. Patient satisfaction data and HRQOL data are routinely collected for a preidentified segment of patients at predetermined intervals, before and after treatment, and the results provide the basis for outcome assessment. A common approach is to begin such a process by collecting data on all patients within a practice. However, this is to be discouraged because it results in the accumulation of data that can be time-consuming to manage and difficult to analyze. This type of nonselective data collection quickly leads to frustration of the office staff members who are responsible for form administration and collection. Patient cooperation and support of these projects, however, is rarely a problem. Patients have been found to be most receptive to completing these types of questionnaires and believe that this process, as well as satisfaction surveys, represents an effort on behalf of the practice to meet their needs.

The best approach in beginning outcomes assessment within a practice is to target a musculoskeletal condition or injury that is frequently treated within that practice. It is best for the clinical and research staff involved in data collection if an eligible patient is seen 8 to 10 times per week. Institutional Review Board approval should be obtained if affiliated with a medical center or from an outside agency (such as In-Touch Research) to ensure compliance with standard ethics and Health Insurance Portability and Accountability Act requirements of consent and follow-up. Patients should be approached before treatment, asked to complete an HRQOL questionnaire, and then notified that they will be contacted at predetermined intervals to complete the same survey. The physicians responsible for the project should decide before enrolling patients which clinical data they need to collect to properly analyze the HRQOL data. Data points involving clinical, demographic, or radiographic assessments should be collected before treatment and at predetermined intervals. The exact timing and interval of data collection is not standardized, and the appropriate time intervals may vary for different musculoskeletal injuries and conditions. A patient with an isolated ankle fracture will return to normal function more quickly than a patient with a tibial plafond fracture, and more frequent data collection may be required. Studies need to be completed that better characterize the rate of functional recovery of patients with a variety of musculoskeletal injuries to better answer patient questions and more accurately respond to work-related and legal issues.

A minimalist approach, in terms of the number of conditions studied, is the most beneficial when starting to assess outcomes in clinical practice. Identifying a condition that is common to the practice (and thus important to the success of the practice) and collecting data on patients with this condition will lead to a product that will be useful for evaluating current practice and planning for changes in the process of care.

The quality of studies in the orthopaedic literature is improving with increased awareness of study design, statistical impact, and adequate follow-up of clinical and functional outcomes. Regional and statewide organizations such as the Maine Medical Assessment Foundation can effectively collect data. The information derived from pooled orthopaedic practice data will be instrumental in improving the quality of musculoskeletal care. It would allow rapid patient enrollment and encourage timely analysis of clinical uncertainties. In community and academic settings, data collection must be done efficiently at minimal cost. The response to cost-benefit analysis of orthopaedic surgery interventions has been quite favorable and will continue to benefit orthopaedists and their patients. This type of analysis helps justify and support orthopaedic medical surgical care as payor/government agencies evaluate the effect of treatment given limited resources.

Patient-based outcome measurement has increased significantly in the past 10 years and is likely to continue. Future clinical research studies will better define the sensitivity of various instruments to change over time. With outcome data, patients' scores can be compared with normal general population scores. This will allow physicians to predict and determine when patients reach their level of maximum improvement. Patient-based outcome measures may improve the ability to identify patients who will score better on classic outcome measurements (such as range of motion, strength, and union) based on their ability to cope or adapt to their injury or disease condition. Orthopaedic research needs to better identify the factors that are outside the control of the orthopaedic surgeon that may have a great effect on outcomes. It is becoming clear that a patient's education level, income, family support, employment, addiction status, and marital status have a significant impact on long-term outcomes and may be more important than the severity of injury or treatment. Intervention in these areas by a health care team, therefore, may be as important as the medical and surgical care provided.

Although language and culture present barriers to assessing patient-based outcome measures for a large percentage of the US population, these barriers will be overcome as outcome instruments are validated in different languages. Technology will also provide significant changes in the ability to perform outcome measurements. Keystroke entry of patient information is relativity inefficient and prone to error. The development of scannable forms, touch screens, and wireless Web-based real-time entry will further improve the quality and efficiency of data collection.

Initially, outcome measurements were designed to assess health care cost, expectations, and the clinical and biologic status of patients. As the outcome measurement movement progresses, it will be easier for investigators to integrate all aspects of a patient's recovery from injury or a disease more clearly and effectively.

Annotated References

1. Codman EA: The product of a hospital. *Surg Gynecol Obstet* 1914;18:491-496.

2. Weinstein JN, Deyo RA: Clinical research: Issues in data collection. *Spine* 2000;25:3104-3109.
   The authors outline all of the issues that contribute to the evaluation of patients to include patient well-being or health status, costs, expectations, and biologic status.

3. Beaton DE, Schemitsch E: Measures of health-related quality of life and physical function. *Clin Orthop* 2003;413:90-105.
   This article reviews the increased use of functional outcome measures in studies published in the orthopaedic medical literature from 1991 to 2001. It reviews use of the SF-36, MFA, DASH, WOMAC, and other joint-specific measures.

4. Hays RD, Morales LS, Reise SP: Item response theory and health outcomes measurement in the 21st century. *Med Care* 2000;38(suppl 9):II28-II42.
   Item response theory has some advantages over classical test theory in assessing self-reported health outcomes. Item response theory is ideally suited for implementing computer adaptive testing, and its methods can be helpful in developing better health outcome measures and in assessing change over time in individual patients.

5. Beaton DE, Katz JN, Fossel AH, et al: Measuring the whole or the parts: Validity, reliability and responsiveness of the DASH outcome measure in different regions of the upper extremity. *J Hand Ther* 2001;14:128-146.
   The purpose of this study was to evaluate the reliability, validity, and responsiveness of the DASH outcome measure in a group of diverse patients and to compare the results with those obtained with joint-specific measures. Two hundred patients with either wrist and hand or shoulder problems were evaluated using questionnaires before treatment, and 172 (86%) were reevaluated 12 weeks after treatment. Evidence was provided of the validity, test-retest reliability, and responsiveness of the DASH outcome measure. This study also demonstrated that the DASH outcome measure had validity and responsiveness in patients with proximal and distal disorders, confirming its usefulness across the whole extremity.

6. Ware JE Jr, Kosinski M, Keller S: *SF-36 Physical and Mental Health Summary Scales: A User's Manual.* Boston, MA, The Health Institute, 1994.

7. Bergner M, Bobbitt RA, Carter WB, et al: The Sickness Impact Profile: Development and final revision of a health status measure. *Med Care* 1981;19:787-805.

8. Kaplan RM, Anderson JP: The Quality of Well-Being scale: Rationale for a single quality of life index, in Walker SR, Rosser R (eds): *Quality of Life: Assessment and Application.* Lancaster, England, MTP Press, 1988, pp 51-77.

9. Engelberg R, Martin DP, Agel J, Obremskey W, Coronado G, Swiontkowski MF: Musculoskeletal Function Assessment instrument: Criterion and construct validity. *J Orthop Res* 1996;14:182-192.

10. Martin DP, Engelberg R, Agel J, Snapp D, Swiontkowski MF: Development of a musculoskeletal extremity health status instrument: The Musculoskeletal Function Assessment instrument. *J Orthop Res* 1996;14:173-181.

11. Engelberg R, Martin DP, Agel J, Swiontkowski MF: Musculoskeletal function assessment: Reference values for patient and non-patient samples. *J Orthop Res* 1999;17:101-109.

12. Swiontkowski MF, Engelberg R, Martin DP, et al: Short Musculoskeletal Function Assessment questionnaire: Validity, reliability and responsiveness. *J Bone Joint Surg Am* 1999;81:1245-1260.

13. Martin DP, Engelberg R, Agel J, Swiontkowski MF: Comparison of the Musculoskeletal Function Assessment questionnaire with the Short Form-36, the Western Ontario and McMaster Universities Osteoarthritis Index, and the Sickness Impact Profile health-status measures. *J Bone Joint Surg Am* 1997;79:1323-1335.

14. Bellamy N, Buchanan WW, Goldsmith CH, Campbell J, Stitt LW: Validation study of WOMAC: A

health status instrument for measuring clinically-important patient-relevant outcomes following total hip or knee arthroplasty in osteoarthritis. *J Rheumatol* 1988;15:1833-1840.

15. Hunsaker FG, Cioffi DA, Amadio PC, Wright JG, Caughlin B: The American Academy of Orthopaedic Surgeons outcomes instruments: Normative data from the general population. *J Bone Joint Surg Am* 2002;84-A:208-215.
    Using panel mail methodology, the AAOS collected normative data on 11 musculoskeletal outcome measures, which can now be used as a benchmark for future studies.

16. Pransky G, Feuerstein M, Himmelstein J, Katz JN, Vickers-Lahti M: Measuring functional outcomes in work-related upper extremity disorders: Development and validation of the Upper Extremity Function Scale. *J Occup Environ Med* 1997;39:1195-1202.

17. Davis AM, Wright JG, Williams JI, Bombardier C, Griffin A, Bell RS: Development of a measure of physical function for patients with bone and soft tissue sarcoma. *Qual Life Res* 1996;5:508-516.

18. Lippitt SB, Harryman DT II, Matsen FA III: A practical tool for evaluating function: The simple shoulder test, in Matsen FA III, Fu FH, Hawkins RJ (eds): *The Shoulder: A Balance of Mobility and Stability*. Rosemont, IL, American Academy of Orthopaedic Surgeons, 1993, pp 501–518.

19. Roland M, Morris R: A study of the natural history of back pain: Part I. Development of a reliable and sensitive measure of disability in low back pain. *Spine* 1983;8:141-144.

20. Merchant TC, Dietz FR: Long-term follow-up after fractures of the tibial and fibular shafts. *J Bone Joint Surg Am* 1989;71:599-606.

Chapter 2

Delivery of Orthopaedic Trauma Care

Samuel G. Agnew, MD, FACS

Jeffrey O. Anglen, MD, FACS

Trauma

Trauma is one of the most significant public health problems in the United States. Although chronic conditions such as cancer and cardiac disease account for more deaths in older age groups, trauma cuts short many productive lives because it is the most common cause of death in Americans age 1 to 44 years. Injury kills more than 150,000 people in the United States each year, and it causes more deaths in young people age 1 to 24 years than all other specific recorded causes combined.[1-3] On average, one American dies of unintentional injury every 6 minutes, and a disabling injury occurs every 2 seconds.[2] The effects of injury are accentuated in rural areas of the country where death rates from unintentional injury are 50% higher than in urban areas. Motor vehicle–related mortality is 1.6 times higher in rural than urban settings.[2,4]

The economic impact of trauma is significant and involves both direct costs of care and lost productivity. Trauma is the leading cause of hospitalization for patients younger than 45 years, and it is responsible for 25% of all emergency department visits. Every year, 25% of all Americans will seek treatment of an injury. Unintentional injury alone costs the nation more than $480 billion annually. Road traffic accidents alone are the second highest cause of disability adjusted life years in American men. Data revealed that the average total medical expenditure cost for individuals hospitalized for lower extremity trauma was $19,748 and that the average comprehensive cost was $349,517.[5,6]

Many areas of the country have organized trauma systems in which specialized hospitals are designated as trauma centers and injured patients are directed to such facilities. These trauma systems have been shown to save lives, reduce preventable deaths, lower disability rates, and decrease costs of care. It has been estimated that 20% to 45% of trauma patients who die after reaching the hospital could have been saved by an organized trauma system. Studies have shown a 30% to 60% reduction in preventable trauma mortality by the introduction of organized trauma care systems that use designated trauma centers in such diverse settings as San Diego, CA; Dade County, FL; Orange County, CA; Portland, OR; and Washington, DC.[2,7-9] However, it is estimated that only 25% of the geographic area of the United States is served by an organized trauma care system. In 1990, 23 states had no state or local trauma care systems in place.[10,11]

Trauma center hospitals have made special, voluntary commitments to providing care to injured persons. They are categorized as Level 1 through Level 4, based on capabilities and resources. Level 1 trauma centers are able to treat the most severely injured patients and must meet stringent criteria in terms of specialist services, diagnostic and surgical capability, and continuous availability. To maintain Level 1 status verification by the American College of Surgeons (ACS), these trauma centers must undergo periodic evaluation and meet high standards of performance in patient care, data collection, research, and teaching.[12] Information about trauma center verification as well as a list of ACS–verified trauma centers is available on the ACS Web site (http://www.facs.org).

Trauma care for severely injured patients can be very expensive. Young adults and the poor have a propensity for injury and make up a disproportionate share of the patient population in a trauma center. The combination of expensive care and adverse patient selection places a financial burden on the trauma center hospital. A conservative estimate is that 12% to 15% of hospital charges for trauma patients in the United States are for care of indigent (uninsured) patients, which translates into more than $1 billion of uncompensated care in a single year.[10,11] More than one third of trauma patients are covered only by government insurance programs, which typically pay rates below costs. As a result, many hospitals have given up trauma center status because of economic pressure. A US General Accounting Office study found that the primary reason for trauma center closure was financial loss from treating underinsured patients. By the mid 1990s, an estimated 100 trauma centers had closed in the United States, leaving large segments of the population without a nearby trauma center. In many instances, poor physician reimbursement for trauma care eroded medical staff commitment to this vital area and increased pressure on the hospital to abandon trauma center status.[10,11]

Although solutions to funding trauma care have continued to be elusive, several states have enacted legislation to support this important aspect of public health. Surcharges on moving violations and on automobile registration have been used to raise public funds for trauma care. In some areas, initiatives such as physician-hospital integrated care delivery organizations have improved efficiencies. Trauma care has been carved out of managed care contracting, resulting in better cost recovery. The crisis, however, continues in many parts of the country. Orthopaedists who are involved in the care of injured patients should help to educate the public and increase awareness of this continuing problem.

Orthopaedic Traumatology

Orthopaedic traumatology is one of the more recent subspecialties to emerge in the continuing evolution of orthopaedics. Most orthopaedists treat fractures, but relatively few make a career of treating traumatic conditions. Isolated, closed, low-energy extremity fractures are treated quite effectively by qualified orthopaedic surgeons who are trained in modern fracture care during the course of their residency. One author has estimated that this type of fracture constitutes approximately 80% of all fracture care.[13,14] Orthopaedic traumatologists may also treat isolated or low-energy fractures, but the subspecialty exists because of the special problems encountered in the treatment of high-energy trauma.[15] These fractures are found in the setting of a multiply injured patient, and they may be multiple, segmental, badly displaced, or associated with disrupted soft tissues. These injuries are estimated to comprise approximately 15% of all fractures, but they have more than 90% of the most costly complications, the most prolonged and significant associated disabilities, and the highest mortality rates. Their treatment requires special training and experience to achieve successful results without excessive complications. This training is commonly obtained in the setting of postresidency fellowships (a listing of such fellowship programs can be found on the Web site of the Orthopaedic Trauma Association [OTA]: http://www.ota.org). The OTA is the specialty organization for orthopaedic traumatologists in North America. The OTA publishes a professional journal devoted exclusively to orthopaedic traumatology, *The Journal of Orthopaedic Trauma* (http://www.jorthotrauma.com).

Orthopaedic Trauma Service and Delivery of Optimal Orthopaedic Trauma Care

Injury to the musculoskeletal system constitutes a major component of trauma. According to the National Health Interview Survey, 28.6 million musculoskeletal injuries were reported in the United States in 1995, including 10 million fractures. The rate of limb injury alone was nearly 70 per 1,000 patients. In the same year, approximately 1 million hospitalizations with fracture as the primary diagnosis were reported. Lower extremity fracture is the leading cause of trauma admission for adults younger than 65 years in the United States. More than half of all hospitalized trauma patients have significant musculoskeletal injuries.[12]

For every hour of completed surgery on a trauma patient by general trauma surgeons in Level 1 and Level 2 trauma centers, the orthopaedic surgeon completes an average of 4 to 6 hours, which does not include delayed procedures such as those required to treat nonunions, infections, contractures, or other common complications. Because of the frequency of musculoskeletal trauma, orthopaedic surgeons are integral members of the trauma team, and they need to be involved in the care of the injured patient from the earliest stages. An ACS–verified Level 1 trauma center must have a surgeon designated as director or liaison to the trauma team who meets the minimum qualifications set forth in *Resources for the Optimal Care of the Injured Patient: 1999*. This publication provides a general description of certain minimal institutional resources that should be available for orthopaedic care in the trauma center, such as flexibility in the operating room and staff scheduling and the availability of individuals to help with tasks such as traction, casting, surgical care, rehabilitation, and discharge planning.

The organization of the general trauma service is believed to affect the quality of care received by the trauma patient. The integrated trauma service concept enhances education and research as well as patient care.[16] One report listed the advantages of an integrated trauma service to include concentration of experience for both house staff and attending physicians, better care coordination, more effective quality assurance, easier research, and improved educational programs.[17] This report also documented a marked decrease in mortality for trauma patients in the intensive care unit after the institution of a trauma service and also identified a decrease in the rates of sepsis, multiple organ failure, complications, length of stay, and preventable death. It is likely that an orthopaedic trauma service would have similar benefits in improving outcomes using the same mechanisms. In other surgical disciplines, increased volume has been related to improved outcomes, which is likely to be true as well for complex fracture procedures.

Separating orthopaedic trauma care from a general or elective orthopaedic practice has advantages for both elective and trauma patients and for the orthopaedic medical staff. In addition, the institution of a dedicated orthopaedic trauma service has benefits to the community and the trauma system. Developing a regionwide plan for both trauma diversion/triage as well as complex orthopaedic diversion/triage is an integral part of attaining and maintaining a region's ability to deliver high-quality care in a timely manner. A comprehensive regional diversion/triage plan for complex orthopaedic injuries should be in place to ensure optimal utilization of regional expertise to improve outcomes and reduce morbidity. The diversion/triage plan should be in place before a regional or central facility participates in diversion. In most states, this type of planning does not exist. Complex orthopaedic injuries, such as pelvis/acetabular fractures and pilon, periarticular, high-energy fractures would be categorized so that all of the referring facilities would know what to do and where to send patients with these injuries at the time of diagnosis. The orthopaedic traumatologist leading a dedicated service should take a proactive role in establishing the facility and regional triage system rather than wait for state officials to understand the need and organize such a system. High-energy injuries with multiple or isolated fractures are the bane of the referral center's existence, and any assistance in the timely egress of these patients to a center of higher care will be embraced.

Although the general surgical trauma team in many trauma centers is organized and structured along guidelines established by the ACS, most orthopaedic trauma services seem to have been developed locally and informally based on interest and ability of the orthopaedic department or group(s) and the nature or needs of the hospital.[18] They span the spectrum from one interested surgeon to entire departments with many surgeons, physicians, residents, nurses, advanced practice nurses, physician assistants, and technicians. They are supported to varying degrees by departments, private groups, hospitals, or medical schools, with no current consensus regarding optimal organization or essential resources. However, recent research and common opinion support the value of a separate designated orthopaedic trauma service.[18-20] The institution of such a service improves financial and clinical productivity of orthopaedic departments, improves resident education, and enhances the job satisfaction of both traumatologists and orthopaedic surgeons who perform elective surgery. The hospital benefits from the provision of organized, high-quality clinical service, quality control, improved efficiency, and effective cost-containment efforts, such as standardized purchasing and the ability to perform more work in less time through specialization. Establishment of such a service facilitates appropriate interservice and intraservice transfers and fosters the development of interdisciplinary protocols and pathways. Predetermined evidence-based treatment algorithms facilitate prompt, smooth, and non-contentious interspecialty care coordination, particularly in patients with multiple injuries such as pelvic fractures with genitourinary damage or hemodynamic instability and fractures with vascular or neurologic disruption.

TABLE 1 | Duties of the Orthopaedic Trauma Director

Administration	Manage the orthopaedic on-call schedule; serve on the trauma committee; oversee operating room and hospital contracting and purchasing for orthopaedic trauma supplies, implants, and instruments; oversee policy development; oversee resource deployment; participate in verification processes; evaluate staff; and participate in community and state trauma system planning.
Education	Set the teaching schedule; organize conferences; organize training and development of staff; develop continuing medical education; teach and evaluate residents and students; and participate in local, national, and international teaching of patients and medical professionals.
Quality assurance and improvement	Monitor quality of care delivered by orthopaedic physicians and staff, including trainees; run morbidity and mortality conferences; and ensure compliance with contractual, state, and federal obligations.
Communication and coordination	Serve as liaison to trauma team and other departments, manage relations with private physicians on the on-call schedule, handle disputes or patient complaints, and make sure phones and consultations are covered continuously.
Research	Perform, review, stimulate, and recruit studies.
Patient care	Participate in surgery and rounds and take over difficult cases.
Other	Participate in marketing, hire and recruit faculty and staff, develop protocols for treatment and transfers, and manage the trauma registry and data collection.

Although some variation in organization exists, certain key components are required in any dedicated orthopaedic trauma service. The general surgical trauma service in a Level 1 trauma center is led by a trauma director, whose salary is usually supported by the institution.[21] An orthopaedic trauma director should be designated as a surgeon leader of that service. The exact duties of this position vary, but they typically involve most of the activities listed in Table 1. This position should be supported with a salary provided by the hospital. It has been reported that part-time orthopaedic trauma directors of fully accredited community programs receive between $30,000 and $200,000 per year.[20]

Other key components of the trauma team include the placement of orthopaedic surgeons on the trauma call panel, two orthopaedic trauma physician assistants for every full-time surgeon, orthopaedic trauma–specific nursing personnel, transfer specialist(s), a research coordinator specializing in trauma and orthopaedic trauma, and adequate support resources.

Although some institutions have enough fellowship-trained orthopaedic traumatologists to fully staff the trauma call panel, most have to rely on general or nontrauma orthopaedic surgeons. Minimal criteria for participation include an unrestricted license, hospital staff privileges, current board certification (with certain exceptions allowed as detailed in the *Resources* publication previously mentioned), and agreement to meet performance standards such as response time, continuing medical education in trauma, participation in quality improvement, and meeting attendance. The hospital should appropriately compensate surgeons with call pay for their service on the trauma call panel. In addition to call pay, institutions should support trauma-related continuing medical education activities and travel for trauma call panel physicians.

The addition of two trauma-specific physician assistants for every full-time surgeon in Level 2 trauma centers is beneficial. The value in time savings, standardization of pathways and protocols, and assistance given to nontrauma call panel physicians well exceeds the cost. Orthopaedic residents may be helpful to the orthopaedic trauma service, depending on the setting and type of hospital. Orthopaedic residents need to be exposed to different tiers of fracture care, orthopaedic traumatology, and complex (isolated) fracture care. Additionally, the virtues of such a career need to be established and made self-evident. With reduced resident work hours and increased faculty-to-resident ratios, the presence of adequate, dependable manpower on the trauma service needs to be ensured.

Orthopaedic trauma–specific nursing personnel (advanced registered nurse practitioners, registered nurse first assistants, certified surgical technologists, and nursing, radiology, and surgical technicians) who are trained specifically for the operating room should also be on the trauma team. These staff members must be experienced and trained in the complexities of orthopaedic trauma care and capable of confronting the varied surgical challenges that occur daily. Because of the variety of surgical approaches and patient positions, the large inventory of equipment and implants, and the duration and intensity of orthopaedic trauma cases, it takes time for staff to acquire the necessary expertise, and this level of expertise should be recognized with pay differentials. As with the catheterization laboratory (interventional radiology) team, for example, the orthopaedic trauma service should be recognized by the institution as a separate specialized unit for which constituent personnel have a dedicated space and are assigned to the same patient population each day until all the care is delivered.

The frequent necessity of arranging transfer into the trauma center for severely injured patients and the complex postdischarge needs of this patient population require the expertise of transfer specialists, full-time staff members who are specifically trained and designated to facilitate timely and appropriate interfacility and intrafacility transfer of care.

A research coordinator specializing in trauma, ideally orthopaedic trauma, is a key component of the trauma team. This person should be proficient in the use of the OTA database and the Trauma Registry Advisory Committee general surgical database, as well as trained in the entry of state registry data. The competent administration of patient outcome instruments for continued participation in national databases must exist on every level of facility to improve orthopaedic trauma care and results. Research coordinators for trauma research studies should be partially funded by the hospital.

In addition to adequate administrative staff, other resources are necessary to support a dedicated orthopaedic trauma service. Adequate operating room time must be made available and protected, not only for acute emergencies (which need 24-hour access every day), but for most orthopaedic trauma cases (which are not immediately life-threatening or limb-threatening, but nonetheless have a time-sensitive component to them). Operating room time can be approximately 60 hours per week in a busy hospital, and this block of time should not be released to competitive posting by elective surgeons until it is clear that the room and staff will not be needed that day. In most instances, that will not be known with certainty until 6:00 am every day, so the release of that room and staff to other services should be under the daily control of the orthopaedic trauma director. Equipment in the operating room, including special tables, C-arms, and instrument and implant sets, must be provided as necessary for the modern practice of fracture surgery. Institutions can further support a viable orthopaedic trauma service by providing computer and information technology services, hardware, internet access, audiovisual equipment, statistical and editorial consultant services, marketing and promotional assistance, contracting and negotiating support, and insurance coverage.

Practice Models and Career Sustainability

The delivery of quality orthopaedic trauma care, education, and research will only take place if a suitable, stable environment is provided in which health care professionals can practice for an extended period of their careers. Classic errors in trauma career development stem from the misconception that the career can be launched and sustained with little assistance from colleagues, chairpersons, and the facility or community for which it was developed. Trauma is often considered a specialty for young surgeons and a way for new, inexperienced surgeons to build a practice. It is also generally believed that surgeons should find specialty niches outside of trauma for long-term financial and lifestyle security. As a result, more surgeons who are experienced in orthopaedic trauma and who are in active practice are needed.

In the past, orthopaedic trauma specialists worked primarily in public or university hospitals, which is typically a demanding clinical job, requiring long hours in the operating room every day. The cases are unpredictable and strenuous. Orthopaedic trauma cases, because they are not scheduled and are rarely immediately life-threatening, commonly are placed on the add-on schedule, leading to evening and night surgery. Orthopaedic trauma patients also often have drug or alcohol abuse problems or personality disorders, and these patients are frequently uninsured. There is also the perception that orthopaedic trauma surgeons are at increased risk of malpractice litigation and viral disease exposure. These conditions negatively impact the lifestyle of orthopaedic trauma surgeons, particularly young surgeons with children. Often, academic departments underappreciate the difficulties of pursuing an academic career under these conditions and do not place enough value on the contributions of those willing to devote their life to this type of work.

It has been difficult to recruit and to retain orthopaedic trauma surgeons in the United States. Fewer than 4% of orthopaedic residents going on to fellowships select trauma and fracture training as their specialty. There were potentially 57 fellowship spots in North America in 1995, but a pool of 40 to 45 applicants. The number of applicants has decreased in recent years, which may be the result of a lack of senior mentors and role models, as well as the negative impact of the lifestyle, which potential applicants may observe in the faculty who are working in this area.

With regard to retention, an OTA survey has shown a 15% attrition rate among orthopaedic traumatologists each year—approximately 39 traumatologists left the specialty each year, whereas only 32 were produced. Again, this trend has worsened in recent years because skilled traumatologists require approximately 3 years of practice after residency and fellowship to become comfortable and efficient with traumatology, but they usually work under these circumstances for only approximately 5 years. They then switch to private general orthopaedic practice, possibly specializing in posttraumatic reconstruction, a field in which they are exceedingly competent and financially successful because of the high level of skill they developed in traumatology. However, their departure represents an enormous loss to the community.

However, in recent years there has been progress in recognizing these problems and creating solutions to make a career in orthopaedic trauma sustainable, even quite rewarding. Several different practice models for the orthopaedic traumatologist have been identified and some organizational solutions to many of the problems have been found in several settings. To some degree, each situation is locally unique and may require solutions incorporating specific local resources, historical factors, and opportunities.

The following five practice models have been identified: academic practice, private group practice, solo practice, hospital-based practice or hospital employment, and a combination practice.

Academic practice is the traditional and familiar mode of practice for those at Level 1 trauma centers with academic affiliation. Problems associated with this practice model include excessive workload, disparate remuneration, limited operating room access, and inadequate time available for academic endeavors. However, when these issues are addressed and controlled, particularly with the support of a strong department chairman, this can be a viable model.

Large multispecialty groups will often recruit, hire, and support a trauma or fracture specialist or group of surgeons in a private group practice. This helps the group as a whole to maintain subspecialty focus and increases efficiency. The elective orthopaedists in the group must recognize and value the contribution of the traumatologists to their own success because they may have to provide some support and give up some operating room time.

Solo practice is difficult to maintain for long, but it has worked in rare situations in which the reimbursement levels are high and other orthopaedic surgeons in the community are supportive.

Hospital-based practice or hospital employment is a new model that is becoming popular in nonacademic Level 1 and Level 2 trauma centers. The traumatologist is typically employed by the hospital, which provides a salary (usually with incentive based on work performed), practice management, billing and collection services, and office space and assistance. The relationship of the traumatologist to other orthopaedic physicians on staff is variable, but it usually involves patient transfer agreements and cross-coverage arrangements.

Components of all of the practice models can be combined to set up creative arrangements, with the ultimate goal of getting the work done and the patients receiving high-quality, sustainable care.

An additional and intriguing idea that has recently surfaced is the creation of a national medical group of orthopaedic traumatologists, similar to the national groups of oncologists and neonatologists (Pediatrix, Inc). With a nationwide company providing negotiation, contracting, and legal, marketing, and business management services, surgeons would be able to concentrate on the clinical practice of orthopaedic traumatology, teaching, and research. Nationwide market value data could be made available, economies of scale and increased purchasing volume discounts could be obtained, and clinical research could be facilitated.

In any of these practice models, two important issues must be managed to make the practice viable over the long term. These issues are workload and compensation.

The average trauma surgeon in a Level 1 facility may produce as many as 12,000 work relative value units (wRVUs) annually, which is the approximate work equivalent of performing 600 total hip replacements, 760 cervical laminectomy-diskectomy procedures, 1,550 arthroscopic meniscectomy procedures, or 4,196 Level 5 examinations. The highest individual producer for three independent private-elective–based multisurgeon billing services recently surveyed averaged 14,000 wRVUs in 1 year (range, 13,500 to 16,100 wRVUs). The Level 2 facility counterpart fracture/trauma surgeons averaged 8,200 wRVUs (range, 7,125 to 10,250 wRVUs) exclusively on a trauma patient population. To accomplish this level of work in tolerable fashion, the service must have access to at least 40 hours of protected first-start operating room time each week per full-time surgeon. If relegated to the add-on schedule, this amount of surgery quickly becomes intolerable. In addition, adequate technical assistance must be provided by the hospital, institution, or group. As previously discussed, this will usually be two physician assistants or advanced practice nurses per full-time surgeon. The hospital or group must be committed to recruitment of an adequate number of surgeons to handle the workload.

Unfortunately, the fee schedules for fracture procedures have been found to be approximately 60% (range, 50% to 73%) of the listed counterparts ($/wRVU) for those regions and facilities studied; additional payment reduction occurs based on multiple procedures performed simultaneously. The reimbursement level becomes significantly disproportionate to the actual work performed. Trying to nurture a traumatology career on a production model is a schematic for career destruction.

The issues and strategies involving both compensation and practice organization for a sustainable, durable career in traumatology are beginning to be studied for general surgeons,[22,23] and similar results are anticipated for orthopaedic surgeons. The value of the orthopaedic trauma surgeon to practice partners, other medical staff, the facility, and the community must be considered when initiating a trauma practice. Value to the hospital results from the traumatologist's ability to control costs and to improve quality and efficiency simultaneously. Value to the nontrauma orthopaedic surgeon results from lessening the burden of stressful and inconvenient fracture and trauma care. Patient care is facilitated, and risk is reduced. To obtain these benefits, compensation to the traumatologist must involve both monetary and lifestyle components; otherwise, the practice of traumatology will overwhelm the practitioners, and both the community and the facility will lose more dedicated trauma surgeons.[24] Financial supplements may include adjustments in fee schedule profiling ($/wRVU equaling that of group subspecialists) or compensation floors established within an acceptable range for an individual expected to perform at the 75th percentile level for wRVUs. Based on comparable regional and national

TABLE 2	Market Value Guideline for Trauma Surgeons

$450,000 annual salary and benefit package (MGMA 70th percentile for fiscal year 2002 data) as base compensation (administrative stipend and clinical base inclusive).

Incentive package when individual wRVU production exceeds 7,000/year; (70th percentile) $60/wRVU above 7,000 annually.

Incentives based on efficiency of service as a whole, including parameters such as decreasing length of patient stay in the intensive care unit or hospital and sharing cost savings as a result of implant or system standardization or volume discounts.

Sharing income received from ancillary services such as diagnostic imaging, therapy, and outpatient surgery. This is analogous to what is occurring with elective orthopaedic surgeons and the development of diagnostic imaging centers, ambulatory surgery centers, and other joint ventures.

data for actual work performed (wRVUs), the corresponding compensation for work performed (compensation/wRVU) from Medical Group Management Association (MGMA) respondent database, the market value guideline in Table 2 was created.

Despite the rigors of a career in orthopaedic traumatology, there are tremendous rewards available to those who dedicate their professional life to caring for injured patients. The OTA Fellowship and Career Choice committee has recently produced a video for residents about the field in which orthopaedic trauma surgeons of all ages from around the country are interviewed. The message is similar from each surgeon. The practice of orthopaedic traumatology offers a stimulating variety of clinical challenges, provides access to a wide spectrum of patients from all walks of life who are tremendously grateful for the skillful care that returns them to an active life, and provides a satisfying and rewarding sense of accomplishment and a unique camaraderie that comes from working with committed, hardworking, excellent surgeons who love what they do. The lifestyle can be difficult, but with advances in understanding on the part of colleagues and administrators and the leadership from those in the field, it is becoming increasingly sustainable. To help promote careers in orthopaedic traumatology, the OTA has recently established a committee to assess and evaluate job opportunities in the field and to help hospitals, departments, and orthopaedic groups set up and organize orthopaedic trauma job situations with sustainable levels of support.

The Emergency Medical Transfer and Active Labor Act and Being On-Call

The Emergency Medical Transfer and Active Labor Act (EMTALA) is federal legislation that was enacted in 1986 in response to a perception that patients were being turned away from some hospitals because of their inability to pay (dumping). The purpose of this legislation was to prevent hospitals from denying service to patients with emergency conditions because they could not pay and to prevent hospitals from transferring people with unstable conditions. The legislation itself is relatively limited and straightforward, but additional regulations issued by the Department of Health and Human Services have provided more specifics regarding hospital obligations. Basically, the statute requires that hospitals must provide a medical screening examination to all individuals seeking emergency services to determine whether an emergency medical condition exists. If such a condition does exist, the hospital must provide stabilizing treatment within its capabilities before discharge or transfer. The hospital cannot transfer an unstable patient unless the patient requests transfer and the transferring physician certifies in writing that the medical benefits of transfer outweigh the risks. In addition, the hospital must maintain an on-call schedule and be responsible for ensuring that on-call physicians respond within a reasonable time. If the on-call physician does not respond in a timely manner, the name and address of the physician must be reported. If a hospital provides specialty services to the public, they should provide those services on an emergent basis through an on-call schedule.

EMTALA violations can be punished with fines, which can range from $25,000 to $50,000, based on hospital size and the nature of the violation. A single incident can result in multiple violations. Ultimately, a hospital could be excluded from Medicare participation for EMTALA violations, but this has occurred fewer than half a dozen times since the legislation was enacted. Individual physicians can also be fined up to $50,000 per violation and excluded from Medicare participation. Individual physician violations specifically mentioned in the statute include signing a certificate stating that the benefits outweigh the risks of transfer when one knows or should know that they in fact do not and misrepresenting the patient's condition or other information to the receiving hospital.

It should be noted that if the screening medical examination provided by a medical professional (not necessarily a physician) determines that no emergent medical condition exists, there are no EMTALA obligations for the hospital or physicians. An emergent medical condition is defined as any medical condition manifesting itself by acute symptoms of sufficient severity (including severe pain) such that the absence of immediate medical attention could reasonably be expected to result in placing the health of the individual in serious jeopardy, serious impairment of bodily functions, or serious dysfunction of an bodily part or organ.

Neither current nor proposed EMTALA regulations require that the physician treating a patient with an emergent condition must provide follow-up care. Physicians are not prohibited from serving on-call at more than one hospital simultaneously as long as there is a plan for handling potential conflicts. The EMTALA does

not prevent surgeons from performing elective surgery while on-call. Additional information about the EMTALA and its impact on orthopaedic surgeons can be found on the Web site of the American Academy of Orthopaedic Surgeons (http://www.aaos.org; under "Health Policy," click on the button for "more" and the EMTALA compendium will be displayed) (Table 3).

The EMTALA does not require any individual physician to be on-call nor does it set any guidelines about how much on-call time is required. It does mandate that the hospital maintain an on-call list consistent with its capabilities (which may not be 24-hour coverage) in a manner that most effectively serves their patient population; for example, The Centers for Medicare and Medicaid Services allows hospitals some local flexibility in how they set up their on-call schedule. On-call obligations for individual surgeons are imposed by medical staff bylaws, hospital rules, or by contract, but not by the EMTALA. However, if a physician is on the on-call list, failure to respond when called is an EMTALA violation.

TABLE 3 | Trauma Web Resources

Injury Statistics

Burden of Musculoskeletal Injury Fact Sheet. Available at: http://www.ota.org/downloads/muscfacts.pdf

Injury Facts. Chicago, IL, National Safety Council, 1999. Available at: http://www.nsc.org

National Center for Health Statistics Web site. Available at: http://www.cdc.gov/nchs/default.htm

National Health Interview Survey. Available at: http://www.cdc.gov/nchs/nhis.htm

National Safety Council Report on Injuries in America. Available at: http://www.nsc.org/library/report_injury_usa.htm

US Department of Health and Human Services, Public Health Services, Centers for Disease Control and Prevention, National Center for Injury Prevention and Control: Web-based interactive access to data and statistics (WISQARS). Available at: http:www.cdc.gov/ncipc/wisqars

EMTALA

American Academy of Orthopaedic Surgeons Web site. Available at: http://www.aaos.org/wordhtml/health.htm

Orthopaedic Trauma Association Web site: Available at: http://www.ota.org. (Follow the "members only" link to the statement on EMTALA, which also contains a discussion of orthopaedic trauma service organization and care delivery.)

Other Organizations

American College of Surgeons Trauma Programs Web site. Available at: http://www.facs.org/trauma/

American Association for Surgery of Trauma (AAST) Web site. Available at: http://www.aast.org

Eastern Association for the Surgery of Trauma (EAST) Web site. Available at: http://www.EAST.org

OTA Position Paper on Orthopaedic Trauma Service Organization. Available at: http://www.ota.org/committees/otso.htm

Historically, physicians have participated in on-call at the hospital or hospitals where they work without additional compensation beyond that which they could collect for services rendered. This was done as a way to support or build a practice because it was mandated by medical staff bylaws or simply because it was traditional. However, being on-call represents a significant amount of work, especially at trauma center hospitals and those facilities with underrepresented subspecialty physicians. It not only takes time away from family and other activities, but being on-call interferes with the ability to pursue a more productive elective practice. The clinical problems encountered are unpredictable, and the physician may be uncomfortable treating fractures and other injuries often on short notice with no ability to prepare. There is a perception that being on-call exposes a physician to increased risk of malpractice allegations, bloodborne diseases, and patients who are underinsured. It is not unreasonable, therefore, to expect that the hospital would provide some compensation to physicians who, by virtue of being on-call, help the hospital to meet its legal and community obligations.

Many hospitals now provide on-call pay to some medical staff members, usually to those in underrepresented subspecialties. This on-call pay may take the form of a flat stipend per period of time, or in other settings it may consist of paying all or part of the fee for billable services performed while on-call. A California Medical Association report found that in 1998, 22% of California hospitals paid for on-call time, with a stipend ranging from $100 to $1,000 per day. One estimate suggests that approximately 40% of Level 1 and 2 trauma centers currently provide on-call pay, usually in the form of a flat fee for 24 hours of coverage. The average compensation is about $1,800 per day, with a range of $300 to $3,500 per day. The rate will vary based on local conditions in the community and hospital. Some factors to consider include the cost of additional insurance, potential loss of other revenue from office and operating room care, expected frequency of phone calls, expected frequency of in-house service requirement, risk of malpractice, cost of unreimbursed services, commute times, and loss of personal time. The daily on-call pay rate can be based on an average of gross daily charges (annual charges divided by days worked), with added premiums based on the intensity of on-call, additional costs, and additional liability risk. Another method suggests calculating the total daily overhead costs for the practice and using that figure for each 8-hour on-call segment. A third method involves a base stipend that is supplemented by a wRVU-based fee scale to encourage those on-call to do as much of the actual work required as possible, rather than saving it all for the traumatologist or dedicated fracture specialist. In any event, although on-call pay may keep orthopaedic surgeons on the on-call schedule, it does not address the issue of quality of care and the need for more trained orthopaedic traumatologists.

Annotated References

1. Baker SP: *The Injury Fact Book*, ed 2. New York, NY, Oxford University Press, 1992.

2. *Fact Sheet on Trauma*. Chicago, IL, American College of Surgeons, 1993.

3. Anderson RN, Smith BL: Deaths: Leading causes for 2001. *Natl Vital Stat Rep* 2003;52:1-85.

4. Norwood S, Myers MB: Outcomes following injury in a predominantly rural-population-based trauma center. *Arch Surg* 1994;129:800-805.

5. Michaud CM, Murray CJL, Bloon BR: Burden of disease: Implications for future research. *JAMA* 2001;285:535-539.
   This article describes the use of disability adjusted life years to compare the burden of major diseases in various areas of the world. Disability adjusted life years represent the total years of productive life lost because of premature mortality or disability, and they are weighted to reflect the higher social value given to young adults in most societies. Road traffic accidents (one specific type of trauma) were the eleventh highest cause of disability adjusted life years in the world in 1999 and the second highest cause of disability adjusted life years in American men in 1996.

6. Bonnie RJ, Fulco CF, Liverman CT (eds): *Reducing the Burden of Injury: Advancing Prevention and Treatment*. Washington, DC, National Academy Press, 1999.

7. Cales RH: Trauma mortality in Orange County: The effect of implementation of a regional trauma system. *Ann Emerg Med* 1984;13:1-10.

8. Mullins RJ, Veum-Stone J, Helfand M, et al: Outcome of hospitalized injured patients after institution of a trauma system in an urban area. *JAMA* 1994;271:1919-1924.

9. Nathens AB, Jurkovich GJ, Maier RV, et al: Relationship between trauma center volumes and outcomes. *JAMA* 2001;285:1164-1171.
   Using mortality and length of stay as outcome measures, the authors compared high-volume trauma centers (> 650 admissions per year with Injury Severity Scores > 15) with low-volume trauma centers (≤ 650 admissions per year) for patients with penetrating abdominal trauma or blunt multisystem trauma. High-volume centers had significantly lower mortality rates for patients in shock or with coma, but not for those without these conditions. Length of stay

was decreased at the high-volume centers for all patients with multisystem blunt trauma.

10. Eastman AB, Bishop GS, Walsh JC, Richardson JD, Rice CL: The economic status of trauma centers on the eve of health care reform. *J Trauma* 1994;36:835-846.

11. Eastman AB, Rice CL, Bishop GS, Richardson JD: An analysis of the critical problem of trauma center reimbursement. *J Trauma* 1991;31:920-926.

12. *Resources of the Optimal Care of the Injured Patient: 1999.* Chicago, IL, American College of Surgeons, 1999.

13. Hansen ST Jr: Socioeconomic aspects of trauma: Fracture care versus traumatology. *Int J Orthop Trauma* 1991;1:31-34.

14. Hansen ST Jr: Orthopaedist as traumatologist. *J Bone Joint Surg Am* 1992;74:306.

15. Ostrum RF: Orthopaedic trauma surgeon: Distinction or extinction. *Am J Orthop* 2003;32(suppl 9):3-4.
    This editorial defines many of the issues confronting those choosing a career in orthopaedic traumatology.

16. Maull KI, Haynes BW Jr: The integrated trauma service concept. *JACEP* 1977;6:497-499.

17. Baker CC, Degutis LC, DeSantis J, Baue AE: Impact of a trauma service on trauma care in a university hospital. *Am J Surg* 1985;149:453-458.

18. Anglen J, Duncan D: Organization of trauma services: A survey of the Orthopaedic Trauma Association. *J Orthop Trauma* 2000;14:433-439.
    In this observational study conducted by the OTA via mailed surveys to all 427 of its members, 51 separate institution responses were studied, three fourths of which were completed by Level 1 trauma centers. Only 29 of the 51 institutions identified a designated Orthopaedic Trauma Service within the framework of the department or institution. Only 26 of the institutions had an orthopaedic trauma director, and only 18 had hospital-funded ancillary personnel assigned to the orthopaedic trauma service.

19. Harris MB, Webb LX, Ruch DS, et al: The viability of an orthopaedic trauma service, in *Proceedings of the Orthopaedic Trauma Association Annual Meeting, October 10, 2003, Salt Lake City, UT.* Available at: http://www.hwbf.org/ota/am/ota03/otapa/OTA03530.htm. Accessed April 16, 2004.
    This is a business evaluation of the opportunities, costs, and potential fiscal benefits from the development of the Orthopaedic Trauma Service within the confines of the Bowman Gray School of Medicine Department of Orthopaedic Surgery. The institution of a dedicated orthopaedic trauma service improved productivity as measured by wRVUs, number of cases, and charges and collections for members of the service and nontrauma faculty as well as the department as a whole. Faculty and resident job satisfaction improved, and trauma and nontrauma faculty reported improved ability to provide subspecialty care and to achieve research goals.

20. Tran D, Frankel H, Rabinovici R: The profile of Level I trauma directors. *J Trauma* 2002;52:835-839.
    Members of the American Association for the Surgery of Trauma were polled via mailed questionnaires, and 72 responded. Demographic data were collected on age, gender, years in practice, training, and practice activity. Approximately one third of respondents' time was spent on average on clinical trauma care and about 20% on administrative activity. Nearly 90% were involved in research. Salary data were collected, and most respondents were earning between $225,000 and $250,000 annually. Salary was derived from clinical revenue (42%), hospital support (37%), and university support (20%). Lack of negotiation skills and information was evident in every respondent.

21. Bray TJ: Design of the Northern Nevada Orthopaedic Trauma Panel: A model, Level-II community-hospital system. *J Bone Joint Surg Am* 2001;83:283-289.
    In this article, the author explains the development of a system of care for the orthopaedic patient population in a busy, rural, Level 2 trauma center. He explains the organization of the orthopaedic medical staff into a trauma panel with specific qualifications, responsibilities, and privileges under the direction of an orthopaedic trauma director. There is a separate trauma on-call and general orthopaedic on-call schedule, with triage performed by the emergency department. Hospital compensation to trauma panel members is discussed, and a minimum of $1,000 per night is suggested. The hospital also provides administrative support.

22. Fakhry SM, Watts DD: What's a trauma surgeon worth? A salary survey of the Eastern Association for the Surgery of Trauma. *J Trauma* 2000;49:833-838.
    An anonymous self-report questionnaire was sent to general surgeon members of the Eastern Association for the Surgery of Trauma. Two hundred and seven questionnaires (53.7%) were returned for evaluation, of which 172 were usable (44% response rate). Eighty percent of the respondents received compensation from more than one source (salary and billing). On-call pay was received by 20% of respondents. The lack of professional assistance in the negotiating process was remarkable. Present trends in health care economics suggest that a more businesslike approach is in the best interest of all parties. This study

represents the first attempt at determining fair market value for a trauma surgeon.

23. Scherer LA, Battistella FD: Trauma and emergency surgery: An evolutionary direction for trauma surgeons. *J Trauma* 2004;56:7-12.

This retrospective review of case logs and activity of surgeons at a university hospital was conducted to determine the ability to recruit and retain young surgeons if an increased volume of emergency (nontrauma) cases were part of the practice profile. In response to decreasing surgical trauma experience, trauma surgeons began participating in emergency general surgery on-call. This approach was undertaken to create surgical niches for the trauma surgeon as a means of improving the surgical volume, compensation, and career longevity.

24. Mileski WJ: Incorporating sustainability into the concept of optimal care. *J Trauma* 2003;54:1020-1023.

The author discusses the manpower crisis in trauma care and some of its underlying causes and argues that it is the willingness of trauma care surgeons to accept the intrinsic professional rewards born of sacrifice, commitment, hard work, and service that has led to their exploitation. He discusses incorporating the concept of sustainability into what is considered optimal in trauma care and managing the human resources of the business in a way that facilitates recruitment and retention. The author concludes that current workload and compensation methods are not sustainable.

Chapter 3

CPT Coding in Orthopaedic Trauma

Robert A. Probe, MD   Marisa Andrews, CPC, CST

Pat Torres, RHIT, CCS, CPC   Bruce Trahan, MHA, CHE

Introduction

Physician compensation for services rendered is an extremely complex process in the United States. The plethora of different payer sources, provider pools, and inconsistent allowances are variables beyond the control of most physicians. What is under the control of physicians is the quantitative reporting of their work via accurate coding. In an office medical practice, this process is usually straightforward. A single level of service by a provider is represented by a single code. Unfortunately, in trauma the application of codes is complicated by multiple problems being addressed simultaneously, by multiple providers participating in treatment of a given patient, and by the delivery of care over multiple periods. Because this system is so complex, physicians often do not put forth the effort to learn how to appropriately report their services. The result is lost revenue for services provided. Therefore, it is important that trauma surgeons understand the entire coding process from the initial trauma patient evaluation through the last reconstructive procedure. It is particularly essential that trauma surgeons have a thorough understanding of evaluation and management (E/M) coding and surgical Current Procedural Terminology (CPT®) codes and their modifiers as they pertain to initial, subsequent, and reconstructive trauma care.

Many of the rules put forward by the CPT editorial panel of the American Medical Association are subject to interpretation. Because differences of opinion and practice are common among physicians and payers, what is reflected in this chapter are coding practices from a single institution that are considered to fairly represent work that is performed in the care of orthopaedic trauma patients.

E/M Codes

Trauma care begins with a provider evaluating a patient. These interactions are reported using E/M codes. Applying the correct E/M code requires defining the level and the type of service. Level of service is determined by defining the level of the following three key components

of the patient encounter: the patient history, physical examination, and medical decision making.[1]

Patient history is classified as problem focused, expanded problem focused, detailed, or comprehensive based on the following four elements: chief complaint; history of present illness; review of systems; and past, family, and social history. The chief complaint is a statement describing the symptom, problem, condition, diagnosis, physician recommended return, or other factor that is the reason for the encounter; it is usually stated by the patient. The medical record must clearly reflect the reason for the visit (chief complaint). The history of present illness is a description of the development of the patient's present illness or injury from the first sign and symptom or from the previous encounter to the present. The review of systems is an inventory of body systems obtained through a series of questions seeking to identify signs and symptoms that the patient may be experiencing or has experienced. The past history includes the patient's past illness, injuries, surgeries, and/or treatments. Family history includes a review of medical events in the patient's family. Social history includes an age-appropriate review of past and current activities (such as drug use).

The second key component of the patient encounter is the physical examination. The levels of E/M services are based on the following four levels of examination: problem focused, expanded problem focused, detailed, or comprehensive examination. Problem focused examination is a limited examination of the affected body area or organ system. Expanded problem focused examination is a limited examination of the affected body area or organ system and any other symptomatic or related body area or organ system(s). Detailed examination is an extended examination of the affected body area or organ system(s) and any other symptomatic or related body areas or organ systems. Comprehensive examination is a general multisystem examination or complete examination of a single organ system.

The third key component of the patient encounter is medical decision making. There are four levels of E/M services for medical decision making: straightforward,

TABLE 1 | 1995 Guidelines for Level 5 Consultation E/M Coding

History	Extended (4 points)
Review of systems	Ten organ systems
Past history	All three (past medical, family, and social)
Multisystem physical examination	Eight of twelve organ systems
High complexity decision making	Threat to limb function

TABLE 2 | 1997 Guidelines for Level 3 Consultation E/M Coding

Chief complaint	Included
History	Extended (four elements)
Review of systems	Two organ systems
Past history	One of past medical, family, or social history
Detailed examination	Twelve bullet points
Moderately complex decision making	Radiographs ordered and reviewed

low complexity, moderate complexity, and high complexity. Medical decision making is based on the number of possible diagnoses and/or the number of management options that must be considered, the amount and/or complexity of medical records, diagnostic tests, and/or other information that must be obtained, reviewed, and analyzed. Also included in medical decision making is the risk of significant complications, morbidity, and/or mortality, as well as comorbidities that are associated with the patient's presenting problems(s), diagnostic procedures(s), and/or possible management options.

There are four levels of risk: minimal, low, moderate, and high. The highest level of risk in any one category (presenting problem, diagnostic procedures, or management options) determines the overall risk. A table for determining the risk of significant complications, morbidities, and mortalities may be found on the Center for Medicare and Medicaid Services (CMS) Web site (http://www.cms.hhs.gov/medlearn/emdoc.asp).[1]

Choice of E/M Level

Level determination, as defined by the CMS, is clearly a complex process that is abstruse and difficult to use. It is useful to work backward from the most common clinical situation, identify the appropriate level for each, and then create documentation that supports this level. Germane to the trauma patient are two situations: the emergency department evaluation and the evaluation of an injury in the outpatient clinic.

The complexity of medical decision making is usually what drives the maximum coding potential for a patient encounter. Trauma patients who require evaluation by an orthopaedic surgeon in the emergency department typically qualify for high-complexity decision making. In many patients, skeletal injury causes a threat to bodily function and must be evaluated with a review of radiographs and laboratory data. The management decisions are also deemed to be complex because orthopaedic surgeons must determine whether surgery is indicated and if so, must decide among different surgical options. This matrix of risk and decision complexity leads to a high rating of medical decision making, which, in turn, qualifies for level 5 consultation billing. In addition, a

multisystem evaluation following advanced trauma life support protocol is critical to identify associated injury. If the orthopaedist performs this service, then this is clearly a situation that is consistent with level 5 work. The CMS uses two sets of guidelines to assess billing (1995 and 1997). As a trauma orthopaedist in the emergency department, this is most easily accomplished using 1995 guidelines. Table 1 summarizes the requirements for a level 5 consultation charge.

If trauma patients are incapable of providing a history, as is common in these patients, this should be noted in the record. Under these circumstances, requirements for history are then waived.

The outpatient evaluation of a single injury is different than a comprehensive emergency department evaluation. The use of the musculoskeletal single-system guidelines from 1997 is generally more appropriate. Although the medical decision making would often rate the complexity as high, the appropriate medical examination is usually restricted to a regional component of the musculoskeletal system and therefore only qualifies as a detailed examination, which correlates with a level 3 new patient/consultation charge. Following this strategy makes it imperative to understand 1997 level 3 requirements (Table 2).

Documentation of a level 3 examination requires that attention be given to the physical examination and documentation of 12 elements from the 1997 musculoskeletal examination. This is usually easily accomplished by commenting on the strength, stability, appearance, and range of motion of the involved area and comparing with that of the opposite side. This provides eight points, thereby allowing the examiner to choose from general appearance, vital signs (at least three), regional nodes, skin appearance, swelling, pulses, temperature, neurologic examination, gait, mood, or orientation for the remaining four points. The 1997 guidelines for all five levels are summarized in Table 3.

Once an appropriate level has been determined for patient history, physical examination, and medical decision making, the setting in which the service is rendered must then be defined. This requires differentiating whether a patient is a new patient, an established patient,

TABLE 3 | 1997 E/M Guidelines

Patient Status	Documentation Guidelines			
New/Consultation History (requires three of three elements; weak link drives the level)		**Examination**	**Level of Medical Decision Making**	**Time (minutes)**
99201/ 99241/ 99251	**Problem focused:** One to three elements (HPI, no ROS, no PFSH)	**Problem focused:** One to five elements	Straightforward	10 New patient 15 Outpatient consultation 20 Inpatient consultation
99202/ 99242/ 99252	**Expanded problem focused:** One to three elements (HPI, 1 ROS, no PFSH)	**Expanded problem focused:** ≥ Six elements	Straightforward	20 New patient 30 Outpatient consultation 40 Inpatient consultation
99203/ 99243/ 99253	**Detailed:** ≥ Four elements (HPI, two to nine ROS, pertinent PFSH in two history areas)	**Detailed:** ≥ Twelve elements from ≥ two areas/systems	Low	30 New patient 40 Outpatient consultation 55 Inpatient consultation
99204/ 99244/ 99254	**Comprehensive:** ≥ Four elements (HPI, 10 ROS, complete PFSH in three history areas)	**Comprehensive:** ≥ Two elements identified by a bullet from nine areas/systems	Moderate	45 New patient 60 Outpatient consultation 80 Inpatient consultation
99205/ 99245/ 99255	**Comprehensive:** ≥ Four elements (HPI, 10 ROS, complete PFSH in three history areas)	**Comprehensive:** ≥ Two elements from nine areas/systems	High	60 New patient 80 Outpatient consultation 110 Inpatient consultation
Established History (requires at least two of the three elements)				
99211	Minimal problem may not require physician			5
99212	**Problem focused:** One to three elements (HPI, no ROS, no PFSH)	**Problem focused:** One to five elements	Straightforward	10
99213	**Expanded problem focused:** One to three elements (HPI, 1 ROS, no PFSH)	**Expanded problem focused:** ≥ Six elements	Low	15
99214	**Detailed:** ≥ Four elements (HPI, two to nine ROS, pertinent PFSH in one history area)	**Detailed:** ≥ Twelve elements from ≥ two areas/systems	Moderate	25
99215	**Comprehensive:** ≥ Four elements (HPI, 10 ROS, complete PFSH in two or three history areas)	**Comprehensive:** ≥ Two elements from nine areas/systems	High	40

HPI = history of present illness, ROS = review of systems, PFSH = past, family, and social history

being seen for consultation, receiving initial hospital care, or receiving subsequent hospital care.

A new patient is one who has not received professional (face-to-face) services from the physician or another physician of the same specialty in the same group practice within the past 3 years. An established patient is one who has received professional services from the physician or another physician of the same specialty in the same group practice within the past 3 years. A patient seen for consultation may be new or established, but other criteria must be met, including (1) a request for a consultation must come from an attending physician or other appropriate source, and medical necessity for the service must be documented in the patient's medical record; (2) the opinion rendered and services ordered or performed must be documented in the patient's medical record; and (3) a report of the findings or opinion must be communicated to the requesting provider via written report.

When evaluating patients in an outpatient setting, use of the consultation group of codes (CPT 99241 to 99245) is desirable when appropriate because it carries the highest level of E/M reimbursement. Physicians may bill for a consultation even if they decide to assume responsibility for continued care. In this instance, all subsequent charges will be of the established patient type because the patient now has been seen within the 3-year guideline. Conversely, if a determination is made before the patient visit to accept care, then this is considered a transfer of care and billing for a consultation is not appropriate. The ability of an orthopaedist to be consulted by another orthopaedist is often questioned. If the intent of the patient visit is to garner an opinion and the three basic criteria for consultation billing are met, then this does qualify as a consultation. If the visit occurs as a result of patient preference or for reasons of geographic convenience, then new patient codes are more appropriate. The following scenarios provide examples to help understand these concepts.

In the first scenario, an orthopaedist has a patient with a healed supramalleolar tibial fracture in 18° of varus. An evaluation by a fellow orthopaedist who is experienced in malunion surgery is requested. After this evaluation occurs, an osteotomy is recommended and performed. In this instance, the initial evaluation by the osteotomy surgeon would be considered a consultation because it meets the true intent of that level of service.

In the second scenario, a patient is seen in the emergency department and a diagnosis of an intra-articular fracture of the calcaneus is made. The emergency department physician discharges the patient with instructions for follow-up care in the office of a local orthopaedist. In this setting, the evaluation by the orthopaedist is not a consultation because the intent of the referring physician is to transfer care of the patient for the treatment of a calcaneal fracture.

The intentions of the referring physician are paramount in making such determinations (Was the intent to transfer care or to receive an opinion?). There are two sets of consultation codes. The first set of codes is used for office or other outpatient consultation (CPT 99241 to 99245). The second set of codes is used for inpatient consultation (CPT 99251 to 99255).

Initial hospital inpatient care codes are used to report admission to a hospital setting. Only one initial hospital inpatient care code should be reported for a single hos-

pital visit. It should be noted that only three initial hospital codes exist (CPT 99221 to 99223). It is generally believed that hospitalization should not be necessary for level 1 or level 2 problems; therefore, a level 1 initial hospital code requires the documentation of a level 3 new patient/consultation code, a level 2 initial hospital code requires the documentation of a level 4 new patient/consultation code, and a level 3 initial hospital code requires the documentation of a level 5 new patient/consultation code.

Subsequent hospital inpatient care codes are used to report each additional follow-up hospital visit after the initial hospital care. Subsequent hospital care codes are per day codes for the evaluation and management of a patient. There are three levels of subsequent hospital inpatient codes (CPT 99231 to 99233), and they require at least two of the three key components of the patient encounter. Subsequent hospital codes are not appropriate for the day before or the day following a surgical procedure without a qualifying modifier because these days are usually covered by the CPT global period.

When a health care provider requests an orthopaedist to evaluate a patient in the emergency department, an opinion is being sought. As such, a consultation code is appropriate, assuming that this request is made in writing. Creation of emergency department documentation is considered to be a written response to the requesting physician. In the event that hospital admission is deemed necessary, the use of an initial consultation code is advantageous because of the associated increase in relative value units (RVUs). For example, the highest hospital admission code returns $151.92 from Medicare, whereas the highest consultation code returns $189.81. For this to be appropriate, the decision for admission must be made by the consulting orthopaedist based on his consultation and not by the requesting physician.

E/M coding is complex, and its many subtleties are beyond the scope of this chapter. Further explanation and details for both the 1995 and 1997 documentation guidelines may be found on the CMS Web site.[1]

CPT Coding for Nonsurgical Fracture Care

Orthopaedists commonly provide nonsurgical treatment of fractures, and there are two coding options for billing for such services. The first option is to follow E/M guidelines and bill for the initial and subsequent visits accordingly. Using this method, additional revenue is received by appropriately charging for application of the initial and subsequent cast or splint (CPT 29000 to 29590). The second option is to bill the CPT code for closed treatment of fractures that corresponds to the particular injury. Subsets of this treatment strategy include fractures treated with manipulation and those treated without manipulation. When using the CPT coding option, the initial cast or splint is bundled with the procedure and cannot

TABLE 4 | E/M Method and Treatment Coding

Diagnosis	ICD-9	Description	
	813.42	Fracture of the radius, lower end	

Date	CPT Code	Descriptions	RVUs
Week 0	99203	New patient	2.54
	29075	Short arm cast	1.93
Week 3	99213	Established patient	1.39
	29075	Short arm cast	1.93
Week 6	99212	Established patient	1.00
	29125	Short arm static splint	1.53
Week 10	99212	Established patient	1.00
Week 16	99212	Established patient	1.00
Total			**12.32**

Date	CPT Code	Descriptions	RVUs
Week 0	25600	Closed treatment of fracture of the distal radius; no manipulation	7.50
Week 3	29075	Short arm cast	1.93
Week 6	29125	Short arm static splint	1.53
Week 10	Global		0.00
Week 16	99212	Established patient	1.00
Total			**11.96**

be billed separately; however, orthopaedists can bill for subsequent cast changes using a 58 modifier.

In general, whenever a fracture reduction is performed by the billing provider, the added work of the manipulation favors the use of the appropriate CPT charge. Additionally, for fractures of larger bones, such as the tibia or humerus, the CPT code almost always results in greater return than coding for each individual visit. This strategy may change as the CPT code drops in value for fractures of smaller bones. The consequences of each strategy are best understood by example. The coding for each strategy for the treatment of a distal radius fracture without manipulation is illustrated in Table 4.

This example does not include an E/M code for the initial patient encounter, which is typically used for a new patient, consultation, or emergency department visit when criteria are met. A 57 modifier is added when a decision regarding treatment is made. As the examples in Table 4 illustrate, the two coding strategies for a distal radius fracture without manipulation result in reimbursement that is approximately equal. If a break-even analysis is performed, the critical variable becomes how many billable follow-up visits will be required in the 90-day global period to outperform the upfront revenue of the CPT coding (for example, treatment of a distal femur would require 17.7 visits to break even, whereas

the break-even point for a phalangeal fracture is only 1.4 visits.)[2]

This analysis suggests that a CPT coding strategy used for more severe fractures can result in a greater return. Additional benefits of this strategy are that dictations do not need to satisfy the criteria for a given E/M level and the largest portion of the bill is entered early. Fractures of the smaller bones, which are likely to require several follow-up visits, may result in a greater return using an E/M strategy as noted previously.

Another common coding dilemma occurs when billing for the treatment of fractures that were reduced by another physician and the patient is now seeing a different physician for subsequent care. In this situation, the billing practice of the subsequent treating physician should be related to the billing provided by the initial physician. If a CPT code for the treatment of a fracture with manipulation and an appended modifier of 54 (surgical care only) were initially used, then the follow-up physician can use the same CPT code with modifier 55 (postoperative management only) appended. This reimburses 21% of the total RVUs for the procedure. Although some physicians bill for such a procedure using the CPT code for closed treatment without manipulation, this is not appropriate because the payer may then be billed twice for treatment of the same fracture. The safest alternative in this instance is to rely on E/M codes as previously described.

CPT Coding

When using a CPT code to bill for a surgical procedure, it generally includes care provided during the 24 hours before the procedure and 90 days subsequent to the procedure. Coding for the care of trauma patients often becomes much more complex because multiple procedures and evaluations are often required, many procedures are not accurately defined by existing codes, multiple procedures are often required during a global period, and multiple providers combine their respective skills in the care of such patients. All of these situations require an understanding of the modifiers that can be applied to basic CPT codes.[3]

Modifier 22 is used to indicate that a procedure has been performed at a greater service than described in the listed code. It is a pricing modifier that is raised at the discretion of the surgeon. There is no consistent policy that dictates what that increase should be. It varies from surgeon to surgeon and from patient to patient. Modifier 22 is only used when another code cannot describe the greater increment of work. There are some issues with Medicare concerning the use of this modifier because of alleged past abuses. When using modifier 22, a cover letter (Table 5) and a separately dictated report should be submitted to explain its use. Some CPT codes also take into consideration whether the surgeon is returning

TABLE 5 | Letter Submitted to Facilitate Reimbursement for Modifier 22 Procedures

Dear Medical Reviewer,

I have attached a modifier 22 to the CPT code of the attached claim because the code does not accurately describe the complexity of the procedure.

I believe that this procedure was ___% more difficult than the similar listed procedure for the following reasons....

I expect an increase in reimbursement of __% for these services.

to an anatomic area that has already been operated on, in which instance the use of modifier 22 would be inappropriate. These codes include malunion and nonunion codes. To facilitate reimbursement, a written bill must be submitted for consideration, and overuse of this modifier can lead to audits. When dictating surgical notes, care should be taken to explain why the procedure required an unusual amount of time, effort, and skill. Specific reasons why this procedure was more difficult should also be provided. General statements, such as "this was a very complex case," should be avoided.

Modifier 24 is used with E/M codes only to indicate that an E/M service was provided to the patient within the defined global period following surgery for a reason unrelated to the original procedure. Modifier 24 is commonly used in the trauma setting when billing for the evaluation of secondary injuries such as ankle sprains in patients receiving surgical care for another injury.

Modifier 25 is used to indicate that a separate E/M service was provided on the same day as a procedure. Modifier 25 is intended to be used for minor procedures. For example, when a physician who evaluates an injured elbow and also provides a therapeutic elbow aspiration, the aspiration would carry a CPT code and the appropriate E/M would have a modifier 25. Full payment should be expected for both procedures.

Modifier 50 is used to indicate that a procedure was done bilaterally. Modifier 50 is a pricing modifier and should always be listed first. Payment for this modifier is based on 150% of the Medicare fee schedule.[4]

Modifier 51 is used when the same physician does multiple procedures at one encounter. This is usually appended to the lesser CPT code and should not be attached to CPT codes that are modifier 51-exempt or add-on codes. In addition, modifier 51 should not be attached to any Medicare claim because such claims are set up to automatically reduce the fee. Payment for modifier 51 is based on the payment adjustment for multiple surgeries (100% and 50% for the next four subsequent surgeries by report) or the actual fee, whichever is lower. This is also a pricing modifier, and it should always be listed first.

Modifier 52 is used to indicate that a procedure has been performed to a lesser degree than desired. It is used when the surgery is terminated or reduced at the discretion of the surgeon for whatever reason. As with modifiers 50 and 51, modifier 52 is a pricing modifier, and it should always be listed first. The payer should be allowed to review the claim and reduce payment accordingly. A separate statement similar to that submitted with the application of modifier 22 should be submitted for review by the payer.

Modifier 53 is used when a procedure is terminated at the risk of a patient's well-being. It is also a pricing modifier and should also be listed first. Modifier 53 is used to indicate that a procedure was started, but it could not be completed because of the patient's health or extenuating circumstances.

Modifier 58 is used when the same physician returns a patient to the operating room within the postoperative period for a staged or related procedure. Modifier 58 is commonly used when billing for the treatment of open fractures. The surgeon performs débridement on day 1; on day 3, the same surgeon performs continued débridement, and on day 5, the same surgeon performs definitive fixation of the fracture. The appropriate modifier for the two subsequent visits on day 3 and day 5 would be modifier 58. All surgical notes regarding the plan to return the patient to the operating room for subsequent treatment should be included with billing submission. Use of modifier 58 should not modify reimbursement.

Modifier 59 is used to indicate a separate, distinct procedural service. It is most commonly used to indicate that a procedure was done at a different site. It is also commonly used to bypass a bundling edit. Bundling edits are clarifications published by the CMS that define procedures intended to be bundled under a single CPT code. The 59 modifier is appropriate if a procedure that is typically bundled is performed during a separate patient encounter.[4]

Several modifiers are used to bill for a return trip to the operating room during the postoperative global period. Modifier 76 is used when the patient must return to the operating room for the same procedure by the same surgeon. Modifier 77 is used when the patient must return to the operating room for the same procedure by a different surgeon. Medicare typically questions the use of these modifiers unless the procedures are performed on the same day; therefore, when reporting repeated procedures, modifier 78 should be used, whether the procedure is done by the same surgeon or not.

Modifier 78 is used to bill for the return of a patient to the operating room for a procedure that was performed during the postoperative period of the initial procedure that is related to the original encounter. A new postoperative period does not begin with the application of modifier 78. Modifier 79 is used to indicate a return trip to the operating room for an unrelated procedure during the postoperative global period. In addition to the modifier, a different *International Classifica-*

tion of Diseases, 9th Edition (ICD-9) diagnosis code should also be reported. A new postoperative period begins with the use of this modifier.

Modifier 82 is used by physicians in teaching institutions to indicate their assistance during surgery. A separate surgical note is not required with the use of modifier 82; however, if separate procedures were performed by either physician, it should be clearly documented as such in separate surgical notes. The use of modifier 82 is contingent on the unavailability of a qualified resident and this should be documented in the body of the note. Exactly what constitutes a qualified resident, however, has not yet been defined. If not in a teaching hospital, then the appropriate modifier for surgical assistance would be modifier 80 rather than 82.

In special circumstances, two different specialties are required to achieve one service. In this instance, modifier 62, which bills for the services of a cosurgeon, is the best one to use. It is attached to the CPT code that best describes the procedure, and it is reported by both surgeons. Payment is usually 62.5% of the fee schedule for each surgeon. When using modifier 62, separate surgical notes need to be dictated to support the work that was performed by the two different physicians. For example, modifier 62 would be used when a general surgeon performs the exposure for an anterior spinal fusion procedure and an orthopaedic surgeon performs the fusion itself. In this instance, both the general surgeon and the orthopaedic surgeon would report the appropriate CPT code with the modifier 62.

Unlisted Procedures

CPT codes are compiled by the American Medical Association. They are updated annually, and existing codes are revised and new codes are introduced. However, in some circumstances, a procedure does not have an established CPT code. When this occurs, it is best to bill for the procedure using the unlisted procedure code. Submission of this code will require a detailed surgical report, and the physician must request a payment amount based on listed procedures of comparable complexity.

Commonly Missed Opportunities

In the course of evaluating and treating multiple trauma patients, attention and coding often focus on major surgical procedures and billing for minor procedure is often forgotten. Although the charges for minor procedures are often small, they can rapidly add up and represent significant revenue. For example, a patient with a 20-cm complex laceration, a stable lateral malleolus fracture, and a both-column acetabular fracture would typically have an evaluation using advanced trauma life support protocol, the laceration closed, and the ankle evaluated and splinted on the day of injury. CT would be done, CT

scans would be reviewed, and the decision to perform acetabular surgery would be made on the second day. The surgery would then be performed on the third day. Table 6 illustrates the possible billing codes for this patient.

Understanding exactly what is being billed for within a given CPT code can also aid surgeons in appropriately reporting their work. Billing for the treatment of a patient with a bimalleolar fracture with syndesmotic injury provides a good example. CPT 27814 is used to bill for the open treatment of a bimalleolar ankle fracture. This injury often requires the additional use of a syndesmotic screw, but this is not part of the code. If this is to be billed, CPT 27829 open treatment of distal tibiofibular joint must be added. Even though modifier 51 will reduce payment, this still returns 8.8 RVUs. The best way to know what is included in a given CPT code is to review the global service data for a code in question.[5]

Attention given to accurate procedure description can often make a significant difference in reimbursement. For example, when using an intramedullary implant to treat a patient with a subtrochanteric fracture, the subtrochanteric fracture can accurately be described as either a proximal femoral shaft fracture or a peritrochanteric fracture. A 3.5 RVU advantage results when identifying this fracture as a peritrochanteric fracture. Knowledge of this difference results in compensation to the surgeon for the recognized complexities of obtaining reduction for subtrochanteric fractures. Another example is provided when performing an arthrotomy to remove debris associated with open wounds. When using débridement codes for open fractures (CPT 11012), a maximum of 14 RVUs are possible; however, when using an arthrotomy for removal of foreign body code (CPT 27331), 20.5 RVUs are returned. Again, the complexity associated with exploring a joint is reflected in reimbursement as long as the coder is cognizant of these differences.

Opportunities for greater reimbursement also exist in accurate coding for the treatment of high-energy articular injuries. Open treatment of a combined femoral neck and femoral shaft fracture would qualify for multiple CPT codes for each. Similarly, an articular fracture with extensive diaphyseal extension that requires extended implants, exposure, and surgery would qualify for description of the articular treatment and the diaphyseal treatment with separate CPT codes; however, the second would be subjected to the appropriate reduction applied to modifier 51. This is true even if both components of the fracture are managed with a single implant. For example, a distal femoral fracture with intra-articular extension and diaphyseal component treated with a submuscular locking plate justifies the use of both CPT 27513 and 27507.

TABLE 6 | Possible Billing Codes for a Patient With a 20-cm Complex Laceration, a Stable Lateral Malleolus Fracture, and a Both-Column Acetabular Fracture

Day 1

99255-57	Initial inpatient consult
27786	Closed treatment of distal fibular fracture without manipulation
13121	Repair, complex 2.6 to 7.5 cm
13122	Each additional 5 cm or less
13122	Each additional 5 cm or less
13122	Each additional 5 cm or less

Day 2

99233-24,57	Subsequent hospital care, level 3 for evaluation of acetabular fracture, CT

Day 3

27228-79	Open treatment of both columns acetabular fracture, unrelated procedure

As this example demonstrates, there are many opportunities to report work that is often unbilled when treating patients with complex injuries.

Smaller Procedures That Are Often Unbilled

CPT Code	Description	RVUs	Modifier 51 Exempt?
20650	Skeletal traction pin	2.23	No
20660	Application of tongs	2.51	Yes
20690	Application of uniplane external fixation	3.52	Yes
20902	Major or large bone graft	7.55	Yes
20974	Electrical stimulation to aid bone healing	0.62	Yes
76006	Manual stress by physician for joint radiography	0.41	Add on

One feature of many of the codes for smaller procedures is the 51 exemption. Normally, modifier 51 suggests to the payer that the value should be diminished by 50% because it is an additional procedure. For those codes that are modifier 51 exempt, no modifier should be applied and no value reduction should occur.

Managing Denials

Avoiding Denials

Health care claim denials present a major problem for providers. Denials can be reprocessed and/or appealed, many times resulting in a decision reversal and subsequent payment. However, this process is time- and resource-consuming, with no guarantee of a positive final outcome. Therefore, attention should first be given to implementing processes that help avoid denials. Most denials are the result of improper claim submissions, which result in part in omission of information that is pertinent to claim processing. Several examples are listed in Table 7.

Appeals Process

Every year thousands of provider claims are denied as a result of what appears to be evidence to support non-payment for services. Many denials go unreviewed and unappealed simply because the provider lacks the resources to pursue an extensive follow-up. Claim denials for services rendered with appropriate documentation should be aggressively pursued. The first step in the appeals process should be writing a letter of appeal. A

TABLE 7 | Examples of Billing Omissions That Can Result in Claim Denials

Incorrect ICD-9-CM diagnosis code

CPT code not supported by the diagnosis code

CPT code bundled with another service performed

Absence of a modifier

Modifier 59 indicates a distinct procedural service performed/reported during or same day the same session of another service

Modifier 76 and 77 indicate repeat procedure, same day, by same or different physician

Modifier 78 and 79 indicate unrelated or related surgery within the global period of another procedure (many surgical procedures have a 90-day global period; specific injections have a 10-day global period)

letter of appeal can be submitted in response to medical necessity denials, precertification denials, timely filing denials, slow payments/payment reductions, and CPT code bundling. The letter of appeal should contain different information for different appeals, but the identification information is typically similar for any letter. A template for a letter of appeal is provided in Table 8.

TABLE 8 | Template for a Letter of Appeal

(Date)

Attn: Claims Management–APPEALS
(Insurance policy carrier)
(Insurance policy address)

Re: *(Patient name)*
(Policy number)
(Subscriber name)
(Dates of service(s)–admission date through discharge date)
(Amount of charges)

Dear Medical Reviewer:

    The above referenced claim was denied by your processing department for *(repeat their written reason for denial)*.

We believe this denial to be incorrect for the following reason(s):

Providers should not fear the appeals process because it can lead to substantial revenue recovery. Physicians must be involved in the appeal process because they are the individuals who are best suited to determine the appropriateness or inappropriateness of a denial. The key to revenue recovery from appealing claim denials is persistence and an attention to detail in each instance. If the first appeal is denied for charges that are clearly supported by documentation, and all billing and coding guidelines have been met, another appeal should be filed. Managing claim denials and mastering the appeals process is vital to cash flow and proper management of the revenue cycle. A hearing with a physician reviewer or hearing officer can be requested and can often take place via conference call.

Summary

Providing service to trauma patients is a complex undertaking. Unfortunately, coding for these services can become equally complex. To receive fair payment for services, providers must understand the nuances of the coding system.

Annotated References

1. *1995/1997 Documentation Guidelines for Evaluation and Management Services.* Baltimore, MD, Centers for Medicare and Medicaid Services. Available at: www.cms.hhs.gov/medlearn/emdoc.asp. Accessed November 8, 2004.

   This portion of the CMS Web site contains PDF downloads that explain in detail each of the components of the history, physical examination, and decision making that must be documented to support a given code. Both the 1995 General Examination Guidelines as well as the 1997 Specialty Examination Guidelines are available.

2. *AAOS Guide to CPT Coding for Orthopaedic Surgery 2000.* Rosemont, IL, American Academy of Orthopaedic Surgeons, 2000.

   This publication is specific to the practice of orthopaedic surgery and covers all of the 20,000 codes as well as the codes for musculoskeletal radiology, the integument system, and spine that are germane to an orthopaedic practice. RVU conversions are provided, which make this an excellent reference to create coding strategy based on reimbursement. In addition to the CPT assistance, E/M guidelines and scenarios are included to assist with clinic coding.

3. *CPT 2003: Current Procedural Terminology (Professional Edition).* Chicago, IL, AMA Press, 2002.

   This reference contains all of the descriptions for a given CPT code. Importantly, it also provides descriptions of modifiers and their uses.

4. *The CMS Online Manual System.* Baltimore, MD, Centers for Medicare & Medicaid Services. Available at: www.cms.hh.gov/manuals. Accessed November 8, 2004.

   Paper publications of CMS rules and regulations are gradually being replaced with electronic versions maintained and available for download from this Web site. Virtually all questions regarding eligibility, benefits, and secondary payers are covered.

5. *Complete Global Service Data for Orthopaedic Surgery, 2005 edition.* Rosemont, IL, American Academy of Orthopaedic Surgeons, 2005.

   This guide, edited by the AAOS Committee on Coding and Classification, details inclusions and exclusions for more than 1,500 musculoskeletal procedures. It dedicates a complete page to each CPT code to fully explain what is bundled into a particular code, its global period, and associated 51 modified codes.

Chapter 4

Evidence-Based Medicine and the Internet

Mohit Bhandari, MD, MSc, FRCSC

Evidence-Based Medicine

The term evidence-based medicine (EBM) first appeared in 1990 in a document for applicants to the Internal Medicine Residency Program at McMaster University that described EBM as an attitude of enlightened skepticism toward the application of diagnostic, therapeutic, and prognostic technologies. As outlined in the journal *Clinical Epidemiology* and first described in the literature in the *ACP Journal Club* in 1991, the EBM approach to practicing medicine relies on an awareness of the evidence on which a clinician's practice is based and the strength of inference permitted by that evidence.[1] The most sophisticated practice of EBM requires, in turn, a clear delineation of relevant clinical questions, a thorough search of the literature relating to the questions, a critical appraisal of available evidence and its applicability to the clinical situation, and a balanced application of the conclusions to the clinical problem. The balanced application of the evidence (the clinical decision making) is the central point of practicing EBM and involves, according to EBM principles, integration of clinical expertise and judgment, patients' and societal values, and the best available research evidence.

How does EBM differ from the traditional approaches to health care provision? According to the traditional paradigm, clinicians evaluate and solve clinical problems by reflecting on their own clinical experience or the underlying biology and pathophysiology or by consulting a textbook or local expert.[2] For many traditional practitioners, reading the introduction and discussion sections of a research article is adequate for gaining relevant information, and observations from day-to-day clinical experience are a valid means of building and maintaining knowledge about patient prognosis, the value of diagnostic tests, and the efficacy of treatment. Because this paradigm places high value on traditional scientific authority and adherence to standard approaches, traditional medical training and common sense provide adequate bases for evaluating new tests and treatments, and content expertise and clinical experience are sufficient to generate guidelines for clinical practice.

EBM posits that although pathophysiology and clinical experience are necessary, they alone are insufficient guides for practice.[3] These evidence sources may lead to inaccurate predictions about the performance of diagnostic tests and the efficacy of treatments. Like the traditional approach to health care, the EBM health care paradigm also assumes that clinical experience and the development of clinical instincts (particularly with respect to diagnosis) are crucial elements of physician competence. However, the EBM approach includes several additional steps. These steps include using experience to identify important knowledge gaps and information needs, formulating answerable questions, identifying potentially relevant research, assessing the validity of evidence and results, developing clinical policies that align research evidence and clinical circumstances, and applying research evidence to individual patients with attention given to their particular experiences, expectations, and values.[3]

Over the past several years, the concepts and ideas attributed to and labeled collectively as EBM have become a part of daily clinical lives, and clinicians increasingly hear about evidence-based guidelines, evidence-based care paths, and evidence-based questions and solutions. The controversy has shifted from whether to implement the new concepts to how to do so sensibly and efficiently, while avoiding potential problems associated with several misconceptions about what EBM is and what it is not. The EBM-related concepts of hierarchy of evidence, meta-analyses, confidence intervals, and study design are so widespread that clinicians willing to use current medical literature with understanding have no choice but to become familiar with EBM principles and methodologies.

Critics of EBM have mistakenly suggested that EBM equates evidence with results of randomized trials, statistical significance with clinical relevance, evidence (of whatever kind) with decisions, and lack of evidence of efficacy with the evidence for the lack of efficacy. Other critics argue that EBM is not a tool for providing optimal patient care, but merely a cost-containment tool. All these statements represent a fundamental mischaracter-

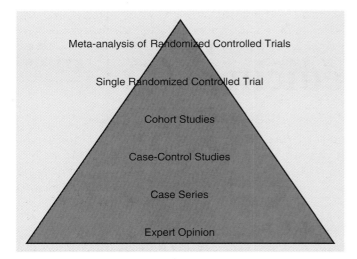

Figure 1 Hierarchy of evidence.

TABLE 1 | Evidence Resources

Publications
Evidence-Based Medicine
Using the Medical Literature
   Journal of the American Medical Association User's Guides
   Canadian Medical Association Journal User's Guides
   Journal of Bone and Joint Surgery User's Guides
   Canadian Journal of Surgery User's Guides

Databases
Best Evidence
Cochrane Library and Cochrane Randomized Trials Register (www.update-software.com/cochrane/)
Database of Abstracts and Reviews of Effectiveness
Internet Database of Evidence-based Abstracts and Articles
MEDLINE/PubMed(www.ncbi.nlm.nih.gov/entrez/query.fcgi)
EMBASE (European equivalent of MEDLINE)
Clinical Evidence (www.clinicalevidence.org/)
SUMsearch (www.sumsearch.uthscsa.edu)
TRIP database (www.tripdatabase.com/)

Electronic Publications
American College of Physicians Journal Club (www.acpjc.org/)
Bandolier: Evidence-Based Healthcare
Evidence-Based Medicine
National Guideline Clearinghouse (Agency of health care policy and research-AHCPR) (www.guidelines.gov)

Internet Resources
Healthweb: Evidence-Based Health Care (www.healthweb.org)
Evidence-Based Medicine from McMaster University (www.hiru.hirunet.mcmaster.ca)
Center for Evidence-Based Medicine (www.cebm.net)
Critically Appraised Topics databank (www.cebm.net/toolbox.asp)
New York Academy of Medicine EBM resource center (www.ebmny.org)
University of Alberta EBM (cebm.med.ualberta.ca/ebm/ebm.htm)
Trauma Links: Edinburgh Orthopaedic Trauma Unit (http://www.trauma.co.uk/traumalinks.htm)

ization of EBM. Although EBM is sometimes perceived as a strict adherence to evidence derived from randomized trials, it more accurately involves the informed and effective use of all types of evidence in patient care, particularly evidence from the medical literature. With the increasing amount of available information, a paradigm shift from traditional practice to one that involves question formulation, validity assessment of available studies, and appropriate application of research evidence to individual patients must be considered.[4]

Hierarchy of Evidence
Among various study designs, a hierarchy of evidence exists, with randomized controlled trials at the top, controlled observational studies in the middle, and uncontrolled studies and opinion at the bottom (Figure 1). Levels of evidence (Levels 1 to 5) have been described, with the findings of high-quality randomized trials (and meta-analyses of randomized trials) constituting Level 1 evidence.[5] The findings of less rigorous randomized controlled trials or prospective cohort (observational studies) are consistent with Level 2 evidence. Case-control studies (retrospective) provide Level 3 evidence. Case series and expert opinion provide Level 4 and Level 5 evidence, respectively.

Finding the Evidence
To be effective EBM practitioners, surgeons must acquire the necessary skills to find the best evidence available to answer clinically important questions. Reading a few articles published in common orthopaedic journals each month is insufficient preparation for answering the questions that emerge in daily practice. There are at least 100 orthopaedic journals indexed by MEDLINE.[6] Given significant clinical demands, surgeons' evidence searches must be time-efficient. Evidence summaries (such as

those published in the *Journal of Orthopaedic Trauma*) and systematic reviews (comprehensive literature reviews) are useful resources for surgeons (Table 1). The most efficient way to find them is by electronic searching of databases and/or the Internet. With time at a premium, it is important to know where to look and how to develop a search strategy, or filter, to identify the evidence most efficiently and effectively.

Cochrane Database of Systematic Reviews
The Cochrane Database of Systematic Reviews (CDSR) contains full-text versions of the regularly updated sys-

TABLE 2 | Highly Sensitive MEDLINE Search Strategy*

Search Terms

controlled.ab.

design.ab.

evidence.ab.

extraction.ab.

randomized controlled trials/

meta-analysis.pt.

review.pt.

sources.ab.

studies.ab.

or/1-9

letter.pt.

comment.pt.

editorial.pt.

or/11-13

(YOUR SUBJECT TERMS)

10 not 14

15 and 16

*Use of these search terms in MEDLINE finds all possible systematic reviews on a topic

tematic reviews prepared by members of the Cochrane Collaboration. The Cochrane Collaboration is an international network of individuals and institutions committed to preparing, maintaining, and disseminating systematic reviews of the effects of health care. Most included reviews are of therapeutic interventions (prevention, treatment, and rehabilitation). The Cochrane Musculoskeletal Injuries Group, Musculoskeletal Group, Back Group, and Injuries Group all prepare and regularly update systematic reviews relevant to orthopaedic surgeons.[6] The CDSR also contains the Cochrane Controlled Trials Register, with more than 300,000 records of controlled trials.

MEDLINE

The most commonly used biomedical database produced by the National Library of Medicine is MEDLINE. Free MEDLINE access is available on the Internet via PubMed. MEDLINE indexes over 4,000 biomedical journals (11 million citations), with coverage from 1966 to the present. Only a small portion of articles in MEDLINE report evidence that can be applied directly to clinical practice. A method of improving the retrieval of high-quality studies applicable to clinical practice is to include search terms that select studies at advanced stages of testing for clinical application (Table 2).

PubMed has a special feature called Clinical Queries, which automatically filters searches on questions of therapy, diagnosis, etiology, or prognosis by looking at the highest levels of evidence in the literature. To access the Clinical Queries search filter, go to the PubMed Web site

(http://www.pubmed.gov) and select "clinical queries." Once in the clinical queries site, choose the type of study (such as therapy or diagnosis) and select "systematic reviews." Keywords can be entered to identify relevant studies.

Critically Appraised Topics Bank

Several medical programs maintain computerized (or Internet-based) logs of studies that meet predefined criteria for validity on a variety of topics as a method of providing a database of current evidence for residents, fellows, and faculty. One popular structured appraisal format for presenting information about a study in a meaningful and succinct manner has been termed Critically Appraised Topics (CATs). Ideally, individuals prepare a CAT before a journal club and post a log of past CATs on a Web site or computer for later referral. A good example of a CAT bank can be found on the Web site of the Center for Evidence-Based Medicine (http://www.cebm.net/toolbox.asp).

SUMsearch

SUMsearch (http://www.sumsearch.uthscsa.edu) searches the Merck Manual of Diagnosis and Therapy, the National Guidelines Clearinghouse (US), the Cochrane Library, and PubMed. This site presents results using a hierarchy of evidence. Guidelines are listed first, with sources of guidelines that are based on systematic reviews. Systematic reviews are listed next, with the CDSR first, followed by PubMed references that are possibly systematic reviews.[5] Finally, PubMed references that are probably randomized controlled trials are listed.

Appraising the Evidence

Once a search for available evidence has yielded relevant articles, surgeons can appraise the work in a few simple steps.[7-12] Table 3 lists these three steps and the criteria for critical appraisal of studies in these fundamental areas of clinical practice. The first factor that can influence physician confidence in research results is systematic error or bias. Bias is directly linked to the design and execution of a study. Thus, the first step is an appraisal of whether results are valid and to what extent bias is present (Are the results of the study valid?). An evaluation of the results follows. The effect of an intervention and how large is the role of random error or chance (What are the results?) must be asked. Finally, it must be determined whether the results are applicable to the real world (patients in health care). Thus, the results must be assessed to help guide decision-making in practice circumstances (How can the results be applied to patient care?).

TABLE 3 | Critical Appraisal of Studies About Prognosis and Therapy or Prevention

Question	Prognosis	Therapy or Prevention
Study design and execution: Evaluation of Bias	**I. Are the results of the study valid?** 1. Was the sample of patients representative? 2. Were the patients sufficiently homogeneous with respect to prognostic risk? 3. Was follow-up sufficiently complete? 4. Were objective and unbiased outcome criteria used?	**I. Are the results of the study valid?** 1. Were patients randomized? 2. Was randomization concealed? 3. Were patients analyzed in the groups to which they were randomized? 4. Were patients in the treatment and control groups similar with respect to known prognostic factors? 5. Were patients aware of group allocation? 6. Were clinicians aware of group allocation? 7. Were outcome assessors aware of group allocation? 8. Was follow-up complete?
Results and random error	**II. What are the results?** 1. How likely are the outcomes over time? 2. Were the patients sufficiently homogeneous with respect to prognostic risk?	**II. What are the results?** 1. How large was the treatment effect? 2. How precise was the estimate of the treatment effect?
Application and uptake	**III. How can the results be applied to patient care?** 1. Were the study patients and their management similar to those in my practice? 2. Was follow-up sufficiently long? 3. Can the results be used in the management of patients?	**III. How can the results be applied to patient care?** 1. Were the study patients similar to my patients? 2. Were all clinically important outcomes considered? 3. Are the likely treatment benefits worth the potential harms and costs?

Access to Evidence in the Orthopaedic Clinic

When clinical questions arise during orthopaedic clinics or ward rounds, significant time can be saved if physicians have computer terminals with Internet access. Online databases, such as PubMed or the CDSR, can be quickly queried to identify current evidence to assist surgeons in resolving questions. Current available technology further includes handheld personal digital assistants (PDAs), which have the capacity for Internet access and the storage of large amounts of information. Evidence resources such as Clinical Evidence are currently available for most commercially available PDAs.[13] Several other available programs for PDAs include: (1) Griffith's 5-Minute Clinical Consult, (2) eMedicine (peer-reviewed synopses of topics in 65 medical specialties), (3) Redi-Reference (clinical practice guidelines), (4) AvantGo (Web information can be downloaded to PDAs), and (5) JournalToGo (provides journal content from medical journals such as the *Journal of the American Medical Association* and *Emergency Medicine*).[13]

Practicing EBM is sometimes challenging. Practitioners must know how to frame a clinical question to facilitate use of the literature in its resolution. Typically, a question should include the population, the intervention, and relevant outcome measures. For example, "What is the role of internal fixation of tibial fractures?" is vague and should be rephrased as "in patients presenting to the emergency department with open tibial diaphyseal fractures (population), what is the effect of external fixators versus nonreamed intramedullary nails (interventions) on reoperation rates (outcome)?"

At first, orthopaedic surgeons may seek a systematic review of randomized trials of treatment alternatives. If a systematic review is not available, they will often look for individual randomized trials and high-quality observational studies of relevant management strategies. If the literature is altogether barren, EBM practitioners will fall back on the underlying biology and pathophysiology and clinical experience.

Consider the treatment of a 70-year-old woman with a displaced fracture of her hip. A surgeon using the traditional approach may choose to perform an arthroplasty of the hip on the basis of previous experience, the opinions of mentors, and/or the patient's preference. A surgeon using an evidence-based approach will ultimately weigh previous experiences, the opinions of experts, and patient preferences in the context of the best available evidence from well-designed clinical studies. In this example, a meta-analysis of randomized trials reports a significant reduction in the risk of reoperation arthroplasty compared with internal fixation of the hip; however, the risk of blood loss, the surgical time, and the risk of hip dislocation are significantly higher with arthroplasty. This surgeon may decide to repair the hip despite current opinion because the patient prefers the risk of revision of her internal fixation over dislocation, increased blood loss, and the possibility of increased mortality.

Summary

Although evidence-based orthopaedics is sometimes perceived as a blinkered adherence to the results of randomized trials, it more accurately involves informed and effective use of all types of evidence (from meta-analysis of randomized trials to individual case series and case reports), but particularly evidence from the medical literature. The Internet provides one efficient method of accessing information to guide clinical practice. Although orthopaedics and orthopaedic trauma surgeons have led the EBM movement in surgery, additional EBM resources and EBM education remain an essential priority in this subspecialty.

Annotated References

1. Guyatt GH: Evidence-based medicine. *ACP J Club* 1991;114:A16.

2. Narayanan UG, Wright JG: Evidence-based medicine: A prescription to change the culture of pediatric orthopaedics. *J Pediatr Orthop* 2002;22:277-278.

    This article describes the traditional paradigm of decision making in pediatric orthopaedics.

3. User's guides to the medical literature, in Guyatt GH, Rennie D (eds): *A Manual for Evidence-Based Clinical Practice*, ed 2. Chicago, IL, American Medical Association Press, 2001.

4. Coomarasamy A, Khan KS: What is the evidence that postgraduate teaching in evidence-based medicine changes anything? A systematic review. *BMJ* 2004;329:1017.

    The authors conducted a systematic review of articles relating the practice of EBM methods. They reported that stand-alone teaching improved knowledge but not skills, attitudes, or behavior and that clinically integrated teaching improved knowledge, skills, attitudes, and behavior. Ultimately, the authors concluded that the teaching of EBM should be moved from classrooms to clinical practice to achieve improvements in substantial outcomes.

5. Sackett DL, Richardson WS, Rosenberg WM, Haynes RB: *Evidence-Based Medicine: How to Practice and Teach EBM*. New York, NY, Churchill Livingstone, 1997.

6. Gillespie LD, Gillespie WJ: Finding current evidence: Search strategies and common databases. *Clin Orthop* 2003;413:133-145.

    This article provides a practical approach to finding useful information to guide orthopaedic practice. The authors first focus on where to find the information by providing details about many useful databases and Web links. Sources for identifying guidelines, systematic reviews, and randomized controlled trials are identified.

7. Schunneman H, Bone L: Evidence-based orthopaedics: A primer. *Clin Orthop* 2003;413:117-132.

    This article describes the critical appraisal of studies related to prognosis and therapy or prevention by building on an example relevant for the clinical orthopaedist. The authors describe how clinicians can apply measures of association and of intervention effects to their practice and patient care. They conclude with a description of the appraisal of systematic reviews, their application to the development of practice guidelines, and the process of guideline development and recommendations.

8. Bhandari M, Guyatt GH, Swiontkowski MF: User's guide to the orthopaedic literature: I. How to use an article about a surgical therapy. *J Bone Joint Surg Am* 2001;83-A:916-927.

    This article is the first in a series designed to help orthopaedic surgeons use the published literature in practice. The authors suggest a three-step approach to using an article from the medical literature to guide patient care. They recommend that surgeons ask whether the study can provide valid results and then review the results and consider how the results can be applied to patients.

9. Bhandari M, Guyatt GH, Swiontkowski MF: User's guide to the orthopaedic literature: How to use an article about prognosis. *J Bone Joint Surg Am* 2001; 83-A:1555-1564.

    When evaluating a study about prognosis the following guides are suggested: Was there a representative sample of patients? Were the patients sufficiently homogeneous with respect to prognostic risk? If not, did investigators provide estimates for all clinically relevant subgroups? Secondary guides include: Was follow-up sufficiently complete? Were objective and unbiased outcome criteria used?

10. Bhandari M, Guyatt GH, Montori V, Devereaux PJ, Swiontkowski MF: User's guide to the orthopaedic literature: How to use a systematic literature review. *J Bone Joint Surg Am* 2002;84-A:1672-1682.

    This article is the third in a series of guides aimed at evaluating the validity of surgical literature and its application to clinical practice. It provides a set of criteria for optimally interpreting systematic literature reviews and applying their results to the care of surgical patients.

11. Bhandari M, Guyatt GH, Montori V, Swiontkowski MF: User's guide to the orthopaedic literature: How to use an article about a diagnostic test. *J Bone Joint Surg Am* 2003;85-A:1133-1140.

    Clinicians frequently confront challenges when ordering and interpreting diagnostic tests. The primary issues to consider when determining the validity of a diagnostic test study are how the authors assembled the patients and whether they used an appropriate reference standard in all patients to determine whether patients did or did not have the target condition. Likelihood ratios are key to the interpretation of diagnostic tests because they link estimates of pretest probability to posttest probability. Sensitivity is the property of the test that describes the proportion of people with the disorder in whom the test result is positive. Specificity is the property of the test that describes the proportion of people without the disorder in whom the test result is negative.

12. Bhandari M, Tornetta P III: Issues in the design, analysis and critical appraisal of clinical orthopaedic research. *Clin Orthop* 2003;413:9-157.

This symposium contains a series of 15 articles that provide information on the design of clinical studies and statistical analysis as it pertains to clinical studies and evidence-based orthopaedics.

13. Adatia F, Bedard PL: Palm reading: 2. Handheld software for physicians. *CMAJ* 2003;168:727-734.

This is a comprehensive review of software and programs available for commercially available handheld PDAs. The advantages and disadvantages of each program are discussed.

Chapter 5

Advances in Imaging and Image-Guided Surgery

David M. Kahler, MD

Cory A. Collinge, MD

Computer-Assisted Orthopaedic Surgery

Computer-assisted surgery is slowly making its way into routine orthopaedic practice. For some time, orthopaedic surgeons have used two-dimensional image data from arthroscopy or fluoroscopy as a tool for optimizing surgical treatment. For the surgical treatment of some injuries, however, these modes of imaging may not be optimal. Injuries in areas such as the pelvis, hips, and spine involve complex anatomy, and surgical errors in these regions may have catastrophic effects. Recently, computer-driven, three-dimensional and single-screen multiplanar imaging systems have become available that may be useful in these instances. Laboratory and early clinical studies indicate that these systems may provide increased surgical accuracy and efficiency.[1-3] In addition, this technology appears useful for minimizing radiation exposure in more straightforward procedures that depend on relatively large amounts of fluoroscopy (for example, hip pinning or intramedullary nailing of long bones).[4-6] Computer-assisted orthopaedic surgery for trauma (synonymous with image-guided surgery or surgical navigation) is a relatively new and rapidly evolving field, and as these systems continue to develop, they may dramatically affect the future practice of orthopaedic surgery.

Surgical navigation circumvents the problems that are inherent in the standard techniques for implant placement. Standard C-arm fluoroscopy provides images that are available in only one plane at a time. This requires that the surgeon position the implant in one view and then obtain additional images in other planes for trial and error placement of guidewires or screws. Significant operating room time is expended while the fluoroscopy technician positions the C-arm to supply the necessary views. This also exposes the patient and the surgical team to significant levels of radiation, especially in areas such as the pelvis where considerable radiation may be necessary to ensure accurate screw placement. In the early 1990s, some surgeons attempted to move the surgical suite to the radiography suite to successfully perform pelvic surgery.[7,8] The logistics of this treatment method proved to be formidable. It was difficult to perform reduction maneuvers and place instrumentation within the confines of the CT scanner, and providing anesthesia in the radiography suite was sometimes problematic. Although improved accuracy was possible, it became clear that these procedures were best suited for the operating room environment.

Surgical navigation systems offer the capability of providing real-time intraoperative guidance in multiple image planes during implant placement. This may improve accuracy and efficiency while minimizing radiation exposure to the surgeon and operating room staff.

Computer-Assisted Surgery Systems

Computer-assisted surgery systems first were used by neurosurgeons in the late 1980s. A three-dimensional CT system became available for spine surgery in the early 1990s, and it was adapted for pelvic and acetabular fracture fixation in 1997. In 1998, a jointly sponsored National Institutes of Health/American Academy of Orthopaedic Surgeons work group convened to identify potential applications that warranted research support. Orthopaedic trauma was identified as one of the key impact areas for this new technology, along with spine and joint arthroplasty surgery.

Three-dimensional CT and virtual fluoroscopy (fluoroscopic navigation) are the two basic types of image-guided surgery. These allow access to either a three-dimensional data set or multiple simultaneously displayed fluoroscopic images, respectively. Using either type of system, images are harvested and stored on a computer workstation. A camera interfacing with the computer then tracks the position of the patient and the surgical instruments relative to one another during the course of the procedure. The predicted position and trajectory of the surgical instrument is superimposed onto the stored images on the computer monitor. This process is known as surgical navigation.

Early experience with the three-dimensional CT-based systems showed them to be useful in the planning and placement of complex screw trajectories about the pelvis.[9-11] One study reported the use of three-dimensional CT technology in the treatment of 21 posterior pelvic ring disruptions between 1997 and 1999.[12] The injured pelvis was provisionally reduced and stabilized with an external fixator, and a preoperative CT scan was obtained. A total of 27 iliosacral screws were placed using the guidance system. The results of this series then were retrospectively compared with those of a study group of pelvis injuries treated with iliosacral screws placed using conventional multiplanar fluoroscopy. All screws were accurately placed in both groups, but surgical time was significantly decreased by 26% and intraoperative radiation exposure was lessened by 86% in the image-guided group.

Although early experience with three-dimensional image-guided surgery was promising, the technique was limited by the inability to update the three-dimensional computer model in the operating room after fracture reduction maneuvers or implant placement. Only minimally displaced fractures or those easily reduced with simple external fixation could be treated with this method. As such, this technology did not gain widespread acceptance.

Fluoroscopic navigation was approved for clinical use in 1999 and has proved to be a more versatile technology for fracture treatment than three-dimensional CT.[4,13,14] The position of special optically tracked surgical instruments or implants may be virtually overlaid onto the fluoroscopic images during implant placement. The ability to update images after fracture manipulation has now expanded the application of computer-assisted surgery to any procedures that traditionally have relied on intraoperative C-arm fluoroscopy. Fluoroscopic navigation has proved to be well suited to a variety of pelvic and acetabular fracture applications, including minimally invasive techniques that were first made possible by the three-dimensional CT technology.[15-19] This technology has also expanded the use of image-guided systems to treat patients with more routine fractures that typically require fluoroscopy such as hip pinning and intramedullary nailing (Table 1).

Four basic steps are performed during a fluoroscopic navigation procedure: (1) attachment of a reference array to the patient's skeleton to allow tracking of the patient during the procedure, (2) harvesting of images with the fluoroscope and transferring them to the computer workstation, (3) calibration (warping) of the fluoroscopic images to make them optically correct, and (4) superimposing the predicted position of the surgical instrument and trajectory onto the acquired images (Figure 1).

In the first step, a reference array of light-emitting diodes or reflectors is attached to the patient's skeletal anatomy to allow tracking of the patient during the procedure. This allows the computer system's camera to

TABLE 1 | Examples of Potential Applications of Virtual Fluoroscopy in Orthopaedic Surgery

Iliosacral screws for posterior pelvic ring disruption

Anterior or iliac pelvic ring disruption

Acetabular fracture (percutaneous and limited open fixation)

Femoral neck and intertrochanteric fracture

Intramedullary nailing (starting point, fracture reduction, and freehand locking)

Osteotomies of long bones and pelvis

Slipped capital femoral epiphysis

Epiphysiodesis

Biopsy or ablation of skeletal neoplasms

track the patient's anatomy during respiration, a shift in position on the operating table, or other movement. The reference array may be attached with a Schanz pin and toothy cannula construct, or alternatively it may be attached to an external fixator, if applicable to the procedure.

A standard analog C-arm fluoroscopy unit is fitted with a calibration device to allow tracking of the C-arm and warping of the image to make it optically correct because significant distortion exists away from the image center. Images are acquired and transferred to the workstation, where they are analyzed by the computer. Any distortion is corrected by automatically warping the image. Typically two to four standard fluoroscopic projections are obtained for display on the workstation.

During navigation, the real-time position of surgical instruments, such as a drill, drill guide, or reduction rod is overlaid onto the stored images. The virtual images are updated several times per second, allowing real-time feedback as the instruments are moved by the surgeon. By convention, the instrument appears as a green line or shape on the screen, and a trajectory of variable length is projected in red ahead of the instrument (Figure 2).

The newest systems are entirely surgeon-driven, using a touch screen interface and a sterile pointer or sterile drape over the touch screen. Replacement of the previous mouse-driven (or so-called "shout and click") interface eliminates the need for an unscrubbed assistant or technical support staff and has led to improved acceptance of this technology in the operating room by surgeons and nursing staff.

Specific Applications of Image-Guided Orthopaedic Surgery

Iliosacral Screws

Virtual fluoroscopy is particularly well suited for the placement of iliosacral screws in patients with posterior pelvic ring disruptions or those with sacroiliac joint,

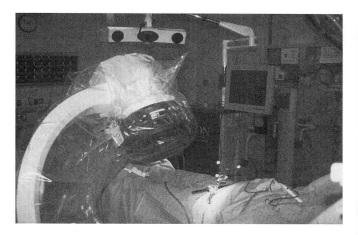

Figure 1 Photograph of the standard operating room setup for fluoroscopic navigation. A calibration target has been attached to a standard C-arm image intensifier. A camera interfaced with the navigation system looks down onto the field and tracks the C-arm, a reference array attached to the patient's external fixator, and special surgical instruments. Images are stored and manipulated by the surgeon using a stylet on the touch screen interface.

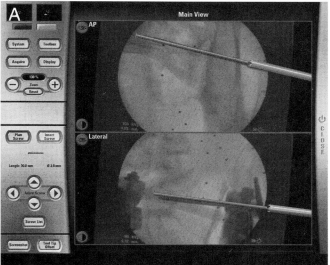

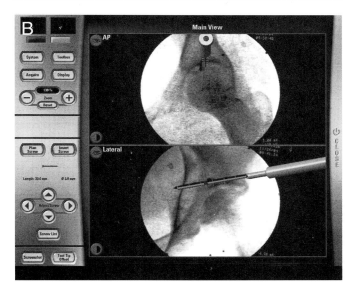

Figure 2 Intraoperative navigation images during iliosacral screw placement for sacroiliac joint disruption **(A)** and lag screw fixation of a posterior column acetabular fracture **(B)**. The predicted position of the drill guide is superimposed on the two stored fluoroscopic images; real-time fluoroscopy is not necessary. A computer-assisted design image of the drill guide and a trajectory ahead of the drill guide with 1-cm gradations are shown.

sacral, or crescent fractures. The surgeon initially reduces the pelvic ring using closed methods (traction, external fixator, or Schanz pin joystick) and confirms adequate reduction with C-arm images. It is helpful to maintain the reduction with either a temporary external fixator or a guidewire from the large cannulated screw set, passed from the ilium into the sacral ala. Multiple images are then harvested and stored on the computer workstation. Two to four images may be used; AP, inlet, outlet, and oblique lateral views for intraoperative guidance are recommended. The trajectory feature is used to identify the optimal starting point on the skin, and the drill guide is passed bluntly down to the ilium through a drill guide. The ideal trajectory into the center of the S1 body is chosen in all views, and a guidewire is inserted to the appropriate depth using the trajectory length feature. Confirmatory images are obtained, and the cannulated screw is then passed over the guidewire. Use of this procedure can result in reductions in fluoroscopic time of well over 50%, and the first pass of the guidewire is typically acceptable in nearly every patient. Despite the requirement for additional setup time (approximately 10 minutes), total surgical time is actually decreased. Rare instances of intraosseous guide pin deflection have been observed and mandate that confirmatory images be obtained before screw passage. No complications or clinically significant screw malpositions have been noted in over 50 individual screw placements using this technique.[18]

Pelvic Ring Disruption
Bony disruption of the pelvic ring either anterior or posterior to the acetabulum may often be managed using a percutaneous technique, provided that an ac-

ceptable reduction can be obtained and maintained during imaging. It has not yet been proved possible to safely stabilize a pure symphyseal disruption with a percutaneous image-guided surgical technique, although the use of endoscopy as an adjunct has been proposed as having the potential to minimize the invasiveness of this procedure. It has often been possible to stabilize other anterior and posterior pelvic ring injuries using large-diameter cannulated screws. This is usually done with the patient in the supine position and by using an antegrade or retrograde anterior column screw for the anterior ring and a lateral compression fracture type II screw for the posterior ring.

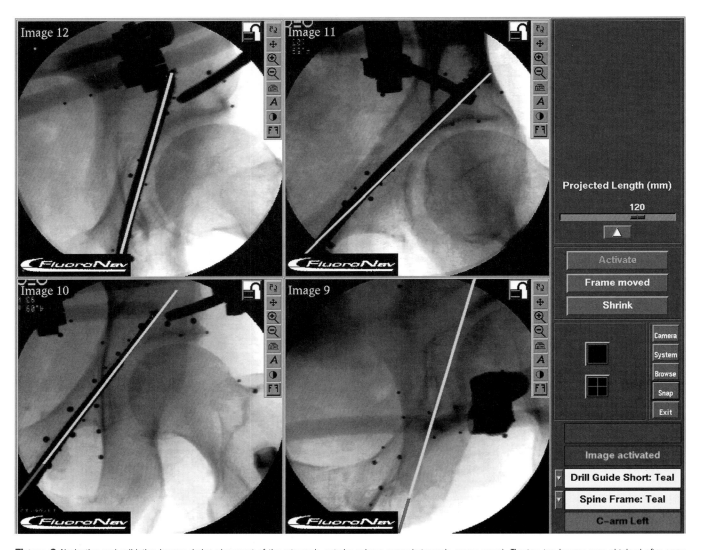

Figure 3 Navigation and validation images during placement of the retrograde anterior column screw (retrograde ramus screw). The two top images were obtained after screw placement, and demonstrate the close correlation between the predicted versus actual position of the screw.

The retrograde anterior column screw (also called the retrograde ramus screw) starts just inferior and lateral to the ipsilateral pubic tubercle, and it courses through the superior pubic ramus across the fracture and just anterior-superior to the hip joint (Figure 3). A 7.3-mm screw can usually be used in male patients. Obturator/ outlet and iliac/inlet views are helpful, although standard Judet views may be adequate for navigation. A true AP view is also used to provide initial orientation in almost all applications.

The lateral compression fracture type II screw starts at the anterior-inferior iliac spine, passes through a broad column of bone just above the acetabulum, courses above the sciatic notch, and terminates near the posterior iliac spine adjacent to the sacroiliac joint. Standard Judet or inlet/outlet views are used for this screw, although an image may be obtained aligned with the planned trajectory of the screw as well.

Acetabular Fractures

A detailed review of acetabular fracture fixation is beyond the scope of this chapter. In general, anterior column, posterior column, transverse, and anterior column/ posterior hemitransverse fractures are best suited for a percutaneous technique, provided a quality closed or limited open articular reduction can be performed. Both-column fractures with good secondary congruity can also be stabilized in situ, particularly in elderly patients. It has not yet been possible to safely reduce and stabilize posterior wall fractures with a percutaneous technique.

The high anterior column acetabular fracture appears to be particularly well suited for closed reduction and percutaneous fixation. This coronal plane fracture generally traverses the weight-bearing dome of the acetabulum and typically displaces proximally with external rotation. Closed reduction is obtained with traction and internal rotation of the large anterior fragment using a temporary external fixator. After confirmation of articular reduction with fluoroscopy, two cannulated screws may be used to provide fixation. Experience has shown that open reduction may be avoided in close to 90% of patients, with a very low complication rate and short hospital stay following percutaneous treatment[19] (Figure 4).

Spine Surgery

Pedicle screws have traditionally been inserted using anatomic landmarks or uniplanar C-arm fluoroscopy. The indications for pedicle screw fixation have been expanded to include the thoracic spine, where pedicle size may be limited and risks for errant screw placement may be considerable. Early reports showed that both three-dimensional CT technology and virtual fluoroscopy decreased the rate of pedicle perforation during insertion of thoracic pedicle screws.[1,13] It was concluded that the treatment was accurate and safe, but these systems had a significant learning curve. A more recent report found that pedicle screws were more accurately and safely placed using virtual fluoroscopy when compared with standard fluoroscopy or CT-based navigation.[20] It was also found that not all navigation systems were equal in terms of accuracy. First-generation systems that used only a single reference marker were reported to be highly inaccurate and unsafe when compared with modern multireference systems.[21,22]

Intramedullary Nailing

Although closed antegrade intramedullary nailing of diaphyseal femoral fractures allows minimally invasive stabilization of these injuries, it may require significant radiation exposure to patients and the surgical team. Multiple C-arm images are usually obtained during the following three critical portions of the procedure: (1) identification of the starting point for reaming, (2) fracture reduction, and (3) insertion of distal locking screws. The total radiation exposure has historically been approximately 4 minutes during these steps, and more than 200 individual images are often obtained. Many of the images must be obtained with the hands of the surgeon in or near the radiation field, particularly during fracture reduction and distal freehand interlocking. Although it is possible for the careful surgeon to avoid most radiation exposure using a conventional technique, many surgeons are less careful when faced with a difficult reduction or locking screw placement.

Virtual fluoroscopy allows the critical portions of the femoral nailing procedure to be done with as few as six individual images and only a few seconds of fluoroscopy time.[4] Furthermore, surgeons can move away from the image intensifier while images are acquired, and no additional imaging is required during virtual guidance.

Fracture Reduction

Recent developments allow fracture reduction to be done under virtual guidance. The fracture is slightly overdistracted by applying traction through the fracture table or femoral distractor, and standard AP and lateral C-arm views of the fracture site are obtained. After navigation for identification of the proper starting point in the proximal femur, the reference array is moved to the distal fracture fragment and attached to the anterolateral metaphysis of the femur. A special navigated reduction rod is inserted into the proximal fragment and advanced to the fracture site under virtual guidance. The position of the reduction rod within the femur is represented as a red line on the stored images. This process defines the axis of the intramedullary canal of the proximal fragment. The fracture is manipulated manually until the virtual axis of the proximal fragment is aligned with the distal fragment. This step is somewhat disconcerting for the untrained observer because the stored images show no change in the displaced position of the fracture fragments. The goal of this task is to align the proximal fragment, as defined by the position of the reduction rod, with the distal fragment being tracked by the reference arc. Fracture reduction is confirmed when the virtual image of the guide rod can be advanced into the distal fracture segment (Figure 5).

All three critical portions of the femoral nailing procedure have been done successfully using virtual fluoroscopic guidance.[4] Moreover, hand radiation exposure and additional imaging during reduction have been eliminated using this technique. In actual practice, several trial fluoroscopic images must be obtained for each step; the optimal images are then chosen and displayed for virtual fluoroscopic guidance. The setup time for the computer has been offset by the surgical time savings during implant placement. Dedicated image-guided surgery instrument sets for specific procedures are likely to improve future use and acceptance of this technology.

Reduction of Radiation Exposure to Patients and Surgeons

Ionizing radiation exposure is probably an underappreciated risk for trauma surgeons and trauma patients. One minute of intraoperative fluoroscopy is equivalent to exposure to 40 mSv (4 rads, 4,000 mrem) of radiation, which is approximately equivalent to the radiation exposure of 250 chest radiographs. The fluoroscopy time required for femoral nailing is routinely reported to be more than 4 minutes.[23] Although careful surgeons absorb very little direct radiation, they are still exposed to scatter radiation from the patient's anatomy; the patient absorbs most of the radiation dose. In actual practice, surgeons frequently place their hands in the radiation beam, especially during fracture reduction and freehand

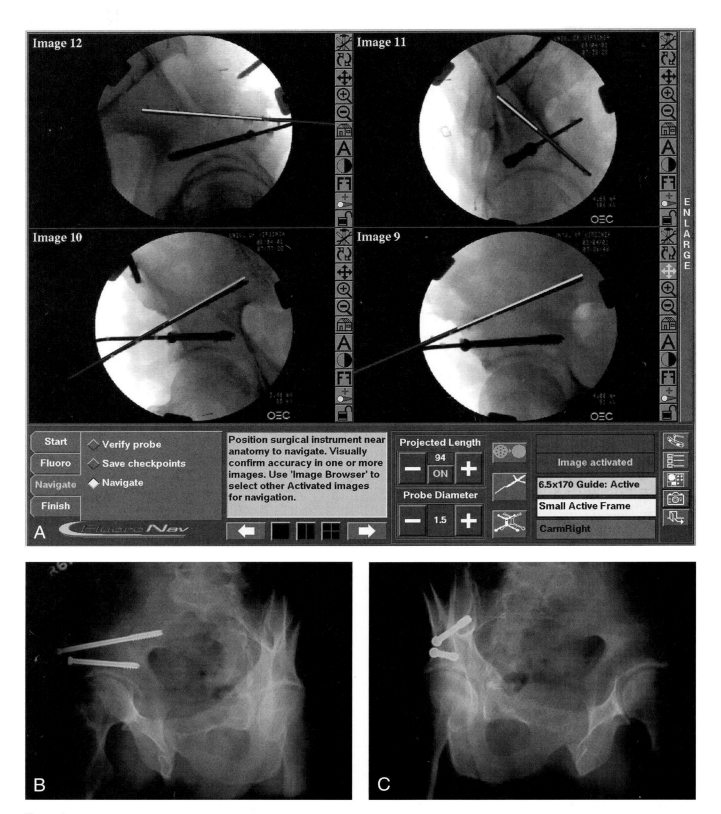

Figure 4 Percutaneous fixation of a high anterior column acetabular fracture. **A,** Navigation images during insertion of two 7.3-mm cannulated screws are shown. The coronal plane fracture line is best seen in the upper left image (iliac oblique). **B** and **C,** Postoperative Judet views are shown.

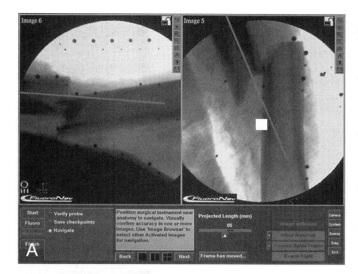

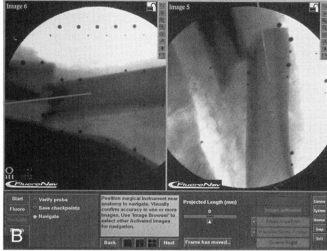

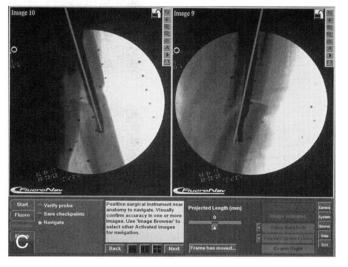

Figure 5 The steps in virtual femoral fracture reduction are illustrated. **A,** Two images of the displaced femoral shaft fracture show the distal fragment tracked by the navigation system, while a reduction rod has been inserted through the proximal fragment to the level of the fracture. The trajectory and length of the reduction rod are shown. **B,** The fracture has been manipulated and the reduction rod has been passed across the fracture line into the distal canal. The fracture does not appear to reduce because the surgeon is using stored images of the displaced fracture; the task is simply to pass the reduction rod into the distal segment. **C,** Confirmatory images shows the reduction rod across the reduced fracture.

locking. The US Occupational Safety and Health Administration's guidelines recommend no more than 50 rem per year of hand exposure, which corresponds to only 12 minutes of fluoroscopy time per year. It is quite possible for orthopaedic trauma surgeons to exceed this threshold.

Measurable health effects can occur with exposure to much lower doses of radiation. For example, air travel above 30,000 feet results in a slight increase in background radiation exposure. Career high-altitude airline pilots receive about 3 to 6 mSv of radiation over environmental background (2 to 8 mSv) per year, which is approximate twice the exposure of the general population. This small additional radiation dose would be equivalent to only 10 to 15 seconds of fluoroscopy time about the pelvis or hip. It is distressing to note that pilots have a fivefold increase in myeloid malignancies and a threefold increase in skin cancers when compared with the population at large. Although the skin cancer risk may be related to increased sun exposure, the small increase in background radiation is thought to be responsible for their hematopoietic malignancies.[24]

Summary

Based on the high visibility of image guidance systems at national orthopaedic meetings, there appears to be great interest in these systems, particularly for total joint replacement applications. Although the potential trauma applications are compelling, the current literature regarding the use of virtual fluoroscopy in orthopaedic surgery is somewhat sparse.

When using virtual fluoroscopy for surgical navigation during implant placement, it is essential that the surgeon take the time to harvest adequate images. The surgeon must be familiar with radiographic anatomy in various customized oblique imaging planes, particularly when working around the pelvis and the columns of the acetabulum. Image quality in pelvic applications sometimes is compromised by patient obesity, bowel gas, or retained intra-abdominal contrast. In many applications, it is logistically difficult to obtain the two ideal orthogonal images perpendicular to the path of intended drilling and fixation, which can lead to increased reliance on nonstandard oblique radiographic projections. In all applications, surgeons must have the diligence to ensure that the images are adequate to proceed safely. In the event that adequate fluoroscopic images cannot be obtained, surgeons must have the discipline to abandon surgical navigation and use an alternative method. Surgeons then have the responsibility to either proceed with formal open reduction using standard technique or consider performing the procedure using a three-dimensional CT technique during a separate surgical sitting.

Surgeons often note several obvious drawbacks in choosing image-guided systems over standard techniques. Those wishing to use this technology must invest some time in learning to use the interfaces and software. The surgeon, scrub nurse, and assistants also must learn to proceed without obstructing the digital camera's view of the surgical field. The operating room must be large enough to accommodate the computer system, camera, and the C-arm unit. Cables connecting the two units may interfere with the mobility of personnel and equipment in the operating suite.

There is inevitably some set-up time involved in interfacing the system with the C-arm and placing a reference array on the patient before obtaining images. The setup process typically adds 10 to 15 minutes at the start of the surgical procedure. Although this time is essentially always recouped during the procedure by gaining increased first-pass accuracy in implant placement, many surgeons find the up-front setup time objectionable.[23]

Image-guided surgery equipment and instruments are costly, and financial considerations likely will hinder widespread acceptance in the short term. Nonetheless, the technology offers substantial potential benefits, including improved accuracy, decreased surgical time, and decreased invasiveness. The greatest benefit, however, may lie in decreasing the orthopaedic surgeon's reliance on intraoperative ionizing radiation for guidance during surgery. Virtual fluoroscopy eliminates direct radiation exposure to the surgeon's body and hands, and it satisfies the goal of keeping patient radiation exposure to an absolute minimum. Fluoroscopic navigation has several real and potential advantages when compared with conventional techniques in orthopaedic trauma surgery. Additional work will help to define the optimal applications for this new technology, and hopefully it will help to justify the expense of these systems.

Annotated References

1. Kim KD, Johnson JP, Bloch BS, Masciopinto JE: Computer-assisted thoracic pedicle screw placement: An in vitro feasibility study. *Spine* 2001;26:360-364.

2. Mirza SK, Wiggins GC, Kuntz C IV, et al: Accuracy of thoracic vertebral body screw placement using standard fluoroscopy, fluoroscopic image guidance, and computed tomographic image guidance: A cadaver study. *Spine* 2003;28:402-413.

   The authors report that fluoroscopic navigation provided improved accuracy (decreased pedicle perforation rates) in the placement of pedicle screws in the thoracic spine. Differences in system accuracy were also demonstrated.

3. Kahler DM: Clinical performance of fluoroscopic navigation in pelvic trauma applications, in Langlotz F, Davies, and Bauer (eds): *Proceedings of the Third Annual Meeting of the International Society for Computer Assisted Orthopaedic Surgery.* Bern, Switzerland, Steinkopf Verlag Damstadt, 2003, p 172.

4. Kahler DM: Virtual fluoroscopy: A tool for decreasing radiation exposure during femoral intramedullary nailing. *Stud Health Technol Inform* 2001;81: 225-228.

5. Slomczykowski MA, Hofstetter R, Sati M, Krettek C, Nolte LP: Novel computer-assisted fluoroscopy system for intraoperative guidance: Feasibility study for distal locking of femoral nails. *J Orthop Trauma* 2001;15:122-131.

   The authors of this feasibility study assessed the effectiveness of an integrated fluoroscopy-based navigation system for placement of distal interlocking screws during femoral nailing. Plastic and cadaver specimens were used, and a single clinical case was presented. The authors reported that 76 consecutive locking screws were placed successfully, using only an average of 1.7 seconds of fluoroscopy per screw. Although the fluoroscopy requirements were extremely low, the system was not compared with standard technique and surgical time was not assessed.

6. Hofstetter R, Slomczykowski M, Krettek C, Koppen G, Sati M, Nolte LP: Computer-assisted fluoroscopy-based reduction of femoral fractures and antetorsion correction. *Comput Aided Surg* 2000;5:311-325.

   The authors of this descriptive study have developed and validated an integrated fluoroscopic navigation system to assess femoral torsion during fracture reduction. They report that this system can be used to successfully measure femoral rotation using two-dimensional projections. The system was validated using a bench study that demonstrated a high degree of precision in the measurement of femoral antetorsion and fracture reduction.

7. Duwelius PJ, Van Allen M, Bray TJ, Nelson D: Computed tomography-guided fixation of unstable posterior pelvic ring disruptions. *J Orthop Trauma* 1992;6:420-426.

8. Gay SB, Sistrom C, Wang G-J, et al: Percutaneous screw fixation of acetabular fractures with CT guidance: Preliminary results of a new technique. *AJR Am J Roentgenol* 1992;158:819-822.

9. Zura RD, Kahler DM: A transverse acetabular nonunion successfully treated with computer-assisted percutaneous internal fixation: A case report. *J Bone Joint Surg Am* 2000;82:219-224.

   This article describes the use of the three-dimensional CT technique for the placement of pelvic internal fixation using an image-guided surgery treatment platform. Tangible benefits (decreased surgical time, decreased radiation exposure to patient, novel screw trajectories) were demonstrated when compared with conventional fluoroscopic technique.

10. Kahler DM: Computer-assisted fixation of acetabular fractures and pelvic ring disruptions. *Tech Orthop* 2000;10:20-24.

11. Kahler DM, Zura R: Evaluation of a computer-assisted surgical technique for percutaneous internal fixation in a transverse acetabular fracture model: Lecture notes. *Comput Sci* 1997;1205:565-572.

12. Kahler DM, Mallik K: Abstract: Computer-assisted iliosacral screw placement compared to standard fluoroscopic technique. *Comput Aided Surg* 1999;4:348.

13. Foley KT, Simon DA, Rampersaud YR: Virtual fluoroscopy: Computer-assisted fluoroscopic navigation. *Spine* 2001;26:347-351.

14. Jane JA Jr, Thapar K, Alden TD, Laws ER Jr: Fluoroscopic frameless stereotaxy for transsphenoidal surgery. *Neurosurgery* 2001;48:1302-1307.

    The basics of fluoroscopic navigation for spine and intracranial surgery are discussed and system accuracy is assessed as well. The authors concluded that fluoroscopic computer-assisted frameless stereotaxy provides accurate real-time information with regard to midline structures and surgical trajectory. Although useful during first-time transseptal transsphenoidal surgery, its primary benefit is realized for recurrent surgery.

15. Kahler DM: Computer-assisted closed techniques of reduction and fixation, in Tile M, Helfet D, Kellam J (eds): *Surgery of the Pelvis and Acetabulum*. Philadelphia, PA, Lippincott Williams & Wilkins, 2003, pp 604-615.

16. Jacob AL, Suhm N, Kaim A, Regazzoni P, Steinbrich W, Messmer P: Coronal acetabular fractures: The anterior approach in computed tomography-navigated minimally invasive percutaneous fixation. *Cardiovasc Intervent Radiol* 2000;23:327-331.

17. Kahler DM: Image guidance: Fluoroscopic navigation. *Clin Orthop* 2004;421:70-76.

18. Kahler DM: Percutaneous screw insertion for acetabular and sacral fractures. *Tech Orthop* 2003;18:174-183.

19. Crowl AC, Kahler DM: Closed reduction and percutaneous fixation of anterior column acetabular fractures. *Comput Aided Surg* 2002;7:169-178.

    In this retrospective analysis of a series of 26 patients treated with percutaneous reduction and fixation of a high anterior column acetabular fracture, several techniques were used for screw placement between 1990 and 2002 during the evolution of computer-assisted surgical techniques. The authors report that adequate closed reduction was obtained in 23 of 26 patients with a high anterior column acetabular fracture. The fractures were then stabilized with two large bore cannulated screws using minimally invasive technique. A low complication rate and excellent outcomes were demonstrated.

20. Schep NW, van Walsum T, De Graaf JS, Broeders IA, van der Werken C: Validation of fluoroscopy-based navigation in the hip region: What you see is what you get? *Comput Aided Surg* 2002;7:279-283.

    The authors of this bench study sought to validate the predicted position of a compound reamer with respect to the actual position during simulated placement of a dynamic hip screw using stored fluoroscopic images. The authors found that the mean difference between the predicted and actual position and depth of the reamer was 1.0 mm. They concluded that an optically tracked fluoroscopic navigation system provided acceptable accuracy for this clinical application.

21. Langlotz F, Bachler R, Berlemann U, Notle LP, Ganz R: Computer assistance for pelvic osteotomies. *Clin Orthop* 1998;354:92-102.

22. Perlick L, Tingart M, Lerch K, Bathis H: Navigation-assisted, minimally invasive implant removal following a triple pelvic osteotomy. *Arch Orthop Trauma Surg* 2004;124:64-66.

    In this case report of minimally invasive image-guided pelvic hardware removal using a fluoroscopic navigation system, the navigation system was used to accurately identify a precise trajectory for successful removal of fixation screws, with minimal soft-tissue damage and radiation exposure to the patient.

23. Mehlman CT, DiPasquale TG: Radiation exposure to the orthopaedic surgical team during fluoroscopy: How far away is far enough? *J Orthop Trauma* 1997; 11:392-398.

24. Gundestrup M, Sturm HH: Radiation-induced acute myeloid leukaemia and other cancers in commercial jet cockpit crew: A population-based cohort study. *Lancet* 1999;354:2029-2031.

Chapter 6

Minimally Invasive Fracture Care

Peter A. Cole, MD

Loren Latta, PE, PhD

Christian Krettek, MD

Introduction

Priority-Driven Evolution of Fracture Care

Treatment of fractures has evolved in recent years toward less invasive strategies for reduction and fixation. Biologically based treatments to stimulate fracture healing continue to be developed and include such techniques as nutritional supplementation, genetic manipulation, biophysiologic stimulation, and new methods of fracture stabilization. This chapter focuses on the strategies for fracture stabilization using less invasive techniques that minimize interference with the fracture healing process. The recent evolution in fracture management emphasizes biologic priorities. This has included changes in surgical approach, methods of fracture reduction, fixation techniques, and even rehabilitation.

Changes in surgical approaches for fracture fixation have been stimulated by comparing fracture healing in conservatively treated patients, those in whom the soft-tissue envelope around the fracture is untouched, and those in whom the soft tissues and attendant vascularity are disrupted by an extensive surgical exposure. The preservation of the soft-tissue envelope around a fracture zone has been reported to have a significant positive influence on the ability of the fracture to heal.[1]

To minimize soft-tissue dissection, direct manipulation of bone fragments has been replaced, when possible, by indirect realignment using traction techniques and percutaneous insertion of an implant (plate or nail) to connect the proximal and distal articulation. These techniques have been described as biologic internal fixation. Other terms that have been used include minimally invasive osteosynthesis, minimally invasive plate osteosynthesis, and minimally invasive percutaneous plate osteosynthesis.[2,3] With these techniques, plates are inserted through small incisions that are often distant from the fracture site in a manner similar to that used to insert intramedullary nails.

For articular fractures, the goal of reduction, anatomic reconstruction, and stable fixation of the articular surface remains unchanged. In metaphyseal and diaphyseal fractures, the goal is proper alignment of the joints on either side of a fracture in a limb where length is properly restored. Although anatomic reconstruction of articular surfaces is paramount, this objective is balanced with a respect for the catastrophic complications associated with poorly timed or executed open approaches to joints, particularly in the lower extremities. Incision and surgical approaches have changed as well. For example, in the distal femur, the conventional standard posterolateral approach makes it difficult to achieve complete joint visualization, particularly with limited soft-tissue stripping. Therefore, a new minimally invasive transarticular approach for use in percutaneous plate osteosynthesis has been developed.[4] This technique uses a lateral parapatellar arthrotomy for direct reduction of the joint surface, and an indirect, submuscular plate insertion technique to fix the articular block to the femoral shaft. Other modifications in approach include more periarticular percutaneous reduction instruments (clamps or joysticks) or keenly placed incisions based on the fracture pattern elucidated by CT. These approaches are aided by improved imaging resolution and in some instances by computer-aided navigation of implant insertion.

Blood Supply

Any disruption of endosteal or periosteal blood supply or inhibition of angiogenesis during fracture healing contributes to the formation of a delayed union or nonunion. Surgical techniques that preserve blood supply should result in improved rates of fracture union, decrease the need for supplemental bone grafting, and decrease the incidence of complications such as infection or refracture.[1,4-7] Research results demonstrate the potential benefits of these techniques. Latex dye injection studies have demonstrated that percutaneously inserted plates cause less disruption of the perforators, nutrient artery, periosteal blood supply, and medullary circulation than conventional open approaches. This suggests that minimally invasive plate osteosynthesis may have advantages for fracture healing.[8-10] These techniques are particularly significant in the lower extremity where outcomes for conventional plate fixation have traditionally included

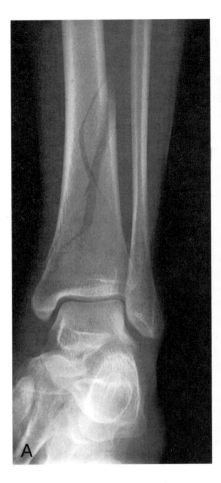

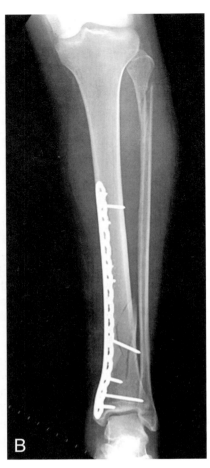

Figure 1 A, AP radiograph of a patient with a distal tibia extra-articular OTA type A fracture. **B,** AP radiograph of the same patient after fixation with a percutaneous plate. Note that conventional and locking screws have been used. The long conventional screw crossing the fracture site was first placed to approximate the fracture. A single conventional screw was then placed in the proximal and distal fragments (longer of the distal and proximal screws) to approximate the bone to the plate, which must be precontoured so as to prevent a malreduction. The shorter unicortical screws were then placed in a locked mode (locked into the plate) on either side of the fracture. The locked screws prevent toggling or loosening at the screw plate interface. Note the extended length of the plate, but the number of cortices purchased by the screws are few, a principle borrowed from experience with external fixation.

higher complication rates. Surgical exposure and soft-tissue stripping are minimized and vascular pedicles are preserved while joint alignment and orientation are restored.

Implants and Surgical Approaches

Limited Plate Contact

In addition to the development of new surgical approaches, fixation technology is also changing. Conventional plates depend on friction between bone and implant for stability. To minimize crushing of the periosteum under the plate, some new plate designs use contours that decrease the area of contact at the bone-implant interface. In one animal study comparing plates with two different contact surface areas, infection rates after 28 days were 63% (12 of 19 animals) for those with plates with greater contact area (dynamic compression plate) compared with 26% (5 of 19 animals) for those with point contact plates ($P = 0.022$). It was concluded that the higher infection resistance was related to the reduced contact area at the bone-implant interface.[11]

The Internal Fixator

Recent additions to the implant armamentarium include plating systems with fixed and stable angles between

screws and the plate, now commonly referred to as locking plates. Locking plates represent an extrapolation of technology from external fixation used to treat extremity fractures and internal fixators used in spine surgery. Because of their angular stability, the plate-screw-bone complex does not depend on the friction at the implant-bone interface. In addition, because screws fixed to the plate cannot loosen and fail sequentially but must pull out together, locking plates obtain better fixation in patients with poor quality bone.

Several different implants have been developed that use this principle of the fixed angle. In some of these implants, the screws deployed are unicortical, self-drilling, and self tapping; thus, screw insertion is done using power drivers and water cooling. All of these systems reduce the need for implant-bone contact. Some systems are being developed to allow a multidirectional screw-to-plate interface. Long spanning constructs (bridge plating) across the fracture zone are advocated for use with these technologies because fewer fixation screws are required for stability. Screw placement simulates the number and spacing of external fixator pins[7] (Figure 1).

Some of the more recently developed implants include plating systems that offer two different kinds of

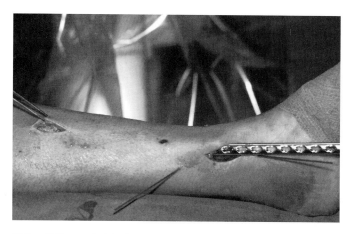

Figure 2 Photograph of the distal medial leg of a patient undergoing fixation for a distal extra-articular fracture. Percutaneous maintenance of reduction was achieved with a Kirschner wire after a percutaneous clamp was used to reduce a 7-day-old fracture.

holes for locked and nonlocked screws, and some designs provide surgeons with the ability to place variable-angled screws. Advocates for the use of such implants point out that they allow versatility in surgical tactics in that they provide surgeons with the advantages of both compression and locking plate fixation techniques. The different mechanical properties of locked and nonlocked screws require a thoughtful sequence for the application of the different screws. For example, the dynamic compression features of the combination screw hole in the plate cannot be used after the use of locked screws in each main fragment.[12] Similarly, lag screws placed through the plate must be placed before locking screws.

Conventional plate fixation relies on friction between a plate and the bone to which it was tightly compressed to achieve absolute stability; therefore, micromovement that could result in loosening of the implant and provide an impedance to healing had to be avoided. New techniques using locked internal fixation, however, seem to tolerate some degree of mobility at the fracture interface, which may in fact be beneficial to indirect bone healing via a callus bridge.[13] The goal of indirect fracture healing, however, requires that a fracture is spanned or bridged and that the overall construct is slightly elastic. Rigid fixation with a gap between main fracture fragments inhibits or prevents callus formation and increases the risk of nonunion.

In its early evolution, percutaneous, submuscular surgical fixation required the use of conventional implants and reduction tools that were perhaps used in an unconventional manner (Figure 2). The necessity for more effective, more efficient, and safer application of these implants less invasively has resulted in the development of a new genre of tools and reduction aids. The development of additional surgical tools is likely to follow as surgical execution meets design innovation.

Arthroscopically Assisted Fixation

Percutaneous reduction and fixation techniques have been widely used to treat patients with unicondylar tibial plateau fractures.[14,15] Because long-term articular prognosis is thought to be affected by the quality of joint reduction, arthroscopy is commonly recommended for visualizing the joint and controlling reduction while depressed fragments are manipulated by bone tamps inserted under the fragments. Arthroscopy can also be used to treat associated injuries such as meniscal lesions or cruciate tears. However, arthroscopy is technically difficult to perform in patients with acute fractures, and significant fluid extravasation may occur. Placement of the hardware usually requires the use of an additional image intensifier.[14,15] Percutaneous manipulation of the fracture under fluoroscopic control with percutaneous osteosynthesis has been used for treatment of unicondylar fractures of the tibia plateau as well.[16] These two techniques differ significantly in the necessary resources and the training of the surgical team. A comparative study analyzed the benefits and disadvantages of both techniques.[14] The authors found arthroscopy demanding because of significant bleeding from fracture clefts, limited visualization of fragmented areas under the lateral meniscus, and fluid extravasation. The routine use of arthroscopy was not believed to provide significant additional information. Additionally, relatively few surgeons teaching fracture fixation techniques are skilled in both arthroscopy and orthopaedic trauma.

This combined skill may be a significant advantage, however, when considering the findings of recent studies on concomitant soft-tissue injuries in patients with tibial plateau fractures. The high number of meniscal lesions that occur in patients with tibial plateau fractures[14,17,18] may justify a greater role for arthroscopic diagnosis and treatment during fracture stabilization. It should be acknowledged, however, that most of these lesions are in the vascularized zone of the meniscus. Early arthroscopic meniscal repair may represent overtreatment because it has been shown that there is a high rate of spontaneous healing of these tears and that stable longitudinal tears of the lateral meniscus are usually asymptomatic.[19] Although joint inspection for the purpose of accurate reduction is important, arthroscopy may be a good surgical adjunct, particularly in those patients who require specific visualization of the joint, for those with fractures of the intercondylar eminence, and for those with fracture types that involve knee ligaments or meniscal injury.[14]

Intramedullary Nailing

The pioneers of intramedullary nailing should be credited for first developing minimally invasive fracture fixation because operating from within the intramedullary cavity of the bone greatly diminishes periosteal stripping and disturbance of the soft-tissue envelope. Modern in-

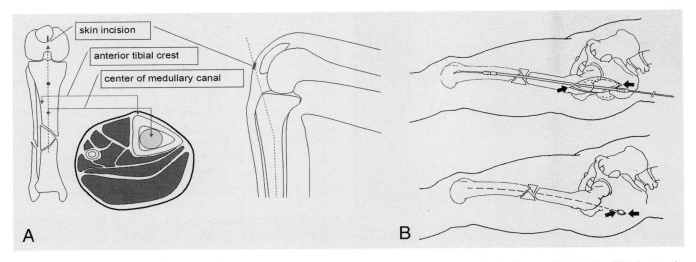

Figure 3 Anatomic considerations for skin incision and starting point selection. The arrows indicate the vector of incision, with the old, conventional technique (**A**) being extensive and in line with the midaxial line of the femur. The newer incision (**B**) represents only the proximal part of the conventional incision, and its vector is now in line with the radius of curvature of the femur.

tramedullary nailing performed without opening the fracture site certainly qualifies as less invasive. Accordingly, it is important to describe some of the techniques that allow surgeons to operate at a distance from the fracture site, manipulate the reduction, and navigate the implant to achieve fixation stability.

A fracture table or radiolucent standard table may be used to position the patient with a long bone fracture. The femoral distractor, in-line traction, and freehand technique with manual traction are all acceptable alternatives for intraoperative fracture reduction. Use of the fracture table or formal distraction will maintain a defined reduction throughout the procedure, which is helpful in the placement of intramedullary nails.[20] However, the fracture table can place perineal skin and neurovascular structures at risk during femur fracture treatment, and the setup time needed is significant.[21] Intramedullary nailing with manual traction and reduction has been shown to significantly reduce setup time, anesthesia time, and operating time.[22,23] Freehand manual reduction also allows for more flexibility in managing certain circumstances common to the multiple trauma patient. For example, ipsilateral or bilateral long bone fractures may be addressed with a single positioning and draping technique.

New approaches to intramedullary nail insertion have been developed to be less invasive. The intramedullary nail starting point is no longer thought to require direct visualization. With well-defined anatomic and radiographic landmarks described for intramedullary nail starting points and with newer instrumentation to accommodate percutaneous nail placement, fluoroscopy is now often used to guide accurate nail placement. Furthermore, soft-tissue protection from the reamer is not necessary, and clinical observation has revealed that only the most proximal portion of these approaches was ac-

tually used. Stab incision techniques have been developed for inserting intramedullary nails to treat fractures of the femur and the tibia.[24] Care must be taken to place the approaches in line with the axis of the medullary cavity but not too close to the starting point on the bone (Figure 3).

When placing an intramedullary nail in the femur of a patient who is in the supine position, flexion and adduction of the hip joint facilitate the approach for antegrade nailing. This decreases the length of the incision, especially in obese patients. When the patient is in the lateral position, a piriformis fossa starting point is more easily accessible. The greater trochanter, lateral condyle, and if possible, the femoral shaft are palpated. A line is extended proximally in a slight curve corresponding to the curvature of the femur. An incision about 3 cm long is made approximately 10 to 15 cm above the tip of the greater trochanter. The surgeon's finger may be used to palpate alongside the implant or guidewire to access the starting point. An incision placed too far posteriorly may harm the abductors, which may manifest in abductor weakness.

When placing intramedullary nails in the tibia, a 15- to 20-mm incision is made in line with the medullary cavity. The knee is flexed greater than 90°. The proximal-anterior edge of the tibia can be easily identified by palpating with the tip of the guide pin. After placing the guide pin through the proximal-anterior edge of the tibia in the direction of the center of the medullary canal, the protective sleeve is inserted through the stab incision directly onto the bone. The central axis of the medullary canal may extend proximally to a position somewhat medial to the middle of the width of the epiphysis. Medial and lateral parapatellar and transpatellar approaches have all been described for this step.[25,26] If there is doubt about the center of the medullary cavity, a

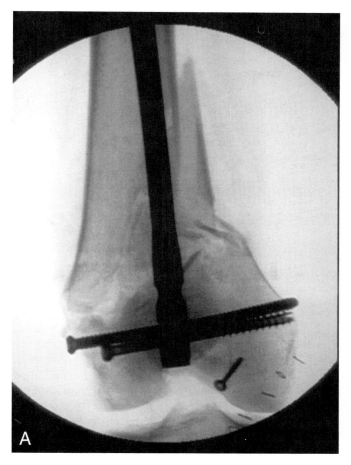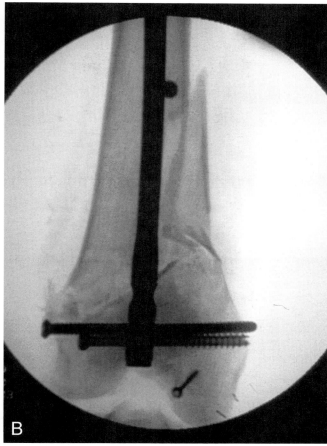

Figure 4 AP intraoperative C-arm images showing the difference in alignment of the distal femur fracture. **A,** The femur without the metaphyseal level A to P blocking screw and the fracture collapses into varus because of the patulous femoral canal relative to the small diameter of the intramedullary nail. **B,** The blocking screw was placed to effectively make the canal narrower so the fracture cannot shift into varus alignment.

20-mm Kirschner wire can be placed in the middle of the shaft at the level of the tibial tubercle under fluoroscopic control. For proximal fractures, it is essential to obtain a starting point exactly in line with the center of the medullary cavity.

When retrograde femoral and antegrade tibial nailing is being done, both insertions can be made through the same skin incision, in which instance the surgeon must be sure that the incision for the retrograde nail is proximal enough (close to the patella).

Reduction of fresh (midshaft long bone) fractures is usually not difficult. Manual reduction alone is usually sufficient. However, in shaft fractures for which treatment is delayed longer than a few days or for patients in whom pharmacologic relaxation is incomplete, reduction becomes more challenging. For these situations, several techniques and tools are available.

The use of temporarily inserted Schanz screws is an effective way to obtain direct, short lever arm control of the bone. For the most effective control, placement of the Schanz screws must be close to the fracture. Furthermore, these screws must either be unicortical or out of the proposed path of the intramedullary nail and ream-

ers. Connecting the Schanz pins to a T-handled chuck will allow for easier manipulation. The visual control of the relative position of both T handles can decrease the use of the C-arm. The tactile control of the main fragments in the sagittal plane may also decrease the need for radiographic visualization. The main indication for the use of a distractor is the need for longitudinal distraction against high resistive forces. Its use is especially helpful in patients for whom treatment has been delayed.[24]

Nailing of metaphyseal fractures is associated with an increase in malalignment caused by strong muscular forces and residual postfixation instability. Because there is a large difference between the implant and metaphyseal diameters with no nail-cortex contact, the nail may translate along the interlocking screws. Blocking screws placed adjacent to the nail can decrease the translation in both the tibia and the femur. These screws, also termed Poller screws, decrease the width of the metaphyseal medullary cavity, physically block transverse nail translation, and increase the mechanical stiffness of the bone-implant construct (Figure 4). Blocking screws can be used as alignment tools, stabilization tools, and/or ma-

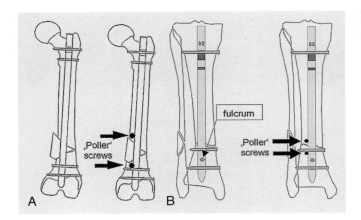

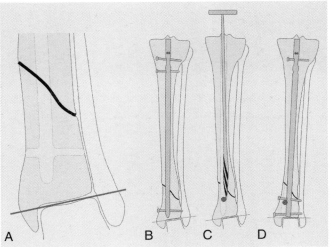

Figure 5 Schematic representation of the Poller screw technique for the prevention of axial deformity. **A,** Comminuted fracture of the distal femoral metaphysis deforms into varus alignment because of instability of the antegrade nail (left), and placement of blocking screws stabilizes fixation in proper alignment (right). **B,** Comminuted metaphyseal fracture of the tibia is displaced into varus after antegrade locked nailing (left), and position of blocking screws corrects and stabilizes alignment (right).

Figure 6 Schematic representation of Poller or blocking screws used to correct a malaligned tibial fracture after nailing. **A,** Oblique distal tibial fracture failed in valgus because of malposition of an antegrade nail. **B,** The eccentric location of the nail in the distal tibial metaphysis results in valgus alignment. **C,** After the nail is removed, a blocking screw is placed to redirect the nail tip laterally. A T-handled awl is then used to create a new tract for the nail. **D,** Alignment is corrected after renailing is done with the blocking screw in place.

nipulation tools (Figures 5 and 6). When placing Poller screws, as with any screw, potential damage to the nail can be done during drilling, and corrosion between nail and screw interface has to be considered. Other potential complications include blockage of the nail by an incorrectly placed Poller screw and screw breakout during nail passage.

In patients with simple midshaft fractures of the femur and tibia, frontal and sagittal plane malalignment is usually not a problem. In patients with complex and/or metaphyseal fractures, however, significant malalignment can occur. The definition of the weight-bearing axis is usually based on long standing radiographs, which are not available intraoperatively. However, the cable technique provides adequate information about the frontal plane axis.[27] With the patella directed anteriorly, the center of the femoral head and ankle joint are visualized fluoroscopically and marked on either the skin or the surgical sheets. The cautery cable is then spanned between these two points with the image intensifier centered on the knee joint. Using the projection of the position of the cable, varus or valgus alignment can be determined. The sagittal alignment is determined using a lateral fluoroscopic image.

External Fixation

External fixation is another minimally invasive fracture treatment technique. It is most often used to stabilize a fractured limb and span the damaged soft-tissue envelope during the staging of treatment. Particularly in the lower extremity, an external fixator may remain in place for weeks while awaiting optimal timing for internal fixation.[28] It is also an effective option for the treatment of severe open fracture wounds, particularly when the surgeon believes that heavy contamination of the wound

precludes internal fixation.[29,30] In patients with open fractures or those who require mangled extremity management, the time spent in an external fixator is useful for the surgeon to obtain consultation with a microvascular surgeon, learn more about the patient's psychosocial resources, and assess limb viability before undertaking extensive reconstruction.

External fixation is occasionally used for the definitive treatment of fractures. If a surgeon deems that it is unsafe to fix a highly comminuted articular fracture because of the risk of infection or soft-tissue loss, external fixation with or without percutaneous internal fixation will control limb length and alignment while limiting surgical trauma. Sacrificing an anatomic articular reduction is better than limb-threatening complications such as deep infection and wound slough. The external fixation may be applied in the mode of a uniplane, ring, or hybrid fixator.[31]

Ring fixators with tensioned wires may be used for stabilizing bone fragments near joints without violating the joint capsule. Such a ring near a joint can be connected to other rings and wires in the diaphyseal bone to bridge the fracture, or it can be connected to half pins to create a hybrid frame.[31] These frames apply traction across the injured site to gain relatively stable control of fragments through ligamentotaxis. When traction is applied across a joint with a fixator, it is called a bridging or spanning frame. This type of frame can be used as a temporary measure to gain control of the fragments until early healing can begin to stabilize the fracture. Additionally, some types of fixator are articulated to allow controlled motion of the joint with the frame in place. A

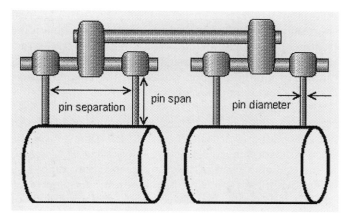

Figure 7 Schematic representation of the concepts used in external fixation technique that are relevant to achieving stability with external fixation constructs.

ring external fixator system can also be used for bone transport to fill a bone defect during an attempt at limb reconstruction or limb salvage.

The external fixator ultimately must provide proper length, alignment, and rotation, as well as provide stability to the fracture site. Fracture stability prevents progressive deformity at the fracture site. Stability may not be related to the rigidity of the fixation device alone. The basic principles of obtaining and maintaining fracture stability address the parameters of fixation: coaptation, compression, neutralization, and tension band wiring and buttressing. The optimal level of stability for healing may not be the same as maximal stability.

Although the most rigid, strong, and visible components in a typical external fixator construct are the connectors from the pins across the bone fragments, the parameters that control neutralization of the fracture are more related to the pins. The parameters over which the surgeon has control include: pin diameter, pin material, pin separation, and pin span (Figure 7).

Plastic and elastic bending of the pins is responsible for most of the fracture site movement. Elastic deformation of the pins in bending affects the pin-bone interface stresses that relate to pin loosening. Bending resistance is related to the fourth power of the diameter. Thus, the bending resistance of a 5-mm pin is 2.5 times greater than a 4-mm pin of the same material. The most common mode of loss of neutralization with external fixators is pin loosening. The stiffness of the pin material is also important. The stiffness of a stainless steel pin is almost two times greater than that of a titanium pin of the same diameter.

Pin span is the distance between the pin-bone interface and the pin-clamp interface. The neutralization of any construct is inversely proportional to the square of the pin spans in the construct. Thus, the closer the pin clamps can be placed to the skin, the stronger and more rigid will be the fixation.

Pin separation is the distance between any two pins within the same bone fragment. This distance provides the leverage by the pin cluster to resist angulation of that fragment in the plane of those pins. Thus, pins widely separated and not all in the same plane improve the neutralization (or strength and rigidity) of the construct on that fragment. Placing a third or additional pins out of the plane of the first two pins significantly reduces the bending of all of the pins, and thus reduces their tendency to loosen. External fixator systems that call for independent pin placement allow the surgeon to more easily achieve strength and rigidity of fixation with a minimum number of components.

Closed, Functional Treatment

The least invasive fracture treatment is that of closed management. Understanding which injuries can be treated with closed functional techniques as well as when and how to treat them requires an understanding of how fractures heal and the role of soft tissues in controlling their position during the mechanical demands of early function.

Two types of motion occur at the fracture site when load is applied to the fragments. Elastic motion is a displacement of the bone fragments in which the fragments completely return to their initial position after the load is relaxed. Plastic motion is a displacement that does not recover after the load is relaxed. A residual malalignment of the fragments results from such a displacement.[32,33]

Elastic motion following rigid fixation (proper plate and screw fixation) will allow motion on the order of microns at the fracture site under normal loading conditions. With this degree of motion, the fracture will heal with direct formation of new bone on the original bone with little or no external callus. With more compliant forms of fixation (intramedullary rods, external fixators, casts, and braces), the elastic motion at the fracture site, even during normal loading associated with functional activities, is at least 1 mm and can be several centimeters. The medullary blood supply will not reconnect across the fracture site until the fragments are stabilized by the callus. With compliant forms of fixation, the peripheral circulation is responsible for the blood supply to the bridging callus. Early limb function is important to provide stimulus to the peripheral circulation, stress to the healing tissues, and to maintain joint motion and muscle tone. It is important to understand how this callus forms and how its mechanical properties provide for elastic motion during normal functional activities and adequate strength to resist plastic deformation.

During closed functional management of fractures, gravity alignment and alignment of the muscle fibers with early function pull the fragments toward their natural anatomic alignment. In the early (soft callus) stage of healing, the patient will be able to begin light exercises and joint motion. The most effective compression mechanism for all compliant forms of fixation is early muscle activity. The muscles that span the fracture site will apply compression to the bone ends. Thus, it is important to allow motion of the joints both above and below the fracture because function of these joints will be activated by muscles that span the fracture site. This same muscle activity is important for stimulating the early blood supply to the bridging callus because the medullary circulation will not be able to cross the fracture site until much later.[32,33] In this way, functional bracing is significantly different physiologically from simple cast immobilization.

Neutralization provides the strength of fixation to a construct. Neutralization with functional braces is accomplished primarily by soft-tissue compression. A circumferential wrap of the soft tissues by any material that can be closely fit to the shape of the limb and adjusted to maintain compression of the tissues throughout treatment will provide the neutralization required for early functional activities. The hardness and rigidity of the material used is less important mechanically than the ability of the device to be adjusted to maintain soft-tissue compression and suspension of the system. Thus, soft, compliant, and comfortable materials can be used successfully. Soft casting materials or thermoplastics applied directly with a custom-fit or compliant prefabricated brace are more comfortable than rigid, hard, or thick thermoplastic sheets. Comfort is important for the early introduction of functional activities. The most rigid materials are plaster and fiberglass reinforced casting materials. Several types of semirigid and soft casting materials are now available that can be used to make casts, splints, and adjustable braces for fracture management. In addition, prefabricated braces made of compliant thermoplastics are also readily available.

With any form of closed treatment, the tension bands are very compliant and are provided by the soft tissues.[33,34] The buttress is provided by bone contact or early callus and the control of fracture movement. The control of fracture movement is influenced by the stage of fracture healing, the soft-tissue compression provided by the brace, and the soft-tissue tethering of the fracture related to the damage of the soft tissues at the time of the injury. Both the buttresses and the tension bands are usually symmetric to provide resistance in all planes of angulation with very compliant but strong resistance to bending.

The indications for closed, functional treatment of tibial fractures include isolated, low-energy closed fractures that are transverse and either nondisplaced or have been reduced and made axially stable.[33,35,36] Although more controversial, relative indications may include axially unstable fractures (such as oblique, spiral, or comminuted fractures) that are less than 12 mm at initial shortening, or segmental fractures with minimal displacement between the fragments and less than 12 mm of shortening. Relative indications of closed, functional treatment also may include type I pediatric open fractures, patients with diaphyseal tibial fractures but intact fibulae, or multiple trauma patients if the other fractures do not preclude ambulation with external support.

In a selected series of 1,000 closed tibial shaft fractures treated in prefabricated braces, the incidence of nonunion was reported to be 1.1%; less than 1% of the fractures experienced refracture, more than 95% healed with less than 12 mm of shortening, and more than 90% healed with less than 6° of angulation in any plane.[35]

The indications for closed, functional treatment of humeral shaft fractures include closed diaphyseal fractures without marked distraction between the fragments, fractures associated with initial radial nerve palsy, and open fractures in children without significant soft-tissue pathology. Surgical treatment of humeral shaft fractures is relatively indicated in patients with bilateral humeral fractures and patients with multiple trauma who are able to assume the erect position early and ambulate with external support on the opposite side.[33,35,37] Closed, functional treatment of ulnar fractures is indicated for patients with isolated diaphyseal fractures that do not demonstrate major displacement between the fragments and no disruption of the distal or proximal radioulnar joints.[35,38]

In a retrospective review that combined 933 patients who were selected for closed, functional treatment with prefabricated braces from two different institutions, 620 were available for complete follow-up. Of these patients, the nonunion rate was 2.6%, and 0.3% of patients required secondary surgery. More than 88% of patients had final angulation of less than 15° in all planes, and 92% had 0 to 10% loss of total shoulder motion.[37]

In a review of 444 selected patients with isolated ulnar fractures that were treated at two different institutions with prefabricated braces, 287 patients had complete follow-up; the incidence of nonunion and synostosis were each 1%, shortening averaged 1.1 mm, and final angulation averaged 5°.[33]

Summary

Orthopaedic surgeons are currently exploring new frontiers of fracture care with a heightened awareness of the importance of less invasive fracture management, which began, at least in part, in the 1980s with the introduction of the concept of "biologic fixation." As new techniques for less invasive fracture management are developed and present challenges to traditional treatment, the evolving technology demands a process of continual updating and critical appraisal by the practicing orthopaedist. Many of these new interventions will likely be discarded as they are tested. Additionally, the newer approaches being developed to accommodate new technology and innovations will eventually be mastered with increased use. Ideally, the advances in minimally invasive fracture care should meld with tried and true principles of fracture care.

Annotated References

1. Baumgaertel F, Buhl M, Rahn BA: Fracture healing in biological plate osteosynthesis. *Injury* 1998;29 (suppl 3):C3-C6.

2. Krettek C, Schandelmaier P, Miclau T, Bertram R, Holmes W, Tscherne H: Transarticular joint reconstruction and indirect plate osteosynthesis for complex distal supracondylar femoral fractures. *Injury* 1997;28(suppl 1):A31-A41.

3. Krettek C, Stephan C, Miclau T: Fracture fixation with minimally invasive percutaneous plate osteosynthesis (MIPPO) using the DCS in the distal femur. *Tech Orthop* 1999;14:209-218.

4. Krettek C, Miclau T, Stephan C: Transarticular approach and retrograde plate osteosynthesis for complex distal intra-articular femur fractures. *Tech Orthop* 1999;14:219-229.

5. Rozbruch SR, Muller U, Gautier E, Ganz R: The evolution of femoral shaft plating technique. *Clin Orthop* 1998;354:195-208.

6. Kregor PJ, Stannard J, Zlowodzki M, Cole PA, Alonso J: Distal femoral fracture fixation utilizing the Less Invasive Stabilization System (LISS): The technique and early results. *Injury* 2001;32(suppl 3): SC32-SC47.

   This article presents the principles, indications, and technique for application of a submuscular plate on the distal femur through minimal surgical exposures. From their early clinical experience in treating 66 patients with this technique, the authors reported that the mean time to full weight bearing was 11 weeks and that the mean range of motion was 2° to 102°. They also reported a union rate of 95%, an infection rate of 3%, and no losses of fixation despite 20 patients being older than 60 years.

7. Cole PA, Zlowodzki M, Kregor PJ: Less Invasive Stabilization System (LISS) for fractures of the proximal tibia: Indications, surgical technique and preliminary results of the UMC Clinical Trial. *Injury* 2003;34(suppl 1):A16-A29.

   This article describes the indications, technique, technical tips, and pitfalls of the Less Invasive Stabilization System when used to treat fractures of the proximal tibia. The early clinical experience with 54 patients is reported. The mean time to full weight bearing was 13.2 weeks and the mean range of motion was 1° to 116°. The authors also reported a union rate of 96%, an infection rate of 4%, and

no late varus collapse or cutout. Malreductions between 6° to 10° occurred in 9% of patients (4 of 5 with apex anterior angular deformity).

8. Farouk O, Krettek C, Miclau T, Schandelmaier P, Guy P, Tscherne H: Minimally invasive plate osteosynthesis: Does percutaneous plating disrupt femoral blood supply less than the traditional technique? *J Orthop Trauma* 1999;13:401-406.

9. Farouk O, Krettek C, Miclau T, Schandelmaier P, Tscherne H: The topography of the perforating vessels of the deep femoral artery. *Clin Orthop* 1999; 368:255-259.

10. Borrelli J Jr, Prickett W, Song E, Becker D, Ricci W: Extraosseous blood supply of the tibia and the effects of different plating techniques: A human cadaveric study. *J Orthop Trauma* 2002;16:691-695.

   This study defines the extraosseous blood supply of the tibia and how plating influences it. Nine matched pairs of human cadaver lower limbs were used. A latex injection to the superficial femoral artery demonstrated a rich vascular supply in both the proximal and distal metaphyseal regions; although the tibial diaphysis was determined to be relatively hypovascular, an anastomic network was found between the anterior and posterior tibial arteries on the medial side. The authors reported that open plating of the distal aspect of the medial tibia caused significant disruption of the vascular supply compared with percutaneous plating.

11. Arens S, Eijer H, Schlegel U, Printzen G, Perren SM, Hansis M: Influence of the design for fixation implants on local infection: Experimental study of dynamic compression plates versus point contact fixators in rabbits. *J Orthop Trauma* 1999;13:470-476.

12. Miclau T, Remiger A, Tepic S, Lindsey R, McIff T: A mechanical comparison of the dynamic compression plate, limited contact-dynamic compression plate, and point contact fixator. *J Orthop Trauma* 1995;9:17-22.

13. Perren SM: Evolution of the internal fixation of long bone fractures: The scientific basis of biological internal fixation. Choosing a new balance between stability and biology. *J Bone Joint Surg Br* 2002;84: 1093-1110.

   The author reviews the changing concepts in internal fixation and explains the evolution from the traditional AO philosophy of rigid internal fixation and anatomic reduction of all fracture fragments to the use of a biologically friendly approach with indirect reduction and less rigid implants. The author describes the notions of stability and bone necrosis and discusses technologic advances that underlie this change in fracture care.

14. Jennings JE: Arthroscopic management of tibial plateau fractures. *Arthroscopy* 1985;1:160-168.

15. Lobenhoffer P, Schulze M, Gerich T, Lattermann C, Tscherne H: Closed reduction/percutaneous fixation of tibial plateau fractures: Arthroscopic versus fluoroscopic control of reduction. *J Orthop Trauma* 1999;13:426-431.

16. Koval KJ, Sanders R, Borrelli J, Helfet D, DiPasquale T, Mast JW: Indirect reduction and percutaneous screw fixation of displaced tibial plateau fractures. *J Orthop Trauma* 1992;6:340-346.

17. Dickson KF, Galland MW, Barrack RL, et al: Magnetic resonance imaging of the knee after ipsilateral femur fracture. *J Orthop Trauma* 2002;16:567-571.

    MRI was used to assess 27 knees after surgical fixation of ipsilateral femoral fractures (1 by open reduction and internal fixation, 19 by antegrade nailing, and 7 by retrograde nailing. Significant injuries to the anterior cruciate ligament (19% of knees), posterior cruciate ligament (7%), medial meniscus (15%), lateral meniscus (26%), medial collateral ligament (41%), and lateral collateral ligament (30%) were discovered. The authors concluded that a thorough physical examination of the knee should be performed after fixation of a femoral shaft fracture to rule out associated soft-tissue injuries and that physicians should have a low threshold for obtaining an MRI scan.

18. Shepherd L, Abdollahi K, Lee J, Vangsness CT Jr: The prevalence of soft tissue injuries in nonoperative tibial plateau fractures as determined by magnetic resonance imaging. *J Orthop Trauma* 2002;16:628-631.

    MRI was performed on 20 consecutive patients who were treated for minimally displaced tibial plateau fractures. Ninety percent of patients had significant injuries to the soft tissues, 80% had a meniscal tear, and 40% had a complete ligament disruption. The clinical significance of these findings is unclear, and the authors caution that the natural history of these lesions during fracture healing is unknown. Many or most patients may heal well without surgery.

19. Fitzgibbons RE, Shelbourne KD: "Aggressive" nontreatment of lateral meniscal tears seen during anterior cruciate ligament reconstruction. *Am J Sports Med* 1995;23:156-159.

20. McFerran MA, Johnson KD: Intramedullary nailing of acute femoral shaft fractures without a fracture table: Technique of using a femoral distractor. *J Orthop Trauma* 1992;6:271-278.

21. Brumback RJ, Ellison TS, Molligan H, Molligan DJ, Mahaffey S, Schmidhauser C: Pudendal nerve palsy complicating intramedullary nailing of the femur. *J Bone Joint Surg Am* 1992;74:1450-1455.

22. McKee MD, Schemitsch EH, Waddell JP, Yoo D: A prospective, randomized clinical trial comparing tibial nailing using fracture table traction versus manual traction. *J Orthop Trauma* 1999;13:463-469.

23. Stephen DJ, Kreder HJ, Schemitsch EH, Conlan LB, Wild L, McKee MD: Femoral intramedullary nailing: Comparison of fracture-table and manual traction. A prospective, randomized study. *J Bone Joint Surg Am* 2002;84-A:1514-1521.

    Eighty-seven consecutive patients with femoral shaft fractures were randomized to undergo fracture-table traction (N = 42) or manual traction (N = 45). All fractures were treated with an intramedullary nail. Malreduction in internal rotation (> 10°) was significantly more common when the fracture table was used (29% versus 7%). Surgical time was shorter by 20 minutes when manual traction was used. Surgeons had an average of two assistants for both groups. The authors concluded that manual traction improves the quality of reduction and decreases surgical time.

24. Dahlen C, Stiletto R, Gotzen L: Techniques of using the AO-Femoral distractor for femoral intramedullary nailing. *J Orthop Trauma* 1994;8:315-321.

25. Vichard P, Garbuio P, Gagneux E, Elias BE: Value of the surgical approach through the patellar tendon for intramedullary nailing of the tibia and the femur [in French]. *Rev Chir Orthop Reparatrice Appar Mot* 1997;83:739-742.

26. Althausen PL, Neiman R, Finkemeier CG, Olson SA: Incision placement for intramedullary tibial nailing: An anatomic study. *J Orthop Trauma* 2002;16:687-690.

27. Krettek C, Miclau T, Grun O, Schandelmaier P, Tscherne H: Intraoperative control of axes, rotation and length in femoral and tibial fractures: Technical note. *Injury* 1998;29(suppl 3):C29-C39.

28. Borrelli J Jr, Catalano L: Open reduction and internal fixation of pilon fractures. *J Orthop Trauma* 1999;13:573-582.

29. Marsh JL: External fixation is the treatment of choice for fractures of the tibial plafond. *J Orthop Trauma* 1999;13:583-585.

30. Hutson JJ Jr, Zych GA: Infections in periarticular fractures of the lower extremity treated with tensioned wire hybrid fixators. *J Orthop Trauma* 1998;12:214-218.

31. Court-Brown CM, Walker C, Garg A, McQueen MM: Half-ring external fixation in the management of tibial plafond fractures. *J Orthop Trauma* 1999;13: 200-206.

32. Latta LL, Sarmiento A, Tarr RR: The rationale of functional bracing of fractures. *Clin Orthop* 1980; 146:28-36.

33. Sarmiento A, Latta L: *Functional Fracture Bracing: A Manual.* Philadelphia, PA, Lippincott Williams & Wilkins, 2002.
     This "how-to-do-it" book on the functional bracing of fractures outlines the indications, contraindications, clinical protocols, and techniques of application of functional braces for selected fractures of the humerus, ulna, and tibia.

34. Ouellette EA, Dennis JJ, Milne EL, Latta LL, Makowski AL: Role of soft tissues in metacarpal fracture fixation. *Clin Orthop* 2003;412:169-175.
     This laboratory study compared the bending characteristics of metacarpal, midshaft osteotomies fixed with external fixators, intramedullary rods, Kirschner wires, plates and screws in denuded human bones versus bones in situ with all the soft tissues present. The authors concluded that the soft tissues play an important mechanical role in the bending support for metacarpal shaft fractures for all types of fixation, but most notably for the less rigid forms of fixation.

35. Sarmiento A, Latta LL: Functional fracture bracing. *J Am Acad Orthop Surg* 1999;7:66-75.

36. Martinez A, Sarmiento A, Latta LL: Closed fractures of the proximal tibia treated with a functional brace. *Clin Orthop* 2003;417:293-302.
     In this clinical study of 108 patients with low-energy, closed fractures of the proximal tibial shaft who underwent closed functional treatment with braces, the authors reported 88% percent of the fractures healed with less than 6° of angular deformity.

37. Sarmiento A, Zagorski JB, Zych GA, Latta LL, Capps CA: Functional bracing for the treatment of fractures of the humeral diaphysis. *J Bone Joint Surg Am* 2000;82:478-486.
     In this retrospective study, the authors combined 933 patients from two different institutions who were selected for closed, functional treatment of fractures of the humeral diaphysis; 620 patients were available for complete follow-up. Although functional braces varied somewhat over the period of the study (early 1970s through the late 1980s), the outcomes varied only slightly. The overall nonunion rate was 2.6% of patients, and 0.3% of fractures required secondary surgery. More than 88% of patients had final angulation less than 15° in all planes; 92% had 0 to 10% loss of total shoulder motion.

38. Sarmiento A, Latta LL, Zych G, McKeever P, Zagorski JP: Isolated ulnar shaft fractures treated with functional braces. *J Orthop Trauma* 1998;12: 420-423.

Chapter 7

Soft-Tissue Injury

David A. Volgas, MD

Introduction

In the early days of modern osteosynthesis, surgeons often approached the treatment of fractures with the overriding goals of achieving anatomic reduction, rigid internal fixation, and early motion. Although soft-tissue injuries were addressed when obvious, the focus of treatment shifted heavily toward treatment of the skeletal injury. As these techniques were employed on a wide scale, a high incidence of complications from the over-aggressive handling of soft tissues during treatment of high-energy fractures was reported. By the 1970s, there was a shift toward external fixation as a definitive treatment of fractures associated with severe soft-tissue injuries. This treatment, however, often caused other problems related to nonunion, malunion, and pin tract and joint infection.

As a result, treatment shifted back toward open reduction and internal fixation, but surgeons began giving more attention to the treatment of soft-tissue injuries. Careful handling, preserving the soft-tissue attachments to bone, and delaying treatment while soft-tissue swelling resolved became more common. The results of this approach have been shown to be superior in many ways to previous treatment methodologies. More recently, techniques such as minimally invasive percutaneous plate osteosynthesis have been developed to minimize additional surgical trauma to the soft tissues.

Despite the advances of the past five decades, the treatment of skin, subcutaneous tissue, and muscle injuries often remains the most difficult problem the orthopaedic trauma surgeon encounters. It has been generally accepted that the health of the soft tissues near the fracture site plays a key role in the prevention of complications such as infection and nonunion. Most trauma surgeons are aware that immediate fixation of high-risk fractures prone to soft-tissue complications may lead to higher complication rates than delayed treatment of those fractures. However, there is general consensus that fracture stability plays a key role in preventing additional damage to soft tissues. As a result, many surgeons will temporize a fracture with an external fixator that bridges the zone of injury and allows time for soft tissues to recover. After soft-tissue swelling has subsided, delayed open reduction and internal fixation may be performed.

In the past few years, there have been four major developments aimed at the management of soft-tissue injuries. Improved surgical instruments and techniques have made a tremendous impact on the additional trauma inflicted by the surgeon on previously injured tissues. Strides are being made to further decrease the additional trauma burden through the use of computer-assisted surgery. Additionally, there has been increased attention given to the basic pathophysiology of wound healing and the role of various growth factors. There has also been renewed interest in the use of local rotational flaps (such as fasciocutaneous flaps) to address soft-tissue defects. Finally, there has been a great deal of work done on skin graft substitutes and biologic dressings.

Surgical Techniques and Instrumentation
Pathophysiology of Wounds

Soft-tissue trauma initiates a complex series of physical and biochemical changes.[1,2] The broad overview of wound healing is well understood.[2] Wounds progress from hematoma to inflammation to proliferation and finally remodeling. Less clear is why some wounds do not heal during this reparative process. Some factors, such as chronic steroid therapy, microvascular disease, and smoking, may affect wound healing. However, even without the presence of these known factors, some wounds fail to heal. The causes of wound healing failure will be better understood as the knowledge about inflammatory mediators, cellular responses, local condition, and their interactions increases.

Injury to the skin and underlying soft tissue triggers a release of a multitude of growth factors, chemotactic factors, and mediators that serve to control hemorrhage and to mobilize repair and defense mechanisms[3] (Table 1).

Cytokines are small peptides or glycopeptides that are produced by most cells. They are characterized by being exceedingly potent in very small concentrations.

TABLE 1 | Significant Inflammatory Mediators in Wound Healing

Inflammatory Mediator	Leukocyte Chemoattraction	Leukocyte Activation	Reepithelialization	Angiogenesis	Wound Fibroplasia
IL-1	+++		+		++
IL-2		+			
IL-4	−				++
IL-6					++
IL-8			++	++	
IL-10	−				
TNF-α	+++				−
TGF-β			++		+++
GM-CSF		+++			
G-CSF		+++			
M-CSF		+++			
MDC	++				
MIP-1	+++				
MCP-1-5	+++				
NAP-2	+++				
IP-10					−
IFNs					−−−
PDGF	+		++	++	+++
PF4					−

IL = interleukin, TNF = tumor necrosis factor, TGF = transforming growth factor, GM-CSF = granulocyte-macrophage colony-stimulating factor, G-CSF = granulocyte colony-stimulating factor, M-CSF = macrophage colony-stimulating factor, MDC = macrophage-derived cytokines, MIP-1 = macrophage inflammatory protein-1, MCP-1-5 = monocyte chemotactic proteins 1-5, NAP-2 = neutrophil-activated protein-2, IP-10 = interferon-inducible protein, IFNs = interferons, PDGF = platelet-derived growth factor, PF4 = platelet factor 4, +++ = strongly positive effect. ++ = moderately positive effect, + = mildly positive effect, −−− = strongly negative effect, - = mildly negative effect. *(Adapted with permission from Henry G, Garner WL: Inflammatory mediators in wound healing. Surg Clin North Am 2003;83(3):483-507.)*

They act within a short distance and exhibit pleiotropism (a single cytokine can trigger different actions on different target cells) and redundancy (several cytokines may have a similar effect on a given cell). Cytokines generally target cells from the hematopoietic system.

Growth factors are typically larger proteins and are present in physiologically active quantities in the general circulation. They tend to target connective tissue.

The temporal nature of inflammatory mediators is outlined in Figure 1. The coagulation cascade normally achieves rapid control of hemorrhage. The platelet α granules then release a myriad of factors that are chemotactic, especially transforming growth factor (TGF)-β, platelet-derived growth factor (PDGF), and platelet factor 4 (PF4). These factors attract macrophages and lymphocytes, which in turn secrete additional cytokines. More inflammatory cells are recruited. Interleukin (IL)-8, tumor necrosis factor-alpha (TNF-α) and IL-1 are active in the cell infiltration phase.

Monocytes are transformed into macrophages under the influence of IL-2, TNF-α, and interferon-γ beginning the first day, and this process peaks about day three. These activated macrophages form the key component of wound healing. They are responsible for secretion of more than 100 factors that regulate the response of the repair cells. Fibroblasts and endothelial cells proliferate during this phase under control of several cytokines and growth factors.

Fibroblasts infiltrate the wound and begin reconstituting the connective tissue matrix. By day four, they are the predominant cell type in the wound. At the same time, epithelial cells begin to migrate in from the wound edges to close the wound.

Initial Wound Management

Traditional teaching about wound management includes the use of high-pressure pulsatile lavage and removal of all nonviable tissue.[4] The ability of high-pressure lavage to reduce bacterial load in open fractures is well established.[5-7] It is less clear what effect high-pressure pulsatile lavage has on bone healing.[8] Animal studies suggest that there is a significant decrease in early bone healing evident, but this effect disappears in later stages of healing.[5] Low-pressure pulsatile lavage has been studied in animal models and appears to have less effect on bone healing, but it is less effective in removing bacteria, especially when débridement is performed more than 3 hours after inoculation with bacteria.[6] The findings of other animal studies using various soaps and detergents

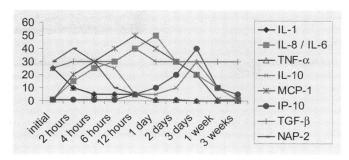

Figure 1 Temporal expression profile of selected inflammatory cytokines throughout the wound healing timeline. This is a graphic representation of the current understanding of wound healing and the effect of inflammatory mediators present in wounds. Of note, tumor necrosis factor alpha (TNF-α) and interleukin 1 (IL-1) are present early in the healing process and are the most important leukocyte chemoattractors. Interleukin 8 (IL-8) release is triggered by TNF-alpha and IL 1 and is responsible for reepithelialization and angiogenesis. Platelet-derived growth factor is important for wound fibroplasia. IL-6 = interleukin 6, IL-10 = interleukin 10, MCP-1 = monocyte chemotactic protein 1, IP-10 = interferon-inducible protein-10, TGF-β = tumor growth factor-beta, and NAP-2 = neutrophil-activated protein-2. *(Reproduced with permission from Henry G, Garner WL: Inflammatory mediators in wound healing.* Surg Clin North Am 2003;83:483-507.)

suggest that low-pressure pulsatile lavage combined with diluted soap solution can be effective in contaminated wounds with less effect on osteoclastic and osteoblastic activity.[9]

The frequency of irrigation may also play a role in fracture healing. A rabbit study found that animals that underwent a lavage of an osteotomy on three consecutive days failed to form callus, whereas those that underwent lavage at day 3 or 4 had decreased callus formation compared with the control group, which had no lavage.[9,10] This was attributed to the disruption of the normal healing cascade. Further study is needed to clarify the role of each type of lavage and to determine which irrigating solution is most appropriate in the treatment of trauma patients.

Flap Coverage

The conventional treatment of exposed bone in the proximal third of the tibia has been a rotational flap using the gastrocnemius, whereas the soleus flap has been used for middle third defects, and free muscle transfers have been used for distal third injuries. The Lower Extremity Assessment Project Study Group published a report that called into question the concept of coverage of proximal third and middle third defects of the leg with rotational muscle flaps.[11] The authors found that complications such as deep infection are common in patients with fractures of the lower leg that require flap coverage. Deep infections occur in approximately 20% of patients with severe lower extremity fractures that were covered with a free flap or rotational flap. Flap necrosis occurs in 8% of these patients, regardless of the type of flap. However, in patients with severe bony injuries (AO C type fractures of the lower leg), rotational flaps have a significantly higher complication rate than free muscle

flaps (44% and 23%, respectively). This is likely caused by the increased severity of injury to the muscle associated with these fractures. Based on the findings of this multicenter study, it is reasonable to consider using a rotational flap for patients with type A and B fractures, but free flaps should be used for patients with more severe bony injuries.

Changes in the approach to the treatment of exposed bone in the lower leg have recently been developed. The major advantage of using local muscle (gastrocnemius-soleus complex or soleus) to cover open fractures is that rotational flaps are less technically demanding and involve less surgical time than free muscle transfers. However, because the muscle belly that is being rotated is often within the zone of injury, the viability of this tissue may be compromised. Free muscle transfers are technically more difficult to perform and require longer surgical times; when successfully done, however, they provide uninjured muscle with a healthier blood supply to the injured area. Free muscle transfers have a relatively steep learning curve, and success rates vary based on the experience of the surgeon. The timing of coverage depends on the availability of a surgeon trained in microvascular techniques.

The timing of flap coverage has been shown to play a role in fracture healing and the development of complications. Coverage within the first 5 days is optimal. However, caution must be used when providing very early coverage because the full extent of the soft-tissue injury, especially the viability of local muscle used for rotational flaps, may not be apparent during the first 48 hours. Flaps that are placed to treat wounds that have been open for more than 30 days have a much higher failure rate (20%) than those placed in the acute setting (1% to 5%).[12] The failure rate is higher in patients with preexisting osteomyelitis (23%) versus patients with chronic wounds who do not have osteomyelitis (13%). A variety of free muscle transfers have been described in the literature, including gracilis, latissimus dorsi, and rectus abdominis transfers.[12-17] All have similar rates of success, with reported flap revision rates of 5% to 10%.

The usefulness of fasciocutaneous flaps (such as the distally-based sural artery flap) has been recently demonstrated.[18-20] This procedure is indicated for patients with distal third soft-tissue injuries up to 10 × 15 cm. The distally based sural artery flap is based on the most distal perforating branch of the peroneal artery that supplies the sural artery. In several series, the flap can be used in many instances in which a free flap would have been required.[18-20] Most series report success rates with this procedure that approach those of free muscle flaps. It cannot be used in patients with damage to the sural nerve or posterior calf. Because it does not require reanastomosis, it may be done much faster than a free flap and does not require a surgical assistant. However, as with free muscle transfers, this option fares less well in patients with preexisting osteomyelitis. Free flap coverage is generally a viable salvage procedure if fasciocutaneous flap coverage fails; however, if a transtibial amputation is being considered, the donor site for this flap may be compromised.

In addition to the ability of rotational muscle flaps to bring in better blood supply to the fracture and close the wound, there is also evidence that they blunt the increase in TNF-α found in open fractures. This effect is significant only in the first 6 days after open fracture occurs, but it can occur even in the presence of bacterial infection.[21] TNF-α is a cytokine that can be cytotoxic at elevated levels; at lower concentrations, however, it stimulates bone and collagen resorption and production of IL-1 and IL-6.

When choosing the appropriate management of a given wound, surgeons must consider the degree of injury to local muscle, their own experience, and patient factors, such as age, smoking history, and systemic illness. Wounds can be temporized with an antibiotic bead pouch or negative-pressure dressing and systemic antibiotics until coverage can be performed.

Antibiotic Bead Pouches

Antibiotics may be incorporated into bone cement and placed on a string to deliver high concentrations of antibiotics locally. This technique may be used to treat open fractures with soft-tissue loss. As much as 4.8 g of tobramycin or 4 g of vancomycin may be used in one package of bone cement. Beads may be placed into a wound that cannot be closed and an adhesive drape can be placed over that to form a pouch. The use of benzoin or colloidin around the wound edge may help prevent maceration of the skin and provide containment of the exudate that will rapidly form.

Negative-Pressure Dressings

Vacuum-assisted wound closure (VAC) has gained widespread acceptance as an adjunct to the management of acute wounds. Despite its widespread use, there are few well-designed studies to evaluate its effectiveness in treating patients with acute trauma. Animal studies suggest that the VAC device dramatically increases the rate of formation of granulation tissue and helps control bacterial counts, but the mechanism by which it does so remains obscure.[22] Anecdotally, many trauma surgeons believe that wound healing is accelerated by VAC closure and therefore use it routinely, even on closed wounds and suture lines. Additional work is needed to further clarify the indications, duration, and limitations of the VAC device. The biologic effect of conventional dressings such as wet-to-dry dressings, Betadine dressings, and various antibiotic-impregnated dressings have not been well studied in the orthopaedic trauma population, but inferences can be made from studies of pa-

tients with burns and diabetic ulcers. Despite the wide variation in opinion, it seems that Betadine can be cytotoxic and should be used with caution in tenuous wounds.[23] Furthermore, wounds heal better when they are kept moist rather than when they are allowed to desiccate.

Skin Graft Substitutes and Other Biologic Dressings

Split-thickness skin grafts are widely used to cover skin defects; however, their use is not without complications.[24] Infection and pain at the donor site, poor cosmesis, and failure of the graft to adhere to the graft site can occur. Patients with large skin defects may also be problematic to treat because skin available for harvest may be limited.

To address these problems, several approaches have been used. Cultured keratinocytes are commercially available that use a small skin biopsy sample as a source for new skin.[25,26] Cultured keratinocytes, however, are expensive and require a prolonged incubation period. Allograft skin may be treated by decellularization and freeze-drying while preserving the matrix.[27] This product offers the advantage of allowing use of a much thinner split-thickness graft, but it has the potential to transmit virus. Another product uses a very thin layer of silicone on a matrix composed of cross-linked bovine collagen and chondroitin-6 sulfate as a temporary skin substitute.[28] After neovascularization of the dermal layer, the silicone layer is removed, and a thin split-thickness skin graft is placed. Although this technique seems to lead to good cosmesis and less wound contraction, wounds treated with this product are prone to infection.

Because of the expense, limited availability of skin available for harvest, and necessity for secondary operations, skin graft substitutes are generally reserved for patients with large defects, such as massive degloving injuries and burns. A useful adjunct to conventional split-thickness skin grafting, especially in irregular wounds, is the placement of a negative-pressure dressing over a porous, nonadherent dressing instead of a bolster.

Compartment Syndrome

Compartment syndrome is an orthopaedic emergency that is challenging to diagnose. The clinical signs that constitute the cornerstone of diagnosis (pain, pallor, paresthesias, paralysis, and pulselessness) are not reliable in trauma patients who are intubated or sedated. As a result, continuous monitoring of compartment pressures with an arterial line transducer has been advocated.[29] Although this has not become a universal standard, the surgeon should maintain a low threshold of suspicion for measuring compartment pressures in obtunded patients. Subtler compartment syndromes occur in the thigh, gluteal region, and foot, and they are frequently ascribed to pain at the fracture site. A high level of suspicion must be maintained when patients report pain that is unrelieved by stabilization.

Summary

Studies are currently underway to help better understand the complex interaction of cytokines and other inflammatory mediators in the healing of soft tissues. As these pathways are defined, interventions may be identified that hasten healing or restart stalled healing. Early research is currently being conducted to assess whether the genetic manipulation of cells can promote the production of the appropriate growth factors needed for wound healing.

Annotated References

1. Cross KJ, Mustoe TA: Growth factors in wound healing. *Surg Clin North Am* 2003;83:531-545.

    The authors of this study review of the role of inflammatory mediators in wound healing.

2. Dubay DA, Franz MG: Acute wound healing: The biology of acute wound failure. *Surg Clin North Am* 2003;83:463-481.

    In this report, the authors provide a comprehensive overview of acute wound healing.

3. Henry G, Garner WL: Inflammatory mediators in wound healing. *Surg Clin North Am* 2003;83:483-507.

    The authors provide a detailed review of the role of cytokines and growth factors in wound healing.

4. Anglen JO: Wound irrigation in musculoskeletal injury. *J Am Acad Orthop Surg* 2001;9:219-226.

    The author discusses wound irrigation débridement in the treatment of patients with musculoskeletal injuries.

5. Adili A, Bhandari M, Schemitsch EH: The biomechanical effect of high-pressure irrigation on diaphyseal fracture healing in vivo. *J Orthop Trauma* 2002;16:413-417.

    In this animal study, the authors demonstrate that high-pressure lavage causes a 37% decrease in peak bending strength and a 32% decrease in stiffness during the first 3 weeks of healing, but this difference disappears at 6 weeks.

6. Bhandari M, Schemitsch EH, Adili A, Lachowski RJ, Shaughnessy SG: High and low pressure pulsatile lavage of contaminated tibial fractures: An in vitro study of bacterial adherence and bone damage. *J Orthop Trauma* 1999;13:526-533.

7. Lee EW, Dirschl DR, Duff G, Dahners LE, Miclau T: High-pressure pulsatile lavage irrigation of fresh intraarticular fractures: effectiveness at removing particulate matter from bone. *J Orthop Trauma* 2002;16:162-165.

    This randomized animal study compared the efficacy of bulb syringe and high-pressure lavage in removing particulate debris from bone. The authors report that the two methods appear to be equally effective in removing particulate debris from metaphyseal bone and does not drive debris into the wound.

8. Dirschl DR, Duff GP, Dahners LE, Edin M, Rahn BA, Miclau T: High pressure pulsatile lavage irrigation of intraarticular fractures: Effects on fracture healing. *J Orthop Trauma* 1998;12:460-463.

9. Bhandari M, Adili A, Schemitsch EH: The efficacy of low-pressure lavage with different irrigating solutions to remove adherent bacteria from bone. *J Bone Joint Surg Am* 2001;83-A:412-419.

    This randomized animal study compared the efficacy of various irrigation solutions in the treatment of contaminated wounds. The authors found soap solution to be the most effective.

10. Park S-H, Silva M, Bahk W-J, McKellop H, Lieberman JR: Effect of repeated irrigation and debridement on fracture healing in an animal model. *J Orthop Res* 2002;20:1197-1204.

    The findings of this randomized animal study suggest that repeated irrigation with a syringe may delay healing.

11. Pollak AN, McCarthy ML, Burgess AR: Short-term wound complications after application of flaps for coverage of traumatic soft-tissue defects about the tibia: The Lower Extremity Assessment Project (LEAP) Study Group. *J Bone Joint Surg Am* 2000; 82:1681-1691.

    The authors of this study found that rotational flaps are inferior to free flaps in the treatment of patients with AO C-type fractures.

12. Gonzalez MH, Tarandy DI, Troy D, Phillips D, Weinzweig N: Free tissue coverage of chronic traumatic wounds of the lower leg. *Plast Reconstr Surg* 2002;109:592-600.

    In this study, 42 free flaps were done in 38 patients, and 34 flaps survived. The authors report that complications were higher in patients with osteomyelitis.

13. Hammert WC, Minarchek J, Trzeciak MA: Free-flap reconstruction of traumatic lower extremity wounds. *Am J Orthop* 2000;29(suppl 9):22-26.

    The authors of this study report that 18 of 20 free flaps used to treat patients with open fractures of the lower extremities were successful.

14. Ninkovič M, Schoeller T, Wechselberger G, Otto A, Sperner G, Anderl H: Primary flap closure in com-

plex limb injuries. *J Reconstr Microsurg* 1997;13:575-583.

15. Redett RJ, Robertson BC, Chang B, Girotto J, Vaughan T: Limb salvage of lower-extremity wounds using free gracilis muscle reconstruction. *Plast Reconstr Surg* 2000;106:1507-1513.

    In this study, 50 patients with lower extremity wounds were treated with free gracilis muscle transfer. The authors report that 3 of 22 flaps that were placed to treat acute defects failed, whereas 2 of 28 that were placed to treat chronic wounds failed.

16. Yajima H, Tamai S, Kobata Y, Murata K, Fukui A, Takakura Y: Vascularized composite tissue transfers for open fractures with massive soft-tissue defects in the lower extremities. *Microsurgery* 2002;22:114-119.

    In this study, 39 patients were treated with cutaneous or osteocutaneous flaps; 9 revisions were required.

17. Zukowski M, Lord J, Ash K, Shouse B, Getz S, Robb G: The gracilis free flap revisited: A review of 25 cases of transfer to traumatic extremity wounds. *Ann Plast Surg* 1998;40:141-144.

18. Fraccalvieri M, Verna G, Dolcet M, et al: The distally based superficial sural flap: Our experience in reconstructing the lower leg and foot. *Ann Plast Surg* 2000;45:132-139.

    In this study, 18 patients were successfully treated with sural artery fasciocutaneous flaps.

19. Price MF, Capizzi PJ, Waterson PA, Lettieri S: Reverse sural artery flap: Caveats for success. *Ann Plast Surg* 2002;48:496-504.

    The authors of this study report that use of a reverse sural artery flap was successful in 11 patients with distal third wounds. The authors also discuss several technical considerations for this procedure.

20. Robotti E, Verna G, Fraccalvieri M, Bocchiotti MA: Distally based fasciocutaneous flaps: A versatile option for coverage of difficult war wounds of the foot and ankle. *Plast Reconstr Surg* 1998;101:1014-1021.

21. Brown SA, Mayberry AJ, Mathy JA, Phillips TM, Klitzman B, Levin LS: The effect of muscle flap transposition to the fracture site on TNFα levels during fracture healing. *Plast Reconstr Surg* 2000; 105:991-998.

    The authors of this case study report that rotational muscle transfer decreases the level of TNF-α in the presence of bacterial contamination during the first 6 days after fracture.

22. Webb LX: New techniques in wound management: vacuum-assisted wound closure. *J Am Acad Orthop Surg* 2002;10:303-311.

    The author reviews the current state of knowledge regarding the use of the VAC device for wound management.

23. Lionelli GT, Lawrence WT: Wound dressings. *Surg Clin North Am* 2003;83:617-638.

    The authors provide a good summary of all types of wound dressings and their indications.

24. Singer AJ, Clark RAF: Cutaneous wound healing. *N Engl J Med* 1999;341:738-746.

25. van den Bogaerdt AJ, van Zuijlen PP, van Galen M, Lamme EN, Middelkoop E: The suitability of cells from different tissues for use in tissue-engineered skin substitutes. *Arch Dermatol Res* 2002;294:135-142.

    The authors report that although dermis, adipose tissue, and eschar can all be used as sources for fibroblasts, dermis is superior for skin substitutes.

26. Boyce ST, Warden GD: Principles and practices for treatment of cutaneous wounds with cultured skin substitutes. *Am J Surg* 2002;183:445-456.

    This review article describes the theory and clinical experience of cultured skin substitutes.

27. Hodde J: Naturally occurring scaffolds for soft tissue repair and regeneration. *Tissue Eng* 2002;8:295-308.

    The authors of this review article discuss various tissues that can be used for cellular ingrowth.

28. Kuroyanagi Y, Yamada N, Yamashita R, Uchinuma E: Tissue-engineered products: Allogeneic cultured dermal substitute composed of spongy collagen with fibroblasts. *Artif Organs* 2001;25:180-186.

    In this study, allogeneic (bovine) collagen with human dermal cells was used successfully to treat 145 patients; 138 patients had no evidence of graft rejection.

29. White TO, Howell GE, Will EM, Court-Brown CM, McQueen MM: Elevated intramuscular compartment pressures do not influence outcome after tibial fractures. *J Trauma* 2003;55:1133-1138.

    In this prospective study comparing the measurements of differential compartment pressures with intramuscular pressures, the authors found that if the differential pressure (diastolic minus compartment pressure) was greater than mm Hg, elevated compartment pressures greater than 30 mm Hg absolute did not affect outcomes.

Chapter 8

The Mangled Lower Extremity

Michael J. Bosse, MD

Ellen J. MacKenzie, PhD

Introduction

The term mangled extremity is used by orthopaedic surgeons to describe a limb injury that is so severe that amputation is a possible outcome. Mangled extremity injuries are typically a result of high-energy trauma with a combination of crush, shear, and bending forces. The skin is often degloved, with large areas of loss secondary to avulsion or ischemia. The fascial compartments are typically incompletely opened by explosion or tear, and the muscle tissues are damaged at local and regional levels by direct and indirect injury. Tissue planes are usually extensively disrupted. If present, contaminants infiltrate all of these planes (Figure 1). The presence of associated fractures with transverse or extensive comminution patterns usually confirm that the injury was the result of high-energy forces (Figure 2). A zone of injury extends proximal and distal from the area of maximal force application, and definition of this zone is critical to understanding and treating the injury.

The modification of passenger restraints in motor vehicles, motor vehicle safety engineering, and legislation requiring seatbelts and air-bag protection in motor vehicles appear to be decreasing the mortality rate associated with motor vehicle crashes. However, the incidence of severe lower extremity trauma may be increasing. Injuries to the lower extremity account for over 250,000 hospital admissions annually for patients age 18 to 54 years. It is estimated that more than half of these admissions result from a high-energy mechanism of injury.[1] Orthopaedic surgeons providing emergency department trauma coverage should understand the historical concepts of the care for these injuries, be aware of recent modification of these concepts based on advances in technology, and have a better understanding of long-term clinical outcomes.

The appropriate management of patients with limb-threatening lower extremity injuries is the subject of extensive debate. Limb injuries that would have required amputation 20 years ago are now routinely treated via complex reconstruction protocols because sophisticated

medical and surgical advances have improved the ability of orthopaedic surgeons to reconstruct severely injured lower extremities. The development of second- and third-generation antibiotics, microsurgical tissue transfers, wound irrigation strategies, and tissue-friendly fracture fixation methods now make initial limb salvage feasible for most patients. Delayed large segment bone defect reconstruction is now routine with the development of autogenous grafts, bone transports, and osteoinductive materials.[2] Although limb salvage is technically feasible, the advisability of the routine use of the limb salvage techniques has been challenged.[3-6]

Because most studies that evaluated the results of the reconstruction protocols consisted of small, retrospective single-center series, the results of the limb salvage efforts are largely unknown. The aggressive application of the limb salvage protocols, however, was associated with a perceived increase in the number of patients with viable but nonfunctioning limbs, which led some investigators to suggest that the functional outcome after a successful limb reconstruction was often poorer than what was achieved more quickly and less expensively with an early amputation and a good prosthesis.[4-12] One study reported a 20.7% mortality rate secondary to lower extremity injury-related sepsis following limb salvage attempts.[3]

Data providing a better understanding of the evaluation, treatment, and outcomes of patients with severe high-energy leg injuries have recently been published.[13] The Lower Extremity Assessment Project (LEAP) Study Group conducted a prospective observational study to assess 601 patients with limb-threatening injuries below the distal femur who were admitted to eight Level 1 trauma centers in the United States. The patients were longitudinally followed for 2 years. A detailed assessment of the demographic, socioeconomic, behavioral, social, and vocational characteristics of each patient was done. The patients' injuries were categorized by a comprehensive scoring of the study limb and of nonstudy injuries. Clinical and functional outcomes were evaluated at 3, 6, 12, and 24 months.

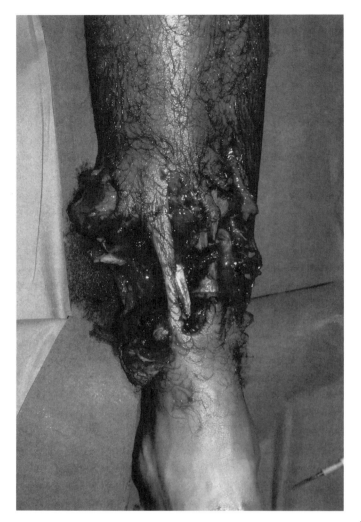

Figure 1 Photograph of a grade IIIB tibial fracture (mangled extremity).

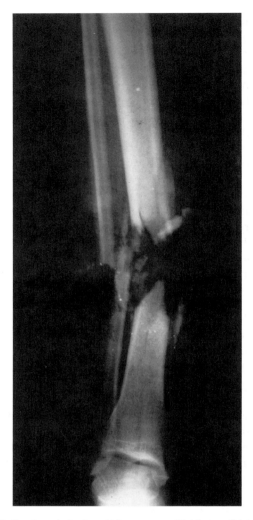

Figure 2 AP radiograph showing a high-energy open tibial fracture. Tibial diaphyseal bone loss was present at the time of hospital admission.

The Patient

Successful treatment of the mangled extremity and return of the patient to the best possible level of function and social interaction depends on the patient's involvement in the treatment regimen, the patient's environment, the extent of the injury, and the treatment course. Understanding the potential impact of elements that are beyond the control of surgeons, the patient, and the patient's environment is critical to the development of a care plan. In the LEAP Study, most of the patients were male (77%), white (72%), and between the ages of 20 and 45 years (71%). Seventy percent were high school graduates compared with 86% nationally ($P < 0.05$). More of the patients lived in households with incomes below the federal poverty line than the national rate (25% versus 16%; $P < 0.05$). This patient cohort also had significantly higher rates of uninsured patients (38%) and had double the national average of heavy drinkers ($P < 0.01$). Patients in this study were found to be slightly more neurotic and extroverted and less open to new experiences when compared with the general population. No significant differences were detected among patients entered into the reconstruction or amputation group.[14]

These findings are important to surgeons who care for patients with mangled lower extremities. Compared with the general population, patients with limb-threatening injuries typically have fewer resources, which may limit their access to rehabilitation services and affect their ability to accommodate residual disabilities. These patients are generally in more physically demanding jobs, which may impede efforts to return to work, and they have poorer health habits, which may complicate recovery. Moreover, it is possible that the personality traits identified in this patient population could predispose these patients to a more difficult recovery.

Treatment Decision Making

High-energy trauma to lower extremities presents both reconstruction and rehabilitation challenges. The decision to amputate or reconstruct a severely injured lower extremity is difficult. Traditionally, retention of a limb that is healed, sensate, and uninfected was considered a successful outcome. Surgeons have reported that the extremity injury must be assessed in the context of the patient's overall injury load and present and predicted physiologic responses.[15,16] Focused assessment of the extremity determines vascular sufficiency, compartment syndrome risk, plantar sensibility, the severity of skin and muscle damage/loss, and the possibility of fracture defect reconstruction. If the vascular supply cannot be established or maintained, reconstruction efforts are futile. The decision to revascularize an ischemic traumatized limb must be a joint decision made by orthopaedic and vascular surgeons. Reconstruction rates for grade IIIC tibial fractures are low, ranging from 25% to 41%.[13,17,18] Efforts wasted to return blood flow to a limb that is beyond reconstructive capacity can potentially harm the patient and the trauma system. Patient factors believed to influence the decision-making process include age, other injuries, and premorbid medical conditions. Recently, the negative effects of smoking on fracture healing and outcome have been recognized.[19]

Factors that influenced the mangled extremity treatment decision-making process have been studied.[20] Orthopaedic surgeons caring for patients with mangled legs were surveyed to determine the factors they typically used to make a decision regarding whether reconstruction or amputation was the best method of treatment. Approximately 33% of 52 orthopaedic surgeons surveyed indicated that plantar sensation was the most important determinant for limb salvage. The severity of the soft-tissue injury and limb ischemia were cited as the next most important determinants by 17% and 15% of orthopaedic surgeons, respectively. No orthopaedic surgeons ranked the Injury Severity Score (ISS) as a critical factor. In contrast, 31% of general trauma surgeons from the same centers ranked the ISS as the most critical determinant, followed by limb ischemia (27%) and plantar sensation (21%). Analysis of patient, injury, and surgeon characteristics determined that the soft-tissue injury (the extent of muscle injury, deep vein injury, skin defects, and contamination) and the absence of plantar sensation were the most important factors that predicted amputation. Patient characteristics and the experience level of the surgeon did not appear to influence the decision-making process. The orthopaedic surgeon was responsible for the initial treatment decision in all instances. The general trauma surgeon participated in the decision-making process 58% of the time, and plastic surgeons participated 26% of the time.

The Significance of Plantar Sensation

It is difficult to trace the origin of the concept that initial plantar sensation is critical to the salvage of an extremity. Articles published before 1980 warn that neuropathic ulcers and chronic complications can be associated with absent plantar sensation. Other authors, however, describe a confirmed avulsion or complete transection of the posterior tibial nerve as their definition of absent plantar sensation.[18,21,22] In most clinical scenarios, however, the injured limb is assessed in the emergency department. Once patients are in the operating room, the additional dissection of the deep posterior compartment is usually considered unwise in an already compromised limb. Therefore, in many centers, the absence of initial plantar sensation is considered to be the same as a physiologic disruption of the nerve. Ischemia, compression, contusion, and stretch can temporarily affect the function of the posterior tibial nerve. Once these factors resolve, nerve function typically returns. In the face of no sensory return, orthopaedic surgeons have demonstrated the ability to care for the insensate foot in other conditions (diabetes or incomplete spinal lesions). Patient education and shoe modifications can be used to treat patients with diabetes. The sciatic nerve can be resected with acceptable results in patients requiring tumor limb salvage.[23]

Although one report supported the inclusion and importance of plantar sensibility in the limb salvage decision-making process,[20] the fact that this was historically an established treatment axiom may have resulted in a self-fulfilling prophecy phenomenon because surgeons once believed that the absence of plantar sensation was an indication for limb amputation and acted accordingly.

One study used the variations in physician practice patterns to explore the outcomes of patients admitted to the LEAP Study in whom plantar sensation was absent.[24] The authors of this report examined the outcomes of a subset of 55 subjects with an insensate extremity at the time of presentation. The 55 patients were divided into two treatment groups: the insensate amputation group (N = 26) and the insensate salvage group (N = 29). In addition, control subjects were identified from the parent cohort so that a comparison could also be made with a group of patients in whom plantar sensation was present and whose limbs were reconstructed: the sensate control group. The sensate control group consisted of 29 subjects who were matched with the 29 patients in the insensate salvage group based on four limb injury severity characteristics (severity of muscle, venous, and bony injury and the presence of an associated foot injury). Patient and injury characteristics as well as functional and health-related quality of life outcomes at 12 and 24 months after injury were compared for patients in the insensate salvage group and those in the other study groups ($P \leq 0.05$ was considered significant).

TABLE 1 | Limb Salvage Score Elements

	Scoring Systems				
	MESS	LSI	PSI	NISSSA	HFS-97
Age	X			X	
Shock	X			X	X
Warm ischemia time	X			X	X
Bone injury		X	X		X
Muscle injury		X	X		
Skin injury		X	X		X
Nerve injury		X		X	X
Deep-vein injury		X			
Skeletal/soft-tissue injury	X			X	
Contamination				X	X
Time to treatment			X		

*MESS = Mangled Extremity Severity Score; LSI = Limb Salvage Index; PSI = Predictive Salvage Index; NISSSA = Nerve Injury, Ischemia, Soft-Tissue Injury, Skeletal Injury, Shock, and Age of Patient Score; HFS-97 = Hanover Fracture Scale (1997 version).
(Reproduced with permission from Bosse MJ, MacKenzie EJ, Kellam JF, et al: A prospective evaluation of the clinical utility of the lower-extremity injury-severity scores. *J Bone Joint Surg Am* 2002;83-A(1):3-14.)

Patients in the insensate salvage group did not report or exhibit significantly worse outcomes at 12 or 24 months after injury compared with patients in the insensate amputation group or sensate control group. Among patients with a salvaged limb (those in the insensate salvage group and sensate control group), an equal proportion (55%) had normal foot sensation 2 years after injury regardless of whether plantar sensation was reported on admission (sensate control group) or absent (insensate salvage group). Pain, weight-bearing status, and the percentage of patients who had returned to work were similar for patients in the insensate salvage group compared with those in the insensate amputation group and sensate control group. Furthermore, there were no significant differences noted in the overall, physical, or psychosocial Sickness Impact Profile scores among subjects without plantar sensation whose limbs were salvaged (insensate salvage group) and those who underwent amputation (insensate amputation group) or subjects with intact sensation whose limbs were salvaged (sensate control group). More than half of patients presenting with an insensate foot treated with limb reconstruction ultimately regain normal sensation at 2-year follow-up. At that time, only two patients (11%) in the insensate salvage group and one patient (5%) in the sensate control group had absent plantar sensation. Initial plantar sensation was not found to be prognostic of long-term plantar sensory status or functional outcomes.

Limb Salvage Scores

The decision to amputate or salvage a severely injured lower extremity is difficult. Attempts to quantify the severity of the trauma and to establish numerical guide-lines for the decision to amputate or salvage a limb have been proposed by several authors. Lower extremity scoring systems include the Mangled Extremity Severity Score (MESS);[21,25] the Predictive Salvage Index (PSI);[22] the Limb Salvage Index (LSI);[18] the Nerve Injury, Ischemia, Soft Tissue Injury, Skeletal Injury, Shock and Age of Patient (NISSSA);[17] and the Hanover Fracture Scale-97 (HFS-97).[26,27] The scores vary in terms of the factors considered relevant to limb salvage (Table 1) and the relative weights assigned to each element. These scoring systems were validated by the developers and demonstrated a high sensitivity and specificity in predicting limb salvage. With the exception of the HFS-97, the development of the lower extremity injury severity scores has been flawed by retrospective design and small sample sizes. In addition, component selection and weighting in all of the indices were affected by the clinical bias of the index developers. The NISSSA, LSI, and HFS-97 weigh the result of the initial plantar neurologic examination. Age, presence of shock, severity of contamination, and time to treatment are included in some of the scoring strategies. For example, the MESS assigns one additional point if the patient is older than 29 years, one additional point for normal perfusion with a diminished pulse, and additional points for transient or persistent hypotension without qualifying cause or response to treatment (Table 2). The suggested MESS threshold for amputation is 7. Using the MESS, for example, a 30-year-old patient (1 point) with a high-energy open tibia fracture (3 points), normal perfusion but a diminished pulse secondary to spasm or compression (1 point), and persistent hypotension before laparotomy related to a spleen injury (2 points) would undergo amputation at the

TABLE 2 Mangled Extremity Severity Score Strategy: ≥ 7 Points	
Skeletal/Soft-Tissue Injury	
Low-energy injury	1
Medium-energy injury	2
High-energy injury	3
Very high-energy injury	4
Limb Ischemia	
Pulse decreased/absent, normal perfusion	1*
Pulseless, decreased capillary fill	2*
Cool, paralyzed, insensate	3*
Shock	
Systolic blood pressure > 90 mm Hg	0
Systolic blood pressure < 90 mm Hg, transiently	1
Systolic blood pressure < 90 mm Hg, persistently	2
Age (years)	
< 30	0
30 to 50	1
> 50	2

*Double value if duration of ischemia > 6 hours

conclusion of the laparotomy despite the fact that the limb perfusion will likely return to normal and a splenectomy and appropriate resuscitation will resolve the patient's hypotension.

Ideally, a trauma limb-salvage index would be 100% sensitive (all patients with amputated limbs will have scores at or above the threshold) and 100% specific (all patients with salvaged limbs will have scores below the threshold). Few clinical tests, however, perform ideally. When making the decision to amputate, high specificity is important to ensure that only a small number of salvageable limbs are incorrectly assigned a score above the amputation decision threshold. Specificity is also important to guard against inappropriate delays in amputation when the limb is ultimately not salvageable.

Researchers who were not directly involved in the development of the limb salvage score systems were not able to duplicate the results reported by the developers. Bonanni and associates[7] retrospectively applied the Mangled Extremity Syndrome Index, MESS, LSI, and PSI limb salvage score strategies to 58 lower limb salvage attempts over a 10-year period. Failure of the reconstruction effort was defined as an amputation or functional failure at 2-year follow-up. A limb was considered to be a functional failure based on the inability of the patient to walk 150 feet without assistance, climb 12 stairs, or independently perform wheelchair transfer. The authors were not able to support utilization of any of the scoring strategies to determine limb treatment.

In an attempt to clarify the clinical utility of any of the limb salvage scoring strategies, one study prospectively captured all of the elements of the MESS, LSI,

PSI, NISSSA, and HFS-97 at the time of each patient's initial assessment and critical decision making regarding limb salvage.[28] The elements were collected so as to not provide the evaluator with a score or impact on the decision-making process. The analysis did not validate the clinical utility of any of the lower extremity injury score strategies. The high specificity of the scores did, however, confirm that low scores could be used to predict limb salvage potential. The converse was not true. The low sensitivity of the indices failed to support the validity of the scores as predictors of amputation (Table 3). The authors concluded that a lower extremity injury score at or above the amputation threshold should be used with caution by surgeons to decide the fate of a mangled lower extremity.

Functional Outcomes: Amputation Versus Reconstruction

The clinical challenge of treating patients with mangled lower extremities is to decide as early as possible the correct treatment pathway for the patient. The surgeon must weigh the fact that for most patients limb reconstruction is possible, given the appropriate application of current techniques and counterbalancing the expected result against that which is possible with an amputation. Prosthetic bioengineering innovations have significantly improved the function and comfort of lower extremity amputees. Most series reporting on the results of limb salvage or amputation were single center, small, and retrospective studies. Their conclusions provided a glimpse of the complexity of the clinical decision-making process, but the results could not be used to guide clinical decision making. Several clinical series reached different conclusions regarding the reconstruction versus amputation dilemma for patients with high-energy open tibial fractures.[4,6,8]

One study retrospectively compared the functional outcomes of 26 patients with grade IIIB tibial fractures that were successfully reconstructed with those of 18 patients who were managed by early below-the-knee amputation.[4] Five patients in the reconstruction group required late amputation secondary to infection complications. The reconstruction patients had more surgical procedures, more complications, and longer hospital stays than patients treated by early below-the-knee amputation. The functional outcomes of the 16 successful reconstructions were compared with those of the early below-the-knee amputation patients. The authors found that the reconstruction patients took more time to achieve full weight bearing and were less willing or less able to return to work. Validated outcomes instruments were used to assess the quality of life for a subset of the patients. Significantly more limb salvage patients considered themselves to be severely disabled and impaired for both occupational and recreational activities. The au-

TABLE 3 | **Clinical Usefulness of Limb Salvage Scores**

	All Gustilo Type III Fractures[†] (N = 357)	Gustilo Type IIIB Fractures[†] (N = 214)	Gustilo Type IIIC Fractures[†] (N = 59)
MESS			
Sensitivity	0.45 (0.35 to 0.55)	0.17 (0.10 to 0.30)	0.78 (0.64 to 0.89)
Specificity	0.93 (0.90 to 0.95)	0.94 (0.89 to 0.97)	0.69 (0.39 to 0.91)
Area under curve	0.78 (0.72 to 0.83)	0.69 (0.62 to 0.78)	0.68 (0.46 to 0.89)
PSI			
Sensitivity	0.47 (0.37 to 0.57)	0.35 (0.22 to 0.51)	0.61 (0.45 to 0.75)
Specificity	0.84 (0.79 to 0.88)	0.85 (0.79 to 0.90)	0.69 (0.39 to 0.91)
Area under curve	0.73[‡] (0.68 to 0.79)	0.68 (0.61 to 0.76)	0.68 (0.50 to 0.86)
LSI			
Sensitivity	0.51 (0.41 to 0.61)	0.15 (0.10 to 0.28)	0.91 (0.79 to 0.98)
Specificity	0.97 (0.94 to 0.99)	0.98 (0.95 to 1.00)	0.69 (0.39 to 0.91)
Area under curve	0.85[§] (0.81 to 0.89)	0.75[‖] (0.69 to 0.83)	0.88[¶] (0.79 to 0.98)
NISSSA			
Sensitivity	0.33 (0.24 to 0.43)	0.13 (0.05 to 0.25)	0.59 (0.43 to 0.73)
Specificity	0.98 (0.96 to 1.00)	1.00 (0.98 to 1.00)	0.77 (0.46 to 0.95)
Area under curve	0.78 (0.78 to 0.83)	0.69 (0.61 to 0.77)	0.72 (0.52 to 0.92)
HFS-97			
Sensitivity	0.37 (0.28 to 0.47)	0.10 (0.04 to 0.23)	0.67 (0.52 to 0.81)
Specificity	0.98 (0.95 to 1.00)	1.00 (0.97 to 1.00)	0.77 (0.46 to 0.95)
Area under curve	0.80 (0.75 to 0.86)	0.71 (0.63 to 0.78)	0.83[#] (0.68 to 0.98)

*MESS = Mangled Extremity Severity Score; LSI = Limb Salvage Index; PSI = Predictive Salvage Index; NISSSA = Nerve Injury, Ischemia, Soft-Tissue Injury, Skeletal Injury, Shock, and Age of Patient Score; HFS-97 = Hanover Fracture Scale (1997 version).
[†]The 95% confidence intervals are in parentheses
[‡]PSI significantly different than HFS-97 ($P < 0.05$)
[§]LSI significantly different than PSI, MESS, HFS-97, and NISSSA ($P < 0.05$)
[‖]LSI significantly different than PSI ($P < 0.05$)
[¶]LSI significantly different than PSI, MESS, and NISSSA ($P < 0.05$)
[#]HFS-97 significantly different than MESS and NISSSA ($P < 0.05$)
(Reproduced with permission from Bosse MJ, MacKenzie EJ, Kellam JF, et al: A prospective evaluation of the clinical utility of the lower-extremity injury-severity scores. *J Bone Joint Surg Am* 2002;83:3-14.)

thors concluded that early below-the-knee amputation resulted in a quicker recovery with less long-term disability.

Another study retrospectively compared 39 patients with complex grade IIIB or IIIC tibial fractures, 18 of whom underwent below-the-knee amputation and 21 underwent reconstruction.[6] Although the authors concluded that limb reconstruction was advisable, the data did not strongly support this conclusion. Reported functional outcome differences were based on the evaluation of pain, range of motion, quadriceps wasting, and walking ability. No patient-based outcomes measure was used. Patients who underwent amputation were reported to have a higher dollar cost to society, a figure that was inflated by adding the estimated cost of permanent disability assigned to an amputee versus that of a patient who underwent reconstruction. Actual medical costs were significantly less for the patients who underwent amputation. Amputees required between three and four interventions and 12 months of rehabilitation. Patients

who underwent reconstruction averaged eight interventions and 30 months of rehabilitation.

Another study retrospectively evaluated 55 patients with IIIB and IIIC tibial fractures who received care over a 12-year period.[8] The Short Form-36 score was used as the primary outcomes measure. Successful salvage patients had significantly better physical subscale scores than the amputees. Both groups had psychological subscores similar to those of a healthy population. Based on their findings, the authors suggested that a below-the-knee amputation was an inferior reconstruction option to a successfully reconstructed leg.

The conclusions reached in these three series are contradictory, which is likely a result of their retrospective design and small sample sizes. The research teams could not adequately assess or control for the injury, treatment, patient, and patient environment variables that could influence the outcome. The LEAP Study was designed to address the shortcomings of previous clinical studies and compare the outcomes of reconstruction and amputation for treating patients with mangled lower extremities.

The LEAP Study prospectively compared the functional outcomes of a large cohort of patients from eight Level 1 trauma centers who underwent reconstruction or amputation. The hypothesis was that after controlling for the severity of the limb injury, the presence and severity of other injuries, and patient characteristics, amputation would prove to have a better functional outcome than reconstruction. Detailed patient, patient environment, injury, and treatment (hospital and outpatient) data were collected on each patient.[14] The Sickness Impact Profile (SIP) (a multidimensional measure of self-reported health status with scores ranging from 0 to 100; scores for the general population average 2 to 3, and scores greater than 10 represent severe disability) was used as the primary outcome measurement. Secondary outcomes included limb status and the presence or absence of a major complication that required rehospitalization. Over 2 years, 569 patients were followed. No significant difference in SIP scores was detected at 2-year follow-up for the amputation and reconstruction groups (12.6 versus 11.8, respectively; $P = 0.53$). After adjustment for the characteristics of the patients and their injuries, patients who underwent amputation had outcomes that were similar to those of patients who underwent limb reconstruction.[13]

The analysis of all patient, injury, treatment, and environmental variables identified several predictors of poorer SIP scores. Negative factors included the rehospitalization of a patient for a major complication, a low education level, nonwhite race, poverty, lack of private health insurance, poor social support network, a low self-efficacy (the patient's confidence in being able to resume life activities), smoking, and involvement in disability-compensation litigation. To underscore the combined influence of these multiple factors on outcome, adjusted SIP scores were estimated for two subgroups of patients. A patient with a high school education or less, poor social support, and rehospitalization for a major complication had a mean adjusted SIP score of 15.8. A comparable score for a patient with some college, strong social support, and an uncomplicated recovery was 8.3. Although patients with substantial economic and social resources and no complications could not function at the level of a healthy adult of similar age and gender (typical SIP score < 4), they were still significantly better off than those without such resources.

The LEAP Study also found that patients who underwent reconstruction were more likely to be rehospitalized than those who underwent amputation (47.6% versus 33.9%, $P = 0.002$). At 2-year follow-up, nonunion was present in 10.9% of the patients who underwent reconstruction and 9.4% had osteomyelitis. Additional surgeries were anticipated for 5% of the patients who underwent amputation and for 19% of the patients who

TABLE 4	Impact of Noninjury Factors on SIP Scores	
High school education or less	Some college
Poor support	Strong support
Low self-efficacy	High self-efficacy
Major complications	No complications
Adjusted SIP score: 15.8	Adjusted SIP score: 8.3

underwent reconstruction. The levels of disability, as measured by SIP scores, were high in both groups. More than 40% of the patients in both treatment groups had SIP scores greater than 10, reflecting severe disability. Except for scores on the psychosocial subscale, there was significant improvement in the SIP scores over time for patients in both treatment groups.[29-32] Return to work success for patients in the LEAP Study was disappointing. At 24 months, 53% of the patients who underwent amputation and 49.4% of those who underwent reconstruction had returned to work ($P = 0.48$).

Clinical Practice Considerations

The findings of the LEAP Study should not be generalized for patient populations that are treated in anything but Level 1 trauma centers. In Level 1 trauma centers, surgeons should advise their patients with mangled lower extremities that the functional outcomes for reconstruction are equivalent to those for amputation. The reconstruction process requires more surgery and more hospitalizations, and it is associated with a higher complication rate. At 2-year follow-up, both patient groups are significantly disabled, and only approximately 48% have returned to work. Patients in both groups have lingering psychosocial disability. Given the "no outcome difference" at 2-year follow-up, patients and surgeons can be comfortable recommending and/or selecting limb preservation surgery. Efforts to minimize complications and hastened fracture union might improve the outcomes of patients who undergo reconstruction.

These results suggest that major improvements in outcomes may require greater emphasis on nonclinical interventions, such as early evaluation by vocational rehabilitation counselors (Table 4). The LEAP Study results also confirm previous research that found both self-efficacy and social support to be important determinants of outcome.[33,34] Interventions aimed at improving support networks and self-efficacy may benefit patients facing a challenging recovery. Surgeons also need to acknowledge the long-term psychosocial disability associated with the mangled lower extremities, regardless of the treatment. Screening for posttraumatic stress disorder and the appropriate referral of patients for therapy may need to become a proactive part of the postoperative treatment plan.[29-32]

For patients undergoing limb amputation, the LEAP Study identified several clinical issues that can be used by the surgeon in planning amputation level and stump coverage. No significant differences in return to work rates, pain, or SIP scores were reported for patients who had either above-the-knee amputations or below-the-knee amputations. Patients with through-the-knee amputation had SIP scores that were 40% higher and physical dimension scores that were 50% higher than those for patients in either the below-the-knee or above-the-knee amputation group ($P = 0.05$ and $P = 0.01$, respectively). Patients with through-the-knee amputation demonstrated significantly lower walking speeds. Physicians were less satisfied with the clinical, cosmetic, and functional recovery of patients with through-the-knee amputation compared with that of the patients in the below-the-knee and above-the-knee amputation groups. In the trauma population, through-the-knee amputation should be avoided. Atypical wound closures, skin grafts, and flaps did not adversely affect the outcome in this study, which suggests that efforts to preserve the knee are worthwhile.[35] Outcomes were not affected by the technical sophistication of the prosthesis, although patients with higher technology prostheses reported being more satisfied. Physicians who currently fit patients with sophisticated (and expensive) prostheses may find these conclusions challenging. The results of the LEAP Study underscore the need for controlled studies that examine the relationship between type of prosthetic device, fit, and functional outcomes.[35,36]

Another study determined the impact of the timing of amputation on outcome and complications.[37] The authors found that patients who underwent amputation after 3 months reported significantly higher levels of disability than those who underwent amputation during the first hospitalization or within the first 3 months. Late amputation usually was done as a result of infection. Patients with mangled extremities undergoing reconstruction appear to be better served if the decision to amputate is not prolonged when they develop significant complications that place the injured limb at risk.

When considering patients with mangled extremities for reconstruction, it is important to consider the timing of treatment, techniques of fracture stabilization, and soft-tissue coverage. One study found no significant differences in the time from admission to first débridement, first débridement to soft-tissue coverage, or injury to first débridement for patients who developed infections within the first 3 months and those who did not.[38] In a different study, the same group of authors found that 27% of high-energy tibial injuries that were treated with a reconstruction protocol had at least one wound complication within the first 6 months after injury.[39] The complication rate differed according to the type of flap coverage. For limbs with the most severe osseous injury (Orthopaedic Trauma Association type C fractures),

treatment with a rotational flap was more than four times more likely to lead to a surgical wound complication than treatment with a free flap. The complication rate for limbs with less severe osseous injuries was not significantly different when assessed according to soft-tissue coverage selection.

Tibial fractures are commonly associated with mangled lower extremities. One study reviewed 162 patients with this combination of injuries.[40] Fifty-one patients underwent early amputation and six (5.4%) required a delayed amputation. One hundred five patients (17 with grade IIIA, 84 with grade IIIB, and 4 with grade IIIC injuries) were available for 2-year follow-up. Patients who had soft-tissue closure without a free flap had significantly better SIP scores than those with a free flap. Definitive treatment with an intramedullary nail yielded better outcomes than external fixation. Patients who were definitively treated with external fixation had an increased likelihood of infection and nonunion.

Summary

With currently available treatment technology and Level 1 trauma center orthopaedic clinical experience and multispecialty support, it appears that the overall 2-year results for leg reconstruction are equal to those for amputation in patients with severe extremity trauma. Continuing efforts to reconstruct severely injured limbs should therefore be encouraged, and patients with these injuries should be directed to experienced limb injury treatment centers. The decision whether to reconstruct or amputate a mangled extremity cannot depend on the limb salvage scores alone because all have proved to have little clinical utility. Strategies to minimize complications (such as infections and delayed unions), address related posttraumatic stress disorder, improve the self-efficacy of patients, and target early vocational retraining for eventual workplace reentry may improve the future outcomes of this patient population.

Annotated References

1. Finkelstein E: *Estimates Based on Health Care Cost and Utilization Project: Inpatient Sample (HCUP NIS)*. Available at: http://www.hcup-us.ahrq.gov/nisoverview.jsp. Accessed December 3, 2004.

2. Govender S, Csimma C, Genant HK, et al: Recombinant human bone morphogenetic protein-2 for treatment of open tibial fractures. *J Bone Joint Surg Am* 2002;84-A(12):2123-2134.

   In this prospective, controlled, randomized study of 450 patients with open tibial fractures, recombinant human bone morphogenetic protein-2 was used in conjunction with intramedullary nail fixation and found to be superior to intramedullary nailing alone. The recombinant human bone morphogenetic protein-2 cohort demonstrated accelerated fracture and wound healing, a reduced infection rate, and required fewer additional surgical procedures.

3. Bondurant FJ, Cotler HB, Buckle R, Miller-Crotchett P, Browner BD: The medical and economic impact of severely injured lower extremities. *J Trauma* 1988;28:1270-1273.

4. Georgiadis GM, Behrens FF, Joyce MJ, Earle AS, Simmons AL: Open tibial fractures with severe soft-tissue loss: Limb salvage compared with below-the-knee amputation. *J Bone Joint Surg Am* 1993;75(10): 1431-1441.

5. Hansen ST: Overview of the severely traumatized lower limb: Reconstruction versus Amputation. *Clin Orthop* 1989;243:17-19.

6. Hertel R, Strebel N, Ganz R: Amputation versus reconstruction in traumatic defects of the leg: Outcomes and costs. *J Orthop Trauma* 1996;10:223-229.

7. Bonanni F, Rhodes M, Lucke JF: The futility of predictive scoring of mangled lower extremities. *J Trauma* 1993;34:99-104.

8. Dagum AB, Best AK, Schemitsch EH, Mahoney JL, Mahomed MN, Blight KR: Salvage after severe lower-extremity trauma: Are the outcomes worth the means? *Plast Reconstr Surg* 1999;103:1212-1220.

9. Fairhurst MJ: The function of the below-knee amputee versus the patient with a salvaged grade III tibial fracture. *Clin Orthop* 1994;301:227-232.

10. Francel TJ: Improving reemployment rates after limb salvage of acute severe tibial fractures by microvascular soft-tissue reconstruction. *Plast Reconstr Surg* 1994;93:1028-1034.

11. Hansen ST Jr: The type-IIIC tibial fracture: Salvage or amputation. *J Bone Joint Surg Am* 1987;69(6):799-800.

12. Hansen ST Jr: Salvage or amputation after complex foot and ankle trauma. *Orthop Clin North Am* 2001; 32:181-186.

13. Bosse MJ, MacKenzie EJ, Kellam JF, et al: An analysis of outcomes of reconstruction or amputation of leg-threatening injuries. *N Engl J Med* 2002;347: 1924-1931.
    This prospective, multicenter longitudinal study assessed the outcomes of 569 patients with limb-threatening lower extremity trauma, and the authors concluded that patients in the limb salvage and the amputation cohorts were severely disabled at 2-year follow-up and had out-

comes (as measured using the SIP) that were similar. The authors also reported that outcomes were affected by numerous patient and environmental factors.

14. MacKenzie EJ, Bosse MJ, Kellam JF, LEAP Study Group: Characterization of the patients undergoing amputation versus limb salvage for severe lower extremity trauma. *J Orthop Trauma* 2000;14:455-466.

15. Bosse MJ, Kellam JF: Orthopaedic management decisions in the multiple-trauma patient, in Browner BD, Jupiter J, Levine A, Trafton P (eds): *Skeletal Trauma: Basic Science, Management and Reconstruction*. Philadelphia, PA, Saunders-Elsevier Science, 2003, pp 133-146.

16. Pape HC, Hildebrand F, Pertschy S, et al: Changes in the management of femoral shaft fractures in polytrauma patients: From early total care to damage control orthopedic surgery. *J Trauma* 2002;53(3): 452-461.

17. McNamara MG, Heckman JD, Corley FG: Severe open fractures of the lower extremity: A retrospective evaluation of the Mangled Extremity Severity Score (MESS). *J Orthop Trauma* 1994;8:81-87.

18. Russell WL, Sailors DM, Whittle TB, Fisher DF, Burns RP: Limb salvage versus amputation: A decision based on a seven-part predictive index. *Ann Surg* 1991;213:473-481.

19. Porter S, Hanley EN: The musculoskeletal effects of smoking. *J Am Acad Orthop Surg* 2001;9(1):9-17.

20. Swiontkowski MF, MacKenzie EJ, Bosse MJ, Jones AL, Travison TG, and the LEAP Study Group: Factors influencing the decision to amputate or reconstruct after high-energy lower extremity trauma. *J Trauma* 2002;52:641-649.
    The authors of this study reported that the severity of soft-tissue injuries had the greatest impact on deciding whether to perform limb-salvage or amputation. The orthopaedic surgeon made the decision in concert with the general surgeon in 42% of the instances.

21. Johansen K, Daines M, Howey T, Helfet D, Hansen ST: Objective criteria accurately predict amputation following lower extremity trauma. *J Trauma* 1990;30: 568-573.

22. Howe HR, Poole GV, Hansen KJ, et al: Salvage of lower extremities following combined orthopaedic and vascular trauma: A predictive salvage index. *Am Surg* 1987;53:205-208.

23. Bickels J, Wittig JC, Kollender Y, Kellar-Graney K, Malawer MM, Meller I: Sciatic nerve resection: Is that truly an indication for amputation? *Clin Orthop* 2002;399:201-204.

24. Jones AL, McCarthy ML, Bosse MJ, et al: The insensate foot: An indication for amputation? in *Final Program of the Orthopaedic Trauma Association 18th Annual Meeting, Toronto, Ontario, October 11-13, 2002.* Rosemont, IL, Orthopaedic Trauma Association, 2002. Available at: http://www.ota.org. Accessed December 3, 2004.

25. Helfet DL, Howey T, Sanders R, Johansen K: Limb salvage versus amputation: Preliminary results of the Mangled Extremity Severity Score. *Clin Orthop* 1990;256:80-86.

26. Suedkamp NP, Barbey N, Veuskens A, et al: The incidence of osteitis in open fractures: An analysis of 948 open fractures (a review of the Hannover experience). *J Orthop Trauma* 1993;7:473-482.

27. Tscherne H, Oestern HJ: A new classification of soft-tissue damage in open and closed fractures. *Unfallheilkunde* 1982;85:111-115.

28. Bosse MJ, MacKenzie EJ, and the LEAP Study Group.: A prospective evaluation of the clinical utility of the lower-extremity Injury-Severity Scores. *J Bone Joint Surg Am* 2001;83-A(1):3-14.

   In this study, prospective limb and patient injury data were collected for 565 patients with severe lower extremity trauma. The sensitivity and specificity were determined for the five commonly used predictive limb injury severity scores. The low sensitivity of the indices failed to support the validity of the scores as predictors of amputation.

29. McCarthy ML, MacKenzie EJ, Edwin D, et al: Psychosocial distress associated with severe lower-limb injury. *J Bone Joint Surg Am* 2003;85-A(9):1689-1697.

30. Michaels AJ, Michaels CE, Moon CH, Zimmerman MA, Peterson C, Rodriguez JL: Psychosocial factors limit outcomes after trauma. *J Trauma* 1998;44:644-648.

31. Michaels AJ, Michaels CE, Moon CH, et al: Post-traumatic stress disorder after injury: Impact on general health outcome and early risk assessment. *J Trauma* 1999;47:460-467.

32. Starr A, Borer DS, Reinert CM, Welch-Mendoza M, Frawley WH: Symptoms of post-traumatic stress disorder after orthopaedic trauma, in *Final Program of the Orthopaedic Trauma Association 18th Annual Meeting, Toronto, Ontario, October 11-13, 2002.* Rosemont, IL, Orthopaedic Trauma Association, 2002. Available at: http://www.ota.org. Accessed December 3, 2004.

33. Ewart CK, Stewart KJ, Gillilan RE, Kelemen MH: Self-efficacy mediates strength gains during circuit weight training in men with coronary artery disease. *Med Sci Sports Exerc* 1986;18:531-540.

34. MacKenzie EJ, Morris JA, Jurkovich GJ, et al: Return to work following injury: The role of economic, social and job-related factors. *Am J Public Health* 1998;88:1630-1637.

35. MacKenzie EJ, Bosse MJ, Castillo RC, et al: Functional outcomes following lower extremity amputation for trauma. *J Bone Joint Surg Am* 2004;86-A(8): 1636-1645.

   The authors of this study reported that patients who underwent knee disarticulation had clinical and functional outcomes that were significantly worse than patients who underwent below-the-knee or above-the-knee amputation. They also found that atypical soft-tissue flap closures, split-thickness skin grafts, and free flaps did not worsen the results of the patients who underwent below-the-knee amputation.

36. Cyril JK, MacKenzie EJ, Smith DG, et al: Prosthetic device satisfaction among patients with lower extremity amputation due to trauma, in *Final Program of the Orthopaedic Trauma Association 18th Annual Meeting, Toronto, Ontario, October 11-13, 2002.* Rosemont, IL, Orthopaedic Trauma Association, 2002. Available at: http://www.ota.org. Accessed December 3, 2004.

37. Smith DG, Castillo RC, MacKenzie EJ, et al: Functional outcomes of patients who have late amputations after trauma is significantly worse than those who have early amputation, in *Final Program of the Orthopaedic Trauma Association 19th Annual Meeting, Salt Lake City, UT, October 9-11, 2003.* Rosemont, IL, Orthopaedic Trauma Association, 2003. Available at: http://www.ota.org. Accessed December 3, 2004.

38. Pollak AN, Castillo RC, Jones AL, Bosse MJ, et al: Time to definitive treatment significantly influences incidence of infection after open high-energy extremity trauma, in *Final Program of the Orthopaedic Trauma Association 19th Annual Meeting, Salt Lake City, UT, October 9-11, 2003.* Rosemont, IL, Orthopaedic Trauma Association, 2003. Available at: http://www.ota.org. Accessed December 3, 2004.

39. Pollak AN, McCarthy ML, Burgess AR, et al: Short-term wound complications after application of flaps

for coverage of traumatic soft-tissue defects about the tibia: The Lower Extremity Assessment Project (LEAP) Study Group. *J Bone Joint Surg Am* 2000; 82-A:1681-1691.

The authors of this study found that free flap transfers were less likely to lead to wound complications that required surgical intervention than rotational flaps when used to treat patients with severe underlying osseous injuries of the limbs.

40. Webb LX, Bosse MJ, Castillo RC, et al: Outcomes in patients with limb-threatening grade III open tibial diaphyseal fractures, in *Final Program of the Orthopaedic Trauma Association 19th Annual Meeting, Salt Lake City, UT, October 9-11, 2003*. Rosemont, IL, Orthopaedic Trauma Association, 2003. Available at: http://www.ota.org. Accessed December 3, 2004.

Chapter 9

Amputations and Prosthetics

Paul J. Dougherty, MD

Douglas G. Smith, MD

Introduction

Amputations typically occur as the result of tumors, trauma, or other medical conditions such as diabetes or infection. Most new amputations in the United States occur among elderly patients with other medical conditions. A smaller group of amputees who undergo amputation secondary to trauma are generally younger and have potentially many years of productive life ahead of them. Treatment goals for this patient population should therefore be oriented toward providing the best possible outcome.

Many factors are involved in achieving a good long-term outcome for amputees. The initial decision to amputate is often difficult. Recent studies have shown that various limb salvage scores are not reliable in predicting who should have an amputation after a traumatic injury (see chapter 8). Factors influencing this decision include the patient's overall medical condition, the patient's wishes, and the severity of injury.

Amputations

Upper Extremity Amputation

Below-Elbow Amputation

The transradial (below-elbow) amputation level can be extremely functional. If it is possible to save a functional elbow joint, even the most extraordinary techniques for providing soft-tissue coverage should be considered. In general, forearm rotation is proportional to the preserved length of the radius and ulna. Volar and dorsal flaps provide optimal padding and enable myodesis (a surgical technique in which muscle is attached directly to bone via suturing through drill holes; myoplasty is when opposing cut muscle groups are sewn together over the distal end of the stump). Myodesis helps avoid the potential creation of a mobile muscle mass that can move over the end of the bone, creating bursal tissue and pain. Stabilized muscle can generate a stronger signal to enhance the use of myoelectric prosthetic devices. The Krukenberg procedure, which is indicated for patients who are blind and those with bilateral forearm amputations, involves separating the radius and ulna into "fingers" that allow the patient to pick up and grasp items.[1]

Elbow Disarticulation and Transhumeral and Shoulder Level Amputation

Elbow disarticulation remains controversial. The advantages include better suspension of the prosthetic device over the condylar flares and improved rotational control of the upper limb prosthetic device. The longer lever arm and full muscle units secured with tenodesis also help improve strength of the upper limb. The disadvantages include a longer and more bulbous socket than a traditional transhumeral prosthetic socket, and the traditional in-line prosthetic elbow creates a disproportionate appearance between the upper versus lower arm segments. The use of external elbow hinges improves segment length, but the devices are also unsightly and can tear clothing. Most surgeons agree that the advantages of elbow disarticulation outweigh the disadvantages; therefore, elbow disarticulation is often done when suitable soft-tissue coverage exists. However, if only very fragile, scarred, or skin-grafted coverage will result, it is better to amputate higher in the upper arm where the soft-tissue coverage will provide better padding. No studies comparing elbow disarticulation to distal transhumeral amputees have been done.

When amputating at the transhumeral (above-elbow) level, bone length should be calculated with utmost respect for the soft-tissue coverage. The biceps and triceps both function across the shoulder and elbow joints, so myodesis to secure these muscles is extremely important to add strength. The most common technique is to secure these muscles via drill holes in the distal humerus and secure the muscle over the end of the bone. For very short transhumeral amputations, the proximal humerus should be saved if there is suitable soft-tissue coverage. Even if the final closure more closely approximates a shoulder disarticulation, saving the humeral head can improve shoulder contour and improve the way clothing will fit. In the ultrashort transhumeral amputation, arthrodesis of the proximal humerus segment to the glenoid has been suggested to prevent the abduction and flexion contracture that occurs in many short transhumeral amputee patients.[2]

Shoulder disarticulation and scapulothoracic amputations are often required in patients with severe proximal injuries. For patients with such injuries, saving the patient's life and establishing hemostasis are the highest initial priorities. Once the patient's life is no longer in jeopardy, the scapula and clavicle should be saved if technically possible. It is not unusual to leave these amputations open initially and then use complex coverage at a later date. Prosthetic fitting for patients with these high-level amputations is often quite frustrating. Even when functional rehabilitation has been obtained, many patients elect not to use their prosthesis because the device is so heavy across the shoulder girdle and a high level of mental energy and concentration is required to use it effectively. Many patients prefer a lighter weight prosthetic arm that provides less function or even a simple shoulder cap to make their shirts and jackets fit more appropriately.

Foot Amputation

Severe foot injuries can result in partial amputation. Crush injuries, frostbite, and lawnmower injuries are the most common causes. Although the patient and the surgeon naturally desire to save as much of the foot as possible, two studies have shown that quality soft-tissue coverage is more important in the ultimate outcome than bone length.[3,4] In patients in whom partial foot amputation is performed in the zone of injury and soft-tissue coverage is not durable, the added length can lead to more pain and functional deficit.

Ankle-Level Disarticulation

The ankle disarticulation and removal of malleolar bone is often referred to as a Syme's amputation.[5] This procedure preserves length and can provide a durable heel pad at the end of the residual limb. In certain instances, this unique combination can enable some weight bearing. Most patients who undergo Syme's amputation need a prosthesis for routine walking. The shape of a Syme's amputation can make prosthetic fitting more difficult.

After removal of the calcaneus, the heel pad must be repositioned and stabilized to provide adequate padding and function. It can be difficult to keep the heel pad centered under the tibia. The heel pad can drift, and if thinner skin is subjected to weight bearing, it becomes susceptible to sores and ulcers. The most durable reattachment seems to be with drill holes in the tibia. Surgical revisions may be needed.[6] Several patients have good use of a Syme's amputation for years, even decades, but eventually they have their amputation revised to the higher transtibial level. Revision of the Syme's amputation procedure can involve repositioning the pad or moving to a higher amputation level.

Some patients have great success with ankle-level disarticulation, whereas others do not. A centered, nontender heel pad that can allow a patient to bear weight generally ensures the best results. If the heel pad is involved in the injury or disease, it may be scarred, tender, and prone to ulcerations or sores. In these instances, saving the damaged heel pad results in more harm than good, leaving a residual limb that is both bulbous and tender.

The correct prosthesis for a typical ankle-level disarticulation takes advantage of some end-bearing potential. If the heel pad is damaged and tender, the end will need protection and will not be useful. Although the Syme's amputation is generally better for end bearing than the transtibial amputation, surgeons should be cautious when treating a patient with a damaged heel pad. A damaged heel pad can cause poor patient outcome in this scenario. If the tradeoff is a residual limb that is painful and/or dysfunctional, skeletal preservation should not be of paramount concern. Another potential problem is heel pad migration, causing difficulty with fitting and end bearing.

An alternative to the Syme's amputation is the Chopart's amputation.[7] The Chopart's amputation is done at the midfoot across the talonavicular joint and calcaneocuboid joint. Advantages include some limited ambulation without a prosthesis and maintenance of a heel height. Disadvantages include equinus deformity that causes pressure sores. This complication can be prevented by attaching the tibialis anterior to the calcaneus and removing the prominence of the anterolateral calcaneus. Prosthetic fitting is done with a Chopart ankle-foot orthosis.

Both the Syme's and the Chopart's amputations are indicated for elderly patients. The Chopart's amputation is also indicated for pediatric patients with congenital deformities.[8] One study of 14 pediatric patients found that the patients who underwent Chopart's or Lisfranc's amputation required more gait adjustment than the Syme's amputation group, but they had less difficulty with activities of daily living and participation in sports activities.

Transtibial Amputation

The transtibial amputation is one of the most frequently performed major limb amputations in patients who experience trauma.[9-17] The timing of definitive amputation, the length of transtibial bone, and the choice of soft-tissue flaps depend on the pattern of injury and the amount of viable soft tissue that remains. At one extreme are the severely mangled foot and ankle injuries in which the calf tissue is intact and out of the zone of injury. With this type of injury, it is not uncommon to perform an immediate, definitive transtibial amputation. Because this injury is confined to the foot area, it is one of the few instances in which the definitive amputation is performed immediately and in one stage. The preferred surgical method for this type of injury is the long posterior flap technique with a tibial bone length approaching one half the length of the tibia. Longer transtibial amputation can be stronger and provide more surface area to transfer the loads of a prosthesis. Amputations in the distal third of the tibia should be avoided because of the lack of soft-tissue padding.

For injuries that involve the calf, the circumstances of amputation are more complex. In patients with calf injuries, it is not uncommon to delay the definitive amputation until the second, third, or even fourth surgical procedure. The surgeon should perform an extensive débridement and remove all devitalized tissue and foreign bodies. The bone should be left long to act as an internal splint during the open period. With injuries involving most of the lower leg, the posterior tissue is often involved in the zone of injury; therefore, a long posterior flap technique cannot be used. When treating patients with this type of injury, surgeons should be open-minded and recognize the potential benefits of other surgical techniques.[9,10,13-15]

The long posterior myocutaneous flap technique has become popular in the United States. This technique provides good distal end padding and leaves the residual limb with a cylindrical shape. The surgeon should measure the length of the flap so that it is equal to the diameter of the limb at the level of bone transection plus 1 cm. The flap should be left long because the center of rotation for this flap is posterior to the calf as opposed to the midcalf location at the corners of the incision.[9,11,15]

The very short transtibial amputation has certain limitations, but it remains the recommended level if the extensor mechanism is intact and the knee joint is sound. Potential problems include less than optimal socket fit, inadequate suspension, pistoning, limited range of motion, and a general lack of comfort. Nonetheless, the value of retaining active power at the knee and enabling the patient to rise from sitting to standing and to advance up stairs makes the very short transtibial level worthwhile in most instances.

Bone reconstruction with the creation of a fusion between the distal tibia and fibula, described by Ertl[16] in 1949, is a surgical technique for some transtibial amputees (Figure 1). Although this is not a new technique, there has been recent interest in using it in young adult amputees as a means of providing a more durable residual limb. Advantages to the technique are purported to be that it allows for more pressure on the distal residual limb (end bearing) and less pain. Disadvantages may include a higher rate of postoperative infection and nonunion. Patients who are candidates for this procedure should have viable soft tissue and a stable residual limb. This kind of bone reconstruction may be performed as staged procedures after the initial procedure is performed. At a recent consensus conference at Walter

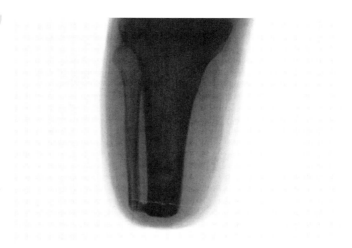

Figure 1 Radiograph of a transtibial amputee with a fusion between the distal tibia and fibula.

Reed Army Medical Center, participants indicated that caution should be used with this procedure within the zone of injury.[17]

Knee Disarticulation and Transfemoral Amputation

Historically, the knee disarticulation has been considered to be a successful amputation level when it is possible to save the full length of the femur and maintain suitable soft-tissue coverage. The advantages of the knee disarticulation over transfemoral level amputation include a longer lever arm, a stronger limb, improved prosthetic function, and, because the muscle bellies are not transected, more balanced thigh muscles. One technique used is preservation of the patella, suturing the patella ligament to the cruciate ligaments to provide stabilization. When the distal tissue coverage is durable and nontender, patients are usually capable of moderate end bearing, which promotes excellent functional results. In general, if a knee can be salvaged and adequate soft-tissue coverage will provide a nontender distal residual limb, disarticulation should be done. However, if soft-tissue coverage remains questionable, conversion to a transfemoral amputation is recommended.

Transfemoral amputation is necessary when there is severe damage to the lower extremity and knee area. In the transfemoral residual limb, the femur is pulled into flexion and abduction because of the proximal attachments of the iliopsoas and the hip abductors. These forces require a secure myodesis of the adductors and the medial hamstrings to balance the femur. Postoperative care of the transfemoral amputee requires placement of the patient in the prone position to stretch the hip and prevent hip flexion contractures. Hip flexion contracture of more that 15° can severely compromise prosthetic fitting.

Hip and Pelvic Level Amputation

Severe proximal trauma can necessitate hip disarticulation and transpelvic amputation. When these proximal amputations are required, preservation of as much bony anatomy as possible for sitting support and future prosthetic fitting is essential. Severe proximal injuries usually require multiple surgical procedures and may require creative and complex soft-tissue coverage.

Prosthetics

Immediate Postoperative Rehabilitation

Postoperative patient care differs with each patient.[9,18] In patients who undergo transtibial amputation, rigid dressings, casting, and prosthetic management are standard elements of immediate postoperative care. In patients who undergo amputation above the zone of injury as a result of trauma, a long leg amputation cast with a supracondylar mold should be applied while the patient is still in the operating room, with care being taken to keep the knee in 3° to 5° of flexion. After casting, a distal pylon and foot should be applied. Preliminary rehabilitation exercises include straight leg raising, gentle towel pulls over the cast, transfer skill activities, and careful weight bearing of 20 to 30 lb.

The first cast change should be done within 5 to 7 days. If healing is progressing as expected, a new long leg amputation cast with pylon and foot should be applied. The patient should then be discharged with instructions to return weekly for outpatient cast changes. Weight bearing should be advanced to approximately 30 lb on a weekly basis until postoperative edema has resolved, wrinkles return to the skin, and the limb volume appears unchanged from the previous week. This usually takes from 4 to 6 weeks. At this point, the limb should be placed in shrinker socks, and the prosthetist should begin fabricating the first prosthesis. Multiple socket modifications and as many as two to three socket changes are usually required during the first 12 to 18 months of patient care. Because this is a time of great volume fluctuation, the initial prosthesis should be made in a modular fashion to allow for socket changes without replacement of all of the components.

In patients who undergo amputation involving the zone of injury as a result of trauma, a rigid dressing prevents knee flexion contractures and protects the limb from outside injury. If open wound care is required, a thermoplastic posterior amputation splint should be applied to allow care and provide splinting, pain alleviation, and contracture prevention. Standard knee immobilizers have also been used successfully to splint the knee joint and protect the end of the amputated limb. When the wound is closed but significant edema is still present, a cast and pylon should be applied. Weight bearing should begin at the standard 20 to 30 lb. If the edema has resolved and wrinkles have returned to the skin, shrinker socks should be worn and the first prosthesis should be fabricated. As mentioned earlier, the initial prosthesis should be made in a modular fashion to allow socket changes without replacement of all of the components.

Newer developments for lower extremity prostheses include the use of a microprocessor for a knee component of transfemoral amputees (Figure 2). Early results show that amputees had improved stair descending and downhill walking. Lower extremity amputees of the Lower Extremity Assessment Project were evaluated using the Sickness Impact Profile comparing prostheses of high, medium, and low technology. The authors found no differences in the Sickness Impact Profile scores, though this scoring system does not evaluate specific functional amputee tasks.[19]

For upper extremity amputees, a myoelectric prosthesis may be indicated for appropriate patients. In general, a patient who has already demonstrated successful use of a body-powered prosthesis and has motor signals to trigger the prosthesis may be a good candidate. The best level for myoelectric use is the transradial amputee.

The First Year of Amputee Care

Surgeons must be familiar with the course of amputee care and the elaborate nature of the prosthetic fitting process. The first year of amputee care is very different from the following years because what is useful in terms of prosthetic technology changes radically after the limb is mature and the patient's activity level has increased. Surgeons should closely supervise prosthetic care and not allow a definitive socket to be made too early. Limb volume is in a state of flux, and as limb volume decreases, the initial prosthesis may no longer fit. Impatience in prosthetic fitting on the part of surgeons or patients can lead to disappointment when prostheses become loose or ill-fitting.

An intermediate period during the first year of amputation is essential while the residual limb changes shape dramatically as a result of the resolution of edema and the change in muscle volume. During this period, many patients need frequent temporary socket modifications and changes. Typically, when a transtibial amputee loses muscle volume, redness and pain at the distal end of the residual limb occur. To modify the fit of the prosthesis, the first step is to increase the ply and number of socks. Because volume loss is not uniform, select regions of the socket must be padded, especially the anteromedial and anterolateral tibial flair regions of the socket or the liner. These are the regions that support the tibia up off the bottom of the socket while simultaneously pushing it back and away from the front of the socket, thus protecting the distal end. It is not uncommon to pad the liner up to four times before fabricating a new socket. Liners that facilitate frequent padding are

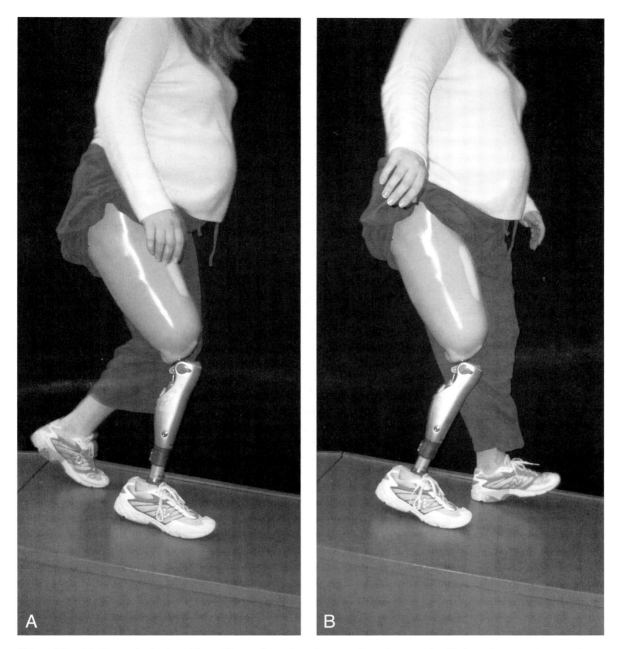

Figure 2 **A** and **B,** Photographs showing a 23-year-old traumatic transfemoral amputee (8 months pregnant) safely descending a ramp in a new microprocessor controlled knee unit. As the patient steps down into a bent knee, the microprocessor knee unit allows a controlled yielding descent. A traditional, nonmicroprocessor knee unit loaded in this position would result in a rapid buckling of the knee unit, leading to collapse and a fall. *(Reproduced with permission from Prosthetics Research Study, Seattle, WA.)*

needed in the first year. Sockets with foam liners are typically easier to pad than sockets with gel liners. These padding techniques save time and money and help maintain a smooth course of rehabilitation that often obviates the need for reauthorizing the fabrication of a new prosthetic limb.

Sometimes a patient has limited funding available for prosthetic care and the funds are used too early in the course of treatment. Patients often purchase definitive prostheses too quickly, and after the drastic volume changes through the healing process, the prostheses no longer fit. In this worst-case scenario, patients have prostheses that look great, but funds are no longer available to make them useful. Surgeons therefore should be patient and encourage financial caution to avoid this predicament.

Many young patients who undergo amputation as a result of trauma are adamant about obtaining the "best" prosthetic components for their prosthesis. Because the prosthesis is going to become a part of their bodies, the desire for the finest components is understandable. However, many of the high-tech components designed for impact activities are too stiff for the first year of amputee care. Less technologically sophisticated components may make adapting to the prosthetic device easier. A new prosthetic prescription should only be generated after the amputee has established a steady symmetric gait, can engage in impact activities, and is ready to advance to a higher level of activity. The amputee should be successful at maneuvering barriers, managing stairs, and negotiating inclines and ramps, which typically does not happen until between 9 and 18 months of prosthesis use. The old prosthesis can be refurbished to become a spare limb or a water limb.

Nerves and Neuromas

Amputation transects all of the major nerves at the amputation level. Any transected nerve will eventually form a neuroma; however, not all neuromas are symptomatic. During amputations, the major nerves should be isolated, drawn down, divided, and allowed to retract away from areas of pressure, scarring, or pulsating vessels. The superficial peroneal, deep peroneal, tibial, saphenous, and sural nerves should be identified during transtibial amputation. After identification, each nerve should be drawn down several centimeters, transected, and allowed to retract up into the soft tissues. There is no definitive evidence that cauterization, ligation, end-loop anastomosis, or nerve capping are more effective than careful resection. During transfemoral amputation, the sciatic nerve should be isolated, drawn down, and ligated before dividing it and allowing it to retract. The sciatic nerve has large blood vessels and is capable of significant bleeding.

When an amputee reports a discrete area of pain, has a palpable nodule, and percussion reveals the presence of Tinel's sign, this indicates the presence of a symptomatic neuroma. If the pain cannot be adequately relieved with prosthetic modification, the neuroma should be resected. In some patients, the entire peroneal nerve can be isolated and transected into the thigh above the level of the socket brim. This technique has occasionally benefited patients with severe dysthesia, pain, and neuromas in the peroneal nerve distribution.

Phantom Pain

Phantom sensation is the feeling that all or a part of the amputated limb is still present.[20-24] Phantom pain manifests as pain in the missing limb and is often described as burning, throbbing, stabbing, shooting, or electrical pain. Although up to 80% of patients who undergo amputation experience some episodes of phantom pain, for many the episodes are infrequent and not severe. Recent research has investigated the prevention of phantom limb pain. Several descriptive studies proposed that perioperative epidural anesthesia or intraneural anesthesia might decrease the incidence of phantom pain.[24,25] How-

ever, other studies, including one randomized trial, have not supported the theory that preemptive measures can truly reduce the frequency or severity of phantom limb pain.[26]

Transcutaneous electrical nerve stimulation (TENS) is a treatment technique that has gained recent acceptance. The TENS system is battery powered and can be incorporated into a prosthesis or kept as an isolated unit worn by the amputee. Although the TENS system can be helpful in the first several months following amputation, it is rare that patients choose to use it for the long term. Therefore, patients should be encouraged to consider renting a TENS system before buying one outright.

Pharmacologic treatment options for pain often began with the use of amitriptyline. However, patients report near universal dissatisfaction with the adverse effects of this drug, which include drowsiness, dry mouth, and alterations in the taste of food. Gabapentin is currently preferred by many physicians to treat phantom pain, but other drugs such as carbamazepine (Tegretol, Novartis Pharmaceuticals, East Hanover, NJ), phenytoin (Dilantin, Parke-Davis, Morris Plains, NJ), and mexiletine may also decrease the frequency and intensity of phantom pain episodes.

Outcomes

Of importance to patients and surgeons is the outcome of a traumatic amputation. Recent studies have evaluated amputees over the long term with regard to function and life measures such as employment and family life. The Lower Extremity Assessment Project Study Group has reported several outcome measures for amputees.[27,28] Patients were evaluated 2 years after amputation, and it was reported that approximately half returned to work. Sickness Impact Profile scores for all amputees suggested severe disability for patients. Sickness Impact Profile scores were similar for transfemoral and transtibial amputees, but they were higher for those with a through-knee amputation. Factors contributing to the poorer outcomes reported with the knee disarticulation group included the use of soft tissue within the zone of injury for coverage, making the residual limb less durable. Satisfaction with a fitted prosthesis was evaluated at 12 and 24 months after injury for 135 patients with transfemoral and transtibial amputations, and approximately 70% of patients reported moderate to high satisfaction with their prostheses. Patients fitted with high-tech prostheses reported significantly higher satisfaction than those fitted with low- or moderate-tech devices; however, no difference was identified between these groups when comparing their Sickness Impact Profile scores. Additionally, significant factors for improved outcome included at least a high school education, being 125% or greater above the poverty level or the head of a household, and reporting better functional status. Factors such as female sex, skin irritation, an atypical flap, and phantom pain were related to poorer satisfaction. In terms of function, the percentage of patients who reached a threshold walking speed (> 4 feet per second) was 62% of patients with transtibial amputations, 21.7% of patients with knee disarticulation, and 43.5% of patients with transfemoral amputations. No functional differences were identified among patients using low-, moderate-, or high-tech prostheses.[28]

Another study evaluating 20 patients who underwent transtibial amputation at an average 5.5-year follow-up showed that all were successful prosthesis wearers, 70% returned to work, and that Medical Outcome Study Short Form 36-Item Health Survey scores were decreased in the areas of physical function, role physical, and pain when compared with published norms.[29]

The results of long-term follow-up of Vietnam War veterans who underwent amputation have also recently been reported.[30,31] Patients who underwent transtibial amputation were followed an average of 28 years after injury. They averaged 15.9 hours per day of prosthesis wear at the time of follow-up and have used an average of 8.34 prostheses since the original fitting. Almost 100% of patients were employed after discharge from the military, and approximately 95% reported being married. Medical Outcome Study Short Form 36-Item Health Survey scores were similar to published norms in the isolated group, but they are significantly less in all categories in patients who had one other major injury, suggesting the presence of at least one other major injury causes long-term disability.

Unilateral transfemoral amputees were also followed for an average of 28 years after initial injury.[31] At follow-up, they reported wearing their prostheses an average of 14.1 hours per day, and 13% reported not currently wearing a prosthesis. Nearly 90% of the patients were employed an average of 20.1 years, and 65.2% had been married an average of 23.1 years at the time of follow-up, which compared favorably with published norms. For both the transfemoral and transtibial groups, the former soldiers sought occupations in the civilian sector that in general were less physically demanding.

Young amputees demonstrate a wide range of capabilities with regard to both employment and sports activities. In general, those with major lower extremity amputations seek occupations other than a heavy laborer and avoid high-impact sports after amputation.

Annotated References

1. Garst RJ: The Krukenberg hand. *J Bone Joint Surg Br* 1991;73:385-388.

2. Baumgartner R: Upper extremity amputations, in DuParc J (ed): *Surgical Techniques in Orthopaedics and Traumatology: Volume 4: Arm, Forearm and Elbow*. Paris, France, Elsevier, 2003.

3. Harris WR, Silverstein EA: Partial amputations of the foot: A follow-up study. *Can J Surg* 1964;41:6-11.

4. Millstein SG, McCowan SA, Hunter GA: Traumatic partial foot amputations in adults: A long-term review. *J Bone Joint Surg Br* 1988;70:251-254.

5. Harris RI: Syme's amputation: The technical details essential for success. *J Bone Joint Surg Br* 1956;38:614-632.

6. Smith DG, Sangeorzan BJ, Hansen ST, Burgess EM: Achilles tendon tenodesis to prevent heel pad migration in the Syme's amputation. *Foot Ankle* 1994;15:14-17.

7. Letts M, Pyper A: The modified Chopart's amputation. *Clin Orthop* 1990;256:44-49.

8. Greene WB, Cary JM: Partial foot amputations in children: A comparison of the several types with the Syme amputation. *J Bone Joint Surg Am* 1982;64:438-443.

9. Burgess EM, Romano RL, Zettl JH: *The Management of Lower-Extremity Amputations*. Washington, DC, US Government Printing Office, 1969. Publication TR 10-6.

10. Alter AH, Moshein J, Elconin KB, Cohen MJ: Below-knee amputation using the sagittal technique: A comparison with the coronal amputation. *Clin Orthop* 1978;131:195-201.

11. Bowker JH: Transtibial amputation, in Smith DG, Michael JW, Bowker JH (eds): *Atlas of Amputations and Limb Deficiencies: Surgical, Prosthetic, and Rehabilitation Principles*, ed 3. Rosemont, IL, American Academy of Orthopaedic Surgeons, 2004, pp 481-501.
   The author of this chapter provides an excellent review of current indications and techniques for transtibial amputees.

12. Fergason JR, Smith DG: Socket considerations for the transtibial amputee. *Clin Orthop* 1999;361:76-84.

13. Humzah MD, Gilbert PM: Fasciocutaneous blood supply in below-knee amputations. *J Bone Joint Surg Br* 1997;79:441-443.

14. Robinson KP, Hoile R, Coddington T: Skew flap myoplastic below-knee amputation: A preliminary report. *Br J Surg* 1982;69:554-557.

15. Smith DG, Fergason JR: Transtibial amputations. *Clin Orthop* 1999;361:108-115.

16. Ertl J: Operationstechik: Dieser Abschnitt solder Veröffentlichung der von einzelnen Chirurgen geübten operativen Technik dienen. Über Amputationsstumpfe. *Chirurg* 1949;20:218-224.

This article (in German) outlines the technique of creating a bone bridge between the distal tibia and fibula for a transtibial amputee. The author provides an illustrated description of the original technique.

17. Smith DG: Amputation techniques in war surgery. *In Motion* 2003;13:42-43.

18. Mooney V, Harvey JP, McBride E, Snelson R: Comparison of postoperative stump management: Plaster versus soft dressings. *J Bone Joint Surg Am* 1971;53:241-249.

19. MacKenzie EJ, Bosse MJ, Castillo RC, et al: Functional outcomes following trauma-related lower-extremity amputation. *J Bone Joint Surg Am* 2004;86:1636-1645.

In this study, 161 patients who underwent amputation because of trauma were followed prospectively for 2 years and evaluated using the Sickness Impact Profile questionnaire, walking speed, independence of transfers, walking, climbing stairs, and pain. As measured by the Sickness Impact Profile questionnaire, severe disability was found to accompany major lower extremity amputation, with through-knee amputees doing significantly worse than transfemoral or transtibial amputees. The through-knee amputation group also had the lowest self-selected walking speeds. The transfemoral amputation group had a slower average walking speed than the transtibial amputation group.

20. Ehde DM, Czerniecki JM, Smith DG, et al: Chronic phantom sensations and pain following lower extremity amputation. *Arch Phys Med Rehabil* 2000;81:1039-1044.

The authors report the responses of 255 lower extremity amputees to a pain questionnaire at 6 months (or longer) after surgery; 79% of the amputees reported phantom limb sensations, 72% reported phantom limb pain, and 74% reported residual limb pain.

21. Ehde DM, Smith DG, Czerniecki JM, Campbell KM, Malchow DM, Robinson LR: Back pain as a secondary disability in persons with lower limb amputations. *Arch Phys Med Rehabil* 2001;82:731-734.

The authors report the responses of 255 lower extremity amputees to a questionnaire designed to assess frequency, intensity, duration, and interference because of back pain. Of the 56% of patients who responded to the questionnaire, 52% reported having persistent, bothersome back pain; 25% of those reporting back pain described it as being of severe intensity, frequent, and interfering with activities.

22. Jensen MP, Smith DG, Ehde DM, Robinson LR: Pain site and the effects of amputation pain: Further clarification on the meaning of mild, moderate, and severe pain. *Pain* 2001;91:317-322.

In this study, 205 patients with acquired amputation and phantom limb and/or back pain were evaluated to determine their average pain intensity and degree of interference with activities. The authors found a nonlinear association between pain intensity and interference, which was similar to that seen in patients with cancer.

23. Smith DG, Ehde DM, Legro MW, Reiber GE, del Aguila M, Boone DA: Pain and sensations in the phantom limb, the residual limb and the back reported by persons with lower extremity amputations. *Clin Orthop* 1999;361:29-38.

24. Bach S, Noreng MF, Tjellden NU: Phantom limb pain in amputees during the first 12 months following limb amputation, after preoperative lumbar epidural blockade. *Pain* 1988;33:297-301.

25. Fisher A, Meller Y: Continuous postoperative regional analgesia by nerve sheath block for amputation surgery: A pilot study. *Anesth Analg* 1991;72:300-303.

26. Elizaga AM, Smith DG, Sharar SR, Edwards WT, Hansen ST: Continuous regional analgesia by nerve sheath block: Effect on postoperative opioid requirements and phantom limb pain following amputation. *J Rehabil Res Dev* 1994;31:179-187.

27. Bosse MJ, MacKenzie EJ, Kellam JF, et al: An analysis of outcomes of reconstruction or amputation of leg-threatening injuries. *N Engl J Med* 2002;347:1924-1931.

This article compares the outcomes of 161 patients who underwent amputation and 384 patients who underwent reconstruction as a result of severe lower extremity trauma. The analysis included patient, injury, and socioeconomic factors. At 2-year follow-up, the authors reported similar outcomes for both groups.

28. Cyril JK, MacKenzie EJ, Smith DG, Bosse MJ: Prosthetic device satisfaction among patients with lower extremity amputation due to trauma, in *Final Program of the Orthopaedic Trauma Association Annual Meeting, Toronto, Canada, October 11, 2002.* Rosemont, IL, Orthopaedic Trauma Association, 2002. Available online at: http://www.ota.org. Accessed November 17, 2004.

29. Smith DG, Horn P, Malchow D, Boone DA, Reiber GE, Hansen ST Jr: Prosthetic history, prosthetic charges, and functional outcome of the isolated traumatic below-knee amputee. *J Trauma* 1995;38:44-47.

30. Dougherty PJ: Long-term follow-up of unilateral transfemoral amputees from the Vietnam War. *J Trauma* 2003;54:718-723.

In this study, 46 patients who underwent unilateral transfemoral amputations as a result of combat wounds were evaluated an average 28-year follow-up. Medical Outcome Study Short Form 36-Item Health Survey scores were lower than age- and gender-matched published norms in all categories except mental health and vitality. Forty patients (87%) wore a prosthesis for an average of 13.5 hours per day.

31. Dougherty PJ: Transtibial amputees from the Vietnam War: Twenty-eight year follow-up. *J Bone Joint Surg Am* 2001;83:383-389.

In this study, 72 patients who underwent transtibial amputation because of combat wounds were evaluated using the Medical Outcome Study Short Form 36-Item Health Survey and a questionnaire at an average 28-year follow-up. Transtibial amputees were divided into two groups: those with isolated injuries and those with at least one other major injury. If the patient had at least one other major injury, there was a significant disability suggested by the Medical Outcome Study Short Form 36-Item Health Survey scores. This group also had a significantly greater reported use of psychologic services. Patients with isolated injuries had scores that were similar to those of age- and gender-matched control subjects.

Section 2

The Polytrauma Patient and Fracture Healing

Section Editor:
Emil H. Schemitsch, MD

Chapter 10

Evaluation of the Polytrauma Patient

Philip R. Wolinsky, MD

Mark A. Lee, MD

Advanced Trauma Life Support

Advanced Trauma Life Support (ATLS) is well established as the standard of care for trauma resuscitation. The ATLS training program has had striking results in improving resuscitation skills and trauma patient outcomes. In 1997, the American College of Surgeons introduced a significant change in the format of its ATLS course with an interactive format and an increased focus on hands-on practical skills. Since the introduction of the new format, course participants have maintained consistently higher performance levels even at 2 years after training.[1] Recent research has evaluated factors associated with the attrition of ATLS-acquired skills, and trauma patient volume is reported to be the most critical determinant of attrition rate of ATLS-acquired skills.[2] Other factors such as age, gender, and practical specialty do not alter the attrition rate.[3]

After the initial assessment and stabilization of the multiply injured patient, multispecialty evaluation and care must be coordinated. The secondary and tertiary surveys are critical elements of the orthopaedic evaluation of the trauma patient because significant injuries can be missed during the initial evaluation. Undetected injuries can lead to significant morbidity. A recent clinical review examined 45 patients with a median Injury Severity Score (ISS) of 26 who were admitted to the intensive care unit; 12 missed injuries were discovered in 10 patients and resulted in three additional surgical procedures.[4] Three quarters of the undetected injuries were orthopaedic. Severely injured patients are at high risk of clinically significant injuries being missed during the primary and secondary surveys. In particular, hand and foot injuries are commonly missed.

Scoring Systems

With the advent of dedicated trauma centers, scoring systems were developed to determine which patients would benefit from treatment at a trauma center. The original scoring systems were developed for patient evaluation in the field. Different scores incorporate the severity of anatomic and physiologic markers of injury as well as preexisting medical conditions and age.[5] Scoring systems have been used for quality assurance, the evaluation of trauma care, research, and reimbursement issues.

Glasgow Coma Scale

The Glasgow Coma Scale (GCS) was developed in 1974 to quantify the severity of closed head injuries.[5] It can be used as an initial assessment tool and to reevaluate injuries. The GCS incorporates three examinations: the best motor response to evaluate the level of central nervous system function, eye opening to evaluate brainstem function, and best verbal score to evaluate integrative ability. It has been shown that the admission GCS is predictive of the severity of injury and mortality for both diffuse and focal neurologic lesions. The field GCS score does not predict outcome as well as the admission GCS, most likely because of the favorable effects of the initial resuscitation on central nervous system function.

Abbreviated Injury Severity Score

The Abbreviated Injury Severity (AIS) instrument was developed in 1974, and it groups injuries into nine anatomic areas: head, face, neck, thorax, abdomen, spine, upper extremity, lower extremity, and external. Each injury is scored on a scale ranging from 0 (minor) to 6 (maximum injury, possibly fatal). The AIS was most recently revised in 1990 (AIS-90).

Injury Severity Score

The ISS was developed in 1977 and is best used as a research tool to evaluate outcomes.[5] It is not meant to be used as a field score. The nine anatomic areas used for the AIS are grouped into the following six anatomic systems for the ISS: head or neck, face, chest, abdomen/pelvis, extremities, and external. Total scores can range from 1 to 75. As with the AIS subscoring, scores range from 0 to 6, where 0 indicates no injury and 5 is a critical injury with uncertain survival. If any anatomic region has a score of 6 (probably fatal injury), a score of 75 is given. Otherwise, the scores from the three most severely injured systems are squared (AIS scores) and added together to obtain the ISS.

The ISS is a predictor of injury severity and mortality. Because it may not be possible to calculate the score on admission, it is typically used for retrospective analysis of treatment.[6] A shortcoming of the ISS is its inability to predict outcomes for patients with multiple injuries to a single area of the body because it allows only the most severe injury to be included. Moreover, the ISS tends to have little relationship to the long-term disability produced by musculoskeletal trauma. The New Injury Severity Score (NISS) addresses these shortcomings by including the three highest scores regardless of the anatomic areas; therefore, it may be more predictive of complications and mortality than the ISS.[7] This has been shown to be true in the subgroup of patients with multiple orthopaedic injuries.[8]

Revised Trauma Score

The Revised Trauma Score (RTS) is a revision of the Trauma Score (TS) developed in 1981.[5] It is based on the concept that death typically results from an injury to the central nervous system, the cardiovascular system, or the respiratory system. A large number of patients were analyzed to determine the best predictors of outcome. The following five variables were then selected: GCS, respiratory rate, respiratory expansion, systolic blood pressure, and capillary refill. This score, used in the field, was found to predict survival.

In 1989, the TS was revised to the RTS. Capillary refill and respiratory expansion were dropped as variables because of difficulty in evaluating them consistently. Each of the three remaining variables is coded from 1 to 4. RTS scores range from 0 to 12, with lower numbers indicating more severe injuries. An RTS of ≤ 11 identifies 97% of severely injured patients. It is widely used as a prehospital field triage test to determine whether patients need to be transported to a trauma center. Its shortcoming, as with the ISS, is underscoring patients with severe injuries to a single anatomic area.

Trauma Injury Severity Score

The Trauma Injury Severity Score method has been used for analyzing unexpected outcomes of trauma care. It combines the anatomic data from the ISS and physiologic data from the RTS.[5] It creates a graph with an isobar for a predicted 50% survival rate. Outliers above the bar (unexpected survivors) or below the bar (unexpected deaths) can be identified and analyzed. Any trauma system can compare its results with those of the Major Trauma Outcome Study database and use the comparative data for quality assurance analysis and the evaluation of new treatment protocols.

Measurement of Outcomes

Trauma registries in which multiple variables are recorded and allow for systematic review are useful for the evaluation of efficiency and quality for each institution's trauma program.[9] Trauma registries typically include timing of prehospital care, mechanism of injury, vital signs in the field and on arrival, and outcome measures such as mortality. There are clear differences of opinion as to which variables are the most important to monitor with trauma registries. As a result, no clear consensus regarding variables exists, and registries demonstrate significant variability in patient data measurements.

Trauma registries collect very generalized data such as ISS or other nonspecific variables.[10] Other details of injury such as fracture classification and procedural details are rarely included. More detailed recording of skeletal and soft-tissue injury information is required for more seamless integration with outcomes assessment tools and outcomes research.

Significant resources are required to maintain an effective trauma registry. Software programs that allow for direct data entry are slowly replacing classic data collection forms. Simplification of the data entry process may improve the quality and quantity of clinical research projects. With increasing complexity and volume of data being recorded, organization and data management are increasingly complicated. Research coordinators are essential for developing and maintaining registry protocols and for ensuring that complete data sets are obtained from each patient.

Outcomes Assessment

Standardized outcomes assessment has only recently been included in modern orthopaedic clinical research.[11] Lack of patient-related data is problematic for studies evaluating efficacy of techniques or implants because assessment of patient function and quality of life measures are necessary. Current clinical studies frequently include arbitrary outcome evaluations that are not based on standardized measures of patient function and wellness and, thus, call into question the ability of these studies to provide reliable and useful information. More recently, normative data comparisons have been incorporated into several outcome studies.[12] These studies compare pretreatment and posttreatment data, and then compare this with data from the general population as a reference.[13] As a requirement of normative comparisons, collection of population-based normative data is required.

Several well-validated health status instruments have been developed and are available for use in assessing patient function. Multiple factors influence the applicability of these instruments for trauma patients, including the time required to administer the questionnaire, language issues, and whether the patient can be interviewed or must complete the questionnaire independently. A further impediment is the requirement that patients recall their level of function before the trauma. Four of the most common instruments are the Medical Outcomes Study Short Form 36-Item Health Survey,[14] the Sickness Impact Profile, the Nottingham Health Profile, and the Quality of Well-Being Scale. All of these instruments evaluate physical, psychologic, and social functioning (and are described in detail in chapter 1).

A necessary shift in focus from appreciation of radiographic and anatomic results to symptom resolution and functional restoration has been a challenging evolution. Multiple outcomes assessment tools are now available, and they should prove extremely useful for the improved measurement of outcomes in orthopaedic trauma surgery.

Emergent Pelvic Fracture Care

Hemodynamically unstable trauma patients with pelvic ring injuries present a diagnostic and therapeutic challenge. They require management by a multidisciplinary team that includes an orthopaedic surgeon. Management of these injuries is discussed in chapter 21.

The Mangled Extremity (Multiple Trauma)

Decision making for the mangled extremity is discussed in depth in chapter 8. It is critical to remember that a prerequisite for attempted limb salvage is a patient who is physiologically able to tolerate the surgery and blood loss that such an attempt requires. A hemodynamically unstable patient requires lifesaving procedures, not limb salvage. For multiply injured patients, the decision whether to proceed with limb salvage should be made in conjunction with the general surgeon and trauma leader. Amputation may be the most appropriate treatment option if survival of the patient is in question.

Geriatric Trauma

The elderly (older than 65 years) population of the United States has increased 21% from 1980 to 1990 and makes up 12% of the current population. It is projected that by 2050, 20% of the population will be elderly. Geriatric patients currently account for 23% of all trauma admissions. This percentage is predicted to increase to 40% by 2050. Numerous studies have demonstrated that the elderly have higher mortality rates, longer lengths of stay, and increased long-term morbidity when compared with younger patients.[15,16] The mortality rate increases almost 7% for each 1-year increase in age after 65 years.[17] Preexisting conditions have a negative effect on survival and the development of complications. Reduced functional outcome after injury has been documented as well.[18] The outcome (mortality and functional outcome) after head injuries has been shown to be worse in this population.[19] However, despite this, studies justify an aggressive approach to trauma in this population.[20]

Annotated References

1. Ali J, Adam R, Butler AK, et al: Trauma outcome improves following the advanced trauma life support program in a developing country. *J Trauma* 1993;34: 890-898.

2. Ali J, Adam R, Pierre I, Bedaysie H, Josa D, Winn J: Comparison of performance 2 years after the old and new (interactive) ATLS courses. *J Surg Res* 2001;97:71-75.

   This study followed two groups of physicians after change to more interactive ATLS training format and demonstrated that physicians had a consistently higher clinical skill performance level at 2 years versus those trained with older format.

3. Ali J, Howard M, Williams JI: Do factors other than trauma volume affect attrition of ATLS-acquired skills? *J Trauma* 2003;54:835-841.

   This study assessed the roles of age, gender, and practice specialty on the attrition of ATLS skills over 8 years. The authors concluded that trauma patient volume is the most critical determinant of attrition rate of ATLS-acquired skills and that age, gender, and practice specialty do not alter this rate.

4. Brooks A, Holroyd B, Riley B: Missed injury in major trauma patients. *Injury* 2004;35:407-410.

   This retrospective study of severely injured patients evaluated the incidence of significant injuries missed during primary surveys. Twelve missed injuries were discovered in 10 patients during intensive care unit admission; three patients required an additional surgical procedure. Three quarters of the undetected injuries were orthopaedic.

5. Senkowski CK, McKenney MG: Trauma scoring systems: A review. *J Am Coll Surg* 1999;189:491-503.

6. Stevenson M, Segui-Gomez M, Lescohier I, et al: An overview of the injury severity score and the new injury severity score. *Inj Prev* 2001;7:10-13.

   The authors of this article provide a description and statistical analysis of the ISS and NISS.

7. Balogh Z, Offner PJ, Moore EE, et al: NISS predicts post injury multiple organ failure better than the ISS. *J Trauma* 2000;48:624-628.

   This study found that the NISS, which takes into account multiple injuries to the same body system, was better than the ISS at predicting the development of multiple organ failure.

8. Balogh ZJ, Varga E, Tomka J, Suveges G, Toth L, Simonka JA: The new injury severity score is a better predictor of extended hospitalization and intensive care unit admission than the injury severity score on

patients with multiple orthopedic injuries. *J Trauma* 2003;17:508-512.

This study showed that the NISS was more predictive of length of stay and intensive care unit admission for patients with multiple orthopaedic injuries than the ISS.

9. Boyd DR: Trauma registries revisited. *J Trauma* 1985;25:186-187.

10. Weddell JM: Registers and registries: A review. *Int J Epidemiol* 1973;2:221-228.

11. Buckholz RW, Heckman JD (eds): *Rockwood and Green's Fractures in Adults*, ed 5. Philadelphia, PA, Lippincott Williams & Wilkins, 2002, p 76.

This book contains a summary chart of outcomes instruments that are appropriate for the assessment of patients with musculoskeletal injuries.

12. Hunsaker FG, Cioffi DA, Amadio PC, Wright JG, Caughlin B: The American Academy of Orthopaedic Surgeons outcomes instruments: Normative values from the general population. *J Bone Joint Surg Am* 2002;84:208-215.

With use of a panel mail methodology, self-reported data on the 11 AAOS musculoskeletal outcomes measures were collected from the general population of the United States. All 11 instruments met study expectations for providing reliable and valid normative data for use in clinical and research settings.

13. Kendall PC, Marrs-Garcia A, Nath SR, Sheldrick RC: Normative comparisons for the evaluation of clinical significance. *J Consult Clin Psychol* 1999;67: 285-299.

14. Temple PC, Travis B, Sachs L, Strasser S, Choban P, Flancbaum L: Functioning and well-being of patients before and after elective surgical procedures. *J Am Coll Surg* 1995;181:17-25.

15. Taylor MD, Tracy JK, Meyer W, et al: Trauma in the elderly: Intensive care unit resource use and outcome. *J Trauma* 2002;53:407-414.

This retrospective study of 26,237 patients revealed that patients older than 65 years had higher mortality rates and longer hospital stays than younger patients.

16. Tornetta P, Mostafavi H, Riina J, et al: Morbidity and mortality in elderly trauma patients. *J Trauma* 1999;46:702-706.

17. Grossman MD, Miller D, Scaff DW, et al: When is an elder old? Effect of pre-existing conditions on mortality in geriatric trauma. *J Trauma* 2002;52:242-246.

This study showed that for every 1-year increase in age after 65 years the mortality rate increased 6.8%. The presence of liver disease, renal dysfunction, and cancer were reported to have had the greatest effect on mortality.

18. Grossman M, Scaff DW, Miller D, Reed J III, Hoey B, Anderson HL III: Functional outcomes in octogenarian trauma. *J Trauma* 2003;55:26-32.

In this study, the authors reported that functional outcomes are worse for octogenarians when compared with geriatric trauma patients (those older than 65 years).

19. Susman M, DiRusso SM, Sullivan T, et al: Traumatic brain injury in the elderly: Increased mortality and worse functional outcome at discharge despite lower injury severity. *J Trauma* 2002;53:219-224.

The authors of this study compared data obtained from a statewide data set for elderly patients (those older than 64 years) who presented with traumatic brain injury with data from nonelderly patients (those older than 15 years and younger than 65 years) with similar injuries. The authors found that elderly traumatic brain injury patients had a poorer mortality rate and functional outcome than nonelderly patients with head injury even though their head injury and overall injuries were seemingly less severe.

20. Battistella F, Din AM, Perez L: Trauma patients 75 years and older: Long term follow-up results justify aggressive management. *J Trauma* 1998;44:618-624.

Chapter 11

Pathophysiology of the Polytrauma Patient

Wolfgang A. Menth-Chiari, MD

Brent Norris, MD

Charles M. Richart, MD

Greg A. Brown, MD, PhD

Roman Ullrich, MD

Introduction

In the United States, trauma remains the most common cause of death during the first three decades of life and ranks as the fourth leading cause of overall mortality, with more than 100,000 deaths each year.[1] Most patients who do not survive a traumatic event either die at the scene or shortly thereafter secondary to severe closed head injury or exsanguination.[1] Those patients who survive the initial traumatic insult and the acute resuscitation period go on to be threatened by subsequent infections, acute respiratory distress syndrome (ARDS), and multiple organ failure.[2-5] Of the surviving trauma patients who subsequently die, approximately 50% die from infection and multiple organ failure.[2-5]

The treatment of patients with traumatic injuries requires adherence to accepted and validated protocols if favorable outcomes are to be realized. The initial resuscitative and evaluation schemes set forth by the American College of Surgeons Committee on Trauma in the form of Advanced Trauma Life Support (ATLS) remain the gold standard of trauma care. The primary survey involving airway, breathing, circulation, disability, and exposure followed by the secondary survey of total patient evaluation (including a detailed history and physical examination) and definitive care remains the required standard.

A fairly predictable physiologic response can be seen in patients with traumatic injury. The many factors that affect the physiologic response can be classified as external or internal. External factors are rather simple and include but are not limited to the type of force implied (blunt versus penetrating), the amount of kinetic energy (KE) imparted (KE = 1/2 mass × velocity²), and the surface area and time frame in which the KE is applied. Other external factors could include exposure to temperature extremes and/or hazardous chemicals or gases. Internal factors are primarily related to the patient's pre-injury medical condition and underlying comorbidities and include but are not limited to underlying cardiac, pulmonary, and renal disease; diabetes; rheumatoid disease; use of prescription medications; and/or the use of illicit drugs. These conditions will not only affect an injured patient's initial response, but they will also greatly affect the treatment provided during resuscitation and follow-up care. Therefore, a thorough understanding of the mechanism of injury and an inventory of the patient's medical history is paramount to assessing a patient's physiologic condition following a major traumatic event.

Physiology of Injury

The basic element of the pathophysiology of the polytrauma patient is shock. Regardless of the class or the state of shock, prompt recognition and management is essential. Shock begets shock, and when left untreated results in a hypoperfused hypoxic state and the greater the likelihood that it will transition from a reversible shock state to an irreversible shock state. This will culminate in the breakdown of the bioenergetic machine at the cellular level, uncoupling of the mitochondria, and ultimately cellular death followed by death of the organism.

ATLS classifies shock into four groups based on blood volume loss, pulse rate, blood pressure, pulse pressure, respiratory rate, urinary output, central nervous system/mental status, and fluid replacement requirements (Table 1). It is equally important to identify the magnitude of shock. An immediately available clinical indication of the magnitude of shock is reflected by the pH and base deficit. Use of the base deficit is recommended simply because of its immediate availability, with arterial blood gases available through point of care testing.

The pathophysiology of acidosis is associated with the fact that the cell depends on the hydrolysis of adenosine triphosphate (ATP) to adenosine diphosphate (ADP) for the production of energy. As ATP is hydrolyzed to ADP, a hydrogen ion is one of the by-products. In the

TABLE 1 | Estimated Fluid and Blood Losses*

	Class I	Class II	Class III	Class IV
Blood loss (mL)	Up to 750	750-1,500	1,500-2,000	> 2,000
Blood loss (% blood volume)	Up to 15%	15%-30%	30%-40%	> 40%
Pulse rate (beats per minute)	< 100	> 100	> 120	> 140
Blood Pressure	Normal	Normal	Decreased	Decreased
Pulse pressure (mm Hg)	Normal or increased	Decreased	Decreased	Decreased
Respiratory rate (breaths per minute)	14-20	20-30	30-40	> 35
Urine output (mL/h)	> 30	20-30	5-15	Negligible
Central nervous system/mental status	Slightly anxious	Mildly anxious	Anxious, confused	Confused, lethargic
Fluid replacement (3:1 rule)	Crystalloid	Crystalloid	Crystalloid and blood	Crystalloid and blood

*Based on initial presentation for a 70-kg man.
The guidelines in Table 1 are based on the 3:1 rule. This rule derives from the empiric observation that most patients in hemorrhagic shock require as much as 300 mL of electrolyte solution for each 100 mL of blood loss. Applied blindly, these guidelines can result in excessive or inadequate fluid administration. For example, patients with a crush injury to the extremity may have hypotension out of proportion to their blood loss and require fluids in excess of the 3:1 guidelines. In contrast, patients whose ongoing blood loss is being replaced by blood transfusion require less than 3:1. The use of bolus therapy with careful monitoring of the patient's response can moderate these extremes.
(Reproduced with permission from Shock, in Advanced Trauma Life Support for the Doctors: Student Course Manual, ed 6. Chicago, IL, American College of Surgeons, 1997, p 108.)

TABLE 2 | Volume Requirements (Lactated Ringer's Solution and Blood) in Base Deficit Groups*

Base Deficit Group	No. of Patients	Hours After Admission			
		1	2	3	4
Mild (2 to -5)	70	2,966 ± 335	4,030 ± 520	5,881 ± 817	7,475 ± 766
Moderate (-6 to -14)	110	3,893 ± 322	7,522 ± 642	8,120 ± 718	13,007 ± 1,078
Severe (< -15)	29	6,110 ± 589 $P < 0.001$	9,800 ± 982 $P < 0.001$	10,909 ± 1,435 $P < 0.008$	16,396 ± 3,252 $P < 0.001$

*Values expressed as mL ± SEM.
(Reproduced with permission from Davis JW, Shackford SR, Mackersie RC, Hoyt DB: Base deficit as a guide to volume resuscitation. J Trauma 1988;28:1464-1467.)

shock state, at the cellular level, when the decrease in oxygen delivery and consumption are severe and prolonged enough, the resultant hypoxemia results in the accumulation of hydrogen ions in the cytosol and ends in cellular acidosis. The oxygen atom picks up these hydrogen ions and produces water. In the shock state, with the resulting cellular hypoxemia, acidosis ensues. The base deficit groups have been classified as mild, moderate, and severe. The resuscitation volumes needed to resuscitate patients in these base deficit groups at 1 hour, 2 hours, 4 hours, and 24 hours after presentation are listed in Table 2.

There have been many descriptions of shock and the shock state.[6] More modern definitions have evolved as the technology to monitor both oxygen delivery and consumption became available. One author described shock as a syndrome precipitated by systemic derange-

ment and perfusion leading to widespread cellular hypoxia and vital organ dysfunction.[7] Another author emphasized the supply and demand mismatch in his definition of shock as a disordered response of the organism to an inappropriate balance of substrate supply and demand at the cellular level.[8]

There are several different classifications of shock. The most accepted classifications are hypovolemic, cardiogenic, extracardiac obstructive, and distributive. The hemodynamic profiles of the shock states are well described in the physiology literature and are summarized in Table 3. Once a polytrauma patient presents for treatment and a shock state is recognized, aggressive fluid resuscitation begins with crystalloids and blood products. There is much controversy in the literature regarding the end points of resuscitation. The optimal immediate goals in resuscitation are best mon-

TABLE 3 | Hemodynamic Profiles of Shock

Diagnosis	Cardiac Output (CO)	Systemic Vascular Resistance (SVR)	Pulmonary Wedge Pressure (PWP)	Central Venous Pressure (CVP)	Mixed Venous Oxygen Saturation (Svo_2)	Comments
Cardiogenic Shock						
Caused by myocardial dysfunction	↓↓	↑	↑↑	↑↑	↓	Usually occurs with evidence of extensive myocardial infarction (> 40% of left ventricular myocardium nonfunctional), severe cardiomyopathy, or myocarditis
Caused by a Mechanical Defect						
Acute ventricular septal defect	Left ventricular CO ↓↓ Right ventricular CO > left ventricular CO	↑	nl or ↑	↑↑	↑ or ↑↑	If shunt is left to right, pulmonary blood flow is greater than systemic blood flow; oxygen saturation "step-up" (≥ 5%) occurs at right ventricular level; ↑ Svo_2 is caused by left to right shunt
Acute mitral regurgitation	Forward CO ↓↓	↑	↑↑	↑ or ↑↑	↓	Large V waves (≥ 10 mm Hg) in PWP tracing
Right ventricular infarction	↓↓	↑	nl or ↑	↑↑	↓	Elevated right atrial and right ventricular filling pressures with low or normal PWPs
Extracardiac Obstructive Shock						
Pericardial tamponade	↓ or ↓↓	↑	↑↑	↑↑	↓	Dip and plateau in right and left ventricular pressure tracings. The right atrial mean, right ventricular end-diastolic, pulmonary end-diastolic, and PWPs are within 5 mm Hg of each other
Massive pulmonary emboli	↓↓	↑	nl or ↓	↑↑	↓	Usual finding is elevated right-sided heart pressures with low or normal PWP
Hypovolemic Shock	↓↓	↑	↓↓	↓↓	↓	Filling pressures may appear normal if hypovolemia occurs in the setting of baseline myocardial compromise
Distributive Shock						
Septic shock	↑↑ or nl, rarely ↓	↓ or ↓↓	↓ or nl	↓ or nl	↑ or ↑↑	The hyperdynamic circulatory state (↑ CO, ↓ SVR) associated with distributive forms of shock is usually dependent on resuscitation with fluids; before such resuscitation, a hypodynamic circulation is typical
Anaphylaxis	↑↑ or nl, rarely ↓	↓ or ↓↓	↓ or nl	↓ or nl	↑ or ↑↑	

↑ = Mild to moderate increase, ↑↑ = Moderate to severe increase, ↓ = Mild to moderate decrease, ↓↓ = moderate to severe decrease, nl = Normal.
(Reproduced with permission from Parillo JE, Dellinger RP: *Critical Care Medicine: Principles of Diagnosis and Management in the Adult,* ed 2. St. Louis, MO, Mosby, 2002.)

itored by assessing a compilation of metabolic and physiologic responses. The polytrauma patient should receive a sufficient volume of crystalloids and blood products to restore blood pressure, restore urine output (0.5 to 1 mL/kg/h), and correct base deficit (restoring a negative base deficit to 0 or to a base excess of 4). A summary of immediate goals of resuscitation (hemodynamic stability, optimization of oxygen delivery, and reversal of organ system dysfunction) is provided in Table 4.

TABLE 4 | General Approach to Shock: Immediate Goals

Hemodynamic stability	Mean arterial pressure > 60 to 65 mm Hg (higher in the presence of coronary artery disease or chronic hypertension) Pulmonary wedge pressure = 12 to 18 mm Hg (may be higher for cardiogenic shock) Cardiac index > 2.1 L/min/m² for cardiogenic and obstructive shock > 3.0 to 3.5 L/min/m² for septic and resuscitated traumatic/hemorrhagic shock
Optimization of oxygen delivery	Hemoglobin > 10 g/dL Arterial saturation > 92% Mixed venous oxygen saturation (Svo₂) > 60% Normalization of serum lactate (to < 2.2 mEq/L)
Reverse organ system dysfunction	Reverse encephalopathy Maintain urine output > 0.5 mL/kg/h

(Reproduced with permission from Parillo JE, Dellinger RP: Critical Care Medicine: Principles of Diagnosis and Management in the Adult, ed 2. St. Louis, MO, Mosby, 2002.)

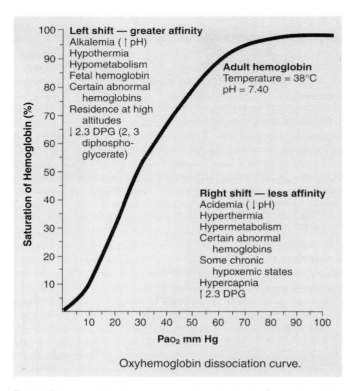

Oxyhemoglobin dissociation curve.

Figure 1 Oxyhemoglobin dissociation curve. *(Reproduced with permission from Parillo JE, Dellinger RP: Critical Care Medicine: Principles of Diagnosis and Management in the Adult, ed 2. St. Louis, MO, Mosby, 2002.)*

In the acute resuscitative phase, in addition to restoration of hemodynamic stability with clearance of base deficit and reestablishment of adequate urine output, it is of paramount importance to avoid hypothermia. Hypothermia secondary to either exposure to the environment or aggressive resuscitation with crystalloids and blood products will eventually add to the ongoing blood loss and oxygen debt through the development of cold coagulopathy.[9,10] Furthermore, hypothermia adds to oxygen debt and cellular hypoxia by shifting the oxyhemoglobin dissociation curve to the left, thereby increasing the affinity of the hemoglobin molecule for oxygen and decreasing the release of oxygen to the tissues (Figure 1).

There is a causal relationship among blunt trauma, hemorrhage, soft-tissue injury, fractures, shock, and the development of immunosuppression. Immunosuppression is followed by the development of infection, sepsis, multiple organ failure, and possibly death. There is a marked depression in cell-mediated immunity that follows hemorrhage, which seems to be the mechanism responsible for the increased susceptibility to subsequent infections and sepsis.[11-14]

The pathophysiologic and inflammatory insult following polytrauma is of a significantly greater magnitude and complexity than that seen in patients with isolated hemorrhagic shock. The release of inflammatory mediators following trauma and hemorrhage are well described in both animal and patient studies.[15-17] The plasma levels of tumor necrosis factor (TNF), interleukin (IL)-6, transforming growth factor-beta (TGF-β), and corticosterone are summarized in Figure 2. In vivo administration of IL-1, IL-6, and TNF-α induce a shocklike syndrome similar to that observed following hemorrhage; it is suggested that these cytokines may play a role in initiating

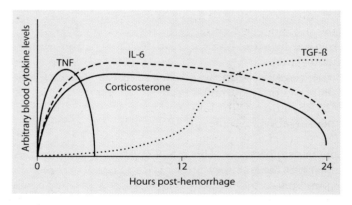

Figure 2 Arbitrary blood cytokine levels during the first 24 hours after trauma-hemorrhage. *(Reproduced with permission from Biffl WL, Moore EE, Moore FA: The two-hit models of MODS, in Deitch EA: Sepsis and Multiple Organ Dysfunction: A Multidisciplinary Approach. London, England, WB Saunders, 2002, p 130.)*

the cascade that leads to the development of multiple organ dysfunction syndrome.

Timing of Surgery: The Second Hit

A two-hit model of multiple organ dysfunction syndrome has been described.[18-21] The unifying hypothesis of the two-hit model of multiple organ failure and multiple organ dysfunction syndrome is that it occurs as a result of a dysfunctional inflammatory response.

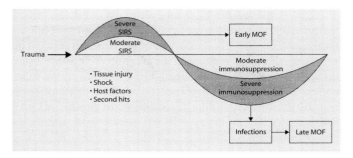

Figure 3 Dysfunctional inflammatory response. MOF = Multiple organ failure. *(Reproduced with permission from Angele MK, Schwacha MG, Ayala A, Irshad H, Chaudry M: The immunoinflammatory response to hemorrhage, in Deitch EA, Vincent JL, Windsor A (eds): Sepsis and Multiple Organ Dysfunction: A Multidisciplinary Approach. London, England, WB Saunders, 2002, p 118.)*

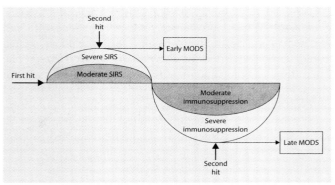

Figure 4 The amplitude and duration of the systemic inflammatory response depends on the magnitude of the initial insult. Later immunosuppression is proportional to the initial inflammatory response. A second hit during the hyperinflammatory phase results in early multiple organ dysfunctions (MODS), whereas a second hit during the immunosuppressive phase results in late, often sepsis-related MODS. *(Reproduced with permission from Moore FA, Moore EE: MODS following trauma, in Deitch EA, Vincent JL, Windsor A (eds): Sepsis and Multiple Organ Dysfunction: A Multidisciplinary Approach. London, England, WB Saunders, 2002, p 29.)*

Following major trauma, tissue injury, fractures, and shock, patients are resuscitated into an early state of systemic hyperinflammation called systemic inflammatory response syndrome (SIRS). The intensity of the SIRS depends on the amount of tissue injury, the degree and duration of shock, and the presence of host factors (specifically age and comorbid disease). A mild to moderate SIRS response is presumed to be beneficial and protective and resolves as the patient recovers. However, if the initial insult is massive (one-hit model), the resultant severe SIRS precipitates early multiple organ failure. If the patient is not exposed to a massive hit, early multiple organ failure can occur as a result of exposure to a secondary inflammatory insult (two-hit model). This second hit may occur if definitive fracture fixation surgery is undertaken in decompensated patients.

A negative feedback system recently described as compensatory anti-inflammatory response syndrome (CARS) attempts to limit certain components of SIRS and thereby limit the autodestructive inflammation.[19] The protective response of CARS may lead to delayed immunosuppression. The intensity of the CARS correlates with the intensity of the SIRS. Therefore, severely injured patients with heightened SIRS/CARS responses are at a high risk for late multiple organ dysfunction syndrome secondary to infections that develop as a result of severe immunosuppression. The dysfunctional inflammatory response model and the two-hit model are summarized in Figures 3 and 4.

The timing of orthopaedic intervention is critical because it may act as a second hit. Patients with severe closed head injury, severe blunt chest trauma with associated severe pulmonary contusion, or those who clearly have experienced a significant initial hit are at risk for the severe SIRS response. Surgical intervention in this patient population, including surgical fracture fixation, may serve as a second hit and induce early multiple organ failure. Orthopaedic surgeons who provide care to this cohort of patients must remain cognizant of this fact and titrate their surgical intervention to facilitate resuscitation but avoid the negative impact of the second hit.

Damage Control Orthopaedics

The advantages of early fixation of femoral shaft fractures using reamed intramedullary nails have been demonstrated.[22] These advantages, including fewer pulmonary complications, fewer intensive care unit days, and shorter hospitalizations, led the American College of Surgeons Committee on Trauma to recommend that all femoral shaft fractures in polytrauma patients be treated within 2 to 12 hours after injury, provided hemodynamic stability has been achieved. Early fracture fixation represents a paradigm shift in the treatment of orthopaedic trauma patients from "this patient is too sick to operate on" to "this patient is too sick not to operate on."

Because intramedullary nails are a definitive treatment of femoral shaft fractures, the concept of early definitive care of fractures in polytrauma patients became more prevalent in the orthopaedic community. However, trauma surgeons noted subgroups of patients with severe pulmonary and/or head injuries that appeared to receive a second hit from surgery, particularly reamed intramedullary nailing. Subsequently, over the past decade numerous studies comparing reamed intramedullary nailing, unreamed intramedullary nailing, and plating of femoral shaft fractures have been done to determine which definitive treatment is best for different subgroups.[23-25] Although the results are conflicting, the general consensus is that early fixation is more important than the type of fixation, and definitive fracture fixation may not be optimal in specific trauma subgroups.

Damage control orthopaedics is a concept developed to provide early fracture fixation and avoid the second hit from prolonged surgical procedures and substantial blood loss.[26,27] External fixation is used for initial femoral shaft fracture fixation in unstable trauma patients and as a bridge to stabilize the fracture until intramedullary nailing could be performed when the patient was stabilized. The mean time to conversion to intramedullary nailing was 4.8 days. The mean operating room times for external fixation and intramedullary nailing were 35 minutes and 135 minutes, respectively; the mean estimated blood losses were 90 mL and 400 mL, respectively. Damage control orthopaedics effectively led to a fourfold reduction in operating room time and estimated blood loss.[26,27]

Reaming and Pulmonary Injury

Intramedullary reaming results in intravasation of fat and bone marrow (fat embolism). Fat embolism has been documented in numerous studies with transesophageal echocardiography.[28,29] However, fat embolism is not unique to reamed intramedullary nailing and occurs during unreamed femoral nailing, femoral component preparation and insertion during total hip arthroplasty, intramedullary instrumentation in total knee arthroplasty, or intramedullary-based femoral shortening osteotomies. Fat embolism syndrome has been shown to occur during the plating of femoral shaft fractures.[30] Based on these observations, it is not clear that reaming and fat embolism alone are sufficient to cause fat embolism syndrome or ARDS.

The debate regarding reaming during femoral shaft intramedullary nailing may never be resolved. ARDS may be the result of a dose-response second hit from embolized marrow elements, the response being a function of the initial pulmonary injury and the patient's pulmonary reserve (age, smoking history, and preexisting pulmonary disease). Alternatively, ARDS may result from proinflammatory cytokines released from the traumatized soft-tissue zone of injury. To understand the effects of reaming, multiple variables must be measured, including pulmonary injury grading, fat embolism volume, soft-tissue injury grading, soft-tissue manipulation during positioning and fixation, and reaming techniques. A well-powered, prospective, randomized trial comparing reamed versus unreamed intramedullary femoral nailing would be difficult to conduct given these clinical variables.

Damage control orthopaedics principles avoid fat embolism and reduce the systemic levels of proinflammatory cytokines. One study measured proinflammatory cytokines in polytrauma patients with femoral shaft fractures.[31] Thirty-five patients were randomized to undergo primary intramedullary nailing within 24 hours of injury or damage control orthopaedics external fixation and secondary intramedullary nailing. IL-6 was measured preoperatively and postoperatively in both groups. IL-6 increased (55 ± 33 pg/dL preoperatively to 254 ± 55 pg/dL 24 hours postoperatively) in the primary intramedullary nailing group ($P = 0.03$) and did not increase in the external fixation (71 ± 42 pg/dL preoperatively to

68 ± 34 pg/dL 24 hours postoperatively) and secondary intramedullary nailing group (36 ± 21 pg/dL preoperatively to 39 ± 25 pg/dL 24 hours postoperatively). The protocol did not state whether reamed or unreamed intramedullary nails were used. However, using the principles of damage control orthopaedics, instrumentation of the intramedullary canal was not done, and proinflammatory cytokines (IL-6) were not increased perioperatively.

Fat intravasation can be decreased by minimizing intramedullary pressure during reaming. The gap equation predicted the intramedullary pressure as a function of the flow past the reamer head.[32] The gap equation was modified by assuming the flow past the reamer head is equal to the frontal area of the reamer head multiplied by the reamer velocity along the longitudinal axis of the femur. The modified gap equation is:

$$\Delta P = 3\mu L d_m v_0 / h^3$$

In this equation, ΔP is intramedullary pressure, μ is bone marrow viscosity, L is reamer head length, d_m is the mean diameter of the intramedullary canal and reamer flute root diameter, v_0 is longitudinal reamer velocity, and h is the gap between the inner cortical diameter and reamer flute root diameter. The modified gap equation suggests reamers should have deep cutting flutes and short reamer heads. The modified gap equation also applies to reamer drive shafts. Reamer drive shafts should have a smaller diameter relative to the reamer head. Intraoperative reaming technique should use an appropriate reamer and slow longitudinal reamer velocity. Fracture location affects intramedullary pressure. Subtrochanteric femoral fractures do not allow venting through the fracture site as the reamer passes through the isthmus of the intramedullary canal. The theoretic maximum intramedullary pressure occurs with reaming at the isthmus because the smallest gap occurs at the isthmus. Therefore, subtrochanteric fractures are at higher risk for increased intramedullary pressure, and venting of the distal intramedullary canal should be considered. These techniques can minimize intramedullary pressure during reaming.

The link between intramedullary reaming and pulmonary injury is complex. The development of pulmonary dysfunction after femoral shaft fracture fixation does not appear to be related to fixation method (reamed intramedullary nailing versus unreamed intramedullary nailing versus plating).[33] Damage control orthopaedics (external fixation) should be considered for hemodynamically unstable patients with pulmonary injuries.

Fracture Fixation and Head Injury

From an evidence-based medicine perspective, there is insufficient knowledge to determine the timing of fracture fixation in polytrauma patients with concomitant

TABLE 5 | Recommended Surgical Intervention Guidelines for Polytrauma Patients

The initial management of all polytrauma patients should be according to ATLS protocols, with fluid resuscitation and rapid hemorrhage control to restore hemodynamic stability and tissue perfusion.

Cavity decompression and temporary fracture stabilization should be performed as soon as possible.

CPP should be maintained at greater than 70 mm Hg during preoperative, intraoperative, and postoperative periods.

Monitoring of cerebral blood flow and tissue oxygenation will provide more information about an individual patient treatment course.

Secondary brain injury can result if fluid resuscitation is inadequate or surgical fracture treatment results in hypotension or low CPP.

Individual patient fracture fixation should be determined by the assessment of each patient's hemodynamic stability and CPP rather than by mandatory time policies.

Orthopaedic injuries should be managed with the assumption that full neurologic recovery will occur.

head injuries. There are no known prospective, randomized studies evaluating the timing of fracture fixation in polytrauma patients with severe head injuries. However, certain physiologic principles can guide the timing of fracture fixation.

Secondary brain injury results from decreased cerebral blood flow and oxygenation. The decreased blood flow can result from hypotension, decreased cerebral perfusion, and/or decreased blood oxygenation from pulmonary dysfunction. Therefore, fracture fixation cannot compromise blood pressure, cerebral blood flow, or pulmonary function with ARDS. Cerebral perfusion pressure (CPP) is defined as the mean arterial pressure (MAP) minus the intracranial pressure (ICP):

$$CPP = MAP - ICP$$

It is recommended that the CPP be kept at greater than 70 mm Hg by maintaining the MAP at greater than 90 mm Hg and the ICP at less than 20 mm Hg.

Fracture fixation can result in a significant blood loss, hypotension, and hemodynamic instability. Patients undergoing surgical femoral fracture fixation within 0 to 2 hours after injury were reported to be eight times more likely to become hypotensive than those who underwent surgical femoral fracture fixation at greater than 24 hours after injury.[34] Delaying surgical intervention until the patient is hemodynamically stable reduces the risk of hypotension. External fixation is an alternative to allow early fracture stabilization. Until further clinical evidence is available, the guidelines listed in Table 5 are recommended.[35]

Fracture and Vascular Injury

In the lower extremity, knee dislocations and supracondylar/distal femur fractures are associated with vascular injuries. In the upper extremity, supracondylar humerus fractures and scapulothoracic dissociations are associated with brachial artery and axillary artery injuries, respectively. These fractures and dislocations, therefore, should raise a high index of suspicion for associated vascular injuries. However, all patients should be evaluated for distal pulses in all four extremities as part of ATLS protocols.

If distal pulses are diminished or absent in any extremity, any joint dislocations should be reduced and any fractures should be aligned with longitudinal traction. If the distal pulse does not return to normal, a vascular surgeon consultation should be obtained. Delineation of the vascular injury depends on the limb ischemia time and other injuries. The limb should be revascularized within 6 hours, and treatment should not be delayed. Temporary or definitive fracture-dislocation stabilization is required before vascular repair to prevent reinjury. Prophylactic fasciotomies may be required to treat reperfusion compartment syndromes.

Monitoring of Resuscitation: How?

Trauma resuscitation is monitored via vital signs and pulse oximetry. Blood pressure can be monitored with automated blood pressure cuffs or arterial lines. Heart rate is most easily monitored with electrocardiography. Core body temperature should be monitored because hypothermia can result in coagulopathy. Tissue oxygenation can be measured with pulse oximetry or tissue probes that are used for plastic surgery tissue transfers. Calculation of the base deficit from the initial blood pH can be used to estimate fluid resuscitation requirements.

ICP monitoring is required for patients with severe head injuries. For these patients, CPP is calculated as noted previously. Intraoperative monitoring of CPP is important because femoral nailing has been shown in one study to decrease intraoperative CPP relative to preoperative and postoperative CPP.[36] In this study, 66% of the patients (10 of 15) had an individual average CPP less than 70 mm Hg. Intraoperative ICP monitoring, therefore, allows intraoperative management of CPP in patients with severe head injuries.

Important Issues

Acute Lung Injury and Acute Respiratory Distress Syndrome

Since its first description in the literature, ARDS has been one of the most important clinical scenarios in the care of critically ill patients; patients with ARDS have a mortality rate of 40% to 50%, and ARDS presents a major therapeutic challenge because no specific therapy is yet available.[37] Patients with ARDS typically have clinical signs of arterial hypoxemia that is unresponsive to oxygen therapy, together with dyspnea and tachypnea; ARDS is also typically accompanied by bilateral infiltrates on an AP chest radiograph[38] (Table 6). The clinical

TABLE 6 | Definition Criteria for Acute Lung Injury and ARDS

Acute onset

Bilateral infiltrates on an AP chest radiograph

Pulmonary capillary occlusion pressure < 18 mm Hg or absence of clinical signs of left atrial hypertension

Arterial hypoxemia (irrespective of positive end-expiratory pressure)

$Pao_2/F_1o_2 < 300$ mm Hg = Acute lung injury

$Pao_2/F_1o_2 < 200$ mm Hg = Acute respiratory distress syndrome

(Adapted with permission from Bernard GR, Artigas A, Brigham KL, et al: The American-European Consensus Conference on ARDS: Definitions, mechanisms, relevant outcomes, and clinical trial coordination. Am J Respir Crit Care Med 1994;149:818-824.)

TABLE 7 | Etiology of ARDS*

ARDS Categories	No. of Patients (%)†	No. of Survivors (%)‡
I. Direct injury		
A. Aspiration	4 (4.8)	3 (75.0)
B. Diffuse pulmonary infection	14 (16.7)	12 (86.0)
C. Near drowning	1 (1.2)	1 (100.0)
D. Toxic inhalation	N/A	N/A
E. Lung contusion	26 (30.9)	23 (88.0)
Subtotal:	45 (53.6)	39 (87.0)
II. Indirect injury		
A. Sepsis syndrome	30 (35.7)	21 (70.0)
B. Severe nonthoracic trauma	4 (4.8)	3 (75.0)
C. Hypertransfusion	3 (3.6)	2 (67.0)
D. Cardiopulmonary bypass	2 (2.4)	2 (100.0)
Subtotal:	39 (46.4)	28 (72.0)
Total	84 (100.0)	67 (80.0)

*Data are from a series of patients from a single referral center (University of Vienna, 1996 to 1998). N/A = not applicable.

†Number (percentage) of patients in the different ARDS categories described by the Report of the American-European Consensus Conference.

‡Number (percentage) of survivors in each ARDS category.

(Adapted with permission from Ullrich R, Lorber C, Roeder G, et al: Controlled airway pressure therapy, nitric oxide inhalation, prone position, and extracorporeal membrane oxygenation (ECMO) as components of an integrated approach to ARDS. Anesthesiology 1999;91:1577-1586.)

course of ARDS is often progressive, with distinctive stages and different histologic and radiographic manifestations. The acute exudative phase is characterized by an acute onset of clinical symptoms and rapid development of an alveolar edema that is clinically indistinguishable from cardiogenic edema. This inflammatory response of the lungs induces diffuse alveolar damage, demonstrating recruitment of neutrophils and macrophages, disruption of the alveolocapillary membrane, alveolar flooding with a proteinaceous edema, and disruption of the alveolar epithelium together with inactivation of surfactant.[39] This diffuse alveolar damage is typically nonhomogeneous in distribution, with predominance of atelectasis formation in the dependent parts of the lungs because of gravitational forces. The loss of alveolar gas-exchanging lung areas produced by atelectasis and alveolar flooding in combination with immunomediated impairment of hypoxic pulmonary vasoconstriction leads to a mismatching of ventilation and perfusion with consequent arterial hypoxemia and increases in alveolar dead space.

If patients survive the acute phase, it is frequently followed by a chronic fibrotic stage, characterized by a fibrosing alveolitis with radiographic diffuse interstitial opacities and clinical signs of persisting hypoxemia and increased alveolar dead space.[39] This chronic fibrotic stage may be perpetuated further or even initiated by the inevitable requirement of mechanical ventilation in most of these patients.[40] Mechanical ventilation itself can induce lung injury that contributes significantly to the morbidity and mortality of patients with acute lung injury and ARDS.[41] Because pulmonary lesions in patients with ARDS are inhomogeneously distributed, the applied high airway pressures and tidal volumes are predominantly distributed to aerated lung areas, thereby imposing considerable mechanical stress on these alveoli. Modern ventilation strategies take these pathophysiologic concepts into account and have been shown to reduce mortality by lowering tidal volumes and maintaining a high end-expiratory positive pressure, thereby minimizing cyclic reopening and collapse.[42] Despite the severity of the disease, all radiologic and clinical symptoms can

resolve, and survivors of ARDS have been shown to return to productive lives with minor limitations in self-related quality of life and near-normal lung function.[43,44]

Acute lung injury and ARDS can be caused by a variety of indirect and direct injuries to the lungs, and various risk factors have been identified[45] (Table 7). Patients who have experienced trauma are especially prone to developing acute lung injury because direct contusion of the lungs and aspiration of gastric contents are common findings in polytrauma patients. Moreover, severe blood loss often results in hemorrhagic shock, with coagulopathy requiring the transfusion of large amounts of blood products; all of these factors have been identified as contributing to the development of acute lung injury. Analysis of CT scans of patients with ARDS has greatly expanded the understanding of the underlying pathophysiology and the changes in respiratory mechanics.[46] Evidence suggests that ARDS caused by direct injury may differ significantly in respect to anatomic distribution and respiratory mechanics when compared with the ARDS caused by indirect injuries, such as sepsis and trauma.[47] Pulmonary ARDS represents diffuse alveolar damage that is more regionally distributed with pronounced basal atelectasis, whereas extrapulmonary ARDS shows a pattern of diffuse distribution within the lungs often in the presence of a considerable increase in intra-abdominal pressure. These findings not only demonstrate different disease patterns but also have significant implications for the use of therapies such as prone positioning and nitric oxide and surfactant inhalation because patients with extrapulmonary and pulmonary ARDS react differently to these therapies.

Sepsis and Multiple Organ Failure

Sepsis is the clinical manifestation of an exaggerated host response to infection or to a noninfectious challenge such as trauma or burns. The beneficial host response becomes amplified and dysregulated to result in an overwhelming inflammatory response.[48] Clinically, the onset is often manifested by an increase in body temperature, mental confusion, hypotension, and reduction in urine output. If untreated, the hypotension becomes unresponsive and is accompanied by disturbances of the coagulation pathway and development of end organ failure, such as respiratory or renal failure. Despite the major insights into the principles governing bacteria-host interactions and the process of inflammatory and proinflammatory immunomodulation, therapies targeted to interfere with these cascades have not yielded beneficial results in respect to mortality. An estimated 740,000 instances of sepsis occur each year in the United States; when accompanied by septic shock, sepsis results in a mortality rate in excess of 50%.[48] The major sources of infection are the lungs, urinary tract, abdominal cavity, and bloodstream; only half of patients with sepsis show a specific infectious pathogen, half of which are gram-positive and gram-negative bacteria.[49,50]

After the initial bacteria-host interaction that is mediated by bacterial cell wall components or exotoxins and communicated through cell surface proteins, such as the toll-like receptor, a strong immune response is triggered, involving both humoral and cellular elements. Proinflammatory cytokines (most importantly, IL-6, IL-1, and TNF-α) and several other cytokines are released by mononuclear cells into the bloodstream[50,51] (Figure 5). These initial cytokines are released within 30 to 90 minutes and induce a second inflammatory reaction mediated by release of chemokines, prostaglandins, leukotrienes, and reactive oxygen species together with an induction of inflammatory cell migration into tissues.[50] Novel early mediators that have been identified and have been shown to protect from experimental lethal sepsis include high-mobility group B1 and macrophage migration inhibitory factor. However, therapies targeted at the inhibition of key mediators such as TNF-α and IL-1 failed to prove beneficial in clinical trials. This may be explained by the early release of these mediators, which are not present any longer when patients come to the intensive care unit.[51]

The inflammatory response also involves a potent activation of procoagulatory and anticoagulatory pathways, which in many patients leads to the most severe

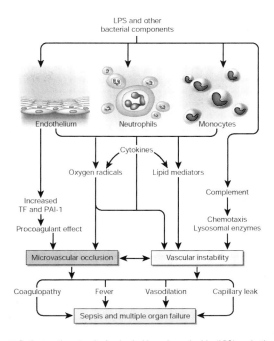

Figure 5 Pathogenetic networks in shock. Lipopolysaccharide (LPS) and other microbial components simultaneously activate multiple parallel cascades that contribute to the pathophysiology of ARDS and shock. The combination of poor myocardial contractility, impaired peripheral vascular tone, and microvascular occlusion leads to tissue hypoperfusion and inadequate oxygenation, and ultimately to organ failure. *(Adapted with permission from Cohen J: The immunopathogenesis of sepsis. Nature 2002; 420:885-891.)*

form of disseminated intravascular coagulation. In general, coagulation is activated and fibrinolysis is impaired during sepsis, resulting in removal of fibrin, microvascular thrombosis with consecutive tissue hypoxia, reduced tissue perfusion, and ultimately end organ failure. The observation that naturally occurring antithrombotic factors such as antithrombin III and protein C are reduced in patients with sepsis has led to clinical trials investigating the effect of substituting these anticoagulants in patients with sepsis.[52] Protein C becomes activated by thrombin complexes and has a potent anti-inflammatory action in addition to its ability to block the coagulation cascade. Substitution of activated protein C has demonstrated a marked effect on survival in patients with sepsis, with an even more pronounced effect on elderly patients with end organ failure.[52] In addition to the proinflammatory cascade, potent anti-inflammatory mediators are released during the course of the disease, including IL-10, soluble TNF-receptor, or IL-1 receptor antagonist. This anti-inflammatory response may also develop into an immunosuppressive, exaggerated host response, leading to susceptibility for further bacterial colonization.

The precise mechanisms governing the pathogenesis of sepsis-induced organ failure remain incompletely understood. However, disturbances of microcirculation and tissue hypoxia resulting from occlusion of microvessels play a major role, together with cellular infiltrates that damage tissue by direct release of lysosomal enzymes and reactive oxygen species. Upregulation of nitric oxide synthases results in excess production of nitric oxide, leading to formation of peroxynitrite and inhibition of mitochondrial respiration that may also contribute to the myocardial depression observed during sepsis.[53] Oxygen debt, activation of the coagulation cascade with consecutive formation of fibrin deposits, strong immunoactivation paralleled by immunosuppression, and release of stress hormones are the key features of sepsis. Interestingly, therapeutic strategies aimed at modulating this response have been recently shown to be beneficial in clinical trials. The optimization of hemodynamic management, including transfusion of blood products, fluid administration, and inotropic support, resulted in better survival rates.[54] Rigorous control of blood glucose levels by administration of insulin lowered mortality rates in one study,[55] and substitution of low-dose glucocorticoids benefited patients in another study.[56] Finally, administration of activated protein C has become the single licensed drug or treatment of patients with sepsis following clinical trials that demonstrated a marked reduction in mortality rates.[52]

Coagulopathy

Uncontrolled bleeding that leads to profound hemorrhagic shock is the major cause of death in polytrauma patients in the prehospital setting or during the first 48 hours following admission to the hospital.[57] When coagulopathy combines with metabolic derangements and hypothermia, it accounts for a significant bleeding-related mortality rate in the postoperative period. Trauma-induced coagulopathy is multifactorial, including hypothermia, consumption of clotting factors, hemodilution, and metabolic effects.[58] For instance, thrombocyte counts are reduced to 40% after replacement of one blood volume. Regular activation of the coagulation cascades requires the presence of intact thrombocytes, and thrombocytopenia is a common feature in polytrauma patients. The large amounts of fluid required for resuscitation result in dilution of coagulation factors and antithrombotic factors, such as antithrombin III and protein C. Together with the loss of coagulation factors resulting from bleeding, this dilutional coagulopathy results in prolonged bleeding times and exaggerated fibrinolysis. Hypothermia has a significant effect on platelet function, leading to increased adhesiveness and aggregation that further aggravates thrombocytopenia together with profound platelet dysfunction. In addition to dilutional coagulopathy, thrombocytopenia, and platelet dysfunction, hypothermia also exerts a direct effect on the coagulation cascade[59] and it directly increases fibrinolysis.[58] Additional factors of trauma-related coagulopathy include the progressive consumption of coagulation factors at the injury site,[59] release of tissue factors after brain injury and pulmonary contusion,[60] and persistent shock.[59] The major treatment goals for trauma-related coagulopathy are the aggressive restoration of in-

travascular volume, transfusion of platelets, fresh-frozen plasma, and coagulation factors and the rigorous correction of hypothermia by any means. Laboratory tests are often of limited value in the primary resuscitation because the tests are time-consuming and represent a single view of a progressive dynamic process. Clinical assessment of ongoing bleeding (oozing from cut surfaces, venous lines, mouth, or nose) in this initial phase is of paramount importance. If intra-abdominal bleeding is present, it can be quickly controlled by surgery, or abdominal packing is performed with rapid transfer to the intensive care unit. After correction of hypothermia and control of bleeding, further administration of coagulation and blood products can be guided by laboratory test results.

Deep Venous Thrombosis and Pulmonary Embolism

Several risk factors have been identified as being associated with the development of deep venous thrombosis (DVT) and pulmonary embolism (PE), including surgery, fractures, immobilization, and coagulopathy, all of which can be present in polytrauma patients.[61] Manifestations of venous thromboembolism (VTE) may range from DVT to frank PE, with an estimated annual incidence of 200,000 and 94,000, respectively, in the United States. Untreated PE is associated with a mortality rate of 30% and imposes a significant risk on the patient.[61] Traditionally, fractures of the pelvis and long bones have been viewed as major risk factors for DVT and PE. However, a recent meta-analysis of the literature suggests that spine fractures and injuries to the spinal cord are the major risk factors for DVT and PE.[62] Increased age, increased Injury Severity Score, and blood transfusion appear to be associated with an increased risk for DVT. However, traditional risk factors such as long bone fractures, pelvic fractures, or head injuries were inconclusive in this meta-analysis. Whereas the occurrence of DVT in polytrauma patients is an accepted fact, controversy exists about the best method of prophylaxis. Low-dose heparin demonstrated no sufficient effect in preventing DVT after trauma.[62] The same finding applies to alternative treatment modalities such as pneumatic compression devices and arteriovenous foot pumps. The mainstay of prophylaxis for VTE remains treatment with low-molecular-weight heparin. Although low-molecular-weight heparin is superior to low-dose heparin in preventing VTE, current recommendations state an indication only for patients with pelvic fractures, complex lower extremity fractures (all requiring surgical fixation and prolonged bed rest), and spinal cord injuries with complete or incomplete paralysis.[62] The benefit of anticoagulation therapy has to be weighed against the increased risk of bleeding in patients with head injuries and patients with an Injury Severity Score greater than 9. In patients with ongoing bleeding or head injuries, insertion of a vena cava filter is an intriguing alternative. Insertion is recommended in patients who cannot receive antico-

TABLE 8	Rules for Predicting the Probability of Embolism	
Variable		**Points**
Risk factors		
Clinical signs and symptoms of deep venous thrombosis		3.0
An alternative diagnosis deemed less likely than pulmonary embolism		3.0
Heart rate > 100 beats per minute		1.5
Immobilization or surgery in the previous 4 weeks		1.5
Previous deep venous thrombosis or embolism		1.5
Hemoptysis		1.0
Cancer		1.0
Clinical probability		
Low		< 2.0
Intermediate		2.0 to 6.0
High		> 6.0

(Adapted with permission from Fedullo PF, Tapson VF: Clinical practice: The evaluation of suspected pulmonary embolism. N Engl J Med 2003;349:1247-1256.)

agulation because of bleeding and/or who present with severe closed head injury, incomplete spinal cord injury, pelvic fractures, or long bone fractures.[63]

Diagnosis of DVT relies on ultrasound imaging by either Doppler ultrasound or duplex ultrasound. Both methods are sensitive and specific in symptomatic patients; however, the accuracy of screening of asymptomatic patients with ultrasound remains uncertain.

PE is suspected clinically and initial symptoms are dyspnea, pleuritic chest pain, and tachycardia.[64] Unfortunately, these signs raise suspicion rather than confirm the diagnosis. Laboratory tests, electrocardiography, and chest radiography all have limited value in ruling out PE.[64] Moreover, D-dimer levels, although suited to rule out PE in patients with a low probability of VTE, are frequently elevated in polytrauma patients with inflammation, which renders the test with a low sensitivity and specificity. Following clinical suspicion, a helical CT or angiography can be used to confirm the diagnosis. The highest accuracy has been achieved with ventilation-perfusion scans; however, their use may be limited in polytrauma patients who are often mechanically ventilated and difficult to transport. Current recommendations for the diagnosis of suspected PE are based on clinical grading in patients with a high, intermediate, and low probability for PE[64] (Table 8). Patients with a high probability demonstrate an incidence of 70% to 90% of PE; when they present with evidence of PE on a CT scan, the incidence is 95%. Patients with an intermediate probability for PE may undergo pulmonary angiography in the case of a negative CT scan because the prevalence of PE with a positive ventilation-perfusion scan is only 88% to 93%, leaving doubt as to the appropriateness of anticoagulation treatment. Patients with a low probabil-

ity of PE only demonstrate an incidence of 5% to 10%, and PE can be ruled out on the basis of a negative D-dimer test result.

Annotated References

1. *Advanced Trauma Life Support*, ed 6. Chicago, IL, American College of Surgeons, 1997.

2. Bone RC: Toward an epidemiology and natural history of SIRS (systemic inflammatory response syndrome). *JAMA* 1992;268:3452-3455.

3. Baue AE: Multiple organ failure, in Baue AE (ed): *Multiple Organ Failure: Patient Care and Prevention.* St. Louis, MO, Mosby Year Book, 1990, pp 421-470.

4. Deitch EA: *Sepsis and Multiple Organ Dysfunction: A Multidisciplinary Approach.* London, England, WB Saunders, 2002.

5. Goris RJA: Sepsis and multiple organ failure: The result of whole body inflammation, in Faist E, Meakins J, Schildberg FW (eds): *Host Defense Dysfunction in Trauma, Shock and Sepsis.* Berlin, Germany, Springer-Verlag, 1993, pp 161-170.

6. Warren JC: *Surgical Pathology and Therapeutics.* Philadelphia, PA, WB Saunders, 1895.

7. Fink MP: Shock: An overview, in Rippe JM, Irwin RS, Alpert JS, et al (eds): *Intensive Care Medicine,* ed 2. Boston, MA, Little, Brown & Co, 1991.

8. Cerra FB: Shock, in Burke JF (ed): *Surgical Physiology.* Philadelphia, PA, WB Saunders, 1983.

9. Steinemann S, Shackford SR, Davis JW: Implications of admission hypothermia in trauma patients. *J Trauma* 1990;30:200-202.

10. Stoner HB: Studies on the mechanism of shock: The impairment of thermoregulation by trauma. *Br J Exp Pathol* 1969;50:125-138.

11. Peitzman AB, Billiar TR, Harbrecht BG, Kelly E, Udekwu AO, Simmons RL: Hemorrhagic shock. *Curr Probl Surg* 1995;32:925-1002.

12. Huynh T, Currin RT, Tanaka Y, Lemasters JJ, Baker CC: Activation of Kupffer cells in vivo following femur fracture. *Arch Surg* 1994;129:1324-1328.

13. Ayala A, Wang P, Ba ZF, Perrin MM, Ertel W, Chaudry IH: Differential alterations in plasma IL-6 and TNF levels after trauma and hemorrhage. *Am J Physiol* 1991;260:R167-R171.

14. Chaundry IH, Ayala A: *Immunological Aspects of Hemorrhage.* Austin, TX, RG Landes Company, 1992.

15. Baue AE: Multiple, progressive, or sequential systems failure. *Arch Surg* 1975;110:779-781.

16. Sauaia A, Moore FA, Moore EE, et al: Epidemiology of trauma deaths: A reassessment. *J Trauma* 1995;38:185-193.

17. Regel G, Lobenhoffer P, Grotz M, Pape HC, Lehmann U, Tscherne H: Treatment results of patients with multiple trauma: An analysis of 3406 cases treated between 1972 and 1991 at a German Level I Trauma Center. *J Trauma* 1995;38:70-78.

18. Eiseman B, Beart R, Norton L: Multiple organ failure. *Surg Gynecol Obstet* 1977;144:323-326.

19. Moore FA, Sauaia A, Moore EE, Haenel JB, Burch JM, Lezotte DC: Postinjury multiple organ failure: A bimodal phenomenon. *J Trauma* 1996;40:501-510.

20. Sauaia A, Moore FA, Moore EE, Lezotte DC: Early risk factors for postinjury multiple organ failure. *World J Surg* 1996;20:392-400.

21. Sauaia A, Moore FA, Moore EE, Norris JM, Lezotte DC, Hamman RF: Multiple organ failure can be predicted as early as 12 hours after injury. *J Trauma* 1998;45:291-301.

22. Bone LB, Johnson KD, Weigelt J, Scheinberg R: Early versus delayed stabilization of fractures. *J Bone Joint Surg Am* 1989;71:336-339.

23. Bosse MJ, MacKenzie EJ, Riemer BL, et al: Adult respiratory syndrome, pneumonia, and mortality following thoracic injury and femoral fracture treated wither with intramedullary nailing with reaming or with a plate: A comparative study. *J Bone Joint Surg Am* 1997;79:799-809.

24. Schemitsch EH, Jain R, Turchin DC, et al: Pulmonary effects of fixation of a fracture with a plate compared with intramedullary nailing. *J Bone Joint Surg Am* 1997;79:984-996.

25. Brumback RJ, Virkus WW: Intramedullary nailing of the femur: Reamed versus nonreamed. *J Am Acad Orthop Surg* 2000;8:83-90.

26. Scalea TM, Boswell SA, Scott JD, et al: External fixation as a bridge to intramedullary nailing for patients with multiple injuries and with femur fractures: Damage control orthopedics. *J Trauma* 2000; 48:613-623.

27. Pape HC, Hildebrand F, Pertschy S, et al: Changes in the management of femoral shaft fractures in polytrauma patients: From early total care to damage control orthopedic surgery. *J Trauma* 2002;53:452-462.

28. Christie J, Robinson CM, Pell ACH, McBirnie J, Burnett R: Transcardiac echocardiography during invasive intramedullary procedures. *J Bone Joint Surg Br* 1995;77:450-455.

29. Coles RE, Clements FM, Lardenoye JW, et al: Transesophageal echocardiography in quantification of emboli during femoral nailing: Reamed versus unreamed techniques. *J South Orthop Assoc* 2000;9: 98-104.
      To quantify the embolic load to the lungs created with two different techniques of femoral nailing, the authors of this study randomized 11 patients with 12 traumatic femur fractures to receive reamed (7 fractures) or unreamed (5 fractures) femoral nails. They report that there was no difference in the presence and similarity of emboli generation with either method and that unreamed intramedullary nails do not necessarily protect patients from pulmonary embolization of marrow contents.

30. Ten Duis HJ, Nijsten MWN, Klasen HJ, Binnendijk B: Fat embolism in patients with an isolated fracture of the femoral shaft. *J Trauma* 1988;28:383-390.

31. Pape HC, Grimme K, van Griensven M, et al: Impact of intramedullary instrumentation versus damage control for femoral fractures on immunoinflammatory parameters: Prospective randomized analysis by the EPOFF study group. *J Trauma* 2003;55:7-13.

32. Sturmer KM: Measurement of intramedullary pressure in an animal experiment and propositions to reduce the pressure increase. *Injury* 1993;24(suppl 3):S7-S21.

33. Schemitsch EH, Jain R, Turchin DC, et al: Pulmonary effects of fixation of a fracture with a plate compared with intramedullary nailing: A canine model of fat embolism and fracture fixation. *J Bone Joint Surg Am* 1997;79:984-996.

34. Townsend RN, Lheureau T, Protech J, et al: Timing fracture repair in patients with severe brain injury. *J Trauma* 1998;44:977-982.

35. Giannoudis PV, Veysi VT, Pape HC, et al: When should we operate on major fractures in patients with severe head injuries? *Am J Surg* 2002;183:261-267.

36. Anglen JO, Luber K, Park T: The effect of femoral nailing on cerebral perfusion pressure in head-injured patients. *J Trauma* 2003;54:1166-1170.

37. Ashbaugh DG, Bigelow DB, Petty TL, Levine BE: Acute respiratory distress in adults. *Lancet* 1967;2: 319-323.

38. Bernard GR, Artigas A, Brigham KL, et al: The American-European Consensus Conference on ARDS: Definitions, mechanisms, relevant outcomes, and clinical trial coordination. *Am J Respir Crit Care Med* 1994;149:818-824.

39. Bachofen M, Weibel ER: Structural alterations of lung parenchyma in the adult respiratory distress syndrome. *Clin Chest Med* 1982;3:35-56.

40. Dreyfuss D, Soler P, Basset G, Saumon G: High inflation pressure pulmonary edema: Respective effects of high airway pressure, high tidal volume, and positive end-expiratory pressure. *Am Rev Respir Dis* 1988;137:1159-1164.

41. Ranieri VM, Suter PM, Tortorella C, et al: Effect of mechanical ventilation on inflammatory mediators in patients with acute respiratory distress syndrome: A randomized controlled trial. *JAMA* 1999;282:54-61.

42. Ventilation with lower tidal volumes as compared with traditional tidal volumes for acute lung injury and the acute respiratory distress syndrome: The Acute Respiratory Distress Syndrome Network. *N Engl J Med* 2000;342:1301-1308.

   The authors conducted a trial to determine whether ventilation with lower tidal volumes would improve the clinical outcomes in patients with acute lung injury and the acute respiratory distress syndrome. It was concluded that mechanical ventilation with a lower tidal volume than is traditionally used for this patient population results in a decreased mortality rate and an increased number of days without ventilator use.

43. Combes A, Costa MA, Trouillet JL, et al: Morbidity, mortality, and quality-of-life outcomes of patients requiring ≥ 14 days of mechanical ventilation. *Crit Care Med* 2003;31:1373-1381.

   The authors conducted this study to determine the outcome and health-related quality of life of 347 patients requiring ≥14 days of mechanical ventilation in the intensive care unit and report that prolonged mechanical ventilation was associated with impaired health-related quality of life compared with that of a matched general population. Nonetheless, 99% of the patients evaluated were independent and living at home 3 years after discharge.

44. Herridge MS, Cheung AM, Tansey CM, et al: One-year outcomes in survivors of the acute respiratory distress syndrome. *N Engl J Med* 2003;348:683-693.

   This study was conducted to assess the long-term outcomes of 109 survivors of ARDS. Patients were evaluated 3, 6, and 12 months after discharge from the intensive care unit, at which time they were interviewed and underwent a physical examination, pulmonary-function testing, a 6-minute-walk test, and a quality-of-life evaluation. The survivors of ARDS were noted to have persistent functional disability 1 year after discharge and most patients had extrapulmonary conditions, such as muscle wasting and weakness.

45. Ullrich R, Lorber C, Roeder G, et al: Controlled airway pressure therapy, nitric oxide inhalation, prone position, and extracorporeal membrane oxygenation (ECMO) as components of an integrated approach to ARDS. *Anesthesiology* 1999;91:1577-1586.

46. Gattinoni L, Presenti A, Bombino M, et al: Relationships between lung computed tomographic density, gas exchange, and PEEP in acute respiratory failure. *Anesthesiology* 1988;69:824-832.

47. Gattinoni L, Pelosi P, Suter PM, Pedoto A, Vercesi P, Lissoni A: Acute respiratory distress syndrome caused by pulmonary and extrapulmonary disease: Different syndromes? *Am J Respir Crit Care Med* 1998;158:3-11.

48. Angus DC, Linde-Zwirble WT, Lidicker J, Clermont G, Carcillo J, Pinsky MR: Epidemiology of severe sepsis in the United States: Analysis of incidence, outcome, and associated costs of care. *Crit Care Med* 2001;29:1303-1310.

   In this seven state study, the authors reviewed data on 192,980 patients with severe sepsis and concluded that it is a common, expensive, and frequently fatal condition, with as many deaths annually as those from acute myocardial infarction. It is especially common in the elderly population and the incidence is likely to increase significantly as the United States population ages.

49. Dinarello CA: Proinflammatory and anti-inflammatory cytokines as mediators in the pathogenesis of septic shock. *Chest* 1997;112(suppl 6):321S-329S.

50. Landry DW, Oliver JA: The pathogenesis of vasodilatory shock. *N Engl J Med* 2001;345:588-595.

51. Cohen J: The immunopathogenesis of sepsis. *Nature* 2002;420:885-891.

   The author of this article discusses the basic principles governing bacterial-host interactions and new opportunities for therapeutic intervention.

52. Bernard GR, Vincent JL, Laterre PF, et al: Efficacy and safety of recombinant human activated protein C for severe sepsis. *N Engl J Med* 2001;344:699-709.

   In this randomized, double-blind, placebo-controlled, multicenter study of 1,690 patients with systemic inflammation and organ failure due to acute infection were randomized to

2eceive an intravenous infusion of either placebo (N = 840 patients) or drotrecogin alfa activated (24 µg/kg of body weight per hour) (N = 850 patients) for a total duration of 96 hours to determine whether treatment with drotrecogin alfa activated reduced the mortality rate among patients with severe sepsis. The authors reported that the mortality rate was 30.8% in the placebo group and 24.7% in the drotrecogin alfa activated group and concluded that although treatment with drotrecogin alfa activated significantly reduced the mortality rate in patients with severe sepsis, it may be associated with an increased risk of bleeding.

53. Ullrich R, Scherrer-Crosbie M, Bloch KD, et al: Congenital deficiency of nitric oxide synthase 2 protects against endotoxin-induced myocardial dysfunction in mice. *Circulation* 2000;102:1440-1446.

54. Rivers E, Nguyen B, Havstad S, et al: Early goal-directed therapy in the treatment of severe sepsis and septic shock. *N Engl J Med* 2001;345:1368-1377.

    This study was conducted to evaluate the efficacy of early goal-directed therapy before admission to the intensive care unit. Of the 263 enrolled patients, 130 were randomly assigned to receive early goal-directed therapy and 133 to receive standard therapy. The authors found no significant differences between the groups with respect to base-line characteristics. In-hospital mortality was 30.5% in the goal-directed therapy group versus 46.5% in the standard therapy group (*P* = 0.009). They concluded that early goal-directed therapy can provide significant benefits regarding outcome in patients with severe sepsis and septic shock.

55. van den Berghe G, Wouters P, Weekers F, et al: Intensive insulin therapy in critically ill patients. *N Engl J Med* 2001;345:1359-1367.

    This prospective, randomized, controlled study was conducted to determine whether the normalization of blood glucose levels with insulin therapy improves the prognosis for 1,548 patients with hyperglycemia and insulin resistance. At 12-month follow-up, intensive insulin therapy reduced mortality during intensive care from 8.0% with conventional treatment to 4.6% (*P* < 0.04, with adjustment for sequential analyses).

56. Annane D, Sebille V, Charpentier C, et al: Effects of treatment with low doses of hydrocortisone and fludrocortisone on mortality in patients with septic shock. *JAMA* 2002;288:862-871.

    This study was conducted to assess whether low doses of corticosteroids improve 28-day survival in 300 patients with septic shock and relative adrenal insufficiency. Patients were randomly assigned to receive either hydrocortisone (50-mg intravenous bolus every 6 hours) and fludrocortisone (50-µg tablet once daily) (N = 151) or matching placebos (N = 149) for 7 days. The authors found that low doses of hydrocorti-

sone and fludrocortisone significantly reduced the risk of death in patients with septic shock and relative adrenal insufficiency without increasing adverse events.

57. Sauaia A, Moore FA, Moore FE, et al: Epidemiology of trauma death: a reassessment. *J Trauma* 1995; 38:185-193.

58. Eddy VA, Morris JA, Cullinane DC, et al: Hypothermia, coagulopathy, acidosis. *Surg Clin North Am* 2000;80:845-854.

59. Gentilello LM, Pierson DJ: Trauma critical care. *Am J Respir Crit Care Med* 2001;163:604-607.

    The authors discuss intensive care unit correction of the triad of hypothermia, acidosis, and coagulopathy, as well as the frequent complication of abdominal compartment syndrome. They argue that prompt correction is required not only to allow expeditious completion of necessary surgical procedures, but because this triad, unless corrected, usually results in death during resuscitation.

60. Goodnight SH, Kennoyer G, Rappaport ST, et al: Defibrination after brain tissue destruction. *N Engl J Med* 1974;290:1043-1047.

61. Carson JL, Kelley MA, Duff A, et al: The clinical course of pulmonary embolism. *N Engl J Med* 1992; 326:1240-1245.

62. Rogers FB, Cipolle MD, Velmahos G, et al: Practice management guidelines for the prevention of venous thromboembolism in trauma patients: The EAST practice management guideline work group. *J Trauma* 2002;53:142-164.

63. Velmahos GC, Kern J, Chan LS, Oder D, Murray JA, Shekelle P: Prevention of venous thromboembolism after trauma: An evidence-based report. Part II: Analysis of risk factors and evaluation of the role of vena cava filters. *J Trauma* 2000;49:140-144.

    The authors performed a literature search and data analysis of the risk factors for venous thromboembolism and the role of vena caval filters in preventing PE and found that spinal injuries, spinal cord injuries, and age are risk factors for development of DVT. Although prophylactic placement of vena caval filters in selected trauma patients may decrease the incidence of PE, future research with well-designed studies is needed to provide definitive answers.

64. Fedullo PF, Tapson VF: Clinical practice: The evaluation of suspected pulmonary embolism. *N Engl J Med* 2003;349:1247-1256.

Chapter 12

Advances in the Enhancement of Bone Healing and Bone Graft Substitutes

Theodore Miclau, MD

Andrew H. Schmidt, MD

Fracture Healing

Fracture healing involves a unique, highly integrated sequence of events in which bone is restored to its pre-injury condition. This capacity for bone to regenerate into tissue identical to that of preinjured bone may be secondary to similarities in the cellular and molecular programs between skeletal formation and regeneration; the events that transpire during the maturation of a fracture callus into bone closely resemble those that occur during development and in the growth plates.[1] Fracture repair is clearly influenced by external factors, including the mechanical environment of the fracture site; motion at the fracture site results in healing primarily through cartilage formation (endochondral ossification), and stability favors the direct formation of bone (intramembranous ossification). Most fractures heal through a combination of intramembranous and endochondral ossification. From a cellular and molecular standpoint, there are at least four components necessary for the repair of skeletal tissues: (1) skeletal progenitor cells at the site of injury that can differentiate into cartilage or bone; (2) an extracellular matrix to provide a scaffold for the cells and a store for cytokines and growth factors; (3) cytokines and growth factors necessary for normal cell signaling; and (4) a blood supply to provide the necessary cells, nutrition, and molecules essential for healing.

After a fracture occurs, the architecture and vascular supply of the bone are disrupted. This results in a loss of mechanical stability, a decrease in the local oxygen tension and available nutrients, and a release of various factors into the site of injury. An inflammatory response is initiated, and macrophages and degranulating platelets infiltrate the fracture site, releasing cytokines, which include platelet-derived growth factor (PDGF), transforming growth factor-beta (TGF-β), and interleukin (IL)-1 and IL-6 (inflammatory stage of repair). These factors likely play a key role in the initiation of the repair process by acting on a variety of cells in the bone marrow, periosteum, and fracture hematoma.

Early after fracture occurs, periosteal preosteoblasts and local osteoblasts, characterized by the expression of osteocalcin, differentiate into new bone. There is an increase in mesenchymal cell proliferation, a phenomenon that is associated with factors such as acidic fibroblast growth factor (also known as FGF-1) and basic fibroblast growth factor (also known as FGF-2). These factors have mitogenic and angiogenic effects on fibroblasts, chondrocytes, and osteoblasts. Coincident with the formation of new bone, mesenchymal cells and fibroblasts proliferate and eventually replace the fracture hematoma. Primitive mesenchymal and osteoprogenitor cells also express several of the bone morphogenetic proteins (BMPs), members of the subfamily of the TGF-β superfamily of polypeptides, which play key roles in cell growth, differentiation, and apoptosis (programmed cell death). Stem cells likely originate from a variety of sources, including the bone marrow, periosteum, local muscle and soft tissues, and vasculature.

As the fracture hematoma becomes more mature, the network of new blood vessels in the healing fracture callus becomes more extensive. These new vessels likely provide a source of progenitor cells and growth factors, which influence the differentiation of mesenchymal cells. The fracture hematoma develops a collagenous matrix composed of various collagen isotypes that may present cytokines such as TGF-β, PDGF, FGF, and BMPs to receptive cells. Type I and type II collagen contribute to the integrity of the noncartilaginous and cartilaginous extracellular matrix, respectively. Mesenchymal cells form aggregates, which express factors such as *Sox9* that upregulate cartilage specific genes, such as type II collagen. These mesenchymal cells differentiate into chondrocytes, which stabilize the fracture through the formation of a cartilaginous callus (soft callus phase of repair). Shortly after the induction of type II collagen, the chondrocytes proliferate and differentiate and are characterized by the expression of genes, such as Indian hedgehog (*Ihh*), which influence these activities. As chondrocytes continue to mature and progress to hypertrophy, the cells begin to express type X collagen and release proteases that degrade the extracellular matrix. Hypertrophic chondrocytes also express factors such as runt-related transcription factor 2, which is essential for ossification and affects cell differentiation by regulating the extracellular matrix proteins osteocalcin and osteopontin.

The conversion of hypertrophic cartilage to bone is a complex, spatially organized phenomenon involving the coordination of terminal chondrocyte differentiation, apoptosis, extracellular matrix degradation, angiogenesis, and osteogenesis. As the hypertrophic chondrocytes undergo differentiation, the cartilage begins to calcify at the junction of the maturing cartilage and newly formed woven bone (hard callus stage of fracture repair). Once the hypertrophic chondrocytes reach terminal differentiation, the cells undergo apoptosis, the extracellular matrix degrades and new blood vessels invade the interface. Although it is not clear whether hypertrophic chondrocyte apoptosis stimulates vascular invasion or angiogenesis stimulates programmed cell death, angiogenesis is likely critical for this coupled event.

Although the regulation of extracellular matrix degradation and angiogenesis is not clear, several molecules, including key angiogenic factors, have been identified in this process. These molecules include TGF-β, FGFs, insulin-like growth factors (IGFs), and vascular endothelial growth factor (VEGF). VEGF, a highly specific mitogen for vascular endothelial cells, binds to receptors expressed in endothelial cells[2] and acts in conjunction with matrix metalloproteinases (MMPs) to degrade the hypertrophic cartilage matrix and stimulate new blood vessel formation. For example, mice deficient in MMP-9 have an abnormal delay in the replacement of hypertrophic cartilage by bone.[3] This delay can be overcome by the delivery of VEGF, suggesting that extracellular matrix degradation is critical for the vascularization of the fracture callus.

As hypertrophic cartilage continues to be replaced by bone, a variety of osteoblast-related factors (BMPs, TGF-β, IGFs, and osteocalcin) and collagen-related factors (types I, V, and XI) continue to be expressed widely in the callus. The newly formed woven bone then undergoes remodeling through organized osteoblast and osteoclast activity (remodeling stage of repair). Ultimately, the mature bone is not distinguishable from the surrounding bone and contains a host of growth factors, including TGF-β, BMPs, and IGFs.

Effects of Fracture Fixation on the Healing Response

Interfragmentary Strain Theory

Fracture healing takes place through a complex cascade of biologic events that occur in a changing mechanical environment. Repair, however, will not progress unless the mechanical environment is also optimal; both rigidly fixed and excessively mobile fractures can lead to non-

union. The interfragmentary strain theory explains one possible link between mechanical forces and biologic events.[4] Mechanically, tissue strain exists when tissue deformation occurs in response to an applied force. Strain is defined as the change in the length of an object divided by its resting length. At the site of a fracture, interfragmentary strain refers to the mechanical strain sustained by tissue in the fracture site, and it is determined by the size of fracture gap and the amount of motion that occurs across the fracture site. When the fracture gap is small (for example, in a transverse fracture with the bone ends approximated together), any motion will result in fairly large strains because all motion that occurs is dissipated across a small distance. In contrast, when the same amount of deformation occurs across a comminuted fracture, the interfragmentary strain is much less because the same motion occurs across a larger area.

This concept is important because endochondral ossification—a key process for fracture repair—likely occurs within a well-defined range of tissue strain. During normal fracture healing, the stiffness of the tissue in the fracture gap increases with time, resulting in progressively lower interfragmentary strain. An appropriate level of strain may then enable the cellular events that govern the production of cartilage, which subsequently ossifies. If tissue strains are too high or too low, endochondral ossification may not occur. If the fracture is rigidly immobilized and the bone ends are directly apposed, the fracture can still heal by the process of primary bone healing. With too much motion, the tissue may remain fibrous (a type of tissue that accommodates large strains), and endochondral ossification may not occur. Although fracture healing is a complex process, this basic concept explains much about the behavior of fractures that are treated surgically or nonsurgically.

Fracture Healing With Plates and Screws

Traditionally, plate fixation of fractures has been associated with absolute fracture stability. In this paradigm, the bone ends are compressed and rigidly fixed. Interfragmentary strains are low, and the healing response is limited to bone formed through intramembranous ossification. As the bone ends undergo normal remodeling, the fracture gap is bridged and primary bone union occurs, particularly in the periosteal and endosteal regions near the site of injury. When fracture fixation is inadequate, increased motion may occur, resulting in excessive interfragmentary strain with the possibility of a nonunion or loss of fixation.

More recently, plates have been applied to bone with a less invasive technique that uses longer plates and fewer screws. The fracture itself is reduced by indirect rather than direct methods. This provides less rigid fixation; however, for a comminuted fracture the interfragmentary strain remains low and the biologic advantages of this approach are tremendous. These advantages include less surgical trauma to the soft tissues, decreased disruption to the blood supply, and avoidance of disruption of the fracture hematoma. Clinically, these minimally invasive plating techniques have resulted in increased callus formation, decreased time to union, and decreased incidences of complications such as infection and delayed healing.

Fracture Healing With Intramedullary Nails

Intramedullary nailing is a commonly used method that is the treatment of choice for many long bone fractures. The intramedullary device splints the bone internally and the implant is inserted through a point distant to the site of injury. The advantages of intramedullary fixation include reliable alignment of the fractured bone and minimal disruption of the soft tissues, fracture hematoma, and external blood vessels. Flexible intramedullary nails and rigid nails locked proximally and distally both have motion at the fracture site that results in the formation of a cartilaginous callus originating primarily at the periosteum. More rigidly fixed fractures are associated with less callus formation. Reamed intramedullary nail insertion is associated with a greater disruption of the endosteal circulation in experimental models. However, clinically there have been no clear differences in healing rates between reamed and nonreamed intramedullary nail insertion. Endosteal circulation can also be influenced by the degree of reaming and the fit of a nonreamed intramedullary nail. Locked intramedullary nails can be dynamized in certain clinical situations, such as in the treatment of transverse fractures, to allow for axial loading at the fracture site.

Fracture Healing With External Fixation

External fixation is a versatile method that allows surgeons a near-infinite number of possibilities for frame construction. Consequently, the relative rigidity of the fixation can be customized by adjusting the placement of unilateral, multiplanar, and circular ring external fixators. External fixator construct stiffness is greater when larger diameter pins are used, pins incorporate a longer segment of bone, more pins are used, pins are placed in multiple planes, and bars are closer to the bone. Furthermore, external fixators may be dynamized during treatment by changing the configuration of the frame to increase its flexibility. Because fractures treated with external fixation tend to have increased motion at the fracture site, union usually occurs via abundant callus formation. Studies indicate that less rigid external fixation tends to promote periosteal new bone formation, whereas more rigid fixation diminishes the periosteal reaction.[5] Axially dynamized external fixation facilitates periosteal bone formation. However, the ideal amount of stability at the fracture site is not known.

TABLE 1 | Properties of Bone Grafts
Characteristic/Type
Source
Autologous
Allogeneic
Form
Powder
Paste/gel
Granular
Fibers
Bulk
Mechanism of action
Osteoconductive
Osteoinductive
Osteogenic

Biologic Enhancement of Fracture Healing

Impaired fracture healing and posttraumatic bone defects are commonly encountered clinical problems. Traditionally, autogenous bone graft derived from local metaphyseal bone or the iliac crest has been the treatment of choice to stimulate healing. Autogenous bone grafting, however, is commonly limited by the amount of available bone and is associated with pain and donor site morbidity (in as many as 30% of patients). Bone grafts and bone graft substitutes are characterized by several properties, including their source, physical form, chemical composition, and biologic potential (Table 1). Purely osteoconductive materials will promote bone formation in a well-vascularized, stable bone defect, whereas osteoinductive or osteogenic material is needed to stimulate bone formation in patients in whom healing is less conducive, such as those undergoing posterolateral spine fusion or patients with a posttraumatic bone defect. Assessment of the relative efficacy of one bone graft preparation over another is limited by a lack of comparative human studies, variability in the physiology of bone grafting among species and among anatomic locations, and the inability to extrapolate animal data directly to humans. A wide variety of bone graft substitutes have been developed for clinical application and include calcium phosphates and coralline ceramics, calcium sulphate, collagen composites, demineralized bone matrix (DBM), and BMPs.

Bone Grafts
Autogenous Cancellous Bone Graft
Autogenous bone has long been considered to represent the best material for bone grafting, but its use is limited by donor site morbidity and the quantity of bone that is available. Commonly, autologous cancellous bone graft is harvested from the iliac crest, distal femur, or proximal

tibia. Autogenous bone contains all of the ingredients that are now known to be necessary to stimulate bone healing, namely an osteoconductive matrix, osteoinductive signaling molecules (including growth factors), and cells capable of responding to these signals. Approximately 80% of the osteogenic capacity of autograft is the result of the presence of mesenchymal stem cells within the harvested bone. These stem cells are capable of differentiating into osteoprogenitor cells in the correct mechanical and biologic conditions. The absence of viable mesenchymal stem cells from most bone graft substitutes is the reason that autograft remains the "gold standard" for bone grafting. Fresh autologous bone has long been the traditional source of bone graft. Autogenous cortical bone is occasionally used, but sources of autogenous cortical bone are usually limited to strips of the iliac crest or segments of the fibula.

Autogenous Bone Marrow

Bone marrow aspirates contain mesenchymal stem cells that are capable of differentiating into bone-forming cells given the appropriate stimulation. These cells have demonstrated osteogenic capacity when placed into non-healing bone defects in both animal models and in human tibial nonunions. The osteogenic potency of a bone marrow aspirate is proportional to the amount of mesenchymal stem cells contained in the aspirate. The concentration of mesenchymal stem cells is optimized by aspirating no more than 2 mL of bone marrow from any one site.[6] The concentration of mesenchymal stem cells in a bone marrow aspirate can be increased by exploiting the ability of mesenchymal stem cells to attach to surfaces, as is done in at least one commercially available system (Cellect, ACE/DePuy Orthobiologics, Warsaw, IN). Bone marrow aspirates may also be combined with osteoconductive materials such as DBM or synthetic bone substitutes.

Cortical Bone Autograft

Autogenous cortical bone is used much less commonly as a source of bone graft because of its more limited osteogenic capacity and its potentially greater donor site morbidity. When cortical bone is harvested, there is, by definition, a cortical bone defect that serves as a mechanical stress riser. There are few bones that are expendable, and the fibula and iliac crest are the primary sources of autogenous cortical bone. Either graft source can be taken with or without a vascular pedicle. Nonvascularized iliac crest grafts have been used for nonunions of the clavicle or small bones of the hands or feet. Vascularized fibular strut grafts have most commonly been used in the treatment of osteonecrosis of the hip or nonunions of the femoral neck, but they have also been used to restore large defects in the humerus, femur, or tibia. Pedicled vascularized grafts from the iliac crest have been used to treat osteonecrosis of the femoral head, whereas similar grafts taken from the volar aspect of the distal radius

have been used in the management of lesions of the hand or forearm, including scaphoid nonunion and Kienböck's disease.

Allogeneic Bone Grafts

Allogeneic bone harvested from tissue donors is a versatile source of bone, and it is available in whole or partial segments of long bones in the form of small cancellous blocks and DBM. Bulk bone grafts may be provided with attached tendons, such as in the Achilles tendon-calcaneal graft or the patella-patellar tendon-tibial tubercle graft. Allogeneic bone is typically used as an alternative to autogenous bone whenever the latter is not warranted. However, frozen or freeze-dried allograft bone is primarily osteoconductive because it does not contain viable cells. Fresh allograft bone, although potentially more osteogenic than processed allograft, is rarely used because of logistic problems with its preparation, maintenance of sterility, and increased potential for disease transmission. Thus, most allograft bone preparations have decreased osteogenic potential with decreased rates of incorporation and remodeling than autologous bone graft. Freeze-drying also degrades the mechanical properties of bone, which further limits the application of allograft bone in situations where structural support is needed. Finally, the use of allograft bone may generate a detrimental immunologic response against the bone graft.

Bone Graft Extenders and Potential Substitutes

A wide range of synthetic bone graft substitutes is available for clinical use and can be broadly categorized into several groups. All synthetic bone graft substitutes are osteoconductive, but vary in their composition, ease of resorption, degree of remodeling, mechanical strength, handling, and cost. These materials have little, if any, osteoinductive activity. These synthetic materials mimic the mineral phase of bone, are typically available in a bottled or paste form, and are variably remodeled into normal bone when inserted into a bone defect. In addition, there are several commercially available bone graft substitutes that represent combination products—typically a mixture of an osteoconductive material with some form of osteoinductive agent.

Calcium Phosphates and Coralline Ceramics

Ceramics comprise a class of compounds with a highly crystalline structure that are made from the sintering of natural mineral salts. Hydroxyapatite is a ceramic that is derived from tricalcium phosphate; it is a very stable biocompatible compound with excellent osteoconductive properties. Because of its highly crystalline form, hydroxyapatite is resorbed from bone very slowly. Hydroxyapatite compounds are synthesized or made from processed coral. Specific species of sea coral contain a calcium carbonate exoskeleton that closely resembles the microstructure of bone. This material can be chemically converted to calcium phosphate, and it is commercially available as blocks of graft with pore sizes of 200 or 500 μm. Although this material has high compressive strength, it is brittle and resorbs very slowly. Its main application has been in the treatment of tibial plateau fractures where it serves as a filler material. Coralline hydroxyapatite can also be used as a carrier for BMPs.

To improve the handling characteristics and resorption of tricalcium phosphate ceramics, calcium phosphate cements were developed. These compounds have a chemical structure similar to dahlite, which is the predominant mineral in bone. These materials are created at the time of use by mixing powdered calcium phosphate and calcium carbonate with liquid sodium phosphate. The resulting paste hardens in an isothermic reaction that forms an osteoconductive compound with excellent compressive strength. A potential disadvantage of calcium phosphate cements is their poor resistance to shear or tensile forces. Furthermore, early clinical experience with these compounds has shown that they are incompletely resorbed in humans.[7]

Calcium Sulfate
Calcium sulfate (plaster of Paris) has been used as a bone void filler for more than 50 years. Calcium sulfate is rapidly resorbed and replaced by bone; in fact, it resorbs so quickly that bone formation may not completely follow. Because calcium sulfate preparations have been inconsistent in their crystallinity, calcium sulfate has unreliable mechanical properties. Presently, a medical grade calcium sulfate preparation is available that is used clinically as an antibiotic depot as well as a filler for stable bone defects, such as a metaphyseal defect resulting from fractures or tumors. Calcium sulfate may be mixed with DBM, and it is also being investigated as a carrier for osteoinductive molecules.

Collagen Composites
Recently, commercial products containing mixtures of different osteoconductive materials have become available, such as mixtures of calcium sulfate and DBM. Although many of these combined products are described as osteoinductive, they are primarily osteoconductive, and no definite advantage to the combined product has been demonstrated over any of the individual components. Another product uses type I collagen, the main component of the bone matrix. Although collagen alone has no potential as a bone graft substitute, the combination of collagen and materials that mimic the mineral phase of bone (such as tricalcium phosphate or hydroxyapatite) results in an osteoconductive material. The further addition of bone marrow or mesenchymal stem cells may result in an osteoinductive and osteogenic material. Several such combined products are available commercially. In one randomized, prospective study, bovine collagen mixed with hydroxyapatite and bone marrow aspirate was compared with autogenous bone graft in 249 fractures treated with internal or external fixation.[8] No significant differences between the composite graft and autogenous bone graft were found with respect to rates of union or functional outcome.

Demineralized Bone Matrix
DBM is obtained from allograft bone using a process of acid extraction, which yields a product containing much of the collagen and noncollagen protein components of bone as well as BMPs. These components are responsible for most of the osteoinductive potential of allograft bone. DBM is highly osteoconductive, but the osteoinductive potency of DBM is low to moderate and varies depending on how it is processed. Bone formation in animal models has been shown to vary among different forms of commercially available DBM, which is available in many forms, including powder, fibers, and pellets. DBM is most often used to treat nonunions, but its use is limited to situations where structural support is not needed or is provided by some other type of graft. DBM is frequently used as a bone graft extender to supplement autogenous bone graft. Because DBM is obtained from allograft bone, it can be a carrier of infectious agents.

Bone Morphogenetic Proteins
The BMPs continue to be of major interest as an osteoinductive factor. The BMPs are present in the bone matrix and are responsible for the osteoinductive ability of whole and demineralized bone preparations. These proteins induce mesenchymal stem cells to differentiate into osteogenic progenitor cells and to proliferate. This is followed by the process of endochondral ossification seen during fracture healing. Recently, many of the individual BMPs have been characterized and can be synthesized using recombinant technology. These recombinant molecules induce bone formation in a dose-dependent fashion and may be given in quantities that vastly exceed their normal amounts. A problem with the application of BMPs is the need for a suitable carrier, typically some type of collagen matrix. Of the more than 20 BMPs available, the BMPs that have been thus far considered for human use include BMP-2, BMP-7, and growth differentiation factor-5, with BMP-2 and BMP-7 being the most osteogenic. Currently, two BMPs are commercially available: BMP-7 (also known as osteogenic protein-1 [OP-1]) and BMP-2. In a human model in which OP-1 was used to treat a critically-sized fibular defect, it has been shown that human recombinant OP-1 caused more rapid bone bridging than a preparation of DBM alone.[9] In another study of 450 patients with open tibial fractures, BMP-2 was found to be better than the standard of care (no bone graft) when added at the time of final wound closure.[10]

Enhancement of Fracture Healing

Numerous hormones and peptides that may influence fracture healing are currently being investigated. Local and systemic administration of these growth factors or signaling molecules that influence the repair process have been reported.[11,12] Methods of administration include direct injection into the fracture, intravenous or intraperitoneal administration, and gene therapy. A wide range of factors have been studied, including those that have been described previously in this chapter. Recent studies have demonstrated osteogenic effects of the BMPs, VEGF, FGF, PDGF, and parathyroid and growth hormones, among other factors, in animal models.[11,13,14]

Autologous growth factors can be isolated from concentrations of platelets, which are contained in the buffy coat of centrifuged blood specimens. When the platelet degranulation process is initiated by the addition of activated thrombin, large quantities of several osteotropic growth factors are released that are active in the bone-healing cascade, including PDGF, FGF, VEGF. Platelet-rich plasma is easily obtained from whole blood using simple, commercially available devices, and it can be mixed with activated thrombin and an osteoconductive compound such as DBM or allograft bone to make a bone graft substitute. This technique is attractive because of its simplicity, low cost, autologous nature, and capacity to apply multiple growth factors simultaneously.

Physical Enhancement of Fracture Healing

The observation that mechanical stimuli can influence bone remodeling (Wolff's law) has formed the basis for the development of physical methods to enhance fracture repair. Ultrasound and electric stimulation are two techniques that use external stimuli to improve the healing response. Both methods continue to be widely studied, and products are commercially available that use each technique.[15]

Ultrasound

Low-intensity ultrasound has been shown to stimulate fracture healing in both animal models and in humans.[16] Although its precise mechanism of action is being investigated, the therapy is based on the application of a high-frequency acoustical pressure wave to transmit mechanical energy to the bone. Ultrasound therapy has been hypothesized to affect multiple stages of fracture repair. In support of this hypothesis, ultrasound has been shown to influence the levels of several growth factors expressed through the different stages of fracture repair, including TGF-β, IL-8, prostaglandin E$_2$, PDGF, FGF-2, and VEGF. Ultrasound therapy has also been shown to result in increased intracellular calcium levels that stimulate proteoglycan synthesis.

Low-intensity ultrasound is directed to the fracture site through a cutaneous transducer. As the rate of energy absorption is proportional to tissue density, bone absorbs a large proportion of the applied energy. Low-intensity ultrasound has been shown to decrease time to healing for radial and tibial fractures treated with casting. A recent meta-analysis demonstrated a significantly positive treatment effect in fractures treated nonsurgically, but the study did not show any additional healing benefit in fractures treated with reamed intramedullary nailing.[17]

Electric Stimulation

Electric stimulation of bone is based on the findings that electric fields can be generated under mechanical strain. The underlying hypothesis is that endogenous strain-generated fields are central to the mechanism of bone remodeling secondary to mechanical stimulation. Electric stimulation devices have been designed to simulate these endogenous electric fields to enhance bone regeneration and repair. The available devices employ inductive coupling, capacitive coupling, and direct current.

Inductive coupling devices use noninvasive external current-carrying coils that are driven by a signal generator to create a secondary electric field at the site of injury. Commonly available inductive coupling devices can generate pulsed electromagnetic fields, which penetrate a cast and create local electric fields. Inductive coupling stimulation potentially acts in multiple stages of fracture repair, including chondrogenesis, osteogenesis, and angiogenesis. Recent publications show that inductive coupling can influence the expression of various growth factors, including BMPs, TGF-β, IGF-2, and FGF-2. Other in vitro studies have demonstrated that osteoblasts respond to inductive coupling with an increase in alkaline phosphatase activity, osteocalcin synthesis, and collagen production. Unfortunately, published clinical studies have investigated the role of inductive coupling in established nonunions, so its effect in enhancing early fracture healing is unknown.

As with inductive coupling, capacitive coupling is noninvasive. The electric field is generated using an external alternative current signal generator and opposing cutaneous electrodes placed at the level of the fracture site. Direct current stimulation is an invasive method whereby surgically implanted electrodes (anode located in the soft tissues and cathode placed at the fracture site) generate a local electric current. Both have been proposed to act by stimulating local bone growth factor expression.

Annotated References

1. Ferguson C, Alpern E, Miclau T, Helms JA: Does adult fracture repair recapitulate embryonic skeletal formation? *Mech Dev* 1999;87:57-66.

2. Gerber HP, Vu TH, Ryan AM, Kowalski J, Werb Z, Ferrara N: VEGF couples hypertrophic cartilage re-

modeling, ossification and angiogenesis during endochondral bone formation. *Nat Med* 1999;5:623-628.

3. Colnot C, Thompson Z, Miclau T, Werb Z, Helms JA: Altered fracture repair in the absence of MMP-9. *Development* 2003;130:4123-4133.

    This study evaluates the role of MMP-9 on fracture healing. Mice lacking MMP-9 were found to have a delay in fracture healing that resembles a hypertrophic nonunion likely caused by a lack of VEGF bioavailability. The authors also reported that MMP-9 may also be a regulator of chondrogenic and osteogenic cell differentiation during early stages of repair.

4. Perren SM: Evolution of the internal fixation of long bone fractures: The scientific basis of biological internal fixation. Choosing a new balance between stability and biology. *J Bone Joint Surg Br* 2002;84: 1093-1110.

    This article synthesizes current thinking about the interplay among mechanical and biologic factors that affect fracture healing. In particular, the author discusses the evolution of fracture fixation devices and introduces the concept of biologic fixation.

5. Thompson Z, Miclau T, Hu D, Helms JA: A model for intramembranous ossification during fracture repair. *J Orthop Res* 2002;20:1091-1098.

6. Muschler GF, Boehm C, Easley K: Aspiration to obtain osteoblast progenitor cells from human bone marrow: The influence of aspirate volume. *J Bone Joint Surg Am* 1997;79:1699-1708.

7. Jansen J, Ooms E, Verdonschot N, Wolke J: Injectable calcium phosphate cement for bone repair and implant fixation. *Orthop Clin North Am* 2005;36:89-95.

    The authors of this review article discuss the efficacy of newly developed calcium phosphate cement when this material is used as a bone defect filler or gap filler around metal implants.

8. Chapman MW, Bucholz R, Cornell C: Treatment of acute fractures with a collagen-calcium phosphate graft material: A randomized clinical trial. *J Bone Joint Surg Am* 1997;79:495-502.

9. Geesink RG, Hoefnagels NHM, Bulstra SK: Osteogenic activity of OP-1 bone morphogenetic protein (BMP-7) in a human fibular defect. *J Bone Joint Surg Br* 1999;81:710-718.

10. Govender S, Csimma C, Genant HK, et al: Recombinant human bone morphogenetic protein-2 for treatment of open tibial fractures: A prospective, controlled, randomized study of four hundred and fifty patients. *J Bone Joint Surg Am* 2002;84-A:2123-2134.

    This is a prospective, randomized multicenter study that evaluated recombinant human BMP-2. The study concludes that recombinant human BMP-2 is safe and, at a dose of 1.5 mg/mL, significantly superior to the standard of care in reducing the frequency of secondary interventions as well as accelerating fracture healing in patients with open tibial fractures.

11. Lieberman JR, Daluiski A, Einhorn TA: The role of growth factors in the repair of bone: Biology and clinical applications. *J Bone Joint Surg Am* 2002;84-A:1032-1044.

    This article provides a comprehensive review of the mechanisms of action, functions, and potential clinical applications of a variety of growth factors during fracture repair.

12. Barnes GL, Kostenuik PJ, Gerstenfeld LC, Einhorn TA: Growth factor regulation of fracture repair. *J Bone Miner Res* 1999;14:1805-1815.

13. Street J, Bao M, deGuzman L, et al: Vascular endothelial growth factor stimulates bone repair by promoting angiogenesis and bone turnover. *Proc Natl Acad Sci USA* 2002;99:9656-9661.

    To determine whether VEGF is required for bone repair, the authors of this study inhibited VEGF activity during secondary bone healing via a cartilage intermediate (endochondral ossification) and during direct bone repair (intramembranous ossification) in a mouse model. They report that inhibition of VEGF dramatically inhibited healing of a tibial cortical bone defect, consistent with the discovery of a direct autocrine role for VEGF in osteoblast differentiation.

14. Andreassen TT, Willick GE, Morley P, Whitfield JF: Treatment with parathyroid hormone hPTH(1-34), hPTH(1-31), and monocyclic hPTH(1-31) enhances fracture strength and callus amount after withdrawal fracture strength and callus mechanical quality continue to increase. *Calcif Tissue Int* 2004;74:351-356.

15. Anglen J: The clinical use of bone stimulators. *J South Orthop Assoc* 2003;12:46-54.

16. Rubin C, Bolander M, Ryaby JP, Hadjiargyrou M: The use of low-intensity ultrasound to accelerate the healing of fractures. *J Bone Joint Surg Am* 2001;83: 259-270.

17. Busse JW, Bhandari M, Kulkarni AV, Tunks E: The effect of low-intensity pulsed ultrasound therapy on time to fracture healing: A meta-analysis. *CMAJ* 2002;166:437-441.

Chapter 13

Nonunions and Malunions

Kevin J. Pugh, MD

S. Robert Rozbruch, MD

Introduction

Nonunions are a significant clinical problem in the United States. It is estimated that 2% to 10% of all tibial fractures do not achieve union. This results in a large number of procedures performed to treat nonhealing fractures, increased morbidity for patients, and significant additional costs.

Fracture union occurs when the bone is repaired to a degree that it is mechanically able to function like the original bone. The patient experiences no pain, and there is clinical stability at the fracture site. Fracture unions are accompanied by radiographic evidence of healing.

A delayed union is a fracture that, although progressing toward union, has not healed in the expected amount of time for a comparable fracture. A nonunion is a fracture that will not heal. A nonunion is the result of an arrest of the repair process and radiographic or clinical evidence of healing has not been seen for months. Nonunions may have some clinical stability because they will have cartilage or fibrous interposition instead of bone. Although nonunions cannot be predicted, some fractures are destined to evolve to nonunion from the beginning of treatment.

Etiology

The etiology of a fracture nonunion is multifactorial. There is an interaction between fracture-related issues, the medical condition and habits of the patient, and the treating surgeon.

Not all fractures are created equally. Fractures result when the energy imparted to the bone during an injury exceeds the mechanical strength of the bone. Fractures disrupt not only the bone and its internal architecture, but the surrounding soft tissues as well. Traumatic stripping of the periosteum and disruption of the surrounding muscle and skin can deprive the fracture of the blood supply essential to healing. The more energy that is imparted to the limb, the greater this disruption.

Fracture Factors

Factors related to the fracture itself include the bone involved and the portion of the bone that is injured. Bones such as the talus, the metaphyseal-diaphyseal junction of the fifth metatarsal, and the scaphoid have well-known blood supplies. Some areas, such as the distal femur, have a robust blood supply, whereas others, such as the distal tibia, are relatively lacking blood supply. Fractures with bone loss, either bone that is lost at the scene of injury or to surgical débridement, are nonunions in evolution, and they require a staged approach to reconstruction. The degree of soft-tissue injury, whether in an open or closed fracture, also plays a role in whether a fracture achieves union. Open fractures are indicative of a high degree of soft-tissue devitalization, and they are a source of contamination and potential infection. High-grade soft-tissue injuries in closed fractures can also result in devitalized bone and altered healing.

Host Factors

Host factors also play a major role in fracture healing. Although young, healthy patients generally heal with little difficulty, those with preexisting medical conditions can have a decreased ability to recover from injury. Patients with chronic disease such as diabetes, heart disease, and chronic obstructive pulmonary disease do not fare as well. Patients who are immunosuppressed, for whatever reason, be it the result of rheumatoid disease, malignancy, malnutrition, human immunovirus, or steroid use will heal slower. Smoking has been shown to decrease the rate of fracture healing in many studies.

Surgical Factors

Surgery also greatly influences the ability of fractures to heal. Fractures require a stable mechanical environment to unite. Fractures treated with constructs that provide relatively nonrigid immobilization such as casts, external fixation, or bridge plating heal via secondary bone healing with the formation of callus.[1] Essential to this form of treatment is stable fixation that allows some motion at the fracture site. Inadequate fracture fixation, whether from a poorly applied cast or a poorly planned external fixator, will lead to too much motion and inadequate healing. Fractures treated with rigid internal fixation rely on primary bone healing to unite. In this type of bone healing, areas of bone undergo direct remodeling by cutting cones, and adequate compression is essential to success. Reductions that leave a gap, malposition the fragments, or leave soft tissue interposed often lead to slow healing. Excessive iatrogenic stripping of the bone adds to the soft-tissue injury inherent in the fracture, leading to a suboptimal biologic environment, slow healing, and possible infection. Infrequent follow-up, premature weight bearing, or surgeon inattention to detail may also contribute to a less desirable result.

For most nonunions, the exact cause is difficult to pinpoint. Most are not the result of one clear-cut cause, but rather a combination of many of the factors discussed previously. The cause of many nonunions is never known. Surgeons who treat these challenging problems should attempt to identify and reverse the contributive factors they can control. Mechanical stability should be provided, soft-tissue envelopes should be respected to preserve blood supply, the biology of the fracture should be augmented when possible, and bone loss should be managed with shortening, grafting, or bone transport techniques.

Evaluation

The evaluation of a patient with a nonunion, just as with a patient with an acute injury, requires a thorough assessment of more than just the fracture pattern and the radiographs. The personality of the fracture must be determined. This involves a complete history of the events of the injury, the fracture, the host, the treating physician, and the institution at which the treatment will occur. Only with this kind of analysis can adequate preoperative planning be done that will optimize the chance for success.

Patient History

A complete patient history is essential. The mechanism of the fracture must be determined as well as that of other associated injuries, such as those involving the head, chest, or abdomen. Was the initial injury open or closed? Was there a high-energy mechanism such as a motorcycle accident or a lower-energy trip and fall? Were there any neurovascular issues present at the time of the initial injury or after treatment? A complete history of the initial treatment and all other previous treatment is necessary. A determination of the type and number of previous surgeries is essential, as is the presence and treatment of previous infection. If there is retained hardware at the fracture site, old surgical notes can be helpful in identifying its type and manufacturer for planned removal.

A complete picture of the patient must also be developed. A thorough past medical and surgical history must be obtained, as well as a list of current medications, allergies, and social habits. Have previous fractures healed in a timely fashion? Patients with recreational drug habits or other substance abuse may have compliance issues. Smokers are at risk because of the well-documented relationship between nicotine use and delayed fracture healing.[2] The occupation of the patient is also important because treatment that requires a non–weight-bearing gait will require more time off from work for a laborer than a patient with a more sedentary occupation.

Physical Examination

A complete musculoskeletal examination is important. Examination of the patient's other extremities will provide clues as to additional disabilities that may play a role in mobility and later rehabilitation. Examination of the nonunited segment includes an inspection for gross deformity and overall limb alignment. Gross limb length can be measured, and if the patient is ambulatory, the gait pattern should be assessed. The skin should be inspected for the presence, location, and healing status of previous open wounds and incisions. The presence or absence of lymphedema or venous stasis should be noted. If previous external fixators have been in place, the condition of the old pin sites should be examined. A complete neurovascular examination should be performed. The presence and character of the pulses should be noted. Patients with suspected dysvascular limbs should undergo more thorough testing, including transcutaneous oxygen tension and ankle-brachial indices. Existing nerve deficits can be examined and tested by electromyography to determine the likelihood of recovery. The fracture site should be checked for tenderness to manual stress, as well as the presence of gross or subtle motion. The motion of adjacent joints should be examined. If joint contracture is present, it should be determined if it is caused by soft-tissue contracture, heterotopic ossification, or both.

Radiographic Evaluation

Radiographic evaluation includes true AP and lateral radiographs of the problem limb segment orthogonal to the "normal" portion of the limb. If deformity or limb length issues are suspected, special radiographs are required. Long leg alignment films and scanograms should be obtained. Comparison films of the contralateral leg are helpful in determining normal alignment, and population norms can be used if the problem is bilateral. Although CT with reconstructions can be helpful in analyzing subtle nonunions, it can be difficult to interpret with fracture fixation devices in place. Plain tomography can be very helpful in these instances. If infection is suspected, a combined bone scan and radiolabeled white cell study can help differentiate bone turnover from active infection. Sinograms can be used to determine whether chronic wounds communicate with the fracture site. MRI can be helpful in the evaluation of bone for infection or the assessment of adjacent joints, but it is not commonly used in the evaluation of nonunions.

Laboratory Evaluation

Laboratory studies can complete the clinical assessment of the patient. In addition to routine preoperative tests and blood cell counts, patients suspected of having infection should have their erythrocyte sedimentation rate and C-reactive protein level assessed. Patients suspected of being malnourished should have a complete nutritional panel drawn, including liver enzymes and total protein and albumin levels.

Preoperative Planning

The last aspect of the evaluation of the personality of the fracture is an assessment of the surgeon and the treating facility. Preoperative planning should include timely and appropriate consultation with plastic or microvascular surgeons if flaps or wound issues are anticipated; vascular surgeons should be consulted if poor vascularity is suspected. The patient's primary care physician can help with the treatment of chronic medical conditions. Surgeons should honestly examine whether they have the training, skill, patience, and experience necessary to treat a complex nonunion. To assess the treating facility, it is important to determine whether the correct equipment is in the hospital or available to be brought in, whether there is experienced nursing and surgical assistance available, and whether the anesthesia staff can address the needs of a sick patient.

At the end of the evaluation, orthopaedic surgeons should create a problem list in anticipation of preoperative planning. This list should include pertinent positive factors about the patient's social condition and history, physical examination, bone, skin, and retained hardware. The consultations required should also be listed, as well as the equipment required for the surgical procedure. A preoperative plan should be prepared and drawn out in detail in all but the simplest of conditions (Figure 1).

Classification

Unlike acute fractures, there is no single definitive classification system for nonunions. Nonunions can be classified on the basis of anatomy, the presence or absence of infection, healing potential, or stiffness. More than one method of describing the nonunion is often helpful in determining a treatment plan.

The first issue to resolve is whether the fracture is a delayed union or a true nonunion. A delayed union may progress to a successful union over time, whereas a true nonunion will require intervention to achieve union. This is not a trivial issue to resolve. Although most nonunions will be diagnosed if the surgeon waits long enough, it is imperative to identify fractures that are falling behind in the healing process as soon as possible to shorten the overall treatment time and restore the patient to full function. Delaying intervention for an arbitrary length of time before calling a fracture a nonunion can result in more disability, more time off work, and greater psychologic stress for the patient. As soon as slow healing is identified, a frank discussion of the possibility of nonunion should be had with the patient about the need for further treatment. Many patients will opt for early intervention when it means an earlier return to work or recreational activities.

Nonunions are also classified by their anatomic location. Diaphyseal nonunions have relatively less biologic potential because they involve cortical bone, but they are amenable to a variety of treatment methods, including intramedullary nails, compression plating, and external fixation. The goal in this instance is to restore length and axial alignment while achieving fracture union. As the nonunion reaches the metaphyseal region, the goals remain the same, but the options for fixation are more limited. Periarticular nonunions may also be associated with stiff or contracted joints that must be accounted for in the preoperative plan. Nonunions of the articular surface are particularly challenging. Defining the extent of the nonunited segment may require multiple radiographs and CT scans. Step-offs, gaps, and injury to the joint surface may lead to local or global arthritis. Treatment may consist of open reduction and rigid fixation, arthrodesis, or arthroplasty.

Nonunions may be aseptic or infected. Although many studies have shown that bone constructs with adequate stability can heal in the face of infection, the general goal is to convert an infected nonunion into a noninfected nonunion, and then proceed with treatment of the fracture. Because many infected nonunions will have skin breakdown, open wounds, and drainage, the diagnosis is not always obvious. Laboratory studies can be helpful, as can nuclear medicine studies. The patient should be counseled that treatment might involve several staged procedures for hardware removal, débridement of dead bone, soft-tissue coverage, and stabilization. A course of intravenous antibiotics based on the results of thorough deep cultures should be followed by definitive reconstruction. Depending on the extent of the infection and bone resected, this may require a period of months. Failed soft-tissue coverage, failure to eradicate the infection, or failure to obtain union may lead to eventual amputation.

Nonunions can be classified on the basis of their biologic potential. Hypertrophic nonunions are characterized by abundant bone formation, and they are often

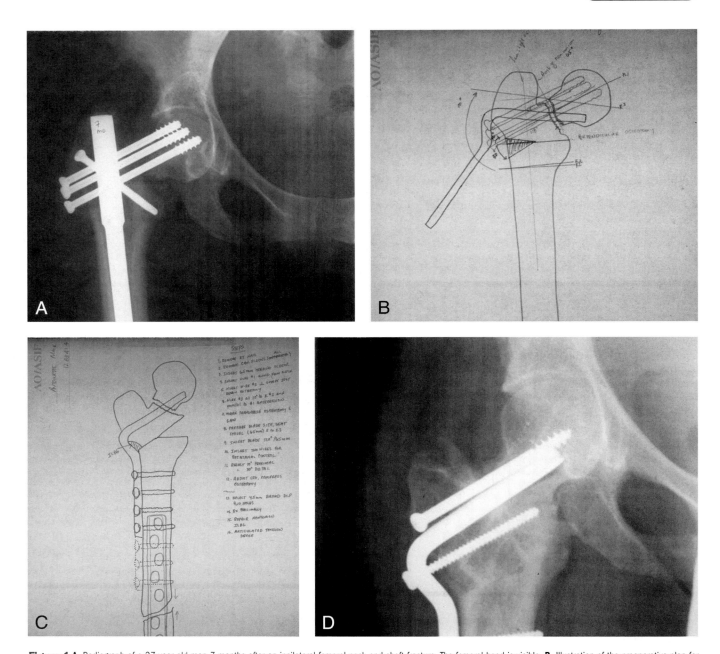

Figure 1 A, Radiograph of a 37-year-old man 7 months after an ipsilateral femoral neck and shaft fracture. The femoral head is visible. **B,** Illustration of the preoperative plan for a valgus-producing intertrochanteric osteotomy. The osteotomy that will convert the shearing forces at the fracture to compressive forces has been calculated. **C,** The final drawing illustrating and listing the step-by-step surgical plan for the osteotomy. By planning on paper preoperatively, orthopaedic surgeons can minimize mistakes and delays at the time of surgery. **D,** Radiograph obtained after the union of the osteotomy. The alignment demonstrated here is essentially that found on the preoperative plan.

referred to as having the appearance of an elephant's foot. In general, they are stiff and relatively stable. Patients are often able to bear weight with pain when they have a hypertrophic nonunion. These nonunions have excellent blood supply and biologic potential and often require only the addition of fracture stability to unite. Atrophic nonunions, conversely, have little biologic potential. Atrophic nonunions are often the result of open fractures or previous surgical procedures that have caused a disruption of the normal vascular supply to the bone. A cessation of the regeneration process has oc-

curred along with resorption of the bone ends and sometimes capping off of the endosteal canal of the bone. These nonunions are mobile; patients usually are unable to bear weight and may require external immobilization for comfort. A special type, the atrophic nonunion, is a true pseudarthrosis in which a false joint has been created between the two ends of the bone. These fractures require biologic stimulation in addition to skeletal stability. Bone grafting and other adjuvants often play a role in their treatment. Oligotrophic nonunions are somewhere in between these two extremes. They have

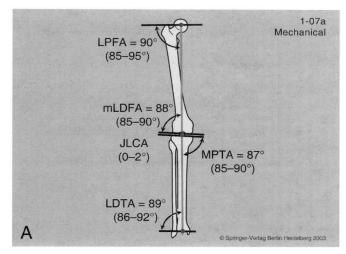

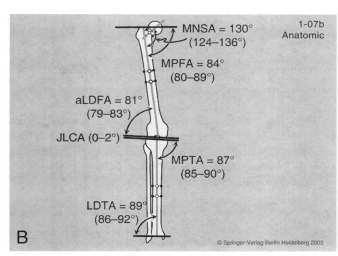

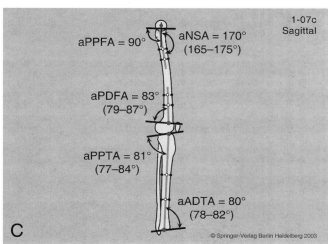

Figure 2 Normal mechanical axis values. **A,** Frontal plane joint orientation angle nomenclature and normal values relative to the mechanical axis. LPFA = lateral proximal femoral angle, mLDFA = lateral distal femoral angle relative to the mechanical axis, JLCA = joint line convergence angle, MPTA = medial proximal tibial angle, LDTA = lateral distal tibial angle. **B,** Frontal plane joint orientation angle nomenclature and normal values relative to the anatomic axis. MNSA = medial neck shaft angle, MPFA = medial proximal femoral angle, aLDFA = lateral distal femoral angle relative to the anatomic axis. **C,** Sagittal plane joint orientation angle nomenclature and normal values relative to the anatomic axis. aPPFA = anatomic posterior proximal femoral angle, aNSA = anatomic neck shaft angle, aPDFA = posterior distal femoral angle relative to the anatomic axis, aPPTA = posterior proximal tibial angle relative to the anatomic axis, aADTA = anterior distal tibial angle relative to the anatomic axis. *(Reproduced with permission from Paley D: Principles of Deformity Correction. Berlin, Germany, Springer-Verlag, 2002.)*

very little callus formation, but the bone ends are vital. They often require both biologic and mechanical augmentation.

Deformity

Deformity is an important issue with regard to both nonunions and malunions. With malunions, the deformity is the sole problem. With nonunions, deformity is often a crucial aspect of the problem. Although with nonunions, the treatment goals are achievement of bony union and correction of the deformity, correction of the deformity is the more central issue. To achieve bony union, the deformity must be corrected first because it is a key mechanical factor that is contributing to the nonunion. In the presence of deformity, the load during weight bearing creates a bending moment at the nonunion site—an unfavorable mechanical situation. With normal limb alignment, weight bearing achieves compression across the nonunion—a favorable mechanical situation.[3-6]

Limb deformity is a more important factor in lower extremities than upper extremities. Studies have sug-

gested that tibial malunions are associated with arthrosis of the knee and ankle.[7] The imprecision of such an analysis is that the absolute amount of angular deformity in the tibia is but one factor. The overall deformity of the limb is affected by the level of deformity, magnitude of angulation, translation, rotation, and shortening. For example, the same 7° angular deformity of the tibia will have a different effect on mechanical axis deviation of the knee and ankle depending on the level of the fracture and any associated translation. In some patients, angulation and translation can have an additive effect and in others they can cancel each other out, resulting in very little limb axis deformity.

Normal mechanical limb alignment is illustrated with a mechanical axis line drawn from the center of the hip to the center of the ankle. The location of this line relative to the center of the knee joint defines the mechanical axis deviation (MAD). Normal coronal plane alignment has a MAD of 0 to 8 mm medial to the center of the knee. The alignment of each bone can then be analyzed with joint orientation angles. Mechanical and/or anatomic analysis can be used (Figure 2). Al-

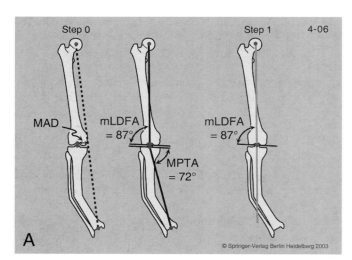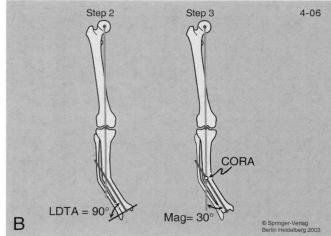

Figure 3 Calculation of diaphyseal deformity. **A,** Step 0: MAD medial to center of knee represents varus deformity. Normal lateral distal femoral angle (LDFA) shows absence of femoral deformity. Abnormal medial proximal tibial angle (MPTA) shows that the tibia is the source of the deformity. Step 1: The proximal mechanical axis line is extended from the normal femur. **B,** Step 2: The distal mechanical axis line is drawn. Step 3: The intersection of the proximal mechanical axis line and the distal mechanical axis line is the center of rotation and angulation (CORA), which identifies the location and magnitude of the deformity in the diaphysis of the tibia. *(Reproduced with permission from Paley D: Principles of Deformity Correction. Berlin, Germany, Springer-Verlag, 2002.)*

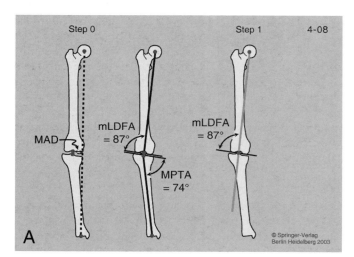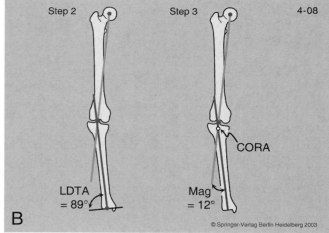

Figure 4 Calculation of metaphyseal deformity. **A,** Step 0: MAD is medial to the center of the knee, showing that there is a varus deformity. The femur has no deformity (normal lateral distal femoral angle [LDFA]). The tibia has varus deformity (abnormal medial proximal tibial angle [MPTA]). Step 1: The proximal mechanical axis line is extended from the normal femur. **B,** Step 2: The distal mechanical axis line is drawn. Step 3: The intersection of the proximal mechanical axis line and the distal mechanical axis line is the center of rotation and angulation (CORA), which identifies the location and magnitude of the deformity in the metaphysis of the proximal tibia. *(Reproduced with permission from Paley D: Principles of Deformity Correction. Berlin, Germany, Springer-Verlag, 2002.)*

though this type of analysis may be useful for a patient with mid-diaphyseal deformities (Figure 3), it is particularly useful for those with metaphyseal deformities or double level deformities (Figure 4). The location and magnitude of the deformity is identified by drawing antegrade and retrograde bone axis lines. The location of the intersection is the center of rotation and angulation. The angle between these lines is the magnitude of the deformity. If the center of rotation and angulation is not located at what seems to be the old fracture site, it usually means that there is associated translation deformity (Figure 5).

Analysis is done in the coronal plane using an AP radiograph and in the sagittal plane using a lateral radiograph. When deformity is present in both planes, it is consistent with an oblique plane deformity. It is actually one deformity in an oblique plane. For example, a tibia with varus and procurvatum has an oblique plane deformity with the apex of deformity in the anterolateral plane (Figure 6). The axis of correction is 90° to that plane. Gradual corrections can be performed with circular frames. Although the classic Ilizarov frame works well in these patients, the Ilizarov/ Taylor Spatial Frame (Smith & Nephew, Memphis,

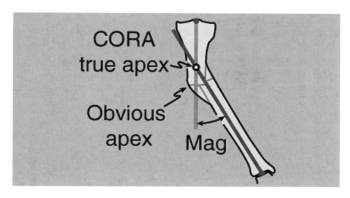

Figure 5 When the center of rotation and angulation (CORA) is not at the obvious malunion site, there is often associated translation deformity. *(Reproduced with permission from Paley D:* Principles of Deformity Correction. *Berlin, Germany, Springer-Verlag, 2002.)*

TN) simplifies the correction with the help of a computer program.[5,8] Acute corrections and internal fixation can also be done to correct deformities.

Limb-length discrepancy and limb alignment can be measured from a weight-bearing long leg radiograph. The short leg is placed on blocks to level the pelvis, and the height of the blocks is recorded. This can be done with the patient using crutches if necessary. A supine scanogram can also be used to measure limb-length discrepancy, but this is not useful for alignment analysis. Rotational deformity is best assessed on clinical examination with the patient in the prone position. Thigh-foot axis is used to assess rotational deformity of the tibia. A rotational profile of the femur is used to assess rotational deformity in the femur. CT can also be used for this purpose. CT cuts at the proximal femur, distal femur, proximal tibia, and distal tibia allow analysis of rotational deformity.[4]

Choosing a Treatment Method

Because the specific treatment of nonunion and malunion of all bones of the skeleton is a vast topic that is beyond the scope of this chapter, treatment principles that can be applied to all bones will be discussed. Each nonunion and malunion has a unique personality that must be understood to choose an appropriate treatment method. The personality of a malunion is defined by the elements of the deformity, which include location, length discrepancy, angulation, translation, and rotation. Additional factors that should be assessed to help determine the personality of a malunion include time since injury, patient symptoms, and patient age and health, previous hardware, and soft-tissue envelope. Assessment of all of these factors will help the orthopaedic surgeon determine the optimal treatment method. Nonsurgical treatment includes the use of a shoe lift. Surgical treatment includes epiphysiodesis in pediatric patients and osteotomy in adults and children. The tools available include

intramedullary rods, plates and screws, and external fixation. The methods include acute or gradual correction.

Epiphysiodesis of a long normal leg can be used to correct limb-length discrepancy in a growing child. A partial growth arrest after trauma leads to progressive angular deformity. To prevent further progressive deformity, the injured growth plate can be completely closed. This procedure can be combined with osteotomy for deformity correction and lengthening as needed.[4]

The personality of the nonunion can be identified by assessing all of the previously discussed factors plus additional characteristics, which include the presence of infection and drainage, bone loss, stability and healing potential of the nonunion, and neurovascular status of the limb. The treatment methods include nonsurgical management with bracing, shoe lift, and noninvasive stimulation with electricity or ultrasound.[9,10] Surgical methods and tools for nonunion repair include bone graft,[11,12] intramedullary rods,[13-19] plates and screws,[20-26] external fixation,[3,5,8,27-32] acute or gradual treatment, and bone transport[3,31] or free fibula grafting.[33-35] Soft-tissue coverage problems can be handled with skin grafts, rotational flaps, free tissue transfer, vacuum-assisted closure device,[36] and soft-tissue transport.[3,31] Amputation reconstruction may also be a primary or secondary treatment option. The experience of the orthopaedic surgeon and the hospital equipment and facilities also help determine treatment.

There are several biologic enhancements to bone healing, including autogenous bone graft, bone graft substitutes,[11] ultrasound, and electricity.[9,10] These are covered in detail in chapter 12. In patients with a delayed union, no infection or deformity, and a stable fixation construct, it is reasonable to try a noninvasive modality such as electricity or ultrasound. Studies have suggested that these modalities enhance bone healing.[9,10]

Bone graft can be used to stimulate the biology of the nonunion.[11,12] In patients with a stable fixation construct and no deformity or infection, bone graft materials can be effective in stimulating union. Bone graft is more typically used in conjunction with surgical repair of the nonunion and stabilization with internal or external fixation. Bone graft should be avoided in patients with infections and should not be used alone in patients with deformities or unstable fixation constructs.

Acute or Gradual Correction

Nonunions or malunions can be treated using either acute or gradual correction. Acute correction can be performed in conjunction with all methods of fixation including plates, intramedullary nails, and external fixation frames. Gradual correction requires the use of special frames or nails. The personality of the problem helps guide the orthopaedic surgeon toward the best method. For example, a tibial malunion with 15° valgus deformity and a 4-cm shortening would be best treated with an

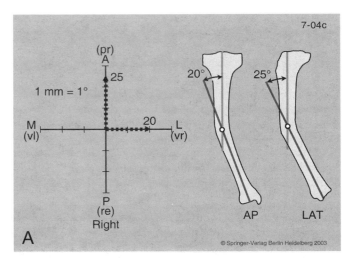

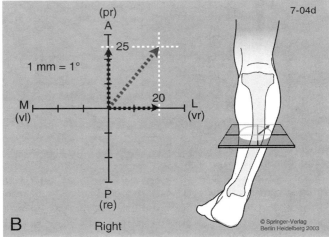

Figure 6 Calculation of oblique plane deformity. **A,** The 20° of varus identified on AP radiograph and the 25° of procurvatum identified on lateral radiograph are graphed as 20 apex lateral and 25 apex anterior. **B,** The resultant vector is the actual magnitude of deformity, with the apex in the anterolateral quadrant. *(Reproduced with permission from Paley D: Principles of Deformity Correction. Berlin, Germany, Springer-Verlag, 2002.)*

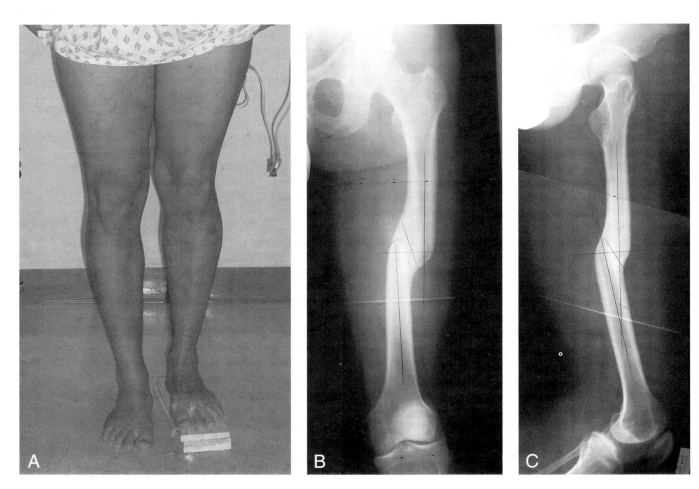

Figure 7 A, Preoperative front view photograph shows a patient with 4-cm lower limb shortening. Preoperative AP **(B)** and lateral **(C)** radiographs of the same patient show femur malunion with angular and translational deformity.

osteotomy to gradually correct the angular deformity and lengthen the bone with a specialized external fixa-

tion frame. The Ilizarov method is used to gradually correct the complete deformity with distraction osteogenesis. The deformity correction and lengthening may be performed at one level if bone regeneration potential is good. Alternatively, a double-level osteotomy may be performed—one level at the center of rotation and angulation for deformity correction and one level for lengthening in the proximal tibia metaphysis. Gradual correction achieves treatment of shortening and carries less risk of peroneal nerve neurapraxia than if attempted with an acute correction.

The use of plates and intramedullary nails requires an acute correction of angular and translational deformities. Acute correction is particularly useful for patients with modest deformities, mobile atrophic nonunions that are surgically approached and bone grafted, and small bone defects that can be acutely shortened. The principal advantage of acute correction is earlier bone contact for healing and a simpler fixation construct. Acute correction is generally better tolerated in the femur and humerus and less well tolerated in the tibia and ankle because of poor quality soft tissues and risk for neurovascular insult.[3,31]

Gradual correction with a specialized frame is useful for patients requiring large deformity correction, associated limb lengthening, bone transport to treat segmental defects,[3,30] and for stiff hypertrophic nonunion repair.[3,5,8,27,32,37] Gradual correction uses the principle of distraction osteogenesis, which is commonly referred to as the Ilizarov method.[3] Bone and soft tissue are gradually distracted at a rate of approximately 1 mm per day in divided increments. Bone growth in the distraction gap is called regenerate. The interval between osteotomy and the start of lengthening is called the latency phase and is usually 7 to 10 days. The correction and lengthening is called the distraction phase. The time from the end of distraction until bony union is called the consolidation phase. Of the phases of the Ilizarov method, the consolidation phase is the most variable and the most affected by patient factors such as age and health. If the structure at risk is a nerve, such as the peroneal nerve in a patient with a proximal tibia valgus deformity or the posterior tibial nerve in a patient with an equinovarus deformity of the ankle, gradual correction may be the safer option. The correction can be planned so that the structure at risk is stretched slowly.[3,4] If nerve symptoms do occur, the correction can be slowed or stopped. Nerve release can be used in selected patients based on the response to gradual correction.[4]

Gradual lengthening after acute correction of deformity can be accomplished with a specialized intramedullary nail that has the capacity for gradual elongation. This process uses the principle of distraction osteogenesis and has the advantage of avoiding external fixation. The principle disadvantage of gradual lengthening is the difficulty with distraction rate control[38] (Figures 7 and 8).

There are hybrid methods that use combinations of internal and external fixation for gradual lengthening

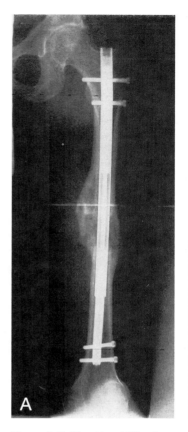
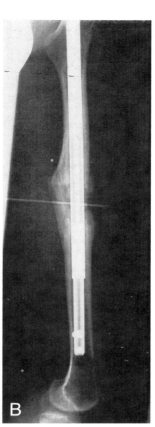

Figure 8 AP **(A)** and lateral **(B)** radiographs of the patient in Figure 7 6 months after surgery show correction of the deformity and lengthening of 4 cm with internal lengthening nail (ISKD, Orthofix, USA) in place.

and correction. With lengthening over a nail, an intramedullary nail is inserted after the osteotomy with only proximal interlocking screws. A frame is applied with no contact between internal and external fixation. The frame is used for distraction over the nail. Once distraction is complete, the nail is locked distally, and the frame is removed. This method has the principal advantage of substantially reducing the time patients must be in the external fixator because the nail supports the regenerate during the consolidation phase. Additional advantages over traditional lengthening include faster return of knee range of motion and protection against refracture.[39]

Another hybrid method is lengthening followed by nailing. A frame is applied with the pins placed so there will be no contact with future intramedullary nailing. The osteotomy is performed and gradual lengthening and correction is performed with distraction osteogenesis. Once distraction is complete, the statically locked intramedullary nail is inserted and the frame is removed. As with lengthening over a nail, the time patients must be in the external fixator is reduced and there is decreased risk of refracture compared with traditional lengthening. In addition, a longer and larger diameter intramedullary nail can be used for a more stable con-

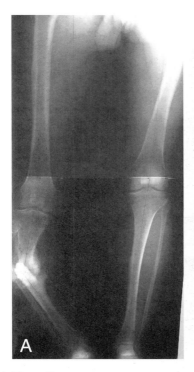
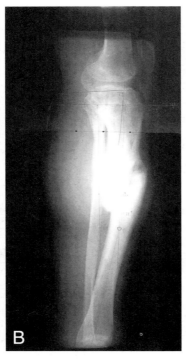
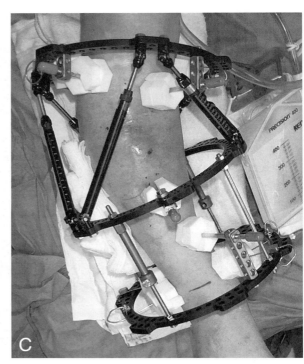

Figure 9 Preoperative AP **(A)** and lateral **(B)** radiographs show a hypertrophic tibia nonunion with deformity and shortening. **C,** Immediate postoperative photograph, frontal view, shows the Ilizarov/Taylor Spatial Frame in place matching the deformity.

struct. Gradual correction of both the deformity and the limb-length discrepancy can be accomplished before the intramedullary nailing procedure. Reaming through the regenerate appears to have a stimulatory effect, and bone healing is rapid.[40] The principal disadvantage of these hybrid methods is the increased risk of deep infection. This risk can be minimized with meticulous technique.

Hypertrophic Nonunion

An excellent application of gradual correction is for patients with a hypertrophic stiff nonunion with deformity. This type of nonunion has fibrocartilage tissue in the nonunion and has the biologic capacity for bony union. It lacks stability and axial alignment. Gradual distraction to achieve normal alignment results in bone formation. The nonunion acts similar to regenerate, and bony healing occurs. Modest lengthening of no more than 1.5 cm should be done through the nonunion. If additional lengthening is needed, a second osteotomy for lengthening is performed. Several studies have confirmed initial success with this technique.[3,5,27,32,37] The principal advantages of using gradual correction to treat patients with a hypertrophic stiff nonunion with deformity are not having to open the nonunion site in patients with poor skin quality and widened callus and gaining length through an opening wedge correction (Figures 9 and 10). This technique is not useful for treating patients with mobile atrophic nonunions and is less applicable to treating those with infected nonunions.

Hypertrophic nonunions can also be treated with internal fixation. Compression plating and intramedullary nailing can be used successfully, especially in patients with a relatively small deformity and healthy soft-tissue envelope.[26] Bone grafting is usually not required in this patient population.

Atrophic and Normotrophic Nonunions

Atrophic nonunions have fibrous tissue at the nonunion site and tend to be mobile. Treatment needs to be directed toward improving both the biology and the mechanical environment to achieve bony union. Normotrophic nonunions have both fibrous and fibrocartilage tissue at the nonunion site and are therefore less mobile than atrophic nonunions. Atrophic and normotrophic nonunions should be exposed, bone ends should be contoured so there is healthy bleeding bone on both sides with good contact, and intramedullary canals should be opened. Stripping of soft tissue should be performed in moderation. Acute correction of deformity should be followed by bone grafting and stable fixation with compression. This can be accomplished with a plate, intramedullary nail, or an external fixation frame depending on surgeon preference and location. Compression plating of aseptic humeral nonunions has been used successfully.[25,26] For diaphyseal nonunions of the humerus,

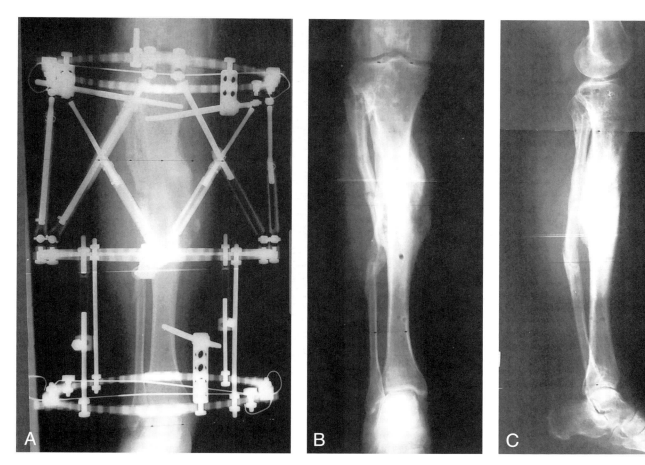

Figure 10 A, AP radiograph of the patient in Figure 9 5 weeks after surgical distraction of the nonunion. Note that no osteotomy and no open approach was performed. AP **(B)** and lateral **(C)** radiographs of the same patient 6 months after surgery show bony union and correction of deformity.

a second plate can be used 90° to the first or an allograft strut can be used if adequate stability is not achieved with one plate.[26] In contrast to acute fracture treatment where rigid stability is not the goal,[41] the goal for stabilization of nonunions should be a relatively rigid construct.[3,25,26]

Several studies have supported the use of reamed intramedullary nailing for the treatment of tibial[18,19] and femoral[13-17] nonunions. This is particularly useful in patients who have undergone previous intramedullary nailing and those with no infection or bone loss. Circular external fixation can also be used to treat atrophic and normotrophic nonunions. In patients with atrophic nonunions, the frame is used for stabilization after acute correction and an open approach. An advantage of using a frame is that in addition to the ability to acutely compress the nonunion in surgery, more compression can be added during the postoperative period. The frame is also stable enough to allow full weight bearing right after surgery.[28,30] Another method for treating recalcitrant normotrophic nonunions after intramedullary nailing in patients without deformity is augmentative Ilizarov frame fixation.[29] This allows intramedullary nail reten-

tion, and additional compression and stabilization is accomplished with the frame.

Normotrophic nonunions can also be treated with gradual correction. The nonunion can be approached in a minimally invasive fashion using 1- to 2-cm incisions. With the aid of intraoperative fluoroscopy, the nonunion can be mobilized with an osteotome, and the intramedullary canals can be opened by using a cannulated drill and curets. Bone graft can then be inserted. The frame is then applied and used to gradually correct the deformity (angulation and translation). Once this is accomplished, axial compression is then performed. Full weight bearing is allowed immediately after surgery. If additional length is needed, an osteotomy for gradual lengthening can be performed at a different site. Lengthening and then nailing techniques can be used in these patients. This provides autogenous bone graft from reaming and protects against refracture.

Nonunions after tibial pilon fractures can result in metaphyseal nonunion combined with ankle arthrosis. Infection, poor soft-tissue quality, and retained hardware often complicate these injuries. Treatment should be directed toward repair of the distal tibia, correction of the deformity, and ankle arthrodesis if necessary. This can be accomplished with internal[22] or external fixation. If bone resection is needed as in the case of infection, then ankle fusion and simultaneous tibial lengthening can be done with the Ilizarov method.[42]

Infection

Infected nonunions are complex injuries that are challenging to treat. Typically, infected nonunions are atrophic and mobile. They can also be stiff and hypertrophic. Infected nonunions are typically approached in an open fashion. The goals of surgery are to remove all dead bone, open the intramedullary canals, appose bleeding bone surfaces, and correct the deformity. The patient should ideally have not been receiving antibiotics for several weeks, and multiple intraoperative cultures and pathology specimens should be sent to the laboratory at the time of surgery. The nonunion is then mechanically stabilized. With the help of an infectious disease consultant, treatment of chronic osteomyelitis is rendered. This usually consists of culture-specific intravenous antibiotics for 6 weeks followed by an oral regimen. Removal of dead bone is needed to eradicate infection. Bone graft should not be used during the primary surgery. Antibiotic beads can be used for dead space management and local antibiotic delivery. Several weeks later, the antibiotic beads can be removed, and the nonunion can be bone grafted. The use of absorbable antibiotic beads made of calcium sulfate has been advocated by some to avoid the need for antibiotic bead removal and subsequent bone grafting.[43] Problems with persistent drainage have been reported using this technique.[43]

Stabilization can be accomplished with a plate, intramedullary rod, or an external frame. The plate and intramedullary rod have the disadvantage of adding foreign material to the infected site.[44] They can, however, be used with caution in patients with a nonpurulent infection of the femur or humerus. The use of internal fixation to treat an infected tibial nonunion or in any purulent infection primarily is fraught with risk. The use of a frame is the preferred approach in most patients with infection. It has the advantage of not adding foreign material to the infection site and can be used to treat more complex situations. If débridement of the nonunion results in a bone defect, the frame can be used for bone transport or acute shortening and gradual lengthening[3,30,31] (Figure 11).

Staging Treatment

Staging the treatment is an important strategy for nonunion management. In patients with infection, antibiotic beads may be removed after several weeks and bone graft inserted. In the patients in whom bone débridement resulted in a bone defect, gradual or acute shortening with a frame may be used. An osteotomy for lengthening

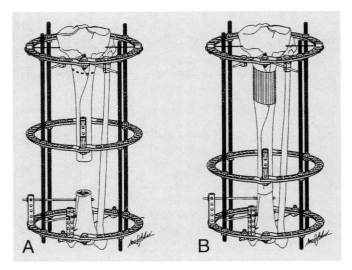

Figure 11 A, Illustration of bone transport used to treat a tibial bone defect. **B,** A proximal tibia osteotomy is shown. *(Reproduced with permission from Paley D:* Principles of Deformity Correction. *Berlin, Germany, Springer-Verlag, 2002.)*

can be done several weeks later, after the infection is cleared and after the patient and surgeon have decided on whether to perform limb lengthening or use a shoe lift. This has the advantage of protecting the osteotomy site from contamination. In addition, it is often difficult to predict the precise amount of bone resection needed. Once this is known, the patient and surgeon can make a more informed decision about limb lengthening.

When bone transport is used to treat a bone defect, the docking site should be prepared when there is a gap of approximately 1 cm. Preparation of the docking site includes débridement of fibrous tissue, realignment of bone ends to maximize bony contact and minimize deformity, and the addition of bone graft. This improves the rate of bony union.[31]

If the soft-tissue coverage is poor, flap coverage may be needed. A staged approach with a plastic surgeon can be helpful. For example, bone and soft tissue may be débrided and a simple frame applied that allows the plastic surgeon access to the wound. After flap coverage has been accomplished, bone transport can be done to treat a bone defect, or the flap can be elevated after several weeks and the nonunion site bone grafted.

Indications for Amputation

Attempts have been made to help determine indications for lower extremity amputation after acute trauma to avoid futile attempts at limb salvage. The indications for amputation after nonunion are complex and ever changing. There is a significant psychologic aspect to this; some patients believe that they have invested so much in saving the limb that they want to keep trying. Others have been worn out by the effort and are ready to move on after amputation. Some patients are not willing to have an amputation even if it is clear that it will improve functional outcome. When possible, below-knee instead of above-knee amputation should be done.

Indications for amputation have changed with the improved ability to reconstruct compromised limbs. Infection, bone loss, deformity, limb-length discrepancy, and poor soft-tissue coverage are no longer absolute indications for amputation. (If these indications were combined with an insensate foot and chronic neuropathic pain, it would be an indication for amputation.) The indications change with the ability of orthopaedic surgeons to successfully reconstruct the nonunion. Nevertheless, the factors that are most problematic are chronic neuropathic pain, lack of sensation on the plantar surface of the foot, and a stiff foot and ankle. The best treatment option for such patients is best determined by assessing all of the features of the nonunion and taking the needs of the individual patient into account.

Annotated References

1. Stoffel K, Dieter U, Stachowiak G, Gachter A, Kuster MS: Biomechanical testing of the LCP: How can stability in locked internal fixators be controlled? *Injury* 2003;34(suppl 2):B11-B19.

   This article discusses the mechanics of newer locked plating constructs. The concept of working length is discussed, as is the optimal screw placement for various fracture configurations.

2. McKee MD, DiPasquale DJ, Wild LM, Stephen DJ, Kreder HJ, Schemitsch EH: The effect of smoking on clinical outcome and complication rates following Ilizarov reconstruction. *J Orthop Trauma* 2003;17: 663-667.

   This study compares the results of Ilizarov reconstruction for nonunions in both smokers and nonsmokers. Nonsmokers had superior radiographic results, fewer complications, and better outcomes.

3. Ilizarov GA: Pseudoarthrosis and defects of long bones, in Ilizarov GA (ed): *Transosseous Osteosynthesis: Theoretical and Clinical Aspects of Regeneration and Growth of Tissue.* Berlin, Germany, Springer-Verlag, 1992, pp 454-494.

4. Paley D: *Principles of Deformity Correction.* Berlin, Germany, Springer-Verlag, 2002.

5. Rozbruch SR, Helfet DL, Blyakher A: Distraction of hypertrophic nonunion of the tibia with deformity using the Ilizarov/Taylor Spatial Frame. *Arch Orthop Trauma Surg* 2002;122:295-298.

   The authors of this study discuss the use of the Ilizarov/Taylor Spatial Frame in two patients with stiff tibial nonunion. The nonunions were not surgically approached. Distraction of the nonunion using the Ilizarov method

   resulted in bony union and correction of the deformity. The Taylor Spatial Frame is used in conjunction with a computer program and facilitates simultaneous correction of angular, translation, and length deformity without the need for modifications of the frame.

6. Milner SA, Davis TR, Muir KR, Greenwood DC, Doherty M: Long-term outcome after tibial shaft fracture: Is malunion important? *J Bone Joint Surg Am* 2002;84-A:971-980.

   The authors of this study reported that although the 30-year outcome after tibial shaft fracture was usually good, mild osteoarthritis was common. Fracture malunion, however, was not the cause of the higher prevalence of symptomatic ankle and subtalar osteoarthritis on the side of the fracture. Although varus malalignment of the lower limb was found to occur occasionally and may cause osteoarthritis in the medial compartment of the knee, other factors were found to be more important in causing osteoarthritis after a tibial shaft fracture.

7. Kettelkamp DB, Hillberry BM, Murrish DE, Heck DA: Degenerative arthritis of the knee secondary to fracture malunion. *Clin Orthop* 1988;234:159-169.

8. Feldman DS, Shin S, Madan S, Koval K: Correction of tibial malunion and nonunion with six-axis analysis deformity correction using the Taylor Spatial Frame. *J Orthop Trauma* 2003;17:549-554.

   In this study, 18 patients with 11 malunions and 7 nonunions were reviewed. These included two infected tibial nonunions, one flap coverage, and one ankle fusion. The authors reported that bony union was achieved with significant correction of deformity in 17 of 18 patients at a mean of 18.5 weeks (range, 12 to 32 weeks).

9. Scott G, King JB: A prospective double-blinded trial of electrical capacitive coupling in the treatment of nonunion of long bones. *J Bone Joint Surg Am* 1994; 76:820-826.

10. Guerkov HH, Lohmann CH, Liu Y, et al: Pulsed electromagnetic fields increase growth factor release by nonunion cells. *Clin Orthop* 2001;384:265-279.

11. Govender S, Csimma C, Genant HK, et al: Recombinant human bone morphogenetic protein-2 for treatment of open tibial fractures: A prospective, controlled, randomized study of four hundred and fifty patients. *J Bone Joint Surg Am* 2002;84-A:2123-2134.

    The authors of this study found the recombinant human bone morphogenetic proteins-2 implant to be safe and, when 1.50 mg/mL was used, significantly superior to the standard of care in reducing the frequency of secondary interventions and the overall invasiveness of the procedures, accelerating fracture and wound healing, and reducing the infection rate in patients with open tibial fractures.

12. Borrelli J Jr, Prickett WD, Ricci WM: Treatment of nonunions and osseous defects with bone graft and calcium sulfate. *Clin Orthop* 2003;411:245-254.

    The authors of this study report that medical-grade calcium sulfate increased the volume of graft material, facilitated bone formation, and was safe in the treatment of nonunions and fractures with osseous defects.

13. Banaszkiewicz PA, Sabboubeh A, McLeod I, Maffulli N: Femoral exchange nailing for aseptic femoral nonunion: Not the end to all problems. *Injury* 2003; 34:349-356.

    In this study, 18 patients with 19 aseptic femoral nonunions underwent exchange nailing. Eleven patients (58%) achieved union in an average of 9 months (range, 3 to 24 months). Five patients did not heal, two developed an infection, and one required dynamization. Eighteen of the 19 nonunions (95%) eventually healed. Eleven had complications requiring further surgery, including four repeat exchange nailings, two Ilizarov frame applications, and five nail removals.

14. Finkemeier CG, Chapman MW: Treatment of femoral diaphyseal nonunions. *Clin Orthop* 2002;398: 223-234.

    The findings of this study support the use of antegrade reamed nailing as a successful technique for treatment of most femoral diaphyseal nonunions.

15. Hak DJ, Lee SS, Goulet JA: Success of exchange reamed intramedullary nailing for femoral shaft nonunion or delayed union. *J Orthop Trauma* 2000;14: 178-182.

    The authors of this article report that reamed intramedullary nailing remains the treatment of choice for most femoral diaphyseal nonunions. Exchange reamed intramedullary nailing has low morbidity, may obviate the need for additional bone grafting, and allows full weight bearing and active rehabilitation. Tobacco use appears to have an adverse effect on nonunion healing after exchange reamed femoral nailing.

16. Pihlajamaki HK, Salminen ST, Bostman OM: The treatment of nonunions following intramedullary nailing of femoral shaft fractures. *J Orthop Trauma* 2002;16:394-402.

    The authors of this study report that exchange nailing without extracortical bone grafting seems to be the most effective method for treating patients with a disturbed union of a femoral shaft fracture after intramedullary nailing. Autogenous extracortical bone grafting alone proved to be insufficient. Dynamization predisposed patients to shortening of the bone.

17. Weresh MJ, Hakanson R, Stover MD, Sims SH, Kellam JF, Bosse MJ: Failure of exchange reamed intramedullary nails for ununited femoral shaft fractures. *J Orthop Trauma* 2000;14:335-358.

    The authors of this study report that routine exchange nailing as the recommended treatment of aseptic femoral delayed union or nonunion may need to be reevaluated because a significant number of patients who undergo reamed exchange nailing will require additional procedures to achieve fracture healing.

18. Court-Brown CM, Keating JF, Christie J, McQueen MM: Exchange intramedullary nailing: Its use in aseptic tibial nonunion. *J Bone Joint Surg Br* 1995; 77:407-411.

19. Templeman D, Thomas M, Vareka T, Kyle R: Exchange reamed intramedullary nailing for delayed union and nonunion of the tibia. *Clin Orthop* 1995; 315:169-175.

20. Bellabarba C, Ricci WM, Bolhofner BR: Indirect reduction and plating of distal femoral nonunions. *J Orthop Trauma* 2002;16:287-296.

    The authors of this study report that contemporary plating techniques are effective in the treatment of distal femoral nonunions. They found that union occurred reliably with few complications, resulting in good or excellent clinical results.

21. Chapman MW, Finkemeier CG: Treatment of supracondylar nonunions of the femur with plate fixation and bone graft. *J Bone Joint Surg Am* 1999;81:1217-1228.

22. Chin KR, Nagarkatti DG, Miranda MA, Santoro VM, Baumgaertner MR, Jupiter JB: Salvage of distal tibia metaphyseal nonunions with the 90 degrees cannulated blade plate. *Clin Orthop* 2003;409:241-249.

    The authors of this study report that the implant proved effective for stable internal fixation of distal tibial metaphyseal nonunions alone or with simultaneous fusion of the tibiotalar joint.

23. Haidukewych GJ, Berry DJ: Salvage of failed internal fixation of intertrochanteric hip fractures. *Clin Orthop* 2003;412:184-188.

    The authors of this study reported that in properly selected patients, revision internal fixation with bone grafting for failed open reduction and internal fixation of intertrochanteric hip fractures can provide a high rate of union and good clinical results with a low rate of complications.

24. Wang JW, Weng LH: Treatment of distal femoral nonunion with internal fixation, cortical allograft struts, and autogenous bone-grafting. *J Bone Joint Surg Am* 2003;85-A:436-440.

The purpose of this retrospective study was to analyze the results of treatment of nonunions of the distal part of the femur with internal fixation combined with cortical allograft struts and autogenous bone grafting. The authors reported that open reduction and internal fixation supplemented with allograft struts and autogenous bone graft was an effective treatment of nonunion of the distal part of the femur.

25. Helfet DL, Kloen P, Anand N, Rosen HS: Open reduction and internal fixation of delayed unions and nonunions of fractures of the distal part of the humerus. *J Bone Joint Surg Am* 2003;85-A:33-40.

The purpose of this retrospective study was to evaluate the results of open reduction and internal fixation of delayed unions and nonunions of fractures of the distal humerus. Open reduction through an extensile exposure and rigid internal fixation consistently resulted in healing of a delayed union or nonunion of the distal humerus. An improved range of motion of the elbow was achieved by securing the site of the nonunion and performing aggressive elbow joint arthrolysis and soft-tissue releases in patients with severe contractures.

26. Rubel IF, Kloen P, Campbell D, et al: Open reduction and internal fixation of humeral nonunions: A biomechanical and clinical study. *J Bone Joint Surg Am* 2002;84-A:1315-1322.

Several studies have compared different methods for fixation of the midpart of the humeral shaft, but there are only scattered data regarding which type of plate construct provides the best fixation for humeral nonunion. The objectives of this study were (1) to obtain objective data on the performance of four different plate constructs used for fixation of humeral nonunion, and (2) to report clinical experience with plate fixation of 37 nonunions of the midpart of the humeral shaft. No significant difference in the healing rate was found between the two clinical groups ($P = 0.4$, $\beta = 0.9$), and the overall healing rate was 92%. However, a two-plate construct with the plates at right angles was found to be mechanically stiffer than a single-plate construct, which might be helpful if rigid stabilization of the humerus at the midshaft level is needed.

27. Kocaoglu M, Eralp L, Sen C, Cakmak M, Dincyurek H, Goksan SB: Management of stiff hypertrophic nonunions by distraction osteogenesis. *J Orthop Trauma* 2003;17:543-548.

In this study, 16 patients with stiff hypertrophic nonunions were reviewed, 5 of which were upper extremity nonunions and 11 were lower extremity nonunions. All patients achieved bony union in a mean of 7.1 months (range, 5 to 10 months). Limb-length discrepancy and deformity were corrected in all patients. There was one recurrence of deformity.

28. Lammens J, Baudin G, Driesen R, et al: Treatment of nonunions of the humerus using the Ilizarov external fixator. *Clin Orthop* 1998;353:223-230.

29. Menon DK, Dougall TW, Pool RD, Simonis RB: Augmentative Ilizarov external fixation after failure of diaphyseal union with intramedullary nailing. *J Orthop Trauma* 2002;16:491-497.

The purpose of this study was to investigate the use of the Ilizarov circular fixator and intramedullary nail retention in treating diaphyseal nonunion following previous intramedullary nailing. The authors reported that there is a role for the use of the Ilizarov fixator with intramedullary nail retention in resistant long bone diaphyseal nonunion in carefully selected patients. This method can achieve high union rates in patients for whom other treatment methods have failed.

30. Ozturkmen Y, Dogrul C, Karli M: Results of the Ilizarov method in the treatment of pseudoarthrosis of the lower extremities. *Acta Orthop Traumatol Turc* 2003;37:9-18.

In this study, 46 patients with 8 femoral and 38 tibial nonunions were reviewed; 7 of these were hypertrophic and 39 were atrophic. Mean bone loss was 7.4 cm (range, 3 to 12 cm). Bony union occurred in 42 patients (91%). The mean time in frame was 208 days (range, 98 to 296 days).

31. Paley D, Maar DC: Ilizarov bone transport treatment for tibial defects. *J Orthop Trauma* 2000;14:76-85.

32. Rozbruch SR, Herzenberg JE, Tetsworth K, Tuten HR, Paley D: Distraction osteogenesis for nonunion after high tibial osteotomy. *Clin Orthop* 2002;394:227-235.

Hypertrophic nonunions with deformity are an unusual complication after Coventry-type high tibial osteotomy. The authors found that these can be treated successfully by gradually distracting the nonunion without an open approach, which results in bony healing, correction of deformity, and increased metaphyseal bone stock; this technique should be helpful if total knee replacement were to become necessary in the future.

33. Duffy GP, Wood MB, Rock MG, Sim FH: Vascularized free fibular transfer combined with autografting for the management of fracture nonunions associated with radiation therapy. *J Bone Joint Surg Am* 2000;82:544-554.

The purpose of this study was to evaluate the functional results, rates of union, and complications associated with vascularized free fibular transfer combined with autografting for the treatment of nonunions in previously irradiated bone. On the basis of this review, microvascular fibular transfer combined with autografting was found to be an appropriate treatment option for difficult nonunions associated with previously irradiated bone.

34. Heitmann C, Erdmann D, Levin LS: Treatment of segmental defects of the humerus with an osteosep-

tocutaneous fibular transplant. *J Bone Joint Surg Am* 2002;84-A:2216-2223.

Because there are limited reconstructive options for the treatment of segmental bone defects of the upper extremity that are greater than 6 cm in length, especially those that are associated with soft-tissue defects, this review was conducted to report on the experience with 15 patients who received an osteoseptocutaneous fibular transplant for reconstruction of a humeral defect. The authors report that the osteoseptocutaneous fibular transplant was an effective treatment of combined segmental osseous and soft-tissue defects of the arm; however, the application of this technique to the arm was more complex than application to the forearm and was associated with a higher rate of complications.

35. LeCroy CM, Rizzo M, Gunneson EE, Urbaniak JR: Free vascularized fibular bone grafting in the management of femoral neck nonunion in patients younger than fifty years. *J Orthop Trauma* 2002;16: 464-472.

Rates for complications, such as nonunion and osteonecrosis, after femoral neck fractures in young patients have been reported to be as high as 86%. Treatments such as osteotomy, muscle-pedicle bone grafting, nonvascularized bone grafting, and vascularized bone grafting have been reported to have variable results. Based on the results reported in this study, vascularized fibular bone grafting compares favorably with a high union rate (91% initially, 100% after secondary procedures), and successful long-term salvage of the femoral head was achieved in 91% of the patients. The authors concluded that free vascularized fibular bone grafting represents a promising solution for this difficult problem.

36. Wongworawat M, Schball SB, Holtom PD, Moon C, Schiller F: Negative pressure dressings as an alternative technique for treatment of infected wounds. *Clin Orthop* 2003;414:45-48.

In this study, 14 patients with open infected wounds were treated with a vacuum-assisted closure system. The authors report that the average wound size was 70 cm^2 (range, 22 to 288 cm^2). After 10 days of treatment, the wound size decreased to 39 cm^2 (range, 10 to 147 cm^2), which was a 43% reduction in wound size.

37. Catagni MA, Guerrischi F, Holman JA, Cattaneo R: Distraction osteogenesis in the treatment of stiff hypertrophic nonunions using the Ilizarov apparatus. *Clin Orthop* 1994;301:159-163.

38. Guichet JM, Deromedis B, Donnan LT, Peretti G, Lascombes P, Bado F: Gradual femoral lengthening with the Albizzia intramedullary nail. *J Bone Joint Surg Am* 2003;85-A:838-848.

This was a review of 41 femora in 31 patients who underwent femoral lengthening with a fully implantable lengthening device. One third of the patients had posttraumatic limb-length discrepancy. The intramedullary nail was inserted antegrade after a femoral osteotomy. The mean gain in length was 3.4 cm (range, 2.0 to 5.5 cm) in the unilateral patients.

39. Paley D, Herzenberg JE, Paremain G, Bhave A: Femoral lengthening over an intramedullary nail: A matched case comparison with Ilizarov femoral lengthening. *J Bone Joint Surg Am* 1997;79:1464-1480.

40. Rozbruch: Blyakher A, Ilizarov S: Distraction of hypertrophic nonunion of the tibia with deformity using the Ilizarov/Taylor Spatial Frame. *Arch Orthop Trauma Surg* 2002;122:295-298.

41. Rozbruch SR, Muller U: Gautier, Ganz R: The evolution of femoral shaft plating technique. *Clin Orthop* 1998;354:195-208.

42. Ilizarov S, Rozbruch SR, Blyakher A: Ankle fusion with simultaneous lengthening by using the Ilizarov method. *Final Program of the Orthopaedic Trauma Association, Salt Lake City, UT, October 9-10, 2003.* Available at: http://www.hwbf.org/ota/am/ota03/otapo/OTP03086.htm. Accessed March 31, 2005.

43. McKee MD, Wild LM, Schemitsch EH, Waddell JP: The use of an antibiotic-impregnated, osteoconductive, bioabsorbable bone substitute in the treatment of infected long bone defects: Early results of a prospective trial. *J Orthop Trauma* 2002;16:622-627.

In this study to assess the use of bioabsorbable, tobramycin-impregnated bone graft substitute in the treatment of 25 patients with infected bony defects and nonunions, the authors found that the bone graft substitute was effective in eradicating bone infection in 23 of the patients.

44. Haidukewych GJ, Sperling JW: Results of treatment of infected humeral nonunions: The Mayo Clinic experience. *Clin Orthop* 2003;414:25-30.

In this study, 10 infected humeral nonunions were treated surgically with external fixation, plating, tension band wiring, and bone grafting. All were débrided and treated with intravenous antibiotics. Bony union was achieved in 7 of 10 patients. The authors concluded that infected humeral nonunions are much more difficult to treat than aseptic nonunions and that additional data are required to determine the best treatment method.

Chapter 14

Infections

Bruce H. Ziran, MD

Nalini Rao, MD

Pathogenesis

The pathogenesis of orthopaedic infections is multifactorial. The body's defense mechanisms usually maintain a symbiotic homeostasis with bacteria. Osteomyelitis can occur with disruption in this homeostasis. An unusually virulent and resistant bacteria or some type of host failure (local or systemic) allows opportunistic bacteria to proliferate. Examples of local host compromise include multiple previous surgeries, conditions that compromise local blood flow, and dead tissue such as necrotic bone caused by reaming or avascular bone fragments caused by a remote fracture. Systemic host compromise can include conditions such as diabetes, vascular insufficiency, and metabolic or nutritional abnormalities. An inert surface such as dead tissue, an implant, or debris can allow some bacteria to colonize and form biofilm that can escape the host defenses as well as antibiotic treatments. If the right combination of conditions occurs with an inciting event, then an infection can be established.[1]

Biofilms

An understanding of biofilm bacteria can help explain the recalcitrant nature of orthopaedic infections. A biofilm is best described as a community of sessile bacteria that is surrounded by a glycocalyx of extracellular matrix. In contrast to free-floating or planktonic bacteria, the sessile colonies exhibit phenotypic changes that mimic a pseudoresistance. One reason for this is the biofilm itself. The antibiotics need to penetrate this film before gaining access to the bacteria.[2] Because this penetration depends on various factors, extremely high concentrations are needed to drive this diffusion-controlled process. Even then, molecules in the biofilm itself may bind the antibiotic, thereby rendering it ineffective.

Biofilms will only form on inert or nonviable surfaces (Figure 1). As orthopaedic implants and other treatment materials are being developed to increasingly minimize the immune response, they are becoming more and more inert. Biofilm has been found to possess primitive methods of communication.[3] As it matures, biofilm signals to other colonies and bacteria to increase its organization.

Get-on and get-off protein signals have been identified that provide a potential method of treatment. In response to the local shedding of bacteria, the body's defenses attempt to eradicate the colonies. However, they are unable to penetrate and disrupt the biofilm, resulting in a "frustrated phagocytosis." The cells release more of their oxidative and degradative enzymes in an effort to burrow through the colony, which depletes much of their resources, and the enzymes can actually harm adjacent local host tissue. The colonies will grow until they either consume the host or until they can be walled off in some manner. If there is local inflammation and access to vascular channels, the colonies can actually break off embolic portions to seek out new locations.

Ultimately, the body tries to control the infection by forming an abscess or involucrum. Alternatively, if a sinus develops, the detritus and bacteria can be dispelled. Eventually, an equilibrium may come to exist in the form of chronic infection. Patients with chronic infection usually have a history of intermittent symptoms and drainage that respond to an antibiotic. The harmful clinical manifestations of infection are generally caused by the toxins released by metabolically active planktonic bacteria. Although these bacteria are quite susceptible to the body's defenses and antibiotics, the continued release of large amounts of toxin into the bloodstream or any weakening of the systemic host will allow ongoing clinical manifestations.

Strategies for the eradication and/or prevention of infection are being developed. From the surgical perspective, an appreciation for thorough débridement is paramount. Other strategies being developed include drugs that may mimic the get-off signal and antagonists to the get-on signal. Acidic surfaces or negatively charged surfaces seem resistant to biofilms. Surface properties on implants or local or systemic drugs may help fight infection.

Classification

There are many classifications of osteomyelitis in the literature. The Waldvogel classification is based on

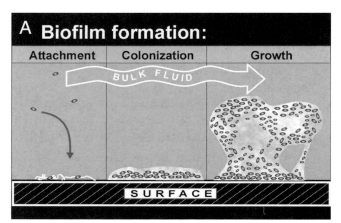

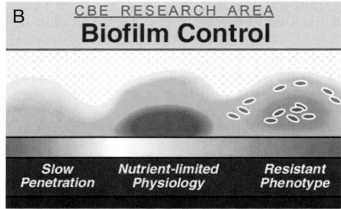

Figure 1 A, Biofilm formation requires an inert surface for the attachment of bacteria. Thereafter, via a complex mechanism, colonization and growth will occur. **B,** The biofilm itself is a barrier to antibiotic penetration. Furthermore, the bacteria within the colony will appear to have pseudoresistance. They undergo phenotypic and metabolic changes that preclude the mechanism of action of most antibiotics.

pathogenesis: type I is hematogenous, type II is secondary to contiguous focus, and type III is associated with vascular disease.[4] The most enduring and useful classification is the Cierny-Mader staging system. This system identifies the extent of infection as well as the condition of the host. Although host parameters are often considered in surgical decision-making, they are infrequently classified or quantified. Clinicians are acutely aware of the differences in outcomes between healthy individuals and those with numerous metabolic conditions.

The Cierny-Mader staging system for osteomyelitis is based on anatomic type and physiologic class of the host. Type I is medullary, type II is superficial, type III is localized, and type IV is diffuse; subtype A indicates little to no compromise, subtype B indicates systemic or local compromise, and subtype C indicates severe compromise. Pairing the four types of osteomyelitis with the three subtypes allows for practical treatment strategies. Type I (medullary) osteomyelitis is confined to the intramedullary region of bone (for example, an infected intramedullary device or such a device used for acute hematogenous seeding in the metaphyseal areas. Type II (superficial) osteomyelitis is defined similarly to contiguous focus osteomyelitis (for example, an exposed infected necrotic surface of bone at the base of a soft-tissue wound). Type III (localized, stable) osteomyelitis is characterized by full-thickness cortical involvement with a permeative infection, but this type of infection does not result in bony instability with resection. Type IV (diffuse) osteomyelitis is a permeative infection that results in either a segmental loss of bone or instability after appropriate débridement (Figure 2). The physiologic class of the host is based on the presence of factors that act either locally or systemically to perpetuate osteomyelitis (Table 1). Factors such as vascular disease, diabetes mellitus, malnutrition, and tobacco use are all systemic detriments to healing. Local factors include multiple surgeries, trauma, vascular disease, or radiation fibrosis.

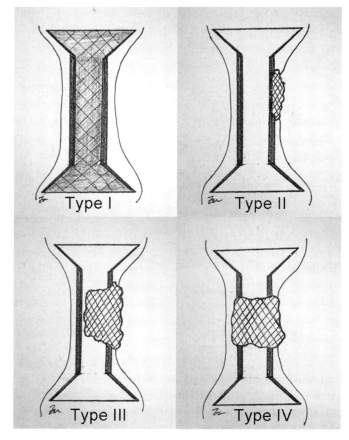

Figure 2 A, Illustration of the Cierny-Mader classification of osteomyelitis. Type I is medullary osteomyelitis (usually hematogenous seeding; intramedullary nail without cortical penetration. Type II is superficial osteomyelitis (external to medullary canal often contiguous with open wound). Type III is invasive/stable osteomyelitis (medullary and external involvement but with axial skeletal stability). Type IV is invasive/unstable osteomyelitis (permeative with unstable segment or segmental loss).

Hosts with subtype A have normal physiologic responses to infection; those with subtype B have either systemically and/or locally active impairment of normal physio-

TABLE 1 | Physiologic Host Classification Used With the Cierny-Mader Osteomyelitis Classification System

Type	Infection Status	Factors Perpetuating Osteomyelitis	Treatment
A	Normal physiologic responses to infection	Little or no systemic or local compromise; minor trauma or surgery to affected part	No contraindications to surgical treatment
B (local)	Locally active impairment of normal physiologic responses to infection	Cellulitis, prior trauma (such as open fracture, compartment syndrome, and free flap), or surgery to area; chronic sinus; free flap	Consider healing potential of soft tissues and bone and anticipate the need for free-tissue transfer and hyperbaric oxygen
B (systemic)	Systemically active impairment of normal physiologic responses to infection	Diabetes, immunosuppression, vascular disease, protein deficiency, or metabolic disease	Consider healing potential of soft-tissues and treat correctable metabolic or nutritional abnormalities
C	Severe infection	Severe systemic compromise and stressors	Because treatment of condition is worse than the condition itself, suppressive treatment or amputation is recommended

logic responses, and those with subtype C are those whose condition is severe enough that the attempted eradication of osteomyelitis is worse than the infection itself (that is, their risk for corrective surgery outweighs other treatment alternatives such as chronic suppression, amputation, or local wound care and coexistence with a chronic stable infection).

With the use of such a staging system, a detailed treatment regimen has also been proposed that defines optimal treatment modalities for each stage. It has been reported that use of this treatment regimen resulted in an overall success rate at 2-year follow-up of 91% for patients in all stages. When broken down by type of lesion and the class of host, class A hosts fared the best, with a success rate of 98%, even in patients with type IV osteomyelitis. For compromised, class B hosts, success rates were significantly lower. Depending on anatomic type, the success rate ranged from 79% to 92%. The success rate plateaued at 8% for class C hosts.[5]

Diagnosis

A history of infection, intercurrent illness, remote surgery, and/or trauma should raise the clinical suspicion for osteomyelitis. Normal signs of inflammation (rubor, calor, dolor, tumor) may be absent; thus, the diagnosis of infection when clinical signs are masked can be difficult. Inflammation resulting from trauma, injury, or surgery can complicate the clinical picture and make the diagnosis of acute osteomyelitis more difficult. Routine blood cultures are of little help unless patients have manifestations of systemic disease. Furthermore, blood cultures that yield coagulase-negative *Staphylococcus*, a common contaminant and pathogen, must be correlated with other clinical findings before any clinical significance can be attributed to them. Sinus tract cultures are notoriously unreliable in isolating the correct pathogen because the sinus tract is polymicrobial. Aspirations, intra-

operative Gram stains, and immunofluorescence all have variable sensitivities and specificities. The best microbiologic test remains the intraoperative culture. However, sampling error from too few sites and too few culture specimens can limit the diagnostic accuracy of this test. It is important that several culture samples be taken from various locations as well as samples of any suspicious tissue.

Laboratory changes include elevations in white blood cell count, C-reactive protein (CRP) level, and erythrocyte sedimentation rate (ESR). Although these levels may also be elevated after surgery and trauma, in the absence of infection, the CRP level rapidly returns to normal within 2 to 3 weeks and the ESR returns to normal within 3 to 6 months after surgery. An elevated ESR and CRP level should not be ignored because an elevation in either increases the likelihood of having infection to greater than eightfold. A negative ESR and CRP level in all but the most indolent of infections decreases the likelihood of a patient having osteomyelitis.

Radiographic findings for osteomyelitis include soft-tissue swelling with obliteration of tissue planes, trabecular destruction, lysis and cortical permeation, periosteal reactions, and involucrum formation. Periosteal reactions are much more common in children, and extensive involucrum and permeation will usually result in pathologic fractures in adults. The hands and feet do not typically exhibit as extensive a periosteal reaction as occurs in the long bones. In general, radiographs are diagnostic for osteomyelitis in as few as 3% to 5% of patients with positive culture results, with a sensitivity of 0.14 and specificity of 0.70. Nonetheless, radiography is the first diagnostic imaging step for assessing most skeletal conditions, and it can help determine whether additional imaging studies are needed.

Radionuclide scintigraphy can be performed in various algorithms. The traditional technetium Tc 99m (^{99m}Tc)/gallium red blood cell bone scan has poor sensitivity and is often used as the only screening test. Because many conditions including healing fractures and nonunions can result in a positive ^{99m}Tc red blood cell bone scan, more specific studies are required. For patients with a positive ^{99m}Tc red blood cell bone scan, a confirmatory imaging test using indium-111 or ^{99m}Tc hexametylpropyleneamine oxime–labeled leukocyte can be useful. The leukocytes migrate to the region of active infection so that the scan can confirm the presence of an active inflammatory reaction. The use of a combined red blood cell and white blood cell scan increases both the sensitivity and specificity significantly and is currently the gold standard of radionuclide testing for infection.

The sensitivity and specificity of MRI for diagnosing osteomyelitis range from 60% to 100% and 50% to 90%, respectively. MRI is especially helpful in diagnosing osteomyelitis in patients with vertebral and diabetic foot conditions because it can identify loci and their relationships to surrounding soft tissues. Unfortunately, MRI has limitations for use in patients with retained surgical instrumentation. T1- and T2-weighted imaging is usually sufficient for this patient population, and fat suppression and short tau inversion recovery sequences may be added to obtain better images of bone marrow and soft-tissue abnormalities.[6] It should be noted that MRI findings can be misleading. Edema patterns suggestive of infection can lead to diagnostic inaccuracies in patients who have experienced trauma and undergone surgery. Gadolinium enhancement should better differentiate postoperative artifact from infection-related bone marrow edema. Gadolinium may be used to better differentiate abscess formation from diffuse inflammatory changes and noninfectious fluid collections.

CT is useful when patients have surgical hardware that is incompatible with MRI and for those with established diagnoses. CT is also useful for evaluating bone healing after reconstruction. In patients who receive bone graft products, CT can help determine graft incorporation. In patients in whom polymethylmethacrylate (PMMA) beads may have migrated or are not easily detectable, CT can help determine their location. In addition, with the increased use of calcium products that have been developed to remodel to bone, CT can determine if troughs filled with such products have actually remodeled.

Ultrasound is not really useful for the diagnosis of infection, but it can be useful in identifying fluid collection that suggests the presence of an abscess or in guiding efforts to aspirate such fluid. Polymerized chain reaction has been used to identify small remnants of bacteria by identifying their nuclear contents. Unfortunately, it cannot easily distinguish living from dead nuclear materials, which increases the likelihood of false-positive results.

Treatment

There is no single method to best treat osteomyelitis. Each patient has unique characteristics and as with patients with tumors, each patient's unique disease characteristics should be classified and staged. The first step involves identifying and optimizing the host and establishing and determining the type of osteomyelitis. The second step involves isolating the infecting organism, if possible. Then a determination should be made regarding one of several treatment algorithms. Attempted ablation and complete cure will often require the tumor treatment equivalent of a wide resection with "clean" margins. In certain patients, incomplete resections may be performed as long as there is rich vasculature, such as involucrum, with the understanding that some bacteria may remain and a small chance of recurrence exists. Amputation is the best option for some patients. Chronic suppression requires either specific antibiotic treatment or broad-spectrum antibiotic treatment as well as possibly requiring local wound care.

If surgical treatment or ablation is undertaken, the hallmark of treatment is débridement. A common error in both fracture treatment and infection surgery is inadequate débridement. All nonviable and inert structures should be débrided to remove potential surfaces for biofilm bacteria. At the same time, every effort should be made not to destabilize the bone structurally. Care must be taken to maintain the structural stability of bone when potentially infected bone that is partially vascularized is present. Although leaving infectious material may result in recurrence, resection and subsequent destabilization can require extensive surgical reconstruction and its associated risks. Therefore, treatment decisions must be made on a case by case basis, taking into account the judgment and experience of the surgeon.

The limits of débridement have classically been determined by the paprika sign, which is characterized by uniform haversian canals or cancellous bleeding. Attention should be given to the soft tissues during débridement. Previous incisions and planes of prior dissection should be used whenever possible. Successful débridement is negated if there is failure to provide healthy soft-tissue coverage. There is often a dense fibrous scar, which is generally avascular. This tissue has little biologic potential, will contribute little to the viability and biology of healing, and can be resected. Monofilament suture material should be used so as not to harbor organisms, and wounds should be closed with the minimal amount of suture material. Although different philosophies regarding closure and drainage exist, in general, the healthier and cleaner the envelope, the safer it is to perform complete closure. When the health and cleanliness of the envelope is in question, closure can be done over a depot of antibiotics, looser closure with wound care can be used, or a wider resection can be performed with microvascular coverage. Again, such treatment decisions are challenging and highly individualized.

Healing by secondary intention is best demonstrated by the open cancellous grafting technique as popularized by Papineau.[7,8] The Papineau technique involves local débridement followed by a period of open management until a healthy granulation tissue covers the wound base, after which fresh autogenous cancellous graft is packed into the defect, followed by frequent dressing changes until the graft becomes incorporated. Split-thickness skin grafting is performed at a later date if needed. This type of management places high metabolic demands on the host because it requires the host to control infection and incorporate bone graft. This method of treatment has been superseded by more successful methods and is usually reserved as an option of last resort in certain patients.

Antibiotic Depot Devices and Techniques

The concept of local antibiotic therapy in the form of antibiotics impregnated in bone cement to treat infected arthroplasties was introduced in the 1970s. On the basis of the success noted in using this method to reduce arthroplasty infections, interest developed in applying antibiotic-impregnated cement as a therapy for osteomyelitis. In 1979, gentamycin-impregnated cement beads were first used to fill the dead space created by débridement of infected bone. A later study reported a 4% infection rate in 53 open tibial fractures treated with tobramycin-impregnated beads.[9] Another study pointed out the significant difference in infection rates with type IIIB fractures with use of aminoglycoside beads plus parenteral antibiotics (6.9% in 112 patients) compared with patients receiving only parenteral antibiotics (40.7% in 27 patients).[10] A recent study demonstrated the equivalence of local antibiotic beads to intravenous antibiotics in a randomized clinical trial of 75 patients with open fractures.[11]

Several antibiotic-impregnated PMMA cements are commercially available, but they have not yet received US Food and Drug Administration (FDA) approval for use in the United States. Most antibiotic cements have been used off-label in the United States, and despite encouraging results from several studies, their FDA approval has been slow. Tobramycin (Nebcin, Eli Lilly, Indianapolis, IN) is usually substituted for gentamicin because it is available as a pharmaceutical-grade powder, whereas gentamicin is not. Its antibiotic release is biphasic, occurring primarily during the first hours to days after implantation; the remaining elution persists for weeks and sometimes years. Other generic compounds may contain carriers and impurities that alter the handling of the cement composite; therefore, alternatives may need to be developed.

Antibiotic depots allow for high local concentrations of antibiotic with little systemic absorption. Other antibiotics that have been used with PMMA include clindamycin, erythromycin, tetracycline, and colistin. Clindamycin elutes well, but is not available as a pharmaceutical-grade powder. Erythromycin was used in some early studies, but a subsequent study demonstrated inadequate elution of erythromycin from Palacos cement.[12] Tetracycline and colistin do not elute from Palacos cement in clinically meaningful quantities. Macrolides and azalides are unavailable, and the use of fluoroquinolones in cement powder has not yet been reported. One problem with PMMA depot systems is that they require removal; in the staged treatments of infections, PMMA spacers can become encased in scar tissue and be difficult to remove. When used to treat open fractures emergently or for short courses of antibiotic therapy, PMMA removal is generally not problematic and has even been described percutaneously.[10,11]

Newer types of resorbable materials that do not require removal are available for local delivery of antibiotics. Calcium sulfate (Osteoset, Wright Medical Technologies, Arlington, TN) has been used in the treatment of both open fractures and infections. Although calcium sulfate products have been promoted for use as a bone graft substitute, there are scant data in the literature regarding this dual function of depot and graft in the treatment of fractures and infections. Another important consideration is that calcium sulfates and carbonates absorb or dissolve independent of bone formation, whereas calcium phosphates tend to be replaced with bone during the resorption process (Figure 3). Furthermore, a large volume of calcium sulfate can result in an osmotic effect that results in fluid accumulation and the potential for seroma formation and wound drainage. When mixed with fluid and blood, calcium drainage resembles bloody pus, which may prompt unnecessary additional surgical treatment. Thus, despite being a seemingly novel treatment concept, these products should be used with caution. Current recommendations suggest limiting the volume of calcium used and performing a tightly sealed closure. With the addition of tobramycin, however, setting times can reach 30 to 45 minutes, which may be impractical.

Gentamicin-impregnated hydroxyapatite ceramic beads simulate bone graft material by serving as an osteoconductive matrix; however, because they are resorbed slowly, they may be identified by the host as foreign bodies and provide inert surfaces with the potential for reinfection. Gentamicin-impregnated polylactide-polyglycolide copolymer implants are biodegradable and may not require removal, but clinical experience with these implants is limited and they can elicit an inflammatory response that may mimic acute infection.

Pulsatile Irrigation

The original goal of pulsatile irrigation was based on early infection study findings that recommended bacteria

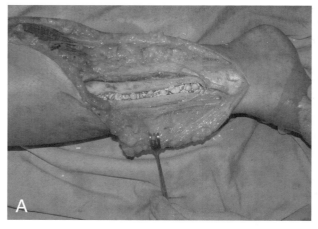
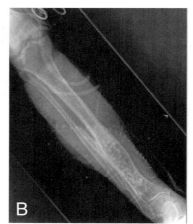
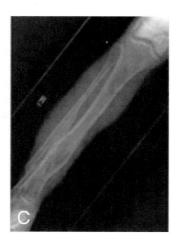
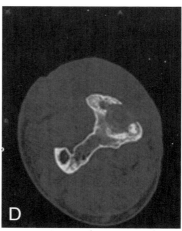
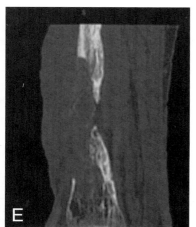

Figure 3 **A,** Intraoperative photograph of a patient with osteomyelitis who had saucerization and implantation of antibiotic-impregnated calcium sulfate. **B,** Radiograph obtained immediately after implantation. **C,** Follow-up radiograph obtained 6 weeks later demonstrating absorption of the calcium. **D** and **E,** CT scans of the same patient at 3-month follow-up demonstrating little bone formation and amorphous calcium in the saucerized trough. Although effective as a depot for antibiotics, calcium sulfates will dissolve in uncontained defects and will not function as a graft substitute in such patients.

be "knocked off" of any surface. Although this method may be effective in patients being treated emergently, mature colonies may not be easily eradicated with this method. Furthermore, evidence suggests that the velocity of the liquid stream may be deleterious to both bone and soft-tissue cells, which is also true for many antiseptics. As a result, surfactant solutions have been recently investigated as a method of disrupting the hydrophobic or electrostatic forces that drive the initial stages of bacterial surface adhesion. Early reports have demonstrated that surfactant irrigation is highly superior to other forms of irrigation.[13,14]

Specific Treatment Strategies

When incompletely healed fractures become infected, physicians must decide whether to treat the infection with the hardware in place or remove the hardware and eradicate the infection. Although these two approaches seem paradoxical, either can be done as long as the physician recognizes the implications. In the first scenario, retaining hardware and treating (suppressing) the infection is an attempt to achieve bony stability. Fractures can heal in the presence of infection, but this "tenet" is unpredictable and the physician must clearly understand that if healing fails to progress, an alternate method must be undertaken. Furthermore, as soon as bony stability (healing) is achieved, the implant and any nidus of biofilm colonization must be removed. Although systemic antibiotics may seem to be effective during treatment with retained implants, the suppression of infection may only be temporary and may recur at a later date, resulting in increased destruction.

The alternative paradigm is to aggressively débride all infected tissue and remove foreign bodies (usually implants), subsequently stabilize and treat with antibiotics, and perform reconstruction at a later date. If bony stability can be maintained with adequate débridement (for example, if bone contact between ends can be preserved), then it should be done to avoid reconstruction of a defect. In some patients, retention of an implant is necessary, but it can be supplemented with the use of antibiotic depots or coated implants such as those used in hip arthroplasty. If the surgeon is so inclined, many defects can be treated with bone transport using the Ilizarov method, which provides several distinct advantages. First, using fine wire fixation results in increased blood flow to the limb. Second, a large volume of bone graft is not needed and the regenerate bone and tissue envelope are well vascularized, thereby decreasing the risk of additional infection (any graft will quickly become an inert surface that is at risk of colonization). Third, the patient can usually ambulate and maintain some function of the limb during the reconstruction. The disadvantages of using the Ilizarov method are that it requires significant skill and attention of the surgeon and major commitment by the patient.

Other Issues

In patients with a destroyed articulation, trauma surgeons generally agree there may be no treatment options available other than fusion or amputation. However, a growing trend toward crossover between trauma surgery and reconstructive surgery has resulted in arthroplasty being increasingly performed by traumatologists. Arthroplasty can also restore function to young patients with a critical articulation (the hip, knee, and elbow typically do not tolerate fusion well). Arthroplasty may not provide longevity, but if the risk of reinfection and implant failure is acceptable, it can greatly improve the short-term quality of life and function in this patient population, particularly if long-term suppression of infection can be achieved until the tissue envelope adequately revascularizes and establishes host defenses.

Hyperbaric oxygen appears to be clinically effective, but none of the studies published in the literature are randomized and controlled. Conflicting reports exist, but most findings support the adjunctive use of hyperbaric oxygen. Unfortunately, it is expensive to use and is not always well tolerated by the patient. Hyperbaric oxygen is used to hyperoxygenate the blood and tissues and thereby increase the diffusion gradient into necrotic tissues. It is currently indicated for the treatment of clostridial infections, crush injuries, necrotizing tissue infections, and refractory osteomyelitis.

No definitive method has yet been identified for the care of open wounds. Treatments range from the application of wet and dry dressings to the use of vacuum systems and algae-based chemical treatments. Although the practice of keeping the wound moist and oxygenated is the established standard of care, general wound care is essentially a practice of trial and error. It is known that strong chemical agents that can actually inflame soft tissues and kill living reparative cells should not be used to treat open wounds because such agents may actually do more harm than good.

Principles of Antimicrobial Therapy

Antimicrobial therapy is often prolonged and requires outpatient management. Antibiotics must possess bone penetration properties and be nontoxic, convenient to administer, and cost-effective. Antibiotics should be administered intravenously at least for the first 2 weeks after surgery to treat patients with osteomyelitis. Selec-

TABLE 2 | Initial Antibiotic Regimens for Patients With Posttraumatic Osteomyelitis

Organism	Antibiotic(s) of First Choice	Alternative Antibiotics
Staphylococcus aureus or coagulase-negative (methicillin-sensitive) *Staphylococcus*	Oxacillin 2 g IV Q 6 h or clindamycin phosphate 900 mg IV Q 8 h	First-generation cephalosporin or vancomycin
S aureus or coagulase-negative (methicillin-resistant) *Staphylococcus*	Vancomycin 1 g IV Q 12 h plus rifampin	Linezolid, trimethoprim-sulfamethoxazole, or minocycline plus rifampin
Varied streptococci (groups A and B β-hemolytic organisms or penicillin-sensitive *Streptococcus pneumoniae*)	Penicillin G 4 million units IV Q 6 h	Clindamycin, erythromycin, vancomycin, or ceftriaxone
Intermediate penicillin-resistant *S pneumoniae*	Ceftriaxone 2 g IV Q 24 h	Erythromycin, clindamycin, or levofloxacin
Penicillin-resistant *S pneumoniae*	Vancomycin 1 g IV Q 12 h	Levofloxacin
Enterococcus species	Ampicillin 2 g IV Q 6 h or vancomycin 1 g IV Q 12 h	Ampicillin-sulbactam, Linezolid
Enteric gram-negative rods	Fluoroquinolone (such as ciprofloxacin 750 mg orally BID)	Third-generation cephalosporin
Serratia species or *Pseudomonas aeruginosa*	Levofloxacin 500 mg IV Q 24 h, cefepime 2 g IV Q 12 h plus Fluoroquinolone	Ertapenem 1 g IV Q 24 h
Anaerobes	Clindamycin 900 mg IV Q 8 h	For gram-negative anaerobes: amoxicillin-clavulanate or metronidazole
Mixed aerobic and anaerobic organisms	Amoxicillin-clavulanate 875 mg and 125 mg, respectively, orally BID	Ertapenem 1 g IV Q 24 h

IV = intravenously, Q = every, BID = twice daily

tion of antibiotics should be based on in vitro susceptibilities of the microorganisms causing the infection. Table 2 lists commonly used regimens for the initial treatment of osteomyelitis. Treatment regimens, however, should be tailored to meet the specific needs of each patient. Because of the increasing complexity of available antibiotics as well as their adverse effects and possible complications, a dedicated infectious disease specialist can greatly facilitate the treatment process. Although early reports suggest such an arrangement may

TABLE 3 | Selected Oral Antimicrobial Agents With Excellent Oral Bioavailability Commonly Used to Treat Patients With Musculoskeletal Infection

Fluoroquinolone
Ciprofloxacin
Levofloxacin
Gatifloxacin
Metronidazole
Linezolid
Rifampin
Trimethoprim-sulfamethoxazole
Azoles
Fluconazole
Itraconazole

improve outcomes, this has yet to be supported by level I evidence-based data.[15]

There is no general consensus regarding the duration of antibiotic treatment for osteomyelitis. Some researchers have recommended as few as 2 weeks of therapy, whereas others have proposed longer-term therapy.[16] Short-term therapy is typically initiated for otherwise healthy patients with excellent débridement and healthy host tissue. Recommendations for longer-term antibiotic treatment are based on biofilm technology data and such recommendations are typically made for patients requiring reconstruction involving a large volume of graft and implants (inert materials). It has been postulated that until complete revascularization takes place, the inert material is a potential site for the colonization of bacteria from the bloodstream or remnants in the tissue bed. Use of an appropriate oral antibiotic can help minimize the risk of bacterial seeding of the reconstruction site, which makes proper selection of antibiotic and monitoring of the antibiotic therapy imperative. Antibiotic agents that are the least toxic, least expensive, and require administration once or twice daily should be selected for convenience and to increase compliance. Table 3 outlines several oral antibiotics with excellent oral bioavailability (drugs that attain similar serum and tissue concentration whether given orally or intravenously) that may be substituted for intravenous antibiotics whenever possible provided the microorganism is susceptible to these agents.

Because increased incidences of vancomycin-resistant *Enterococcus*, particularly in intensive care units, and vancomycin-resistant *Staphylococcus aureus* have been recently reported, vancomycin should be used only if there is a high rate of infection caused by methicillin-resistant *S aureus* or methicillin-resistant *Staphylococcus epidermidis*. A single dose of vancomycin administered immediately before surgery and followed by two or three doses postoperatively should provide adequate perioperative prophylaxis. Vancomycin should only be used for

patients with type 1 hypersensitivity to cephalosporins, which includes those with urticaria, laryngeal edema, and bronchospasm with or without cardiovascular shock. Clindamycin is a good alternative to cefazolin.

Suppressive Antibiotic Therapy

When radical surgical débridement procedures cannot be performed (class C hosts), if hardware has been left in place to maintain stability (patients with acute infection), or if the patient refuses surgical treatment, eradication of infection is unlikely. In such instances, use of suppressive antibiotic therapy may be in order, which typically involves the long-term administration of oral antibiotics. Microbiologic diagnosis must be attempted before initiating suppressive antibiotic therapy, and the patient must be compliant. Even in this scenario, the duration of suppressive antibiotic therapy is not clearly defined. A 6-month course is typically administered to contain (but not eradicate) the infection. In patients with fractures, suppressive antibiotic therapy until healing occurs followed by removal of hardware, débridement, and a subsequent short course of antibiotics is recommended. If it appears that suppressive antibiotic therapy is not working, then hardware removal, débridement, and staged reconstruction should be undertaken. In some patients, suppressive antibiotic therapy must be continued indefinitely.

Annotated References

1. Cardozo Blum Y, Esterhai J: The history of the treatment of orthopedic infections. *Op Tech Orthop* 2003;12:226-231.

   This is a comprehensive historic review of the treatment of infections from ancient times to the present.

2. Stewart PS, Costerton JW: Antibiotic resistance of bacteria in biofilms. *Lancet* 2001;358:135-138.

   The authors of this article report that bacteria that adhere to implanted medical devices or damaged tissue can encase themselves in a hydrated matrix of polysaccharide and protein and form a slimy layer known as a biofilm. Antibiotic resistance of bacteria in the biofilm mode of growth can contribute to the chronicity of infections such as those associated with implanted medical devices. The mechanisms of resistance in biofilms are different from the now familiar plasmids, transposons, and mutations that confer innate resistance to individual bacterial cells. In biofilms, resistance seems to depend on multicellular strategies.

3. Donlan RM, Costerton JW: Biofilms: Survival mechanisms of clinically relevant microorganisms. *Clin Microbiol Rev* 2002;15:167-193.

   This article outlines the universal occurrence of biofilms in aquatic and industrial water systems as well as a large number of environments and medical devices relevant for public health. The authors report that biofilms are not unstructured, homogeneous deposits of cells and accumulated slime, but rather complex communities of surface-associated cells enclosed in a polymer matrix. Microorganisms growing in a biofilm are highly resistant to antimicrobial agents by one or more mechanisms. Detachment of cells or cell aggregates, production of endotoxin, increased resistance to the host immune system, and provision of a niche for the generation of resistant organisms are all biofilm processes that could initiate the disease process. Current intervention strategies are designed to prevent initial device colonization, minimize microbial cell attachment to the device, penetrate the biofilm matrix and kill the associated cells, or remove the device from the patient. In the future, treatments may be based on inhibition of genes involved in cell attachment and biofilm formation.

4. Waldvogel FA, Medoff G, Swartz MN: Osteomyelitis: A review of clinical features, therapeutic considerations and unusual aspects. *N Engl J Med* 1970; 282:198-206.

5. Rao N, Santa E: Anti-infective therapy in orthopedics. *Op Tech Orthop* 2002;12:247-252.

6. Tehranzadeh J, Wong E, Wang F, Sadighpour M: Imaging of osteomyelitis in the mature skeleton. *Radiol Clin North Am* 2001;39:223-250.

   The authors of this article report that the diagnosis of acute osteomyelitis is often challenging but can be made using plain radiography, bone scanning, or MRI. Diagnosis, however, may be more problematic in small bones, immediately after trauma, and in patients with diabetes, compromised immune systems, previous surgery, preexisting bone marrow conditions, associated soft-tissue infections, and in those who have been only partially treated. CT is the modality of choice for revealing sequestra and cortical erosions in patients with chronic osteomyelitis. Nonenhanced and enhanced short tau inversion recovery or fat-saturated sequences are essential to reveal bone marrow abnormality and its extension for patients with subtle evidence of osteomyelitis and those with neuropathic or other associated conditions. Combined radionuclide scintigraphy becomes necessary in complicated situations.

7. Cierny G, Mader JT: Adult chronic osteomyelitis: An overview. *Orthopedics* 1984;7:1557-1564.

8. Cierny G III, Mader JT: Approach to adult osteomyelitis. *Orthop Rev* 1987;16:259-270.

9. Keating JF, Blachut PA, O'Brien PJ, Meek RN, Broekhuyse H: Reamed nailing of open tibial fractures: Does the antibiotic bead pouch reduce the deep infection rate? *J Orthop Trauma* 1996;10:298-303.

10. Ostermann PA, Seligson D, Henry SL: Local antibiotic therapy for severe open fractures: A review of 1085 consecutive cases. *J Bone Joint Surg Br* 1995; 77:93-97.

11. Moehring HD, Gravel C, Chapman MW, Olson SA: Comparison of antibiotic beads and intravenous antibiotics in open fractures. *Clin Orthop* 2000;372:254-261.

    The authors of this prospective randomized study compared the efficacy of antibiotic-impregnated beads and conventional intravenous antibiotics in the treatment of 67 patients with 75 open fractures. Infection occurred in 8.3% of patients treated with antibiotic-impregnated beads alone and in 5.3% of patients treated with conventional intravenous antibiotics. Infection ultimately resolved in all patients who were treated with antibiotic-impregnated beads alone or antibiotic beads in conjunction with conventional intravenous antibiotics.

12. Wininger DA, Fass RJ: Antibiotic-impregnated cement and beads for orthopedic infections. *Antimicrob Agents Chemother* 1996;40:2675-2679.

13. Anglen JO: Wound Irrigation in Musculoskeletal Injury. *J Am Acad Orthop Surg* 2001;9:219-226.

14. Conroy BP, Anglen JO, Simpson WA, et al: Comparison of castile soap, benzalkonium chloride, and bacitracin as irrigation solutions for complex contaminated orthopaedic wounds. *J Orthop Trauma* 1999;13:332-337.

15. Ziran B, Rao N: Treatment of orthopedic infections. *Op Tech Orthop* 2003;12:225-314.

    This is a compendium of articles that focuses on the diagnosis, treatment, and management of orthopaedic infections.

16. Osmon DR, Berbari E: Outpatient intravenous antimicrobial therapy for the practicing orthopaedic surgeon. *Clin Orthop* 2002;403:80-86.

Chapter 15

Long-Term Retention Versus Removal of Orthopaedic Trauma Fixation Implants

Ronald W. Lindsey, MD

Zbigniew Gugala, MD, PhD

Roger Torga-Spak, MD

Introduction

The merits of whether, when, and how to remove internal fixation devices after they have successfully fulfilled their function are poorly defined. Direct implant-related complaints or complications (such as pain and infection) are commonly accepted indications for hardware removal; however, the rationale for elective removal of the asymptomatic retained hardware remains unclear.

The inherent intraoperative and postoperative risks of implant removal will frequently favor implant retention by default. Moreover, a patient's reluctance to consent to yet another surgical procedure and the costs of additional surgery may culminate in a passive acceptance of hardware retention. The principal premise for implant removal is that the patient is completely restored to preinjury physical and functional status. Factors favoring implant removal include pain at the implant site, late infections, implant dislodgement and/or migration, stress-protection bone atrophy, implant corrosion, implant-induced hypersensitivity, and tumorigenesis. Although well appreciated, the extent and/or incidence that these factors constitute a risk are not well substantiated by existing scientific literature to clearly justify routine explantation.

Factors Determining Retention or Removal of Implants

Removal Surgery

The removal of orthopaedic fixation devices, although often considered a benign procedure, is not exempt from numerous potential soft-tissue complications. Although not frequently discussed in the literature, the risk of infection, wound hematoma, heterotopic ossification, soft-tissue scarring, and periwound dysesthesia can be significant. These complications have been reported to occur in up to 40% of patients.[1] The scar tissue associated with secondary explantation surgery can also result in a longer time to full functional recovery.

The removal of fracture fixation hardware may be exceedingly challenging. Smaller implants such as screws and pins can be extremely difficult to localize, whereas larger implants such as intramedullary nails and plates can be obscured by callus or bony overgrowth. Even when they are successfully localized, screws and/or pins may break while embedded in bone during attempted removal (Figure 1). If larger implants are associated with significant bone overgrowth, new bone excision may compromise the structural integrity of the bone and enhance its susceptibility to refracture. Scarring from the previous surgery often alters the anatomic position or mobility of neurovascular structures and increases the likelihood of injury.

The literature has especially recognized technical difficulties during attempted removal of intramedullary nails.[1-3] Most problems can be attributed to intramedullary nail design or excessive bone ingrowth in younger patients when hardware removal is attempted several years after insertion. Regardless of the type of implant, surgeons should anticipate technical difficulties in their preoperative plan for explantation and have an assortment of equipment (such as fluoroscopy, drills/burrs, osteotomes, and broken screw/pin extractors) available.

In this era of cost-efficient health care, the additional expenses incurred from implant removal surgery cannot be ignored. In light of the absence of scientific evidence supporting explantation, many medical insurers refuse to cover these procedures. Furthermore, patients are often reluctant to assume this financial burden.

Implantation Site

The anatomic site of implantation should also be considered in the retention versus removal decision-making process. Devices that are not easily accessed (such as the pelvis, spine, and scapula) rarely warrant elective removal. Lower extremities, as opposed to upper extremities, are subjected to greater loads and risk of greater alteration of bone mass, thereby making implant reten-

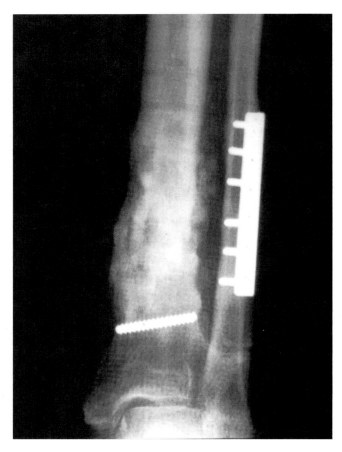

Figure 1 Radiograph of a healed distal tibial fracture with a retained broken screw following plate removal.

tion less appealing. Furthermore, the incidence of complications after implant removal is greater in the upper extremity. Finally, metaphyseal or juxta-articular devices may exhibit adverse effects on joint function, whereas the removal of diaphyseal implants is more prone to cause refractures.

Implant Type

The degree of surgical difficulty is greatly influenced by the implant design and its anatomic placement. Intramedullary devices may be extracted with minimal soft-tissue trauma at the site of injury; however, if the nail extraction threads are obliterated, a locking cap becomes jammed in the nail, or an interlocking screw is broken, intramedullary nail removal becomes extremely challenging. Additionally, titanium intramedullary devices can firmly integrate with the host bone and resist explantation if retained for an extended period. Finally, the more distal the fracture, the more exuberant the callus formation and the more likely that nail extraction will be difficult.

All extramedullary devices requiring removal result in some degree of soft-tissue surgical disruption at the site of implantation. Pins and wires can break, migrate,

or become embedded in scar to complicate their removal. Screws heads can become distorted, screws can break, or screw threads can become stripped. Plates may require reexploration of the entire wound, can be overgrown with new bone, and frequently the extent of fracture healing cannot be reliably determined before plate removal.

Implant-Related Pain

Residual implant pain and tenderness are relatively common problems, but their actual incidence and causes are unknown. Symptoms related to hardware retention can be caused and/or aggravated by meteorologic changes or by distinct pressure on superficially placed implants in anatomic regions. Tendons may rub against prominent hardware and account for symptoms. Prominent implants in the ankle or tibia can be aggravated by high-top shoes such as ski boots.[4] Retained implant pain has even been attributed to implant resonance with concert music (which completely resolved with implant removal).[5]

Hardware pain or discomfort may occur with failure or migration of the fixation device.[6] Migration of intramedullary nails or plates has been reported to cause synovitis, bursitis, myositis, and irritation of the surrounding soft tissue. Acute knee synovitis has been reported after intra-articular penetration by the migration of a flexible intramedullary nail.[7] Distal migration of an unlocked tibial intramedullary nail was reported 16 years after fracture healing.[8] Dislodgement, migration, and spontaneous expulsion of screws have also been reported.[9-11] Screw expulsion via the gastrointestinal tract has been reported following anterior cervical spine osteosynthesis.[10,11] One article reported a patient with a missing anterior cervical plate and screws that were presumed to have passed without notice through the gastrointestinal tract.[11] Expulsion of a screw during urination was reported in a patient 9 years after pubic symphysis internal fixation.[12]

Diminution of Bone Mass

The long-term effect of fixation devices on limb bone mass can greatly influence implant management regardless of the presence or absence of symptoms. Several authors[13-15] have noted long-term cortical atrophy beneath rigid plates resulting from stress shielding. This phenomenon has been documented in small animals;[15,16] however, in larger animals, the findings were inconclusive. Impaired cortical vascularization has also been postulated to cause bone porosis beneath plates.[17-19] Cortical atrophy prompted the development of plates with limited bone contact, which theoretically can reduce bone atrophy by preserving the blood supply.[19]

Although bone porosity under rigid plates has been shown in animals,[20] only one human study has demonstrated plate-induced osteopenia.[21] One group of authors reported that bone mineral density could be well pre-

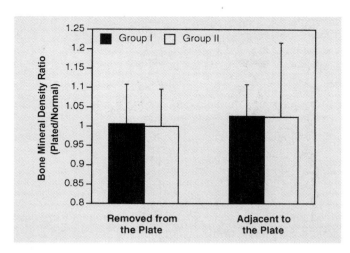

Figure 2 Graphic representation of mean bone mineral density ratios (plated/normal) of sites removed from and adjacent to the plate for patients 2 to 5 years after implantation (Group I) and those more than 5 years after implantation (Group II). *(Reproduced with permission from Lindsey RW, Fenison AT, Doherty BJ, Law P, LeBlanc A: Effects of retained diaphyseal plates on forearm bone density and grip strength. J Orthop Trauma 1994;8:462-467.)*

served long-term under retained forearm plates[13] (Figure 2). Another group of authors reported evidence of cortical atrophy in only one patient in whom the plates had been removed prematurely, further suggesting that stress shielding is probably not a problem for retained plates in the upper extremity.[22]

Although several reports have demonstrated the effect of plates on bone mass,[23-25] only a few studies have analyzed the bone mass effect of intramedullary nails. In one such study, CT scans were obtained from 10 patients after removal of an intramedullary femoral nail.[23] The authors noted a small reduction in diaphysis cortical density and thickness (4% and 7%, respectively) outside the fracture area. Furthermore, a distinct reduction in trabecular density was observed in the ipsilateral femoral and tibial condyles (19% and 17%, respectively). Another study analyzed bone mineral density after successful treatment of femoral shaft fractures with retained locked intramedullary nails in 17 patients at an average of 3.7 years.[24] The authors found an average reduction in bone mineral density of 9% in the femoral neck, 20% in the medial cortex, and 12% in the lateral cortex when compared with the nonimplanted site (Table 1). Both studies suggest that isolated femoral and tibial shaft fractures successfully treated with intramedullary nails may result in long-term adverse effects on limb bone mineral density if the implant is retained. Furthermore, the decreased bone mineral density of the stabilized fractured limb appears to correct following implant removal. One study measured the bone mineral density in femurs and tibias at the time of intramedullary nail removal and at 13-month follow-up.[25] The authors observed 3% to 11% lower bone mineral density in the proximal femur and tibia compared with the uninjured side. The greatest

bone loss was found at the distal tibia of patients with healed tibial shaft fractures that were treated with intramedullary nails. Hence, bone mineral density of the fractured tibia reached the level of the contralateral intact side within 12 months following intramedullary nail removal.

Refracture Risk

The risk of refracture after implant removal is well known and most prevalent in the diaphysis following plate fixation (Figure 3). Most articles that discuss refracture risk refer to plate removal in forearms, where the incidence can be as high as 20% of patients.[26,27] Although most forearm refractures in these studies were associated with high-energy trauma or inadequate plating techniques, the time from plate insertion to removal did not correlate with a refracture risk.[27,28] One study noted a lower incidence of refracture following plate removal from the metaphysis compared with removal from the diaphysis of the radius.[29] The influence of plate size was demonstrated in a retrospective study that reported a significantly greater frequency of refractures after removal of narrow, large-fragment dynamic compression plates than after removal of either small-fragment dynamic compression plates or tubular plates.[30]

The effects of long-term forearm plate retention appear to be innocuous. One study reported a long-term (mean, 4 years) follow-up of patients with plated forearm fractures.[6] The study demonstrated a 16% complication rate following implant removal, whereas the complication rate for retained hardware was 4.4%. If hardware explantation is selected, it has been proposed that plate removal generally should not occur prior to 18 to 24 months after fracture fixation.[13,31] However, this recommendation has not been validated.

Furthermore, precautionary postoperative forearm immobilization in a cast or splint for 6 weeks after plate removal is not a reliable solution for this problem. This was corroborated in a study that demonstrated no reduction in the rate of refractures despite immobilization.[32] However, most authors continue to support a restriction of athletic activities and heavy lifting with the affected forearm for 6 to 12 weeks.

Refracture can also occur after screw removal. Long bones with retained screws gradually regain normal strength; in femurs this process could take approximately 8 to 12 weeks.[33] However, removal of screws created holes that weakened the mechanical properties of bone. Unicortical and bicortical screw holes have been reported to reduce the torsional strength of diaphyseal intact bone by 21.6% and 31.4%, respectively.[34] This phenomenon often accounts for refracture after plate removal.[35]

Late fractures have been reported 20 to 60 years after the implantation of metallic devices.[36] It has been suggested that these long-term retained implants may po-

TABLE 1	Mean Regional Bone Mineral Density of Intramedullary Nail-Treated Versus Contralateral Intact Femurs			
Region	Intramedullary Nail Femur (g/cm^2)	Control Femur (g/cm^2)	Reduction in Bone Mineral Density (%)	P Value
Femoral neck	0.93 ± 0.04	1.02 ± 0.04	9	0.0013
Medial cortex	1.49 ± 0.08	1.78 ± 0.09	20	0.0006
Lateral cortex	1.60 ± 0.09	1.80 ± 0.08	13	0.0458

(Adapted with permission from Kapp W, Lindsey RW, Noble PC, Rudersdorf T, Henry P: Long-term residual musculoskeletal deficits after femoral shaft fractures treated with intramedullary nailing. J Trauma 2000;49:446-449.)

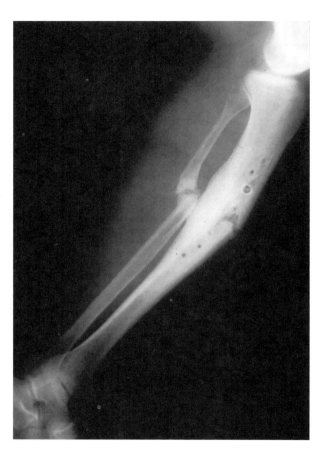

Figure 3 Lateral radiograph of a healed diaphyseal tibial fracture after elective plate removal.

tentially act as stress risers, especially retained screws.[28,37] Fractures about retained hardware in the proximal femurs of elderly patients have also been a concern.[38] Additionally, with the advent of retrograde intramedullary nails, fractures at the proximal end of the nails have also been observed.[39]

Infection Susceptibility

All metallic implant surfaces represent excellent substrata for bacteria colonization (Figure 4). The susceptibility of a retained internal fixation device to coloniza-

tion and/or infection is determined by the host's systemic (nutrition, comorbidities, competency of immune system) and local (vascularity, micromotion, soft-tissue coverage) factors. Additionally, the extent of the surgical approach as well as the implant design, material, and surface characteristics affect the susceptibility to bacterial colonization and subsequent infection.

Differences in biofilm adhesion among implants made from different metals have been demonstrated in a rabbit model. After bacterial inoculation, adhesion to stainless steel was 1.5 times greater than adhesion to titanium.[40] One study reported a 75% higher infection rate for stainless steel plates than titanium plates after percutaneous inoculation with *Staphylococcus aureus*.[41] The design of the implant used may also influence its susceptibility to infection. Another study compared slotted versus solid intramedullary nails in the infected environment and determined that a significantly higher rate of infection occurs in the former.[42]

The risk for late infections resulting from systemic sources has been used by some authors to justify routine implant removal. One study reported six late implant infections at 7 to 24 months after implantation.[43] It has been hypothesized that soft-tissue reaction to the hardware caused by the presence of corrosion particles may promote an environment that is conducive to the growth of bacterial organisms.[44,45] This increased soft-tissue reaction has been particularly evident after instrumented spine surgery because of the modular design of modern spine implants, which can exhibit excessive fretting corrosion. Although undisputed in the presence of active infection, the indications for elective implant removal to prevent late infections remain controversial.

Implant Corrosion

Corrosion constitutes a major long-term concern with all retained metallic implants. All implanted materials corrode, thereby releasing varying amounts of biologically active metal ions into the surrounding tissue.[46-48] Implant corrosion may be precipitated by electrochemical dissolution, wear, or a combination of both processes.[49] This implant degradation results in two unfavorable local outcomes: first, it reduces the implant's mechanical integrity,

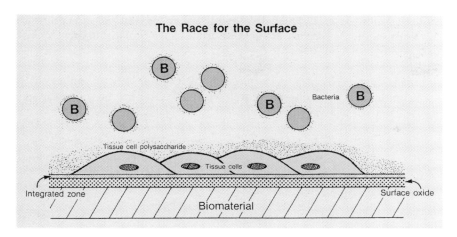

Figure 4 Schematic illustration showing that immediately after the surgery an implant provides a ready surface for bacteria (B). Host tissue attachment and/or the integration of an implant with the surrounding bone limits the accessibility of bacteria to implant surface (race for surface). In contrast, fibrous capsule formation creates a third zone that is ideal for bacterial colonization and limited access to systemic antibiotics. *(Reproduced with permission from Gristina AG: Bacterial-centered infection: Microbial adhesion versus tissue integration. Science 1987;273:1588-1595.)*

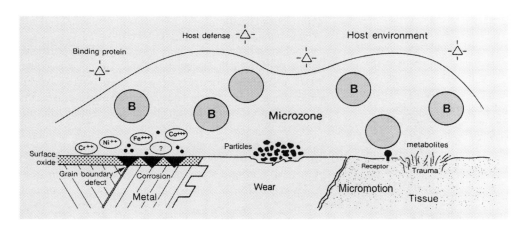

Figure 5 Schematic illustration showing the local and systemic biologic sequelae of excessive metallic implant corrosion. The process includes the release of fretting particles and metal ions, which have an inhibitory effect on the host immunity. B = bacteria. *(Reproduced with permission from Gristina AG: Bacterial-centered infection: Microbial adhesion versus tissue integration. Science 1987;273:1588-1595.)*

thereby exposing it to micromotion and subsequent failure;[50,51] second, the released metal debris causes a myriad of undesirable biologic reactions that include acute inflammation and the formation of granulation tissue leading to local tissue necrosis.[50,52,53] Pronounced systemic effects of corrosion may also occur; released metal ions can diminish the competence of the host immune system and thereby exhibit bacteriologic and oncogenic susceptibility[54] (Figure 5). A direct correlation has been established between the extent of tissue reaction and the locally released metallic products.[46,48,50]

Allergic Reactions

Systemically released degradation products from metallic implants have been associated with allergic reactions such as dermatitis, urticaria, and vasculitis.[55-57] Implant-related hypersensitivity reactions are generally a delayed cell-mediated response (type IV hypersensitivity).[57,58] If cutaneous signs consistent with an allergic response appear after metal implantation, metal sensitivity should be considered, and the implant may warrant removal.

Implant-Related Tumorigenesis

Although the materials used in orthopaedic implants are generally considered to be nontoxic, some of the constit-

uent materials have been reported to be potentially carcinogenic in laboratory animal studies.[59-63] In humans, the development of an implant-associated malignancy is a well-recognized albeit rare complication. A review of all implant-related carcinogenic reports to date identified 38 instances of implant-related sarcoma[64] and 2 instances of implant-related lymphoma in humans.[65] Most of the reported sarcomas have been associated with total joint arthroplasties, whereas only 13 of 40 instances were associated with internal fixation devices. Compared with the number and duration of retained implants in the population in general, these occurrences alone do not justify the routine elective removal of implants. Although there may be an association between retained metallic implants and sarcomas, the past 40 years have failed to establish a clear cause and effect relationship between implants and tumors.

Patient's Age and Lifestyle

Occasionally, elective implant removal may be indicated despite the absence of medical symptoms. Young, active patients would experience longer implant exposure and be subjected to a greater risk for peri-implant fractures or the ill effects of corrosion. In this patient population, elective removal is usually considered reasonable. Sedentary, older patients with osteopenic bone may exhibit a greater discrepancy in bone-implant stiffness and strength, which could culminate in stress risers. In this patient population, implants that reinforce the entire length of the bone (such as intramedullary nails) are typically well tolerated, whereas short-segment implants are less well tolerated. Nonetheless, the optimal elective approach for this patient population has not been determined.

Summary

A review of the orthopaedic literature revealed that there is currently no consensus for justifying elective removal of an asymptomatic orthopaedic fixation implant. Implant removal surgery has all the inherent risks of an additional surgical procedure (infection, hematoma, scarring, and neurovascular structure injury) as well as those risks germane to hardware removal (difficult explantation and refractures). Furthermore, the monetary and functional costs of the removal procedure cannot be ignored. Implant removal is rarely justified for a patient with a sedentary lifestyle, older age, and no implant-related symptoms. In young, physically active patients, the compelling rationale for asymptomatic implant removal involves the perceived increased risk for long-term implant-related complications (increased susceptibility to infection, diminution of bone stock, and metal corrosion). The future of trauma fixation mandates that researchers strive to understand the effects of implants after they have achieved their intended objectives as thoroughly as the benefits of their applications are understood.

References

1. Miller R, Renwick SE, DeCoster TA, Shonnard P, Jabczenski F: Removal of intramedullary rods after femoral shaft fracture. *J Orthop Trauma* 1992;6:460-463.

2. Seligson D, Howard PA, Martin R: Difficulty in removal of certain intramedullary nails. *Clin Orthop* 1997;340:202-206.

3. Star AM, Whittaker RP, Shuster HM, Duda J, Menkowitz E: Difficulties during removal of fluted femoral intramedullary rods. *J Bone Joint Surg Am* 1989; 71-A:341-344.

4. Jacobsen S, de Lichtenberg HM, Jensen CM, Torholm C: Removal of internal fixation: The effect on patients' complaints. A study of 66 cases of removal of internal fixation after malleolar fractures. *Foot Ankle Int* 1994;15:170-171.

5. Lindeck JF, Crichlow TP: An unusual indication for removal of an internal fixation plate. *Injury* 1993;24: 204.

6. Mih AD, Cooney WP, Idler RS, Lewallen DG: Long-term follow-up of forearm bone diaphyseal plating. *Clin Orthop* 1994;299:256-258.

7. Rohde RS, Mendelson SA, Grudziak JS: Acute synovitis of the knee resulting from intra-articular knee penetration as a complication of flexible intramedullary nailing of pediatric femur fractures: Report of two cases. *J Pediatr Orthop* 2003;23:635-638.

8. Razafimahandry HJ, Rakoto-Ratsimba HN, Samison LH, Rakotozafy G: Talo-crural migration of a Kuntscher tibial nail: A case report. *Rev Chir Orthop Reparatrice Appar Mot* 2003;89:648-650.

9. Pompili A, Canitano S, Caroli F, et al: Asymptomatic esophageal perforation caused by late screw migration after anterior cervical plating: Report of a case and review of relevant literature. *Spine* 2002;27: E499-E502.

10. Geyer TE, Foy MA: Oral extrusion of a screw after anterior cervical spine plating. *Spine* 2001;26:1814-1816.

11. Fujibayashi S, Shikata J, Kamiya N, Tanaka C: Missing anterior cervical plate and screws: A case report. *Spine* 2000;25:2258-2261.

12. Heetveld MJ, Poolman RW, Heldeweg EA, Ultee JM: Spontaneous expulsion of a screw during urination: An unusual complication 9 years after internal fixation of pubic symphysis diastasis. *Urology* 2003; 61:645.

13. Lindsey RW, Fenison AT, Doherty BJ, Law P, LeBlanc A: Effects of retained diaphyseal plates on forearm bone density and grip strength. *J Orthop Trauma* 1994;8:462-467.

14. Woo SL, Akeson WH, Coutts RD, et al: A comparison of cortical bone atrophy secondary to fixation with plates with large differences in bending stiffness. *J Bone Joint Surg Am* 1976;58-A:190-195.

15. Terjesen T, Benum P: The stress-protecting effect of metal plates on the intact rabbit tibia. *Acta Orthop Scand* 1983;54:810-818.

16. Tonino AJ, Davidson CL, Klopper PJ, Linclau LA: Protection from stress in bone and its effects: Experiments with stainless steel and plastic plates in dogs. *J Bone Joint Surg Br* 1976;58-B:107-113.

17. Cordey J, Schwyzer HK, Brun S, Matter P, Perren SM: Bone loss following plate fixation of fractures? Quantitative determination in human tibiae using computed tomography. *Helv Chir Acta* 1985;52:181-184.

18. Klaue K, Fengels I, Perren SM: Long-term effects of plate osteosynthesis: Comparison of four different plates. *Injury* 2000;31(suppl 2):SB51-SB62.

19. Perren SM, Cordey J, Rahn BA, Gautier E, Schneider E: Early temporary porosis of bone induced by internal fixation implants: A reaction to necrosis, not to stress protection? *Clin Orthop* 1988;232:139-151.

20. Terjesen T, Apalset K: The influence of different degrees of stiffness of fixation plates on experimental bone healing. *J Orthop Res* 1988;6:293-299.

21. Kettunen J, Kroger H, Bowditch M, Joukainen J, Suomalainen O: Bone mineral density after removal of rigid plates from forearm fractures: Preliminary report. *J Orthop Sci* 2003;8:772-776.

22. Rosson JW, Petley GW, Shearer JR: Bone structure after removal of internal fixation plates. *J Bone Joint Surg Br* 1991;73-B:65-67.

23. Braten M, Nordby A, Terjesen T, Rossvoll I: Bone loss after locked intramedullary nailing: Computed tomography of the femur and tibia in 10 cases. *Acta Orthop Scand* 1992;63:310-314.

24. Kapp W, Lindsey RW, Noble PC, Rudersdorf T, Henry P: Long-term residual musculoskeletal deficits after femoral shaft fractures treated with intramedullary nailing. *J Trauma* 2000;49:446-449.

25. Kroger H, Kettunen J, Bowditch M, Joukainen J, Suomalainen O, Alhava E: Bone mineral density after the removal of intramedullary nails: A cross-sectional and longitudinal study. *J Orthop Sci* 2002;7:325-330.

26. Hidaka S, Gustilo RB: Refracture of bones of the forearm after plate removal. *J Bone Joint Surg Am* 1984;66-A:1241-1243.

27. Deluca PA, Lindsey RW, Ruwe PA: Refracture of bones of the forearm after the removal of compression plates. *J Bone Joint Surg Am* 1988;70-A:1372-1376.

28. Rumball K, Finnegan M: Refractures after forearm plate removal. *J Orthop Trauma* 1990;4:124-129.

29. Houle JB, Tabrizi P, Giachino AA, Benoit MY, Richards RS, Grabowski J: Refracture rate after plate removal from the radial metaphysis. *Can J Surg* 2002;45:53-56.

30. Beaupre GS, Csongradi JJ: Refracture risk after plate removal in the forearm. *J Orthop Trauma* 1996;10:87-92.

31. Labosky DA, Cermak MB, Waggy CA: Forearm fracture plates: To remove or not to remove. *J Hand Surg [Am]* 1990;15:294-301.

32. Rosson JW, Shearer JR: Refracture after the removal of plates from the forearm: An avoidable complication. *J Bone Joint Surg Br* 1991;73-B:415-417.

33. Burstein AH, Currey J, Frankel VH, Heiple KG, Lunseth P, Vessely JC: Bone strength: The effect of screw holes. *J Bone Joint Surg Am* 1972;54-A:1143-1156.

34. Remiger AR, Miclau T, Lindsey RW: The torsional strength of bones with residual screw holes from plates with unicortical and bicortical purchase. *Clin Biomechan* 1997;12:71-73.

35. Davison BL: Refracture following plate removal in supracondylar-intercondylar femur fractures. *Orthopedics* 2003;26:157-159.

36. Bransby-Zachary MA, MacDonald DA, Singh I, Newman RJ: Late fracture associated with retained internal fixation. *J Bone Joint Surg Br* 1989;71:539.

37. Brooks DB, Burstein AH, Frankel VH: The biomechanics of torsional fractures: The stress concentration effect of a drill hole. *J Bone Joint Surg Am* 1970;52-A:507-514.

38. DiMaio FR, Haher TR, Splain SH, Mani VJ: Stress-riser fractures of the hip after sliding screw plate fixation. *Orthop Rev* 1992;21:1229-1231.

39. Leibner ED, Mosheiff R, Safran O, Abu-Snieneh K, Liebergall M: Femoral fracture at the proximal end of an intramedullary supracondylar nail: A case report. *Am J Orthop* 1999;28:53-55.

40. Sheehan E, McKenna J, Mulhall KJ, Marks P, McCormack D: Adhesion of Staphylococcus to orthopaedic metals: An in vivo study. *J Orthop Res* 2004;22:39-43.

41. Arens S, Schlegel U, Printzen G, Ziegler WJ, Perren SM, Hansis M: Influence of materials for fixation

implants on local infection: An experimental study of steel versus titanium DCP in rabbits. *J Bone Joint Surg Br* 1996;78-B:647-651.

42. Melcher GA, Claudi B, Schlegel U, Perren SM, Printzen G, Munzinger J: Influence of type of medullary nail on the development of local infection: An experimental study of solid and slotted nails in rabbits. *J Bone Joint Surg Br* 1994;76-B:955-959.

43. Highland TR, LaMont RL: Deep, late infections associated with internal fixation in children. *J Pediatr Orthop* 1985;5:59-64.

44. Richards BR, Emara KM: Delayed infections after posterior TSRH spinal instrumentation for idiopathic scoliosis: Revisited. *Spine* 2001;26:1990-1996.

45. Bose B: Delayed infection after instrumented spine surgery: Case reports and review of the literature. *Spine J* 2003;3:394-399.

46. Thomas KA, Cook SD, Harding AF, Haddad RJ: Tissue reaction to implant corrosion in 38 internal fixation devices. *Orthopedics* 1988;11:441-451.

47. Cook SD, Thomas KA, Harding AF, et al: The in vivo performance of 250 internal fixation devices: A follow-up study. *Biomaterials* 1987;8:177-184.

48. Steinemann SG: Metal implants and surface reactions. *Injury* 1996;27(suppl 3):SC16-SC22.

49. Jacobs JJ, Gilbert JL, Urban RM: Corrosion of metal orthopaedic implants. *J Bone Joint Surg Am* 1998; 80-A:268-282.

50. Haynes DR, Crotti TN, Haywood MR: Corrosion of and changes in biological effects of cobalt chrome alloy and 316L stainless steel prosthetic particles with age. *J Biomed Mater Res* 2000;49:167-175.

51. Naidu SH, Warner CP, Laird C: Mechanical stamping: a cause of fatigue fracture. *Clin Orthop* 1996;328: 261-267.

52. Gotman I: Characteristics of metals used in implants. *J Endourol* 1997;11:383-389.

53. Voggenreiter G, Leiting S, Brauer H, et al: Immuno-inflammatory tissue reaction to stainless-steel and titanium plates used for internal fixation of long bones. *Biomaterials* 2003;24:247-254.

54. Woodman JL, Jacobs JJ, Galante JO, Urban RM: Metal ion release from titanium-based prosthetic segmental replacements of long bones in baboons: A long-term study. *J Orthop Res* 1984;1:421-430.

55. McKenzie AW, Aitken CV, Ridsdill-Smith R: Urticaria after insertion of Smith-Petersen Vitallium nail. *Br Med J* 1967;4:36.

56. Barranco VP, Solomon H: Eczematous dermatitis caused by internal exposure to nickel. *South Med J* 1973;66:447-448.

57. Cramers M, Lucht U: Metal sensitivity in patients treated for tibial fractures with plates of stainless steel. *Acta Orthop Scand* 1977;48:245-249.

58. Hallab N, Merritt K, Jacobs JJ: Metal sensitivity in patients with orthopaedic implants. *J Bone Joint Surg Am* 2001;83-A:428-436.

59. Heath JC, Freeman MA, Swanson SA: Carcinogenic properties of wear particles from prostheses made in cobalt-chromium alloy. *Lancet* 1971;1(7699):564-566.

60. Kirkpatrick CJ, Alves A, Kohler H, et al: Biomaterial-induced sarcoma: A novel model to study preneoplastic change. *Am J Pathol* 2000;156:1455-1467.

61. Memoli VA, Urban RM, Alroy J, Galante JO: Malignant neoplasms associated with orthopedic implant materials in rats. *J Orthop Res* 1986;4:346-355.

62. Sunderman FW: Metal carcinogenesis in experimental animals. *Food Cosmet Toxicol* 1971;9:105-120.

63. Sinibaldi K, Rosen H, Liu SK, DeAngelis M: Tumors associated with metallic implants in animals. *Clin Orthop* 1976;118:257-266.

64. McDonald DJ, Enneking WF, Sundaram M: Metal-associated angiosarcoma of bone: Report of two cases and review of the literature. *Clin Orthop* 2002; 396:206-214.

65. McDonald I: Malignant lymphoma associated with internal fixation of a fractured tibia. *Cancer* 1981;48: 1009-1011.

Section 3

Upper Extremity

Section Editor:
Andrew H. Schmidt, MD

Chapter 16

Shoulder Trauma

Andrew H. Schmidt, MD

Introduction

The shoulder girdle consists of the scapula, clavicle, and proximal humerus as well as the numerous and complex articulations of these structures with each other and with the chest wall. Thus, the sternoclavicular, acromioclavicular, glenohumeral, and scapulothoracic joints are important parts of the shoulder girdle, and injury to any one or more of these structures can cause impairment of upper extremity function. Trauma to the shoulder girdle frequently occurs as a result of blunt high-energy trauma and is frequently associated with injuries to the chest wall, neurovascular structures in the neck and axilla, lungs, and cardiovascular system. Displaced fractures or dislocations of the glenoid can lead to shoulder pain and traumatic arthritis. Fractures of the clavicle are generally considered to be benign injuries and are most often treated with comfort measures only. However, recent evidence suggests that displaced fractures of the middle third of the clavicle are more prone to healing complications and that malunion of the clavicle resulting in more than 2 cm of shortening may cause chronic shoulder dysfunction. Similarly, injuries to the acromioclavicular or sternoclavicular joint are often benign but occasionally cause significant problems in management. Careful initial evaluation of these injuries is mandatory to recognize those uncommon injuries that demand more aggressive initial management.

Scapular Fractures

Assessment

Scapular fractures are relatively uncommon, representing approximately 1% of all fractures and 5% of fractures about the shoulder. Nearly one half of scapular fractures occur in the body, but 25% involve the glenoid neck. Intra-articular fractures of the glenoid fossa only account for 10% of scapular fractures; injuries to the scapular spine, coracoid, or acromion are even less common.[1] A patient with a scapular fracture has typically experienced significant trauma, and these injuries are often associated with serious thoracic injury. Except for serving as a marker for possible injury to the underlying chest, isolated scapular body fractures are of little importance and do not require specific treatment other than early shoulder motion exercises. In contrast, intra-articular fractures of the glenoid process and unstable fractures of the glenoid neck, coracoid, or acromion should be considered for open reduction and internal fixation. Diagnosis of scapular injuries is most often made radiographically. Although the diagnosis is frequently made initially on a screening chest radiograph, it can be overlooked on this examination. Scapular fractures are best evaluated using the standard shoulder trauma series (Figure 1). When intra-articular involvement of the shoulder joint is suspected, CT is beneficial in determining the presence and severity of articular injury or the degree of fracture displacement. However, it has been demonstrated that assessment of the degree of displacement and angulation of the scapular neck is not improved with axial CT images compared with plain radiography alone.[2] Although it seems that three-dimensional CT would improve the diagnosis of complex scapular fractures, its role has not been systematically evaluated.

[handwritten margin note: AP, Axillary Scap Y]

Scapulothoracic Dissociation

A potentially life-threatening upper extremity injury is scapulothoracic dissociation, which represents a closed avulsion of the arm and is usually associated with axillary artery and brachial plexus injury. The hallmark of this injury is lateral displacement of the scapula on a nonrotated chest radiograph, which may be missed if not specifically looked for. Patients with scapulothoracic dissociation usually present with massive swelling of the arm, and most have an obvious neurologic injury. The outcome of scapulothoracic dissociation is dismal, with just over half of patients having a flail limb and 21% undergoing amputation. The mortality rate following scapulothoracic dissociation is nearly 10%. Essentially all patients presenting with a complete brachial plexopathy have a permanently flail upper extremity.[3,4]

Scapulothoracic dissociation should be considered in any patient with a traumatic upper extremity neurologic

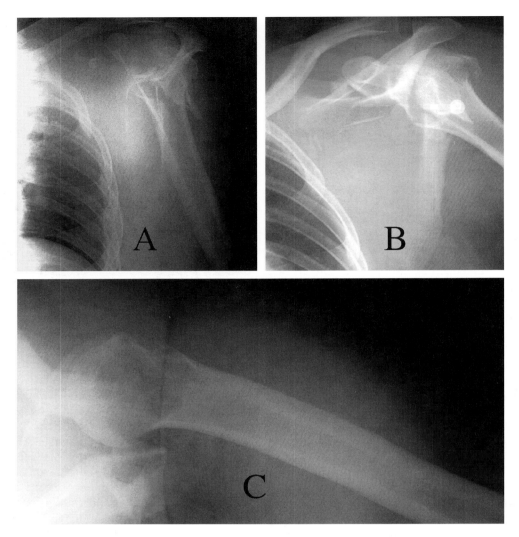

Figure 1 The shoulder trauma series, consisting of scapular lateral **(A)**, AP **(B)**, and axillary lateral **(C)** views of a scapular fracture involving the base of the glenoid neck. The AP view **(B)** shows possible involvement of the inferior glenoid. The scapular lateral view **(A)** demonstrates significant displacement of the scapular body. The axillary lateral view **(C)** shows that the glenoid is significantly anteverted.

and/or vascular lesion. Although most patients have a musculoskeletal injury, clavicle fractures are the most common and occur in nearly half of patients with scapulothoracic dissociation. Acromioclavicular and sternoclavicular joint injury each occur in about one fourth of patients and may be difficult to diagnose. Neurologic injury is present in more than 90% of patients, and it is most often a complete plexopathy. The diagnosis is made when the distance from the center of the spine to the medial border of the scapula is more than 1.07 times greater than the same distance in the uninjured side, as measured on a nonrotated AP or PA chest radiograph. If CT and/or MRI is done, lateral displacement of the scapula will also be identified along with massive injury to the periscapular soft tissues.[4]

The treatment of scapulothoracic dissociation is primarily based on emergent management of any associated vascular injury. Angiography may be performed to diagnose the location and type of vascular injury that is present, which is usually injury of the axillary or subclavian artery. Immediate vascular repair is usually performed to control bleeding, and it is necessary to ensure perfusion of the arm or the residual stump if amputation is needed. At the time of surgical exploration, it is recommended that the brachial plexus also be explored to determine the nature of the neurologic injury. Stabilization of any associated musculoskeletal injuries protects the vascular repair and is recommended.

Complications from revascularization of the arm are very common and include graft thrombosis, compartment syndrome, hyperkalemia, rhabdomyolysis, and myoglobinuria. Because of the potential morbidity of revascularization in these injuries and of a permanently flail limb, serious consideration should be given to primary amputation if a lacerated brachial plexus is found at the time of surgical exploration because there is no chance of any neurologic recovery. Patients with flail upper limbs sometimes benefit from shoulder arthrodesis or above-elbow amputation.

Scapular Body Fractures

Fractures of the body of the scapula are relatively common in patients who experience blunt trauma to the shoulder girdle. Scapular fractures are often diagnosed on plain radiographs or chest CT scans that are done as part of the initial assessment of a trauma patient. Fractures of the scapular body are classified by their anatomic location, pattern, and degree of displacement. Fractures of the scapular body may occur in isolation or be associated with other fractures of the shoulder girdle. When fractures of the glenoid neck are associated with other injuries to the shoulder girdle (most commonly clavicle fractures or acromioclavicular joint dislocations), the shoulder is potentially destabilized. These floating shoulder injuries are discussed in more detail in a following section.

Isolated fractures of the scapular body are treated with a supportive arm sling, which allows use of the arm as tolerated. Although bone union usually occurs rapidly, full recovery of shoulder function can take up to 1 year. Although the outcomes after a scapular fracture are generally good, complications related to these injures include symptomatic nonunion, chronic scapulothoracic pain, and shoulder weakness.[5]

Glenoid Fractures

Fractures that involve the glenoid neck or glenoid fossa deserve special consideration. Fractures of the glenoid neck may be significantly displaced or angulated, especially when they are associated with other injuries to the shoulder girdle. It is especially difficult to assess the degree of displacement of the scapular neck and it has been shown that CT does not improve the interobserver agreement of scapular neck displacement.[2] Significant medial or inferior displacement of the glenoid fossa caused by a displaced glenoid neck fracture has been considered to be a problem that could interfere with shoulder biomechanics. The glenopolar angle is defined on a true AP radiograph of the scapula as the angle between a line connecting the most cranial and most caudal point of the glenoid with another line from the top of the glenoid to the inferior tip of the scapula (Figure 2). This angle is normally between 30° and 45°, and values less than 20° are indicative of severe rotational malalignment of the glenoid. Patients with glenopolar angles of less than 20° following fracture of the scapula have an increased risk of a poor clinical outcome. In one clinical series, half of the patients with glenopolar angles less than 20° had associated clavicle or acromioclavicular joint injuries and half did not.[6]

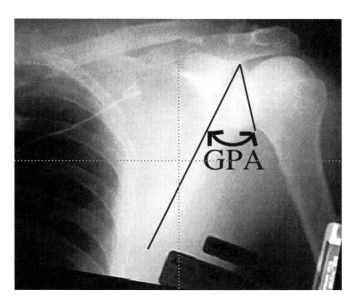

Figure 2 The glenopolar angle (GPA) is the angle between the lines representing the face of the glenoid and the vertical length of the scapula, both of which are measured from the same point at the top of the glenoid process. The normal glenopolar angle is between 30° and 45°.

Intra-articular glenoid fractures can involve the anterior or posterior glenoid rim or represent horizontal transverse fractures of the scapula that separate the glenoid into cranial and caudal fragments. CT is typically used to quantify the degree of displacement and the location of the fracture within the glenoid. Fractures of the glenoid rim are typically associated with shoulder instability and are generally repaired along with injured capsulolabral structures. Displaced intra-articular fractures of the glenoid fossa have classically been considered an indication for surgical treatment. Although reports have been published showing relatively good results after open reduction and internal fixation of glenoid fossa fractures,[7] a small comparative study showed good results with both surgical and nonsurgical management.[8] Therefore, the indications for surgical treatment of glenoid fossa fractures are not fully understood, and the management of each patient must be individualized. Currently, displacement of more than 5 mm or humeral head subluxation represents reasonable surgical indications.

Floating Shoulder

Fractures of the scapular neck in association with an injury to the clavicle have been described as floating shoulder injuries. The term superior shoulder suspensory complex was introduced specifically to describe the supportive bone and soft-tissue aspects of the shoulder girdle.[9] The superior shoulder suspensory complex is a bone and ligamentous ring consisting of the glenoid, coracoid process, coracoclavicular ligaments, distal clavicle,

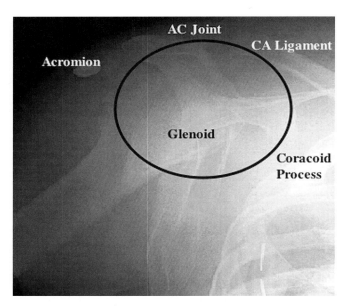

Figure 3 The superior shoulder suspensory complex consists of the glenoid, coracoid process, coracoclavicular (CA) ligament, distal clavicle, acromioclavicular (AC) joint, and acromion. This complex is supported by the clavicle anteriorly and the spine of the scapula posteriorly.

acromioclavicular joint, and acromion (Figure 3). This ring is supported in space by the clavicle anteriorly and superiorly and the scapular body and spine posteriorly and inferiorly. An injury to any two or more of the components of the superior shoulder suspensory complex could cause loss of stability of the shoulder and potentially lead to malunion, impingement, altered shoulder mechanics, arthritis, and/or neurovascular compromise. Fixation of at least one of the components of this injury (typically the clavicle) is thought to restore the anatomy and biomechanics of the shoulder (Figure 4).

Recently, the concept of the floating shoulder has been studied in both biomechanical and clinical studies. In a cadaver model, loss of resistance to medial glenoid displacement did not occur unless there was disruption of the coracoacromial and acromioclavicular ligaments in additional to scapular neck and clavicular fractures.[10] Several articles have compared the results of treating patients with floating shoulder injuries surgically or nonsurgically.[11-13] Interestingly, most of these studies did not find appreciable differences in outcome among patients treated surgically and those treated nonsurgically. However, one study found that patients with caudal displacement of the glenoid who were treated nonsurgically had notably poorer results than other patients, suggesting that this pattern of displacement in particular portends a poor prognosis unless the displacement is corrected.[13] Another study found better results with surgical treatment, but the study design had a strong selection bias because patients treated nonsurgically were medically unfit for surgery.

Surgical Approaches to the Scapula

Most fractures of the scapular body and glenoid are approached posteriorly. The exception to this is the isolated anterior glenoid rim fracture (osseous Bankart lesion), which is repaired via a standard anterior deltopectoral approach. Fractures of the posterior glenoid rim and most glenoid fossa fractures are repaired via a standard posterior shoulder approach. Extensile approaches to the scapula have been described.[14,15] Internal fixation with small or minifragment plates and screws may be applied to the lateral border of the scapula, glenoid neck, and/or scapular spine.

Fractures of the Clavicle

Fractures of the clavicle commonly result from blunt trauma to the shoulder. Recent reports have characterized the epidemiology of clavicular fractures.[16] Although clavicular fractures are traditionally treated nonsurgically (except for specific indications discussed in the following section), there is mounting evidence that displaced fractures may lead to permanent shoulder dysfunction. Deformity of the clavicle occurs frequently and is caused by a combination of angulation and overlapping of the medial and lateral fragments.[17] After middle-third fractures, healing typically occurs in more than 95% of patients.

Clavicular fractures are often diagnosed on clinical examination or found incidentally on a chest radiograph. Careful physical examination of the chest and upper extremity is necessary to find possible associated injuries. Suggested additional radiographic evaluation uses an AP shoulder radiograph and 15° cephalad-oblique radiograph. It is difficult to precisely assess clavicular displacement (angulation and/or shortening) on plain radiographs. It has been recently shown that a PA radiograph angled caudad view allows more accurate assessment of true clavicular length than the corresponding AP view.[18] A recent review of 1,000 adult clavicular fractures identified five groups: patients with fractures of the medial fifth, those with displaced or nondisplaced diaphyseal fractures, and those with displaced or nondisplaced fractures of the outer lateral fifth.[16]

Most clavicular fractures can be treated with a simple sling. One comparative study found no advantage to the use of a figure-of-8 bandage.[19] After 2 to 4 weeks, range-of-motion exercises are begun. Surgery is usually reserved for patients with open clavicular fractures, fractures associated with impending skin necrosis or neurovascular injury, displaced lateral fifth fractures, and nonunions. Reduction and internal fixation of displaced middle-third fractures has recently been recommended on the basis of poor results and increased risk of nonunion in patients with fractures with greater than 2 cm of shortening at presentation.[20,21] Fractures of the lateral end of the clavicle have a high incidence of problems.

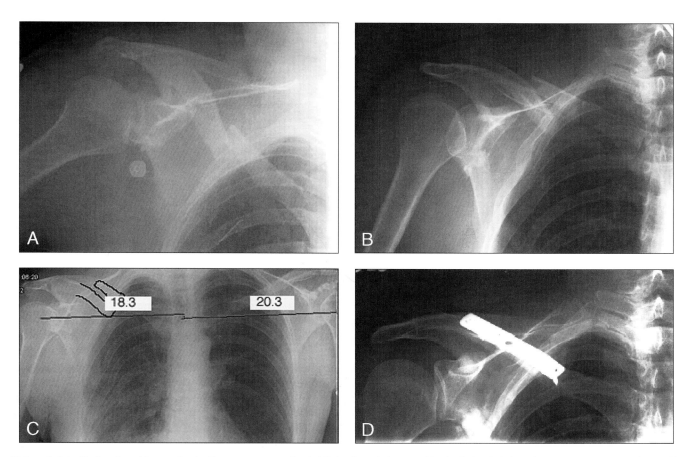

Figure 4 A double disruption of the superior shoulder suspensory complex. **A,** Initial radiograph shows a minimally displaced clavicular fracture and scapular neck fracture. The patient had few complaints at this time. Several days later, the patient presented with a drooped arm, a significant increase in pain, and paresthesias in the ipsilateral arm. **B,** Repeat radiograph shows an increase in the displacement of the clavicular fracture. **C,** Chest radiograph shows medialization of the right shoulder. **D,** After open reduction and internal fixation of the clavicle, the patient's neurologic symptoms improved and pain was reduced.

Displaced fractures that occur between the coracoclavicular ligaments have an especially high rate of nonunion and require close clinical follow-up. Although surgical stabilization of displaced fractures of the lateral clavicle results in a high rate of union,[22] one recent retrospective comparative study found no functional differences between patients treated surgically or nonsurgically despite the high incidence of nonunion in the patients treated nonsurgically.[23]

Clavicular fractures that require surgery are usually treated with open reduction and plate fixation.[24] The plate can be applied to the superior, anterior, or anteroinferior surfaces. Although anteroinferior plating results in better cosmesis, superior application of a limited-contact dynamic compression plate has biomechanical advantages.[25] Bone grafting is recommended for the treatment of atrophic nonunion, but it is not necessary for the treatment of acute fractures.

Intramedullary fixation is an alternative to plating and can be done with either 4.5-mm to 6.5-mm partially threaded screws or flexible titanium nails. With the fracture site opened, a guide pin can be inserted in retrograde fashion, pulled out laterally until the medial end is in the lateral fragment, and then driven back across the reduced fracture. With the fracture thus reduced, a cannulated screw can be placed from lateral to medial over the guide pin, which is then removed. There are very few published reports that detail the results of intramedullary fixation of clavicle fractures. One recent review of midclavicular fractures compared intramedullary fixation with a 2.5-mm threaded pin to nonsurgical management and found that nonsurgical management was associated with faster return of function and no complications, although the average shoulder score and proportion of satisfied patients were the same at final follow-up.[26] Alternatively, flexible titanium nails (such as those used for pediatric femur fractures) can be inserted from a percutaneous medial portal and advanced laterally across the fracture.[27] Resistance to interfragmentary motion and implant migration is afforded by three-point fixation of the flexible nail within the clavicle.

Current information indicates that outcomes of clavicular fracture treatment are mostly related to the degree of displacement.[20,21] It has been shown that patients with malunited fractures (those with > 2 cm of shortening) have a greater risk of having long-term shoulder problems. Patients with clavicular nonunion often have pain, weakness, and motion at the fracture site. These symptoms typically resolve after plate fixation with or without bone grafting.[28,29] Neurologic symptoms can result from residual deformity of the clavicle or hypertrophic callus causing thoracic outlet syndrome. Surgical intervention may include excision of callus, neurolysis, osteotomy, and internal fixation, and generally leads to improved outcomes, although residual symptoms remain common.

Acromioclavicular and Sternoclavicular Joint Injuries

The acromioclavicular and less commonly the sternoclavicular joints may be injured with trauma to the shoulder girdle. Both are diarthrodial joints that are stabilized by a joint capsule and surrounding ligaments. The deltotrapezial fascia and two separate coracoclavicular ligaments stabilize the distal clavicle. Because displacement of the acromioclavicular joint depends on progressive degrees of injury to these structures, the pathology can typically be determined by carefully assessing the degree of displacement. The sternoclavicular joint is stabilized by its capsule, the interclavicular ligament, and costoclavicular ligaments. The anterior portion of the sternoclavicular joint capsule is much stronger than its posterior counterpart. Acromioclavicular joint injuries occur as a result of force applied to the superior shoulder with the arm at the side and are classified by the amount and direction of displacement. Sternoclavicular joint injuries occur when an axial load is applied to the abducted arm. Because the medial clavicular growth plate fuses early in the third decade of life, many apparent sternoclavicular dislocations are actually physeal injuries.

Injuries to the acromioclavicular and sternoclavicular joints are usually apparent clinically because of deformity and pain. Careful neurovascular assessment is necessary because either injury can be associated with significant neurologic or vascular damage. Acromioclavicular joint injuries can occur with scapulothoracic dissociation, and posterior sternoclavicular joint injuries may compress the mediastinum. The true amount of displacement of these injuries can be difficult to determine on plain radiographs. It is well-known that the radiographic evaluation of the acromioclavicular joint is improved with the use of specialized views. The Zanca view is an AP view of the acromioclavicular joint angled 20° cephalad and given less exposure than a standard shoulder radiograph. Additionally, 45° oblique superior and inferior views (Quesana views) provide better assessment of deformity. CT is usually necessary to evaluate displacement of the medial clavicle.

Acromioclavicular Joint Injuries

Most acromioclavicular joint injuries are treated nonsurgically with a sling for comfort for 7 to 10 days, followed by shoulder exercises. Good functional results are expected despite residual prominence of the distal clavicle, although symptoms may persist for more than 6 months in 40% of patients.[30] Acromioclavicular joint injuries with significant cranial (Rockwood type V), inferior (Rockwood type IV), or posterior (Rockwood type VI) injuries are considered for surgical repair. Rockwood type III injuries are more controversial, but current evidence argues for initial nonsurgical management in all patients.[31] There is no apparent relationship between correction of the subluxation and improvements in pain, strength, or motion of the shoulder. Patients usually are able to return to full athletic activities with no deficits after acromioclavicular joint injury with appropriate rehabilitation. Those few patients with continued symptoms after conservative management may be successfully treated surgically.

There are many options for repair of acromioclavicular joint separations. In general, suture fixation is adequate and should include repair of the capsule, deltotrapezial fascia, and coracoclavicular fixation. Biomechanical studies have shown that suture anchors placed in the base of the coracoid provide equivalent fixation to sutures passed around the base of the coracoid process, and suture anchors may be safer to insert.[32] A dorsal tension-band suture has been shown to provide good results.[33] Recently, a clavicular hook-plate has been shown to provide reliable fixation of acromioclavicular and distal clavicle injuries.[22] One potential problem with fixation techniques is that anchoring the clavicle to the coracoid process results in anterior displacement of the clavicle in relation to the scapula. In a cadaver model, the use of an anterior hole in the clavicle and fixation to the base of the coracoid process with suture anchors restored anatomy the best.[34]

Sternoclavicular Joint Injuries

All patients with suspected posterior sternoclavicular dislocation should be carefully examined for dysphagia, dyspnea, venous congestion of the upper limb, and carotid bruit, and their distal pulses should be assessed.

Treatment of sternoclavicular joint subluxation depends on the direction of displacement. Anterior dislocations of the sternoclavicular joint are far more common than posterior dislocations. Anterior subluxation of the medial clavicle almost always recurs after reduction, but fortunately anterior subluxation rarely results in significant disability, and any deformity resulting from the anteriorly displaced medial clavicle is usually asymptomatic. In contrast to the benign behavior of anterior sternoclavicular dislocations, 30% of patients with acute posterior sternoclavicular dislocations experience serious complications such as compression of the trachea, esophagus, brachial plexus, or great vessels.[35] Closed reduction of acute posterior sternoclavicular subluxation should be attempted, and the medial clavicle is usually stable after reduction. Closed reduction of posterior subluxation of the sternoclavicular joint is done with the patient supine with a support between the scapulae by applying traction to the arm, which is abducted 90° and slightly extended at the shoulder. Posterior pressure on both anterior shoulder regions distracts the dislocated joint. Anterior traction on the medial clavicle with a percutaneously applied towel clip may help. Intraoperative ultrasound has been advocated as a simple means of accurately assessing the reduction of posterior sternoclavicular dislocation.[36] If a patient presents with a posterior sternoclavicular dislocation more than 7 days after injury, closed reduction should be avoided because of possible adhesions of retrosternal structures. If open reduction of an irreducible or late dislocation is necessary, the assistance of a cardiothoracic surgeon will be valuable.

Glenohumeral Dislocations

Dislocations of the glenohumeral joint are common in all age groups. The pathology may differ depending on the age of the patients. Young patients most often have capsulolabral avulsions (classic Bankart-Perthes lesions), whereas patients older than 40 years may have an associated rotator cuff tear.[37] Patients with anterior shoulder dislocations report pain and deformity. Posterior dislocations are less common and are missed in up to 50% of patients. Radiographs (AP, scapular Y, and axillary lateral views) are essential to diagnose the dislocation and any associated fractures. Shoulder dislocations should be reduced promptly after evaluation and radiographic confirmation, using relaxation and traction in line with the humeral shaft. When compared with intravenous sedation, intra-articular lidocaine is safe, effective, and relatively inexpensive and requires less time and nursing resources. The goal of treatment for patients with this type of injury is a stable shoulder reduction with recovery of normal function. Despite the common nature of this injury, recent reports have shown that considerable variability in the management of shoulder dislocation exists, which testifies to the lack of generally agreed upon treatment guidelines.[38]

The natural history of shoulder dislocation with respect to the risk of recurrent dislocation is still being defined. Young patients with traumatic dislocations have the greatest risk of recurrent dislocation. Arthroscopic evaluation and/or early MRI may play a role in defining lesions associated with late instability and may allow for early repair, potentially reducing morbidity from chronic instability. Elderly patients often have an associated in-

jury to the rotator cuff; if present, surgical repair should be considered.

Early MRI appears to be better than delayed MRI in defining the presence of intra-articular pathology. CT allows determination of glenoid morphology and quantification of bone loss. Flattening of the anterior glenoid is common after anterior shoulder dislocation, but it is rare in patients without such a history; the amount of flattening correlates with an increasing number of dislocations. The role of primary arthroscopy is also still being defined. Arthroscopy has been shown to cause a more rapid loss of joint effusion in the shoulder after dislocation, perhaps affording a sounder adaptation and healing of the soft tissues. The factors associated with an increased risk of recurrent dislocation are younger age of the patient, higher-energy injury, and damage to the anterior labrum and capsular attachments. Arthroscopic examination soon after acute dislocation may help identify those patients with high-risk lesions, allowing early repair and less long-term disability.

Acute anterior dislocation is managed by immediate, gentle closed reduction. Although postreduction radiographs are routinely ordered, one recent study suggested that routine radiographs are not necessary.[39] The need for immobilization after reduction remains controversial. Reports suggest that the duration of immobilization after the initial dislocation is not related to the risk of recurrent dislocation.[40] Surgical repair is usually done in patients with recurrent dislocation. Early surgery may be considered for young, high-demand patients who are unwilling to modify their lifestyle and who are considered to be at high risk for recurrent dislocation. A recent prospective randomized trial compared arthroscopic Bankart repair with a bioabsorbable tack versus immobilization for 4 weeks in a small number of young athletic patients, and demonstrated a reduction in recurrent dislocation from 75% after immobilization to 11% in patients who were treated surgically.[41] Another nonrandomized study of patients between ages 17 and 27 years reported recurrent dislocation in 17 of 18 patients treated nonsurgically compared with just 1 of 28 patients treated with arthroscopic repair following an acute first dislocation.[42] Early surgical intervention is justifiable in patients younger than 30 years who participate in high-demand activities and who do not want to risk another dislocation.

Complications such as neurologic injury (particularly to the axillary nerve) are common after shoulder dislocation. Lateral shoulder sensation and contraction of the deltoid muscle must be evaluated in all patients. Avulsion fracture of the greater tuberosity may be associated with anterior shoulder dislocation. The amount of greater tuberosity displacement that is acceptable remains unknown. A biomechanical study found that greater tuberosity displacement of less than 1 cm alters the forces needed to elevate the arm.[43] Furthermore, residual superior or posterior displacement of the greater tuberosity may result in subacromial impingement. When surgery is indicated, the greater tuberosity is approached through a lateral deltoid-splitting incision and repaired to its bed with transosseous sutures. Any associated tearing of the rotator cuff tendons should also be repaired.

Posterior dislocations of the glenohumeral joint must always be considered in any patient with a shoulder injury. In patients with a posterior dislocation, the AP radiograph may appear unremarkable because medial displacement of the humeral head is slight. An axillary lateral or transscapular lateral radiograph will confirm or disprove this diagnosis, which must be considered whenever a patient lacks normal external rotation of the shoulder. Locked posterior dislocations represent an especially difficult situation. Open reduction may be required if the dislocation is subacute or chronic. If there is a small reverse Hill-Sachs lesion, transfer of the lesser tuberosity into the defect is appropriate. If there is extensive damage to the articular cartilage, a reverse Hill-Sachs lesion of more than 45% of the humeral head, or duration of dislocation longer than 6 months, then total shoulder arthroplasty is indicated.

Summary

Trauma to the shoulder girdle is associated with many potential complications. Careful physical examination and appropriate imaging leads to the correct diagnosis in most patients. Although many scapular, clavicular, and glenohumeral fractures or dislocations may be treated nonsurgically, specific injuries may be best treated surgically. These include displaced glenoid fossa fractures, certain displaced fractures of the clavicle, and significantly displaced injuries of the acromioclavicular joint. With any injury to the shoulder girdle, early institution of range-of-motion exercises is paramount regardless of how the injury is initially treated.

Annotated References

1. Goss TP: Scapular fractures and dislocations: Diagnosis and treatment. *J Am Acad Orthop Surg* 1995; 3:22-33.

2. McAdams TR, Blevins FT, Martin TP, De Coster TA: The role of plain films and computed tomography in the evaluation of scapular neck fractures. *J Orthop Trauma* 2002;16:7-11.
   The interobserver variability in the assessment of the pattern, displacement, and angulation of scapular neck fractures was assessed in this study. Moderate agreement was found when plain radiographs were used. The addition of axial CT images actually confused the assessment and resulted in more interobserver variability than was found when radiographs alone were used.

3. Clements RH, Reisser JR: Scapulothoracic dissociation: A devastating injury. *J Trauma* 1996;40:146-149.

4. Damschen DD, Cogbill TH, Siegel MJ: Scapulothoracic dissociation caused by blunt trauma. *J Trauma* 1997;42:537-540.

5. Michael D, Fazal MA, Cohen B: Nonunion of a fracture of the body of the scapula: Case report and literature review. *J Shoulder Elbow Surg* 2001;10: 385-386.

6. Romero J, Schai P, Imhoff AB: Scapular neck fracture: The influence of permanent malalignment of the glenoid neck on clinical outcome. *Arch Orthop Trauma Surg* 2001;121:313-316.
   This article defines the glenopolar angle and reports that a glenopolar angle less than 20° can predict a poor outcome in patients with scapular fractures.

7. Schandelmaier P, Blauth M, Schneider C, Krettek C: Fractures of the glenoid treated by operation: A 5- to 23-year follow-up of 22 cases. *J Bone Joint Surg Br* 2002;84:173-177.
   This article reports the results of a series of patients who underwent surgical treatment of intra-articular glenoid fractures. An anterior approach to the shoulder was used for patients with fractures of the anterior or inferior glenoid rim, whereas a posterior approach was used for the others. After long-term follow-up, the median Constant score was 94% of that of the uninjured shoulder.

8. Kligman M, Roffman M: Glenoid fracture: conservative treatment versus surgical treatment. *J South Orthop Assoc* 1998;7:1-5.

9. Goss TP: Double disruptions of the superior shoulder suspensory complex. *J Orthop Trauma* 1993;7: 99-106.

10. Williams GR, Naranja J, Klimkiewicz J, Karduna A, Iannotti JP, Ramsey M: The floating shoulder: A biomechanical basis for classification and management. *J Bone Joint Surg Am* 2001;83-A:1182-1187.

11. Edwards SG, Whittle AP, Wood GW: Nonoperative treatment of ipsilateral fractures of the scapula and clavicle. *J Bone Joint Surg Am* 2000;82:774-780.
    In this study, 20 patients with a floating shoulder injury were treated with either a sling or a shoulder immobilizer, and the outcome was determined by shoulder range of motion, abduction strength, and the use of three scoring systems. Eleven patients had displaced clavicular fractures, and five had displaced scapular fractures. Physical therapy was begun within 2 weeks of the injury. Nineteen of the 20 pairs of fractures united. The only clavicular nonunion was associated with segmental bone loss. In all patients, the

strength of the injured extremity was equal to the uninjured arm. Eighteen patients had a full, symmetric range of shoulder motion, and the shoulder scores were excellent in 17 patients. These data indicate that many patients can achieve excellent outcomes with the nonsurgical management of floating shoulder. However, most patients in this series did not have significant displacement of the scapulae, which might portend a worse prognosis when present.

12. Egol KA, Connor PM, Karunakar MA, Sims SH, Bosse MJ, Kellam JF: The floating shoulder: Clinical and functional results. *J Bone Joint Surg Am* 2001; 83-A:1188-1194.

    In this study, 19 patients with floating shoulder (displaced glenoid neck fractures and ipsilateral clavicular fractures or acromioclavicular joint injuries) were evaluated with three outcome scores, isokinetic strength testing, and radiographs. Twelve patients were treated nonsurgically and seven had surgery; four of the seven surgically treated patients also had an intra-articular glenoid fracture. Despite this potential selection bias, there was no significant difference between the surgically and nonsurgically treated patients with respect to any of the three functional outcome scores. Although the surgically treated shoulders had greater forward flexion than those of patients who received nonsurgical treatment, they had significantly less internal and external rotation. Although the small number of patients and retrospective design temper the conclusions of this article, it is the first to directly compare the outcomes of surgery and nonsurgical management and to use multiple standardized outcomes scores.

13. van Noort A, te Slaa RL, Marti RK, van der Werken C: The floating shoulder: A multicentre study. *J Bone Joint Surg Br* 2001;83:795-798.

    In this article, the outcomes of 35 patients who underwent treatment for ipsilateral scapular neck and clavicular fractures were determined retrospectively. Only four patients were treated surgically. Of those treated nonsurgically, the presence of caudal dislocation of the glenoid at the end of treatment was associated with a worse outcome as determined by the Constant score.

14. Ebraheim NA, Mekhail AO, Padanilum TG, Yeasting RA: Anatomic considerations for a modified posterior approach to the scapula. *Clin Orthop* 1997;334: 136-143.

15. Kligman M, Roffman M: Posterior approach for glenoid fracture. *J Trauma* 1997;42:733-735.

16. Robinson CM: Fractures of the clavicle in the adult: Epidemiology and classification. *J Bone Joint Surg Br* 1998;80:476-484.

    The author reviewed 1,000 consecutive clavicular fractures in adults and identified how the outcome related to fracture pattern and location. A new classification of clavicular fractures is proposed. Displaced fractures of the

middle-third and lateral-fifth clavicle were noted to have a high rate of complications.

17. Edelson JG: The bony anatomy of clavicular malunions. *J Shoulder Elbow Surg* 2003;12:173-178.

    In a series of museum specimens, 73 clavicular fractures were identified. Fifty-four of these were malunited, and all malunions exhibited a characteristic pattern of anterior angulation of the distal fragment combined with overlapping because of anterior displacement of the medial fragment in front of the lateral fragment. The authors concluded that the combination of angulation and overlapping contributes to the apparent shortening of displaced clavicular fractures.

18. Sharr JR, Mohammed KD: Optimizing the radiographic technique in clavicular fractures. *J Shoulder Elbow Surg* 2003;12:170-172.

19. Andersen K, Jensen PO, Lauritzen J: Treatment of clavicular fractures: Figure-of-eight bandage versus a simple sling. *Acta Orthop Scand* 1987;58:71-74.

20. Hill JM, McGuire MH, Crosby LA: Closed treatment of displaced middle-third fractures of the clavicle gives poor results. *J Bone Joint Surg Br* 1997;79: 537-539.

21. Nordqvist A, Redlund-Johnell I, von Scheele A, Petersson CJ: Shortening of the clavicle: Incidence and clinical significance. A 5-year follow-up of 85 patients. *Acta Orthop Scand* 1997;68:349-351.

22. Flinkkila T, Ristiniemi J, Hyvonen P, Hamalainen M: Surgical treatment of unstable fractures of the distal clavicle: A comparative study of Kirschner wire and clavicular hook plate fixation. *Acta Orthop Scand* 2002;73:50-53.

23. Rokito AS, Zuckerman JD, Shaari JM, Eisenberg DP, Cuomo F, Gallagher MA: A comparison of nonoperative and operative treatment of type II distal clavicle fractures. *Bull Hosp Jt Dis* 2002-2003;61: 32-39.

24. Shen WJ, Liu TJ, Shen YS: Plate fixation of fresh displaced midshaft clavicle fractures. *Injury* 1999;30: 497-500.

25. Iannotti MR, Crosby LA, Stafford P, Grayson G, Goulet R: Effects of plate location and selection on the stability of midshaft clavicle osteotomies: A biomechanical study. *J Shoulder Elbow Surg* 2002;11: 457-462.

26. Grassi FA, Tajana MS, D'Angelo F: Management of midclavicular fractures: Comparison between non-

operative treatment and open intramedullary fixation in 80 patients. *J Trauma* 2001;50:1096-1100.

In this study, fixation of midclavicular fractures with a single 2.5-mm threaded pin was associated with a significantly longer time to return to usual daily activities (41 days versus 17 days) and more frequent complications (37.5% versus 0) than treatment with a figure-of-8 bandage. The authors concluded that although intramedullary fixation may be appropriate in certain circumstances, a 2.5-mm pin may be too small, and in the absence of other evidence this method should be considered inferior to plate fixation.

27. Jubel A, Andermahr J, Schiffer G, Tsironis K, Rehm KE: Elastic stable intramedullary nailing of midclavicular fractures with a titanium nail. *Clin Orthop* 2003;408:279-285.

28. Kitsis CK, Marino AJ, Krikler SJ, Birch R: Late complications following clavicular fractures and their operative management. *Injury* 2003;34:69-74.

29. McKee MD, Wild LM, Schemitsch EH: Midshaft malunions of the clavicle. *J Bone Joint Surg Am* 2003;85-A:790-797.

   In this study, 15 patients with symptomatic malunion of the clavicle underwent corrective osteotomy through the malunion and internal fixation; 14 of the malunions united, and all of these patients had significant improvements in shoulder function.

30. Shaw MB, McInerney JJ, Dias JJ, Evans PA: Acromioclavicular joint sprains: The post-injury recovery interval. *Injury* 2003;34:438-442.

   The authors describe the natural history of grade I or II acromioclavicular sprains in 47 patients who answered questionnaires at least 1 year after injury. Pain was reported to be present 6 months after injury by 40% of patients; 14% reported pain to be present 1 year after injury. One year following injury, 9% of patients had residual symptoms that were severe enough to affect their ability to perform activities of daily living and 6% had to change athletic activities. These data serve as a useful benchmark for the outcome of less severe acromioclavicular joint injuries.

31. Schlegel TF, Burks RT, Marcus RL, Dunn HK: A prospective evaluation of untreated acute grade III acromioclavicular separations. *Am J Sports Med* 2001;29:699-703.

   In this study, 25 patients with acute grade III acromioclavicular separations were treated with a sling and early range-of-motion exercises; the patients were assessed at 6, 12, 24, 36, and 52 weeks. Follow-up assessments included a questionnaire and strength testing. Twenty patients completed a 1-year follow-up. Of these, four patients (20%) reported that they were not satisfied with the outcome. Objective evaluation did not reveal any limitations in shoulder motion or in rotational strength. The injured shoulder was reported to be 17% weaker in bench press testing at 1-year follow-up.

32. Breslow MJ, Jazrawi LM, Bernstein AD, Kummer FJ, Rokito AS: Treatment of acromioclavicular joint separation: suture or suture anchors? *J Shoulder Elbow Surg* 2002;11:225-229.

33. Hessmann M, Kirchner R, Baumgaertel F, et al: Treatment of unstable distal clavicular fractures with and without lesions of the acromioclavicular joint. *Injury* 1996;27:47-52.

34. Jerosch J, Filler T, Peuker E, Greig M, Siewering U: Which stabilization technique corrects anatomy best in patients with AC-separation? An experimental study. *Knee Surg Sports Traumatol Arthrosc* 1999;7: 365-372.

35. Ono K, Inagawa H, Kiyota K, Terada T, Suzuki S, Maekawa K: Posterior dislocation of the sternoclavicular joint with obstruction of the innominate vein: Case report. *J Trauma* 1998;44:381-383.

36. Siddiqui AA, Turner SM: Posterior sternoclavicular joint dislocation: The value of intra-operative ultrasound. *Injury* 2003;34:448-453.

37. Pevny T, Hunter RE, Freeman JR: Primary traumatic anterior shoulder dislocation in patients 40 years of age and older. *Arthroscopy* 1998;14:289-294.

38. te Slaa RL, Wijffels MP, Marti RK: Questionnaire reveals variations in the management of acute first time shoulder dislocations in the Netherlands. *Eur J Emerg Med* 2003;10:58-61.

39. Hendey GW, Kinlaw K: Clinically significant abnormalities in postreduction radiographs after anterior shoulder dislocation. *Ann Emerg Med* 1996;28:399-402.

40. Hovelius L, Augustini BG, Fredin H, Johansson O, Norlin R, Thorling J: Primary anterior dislocation of the shoulder in young patients: A ten-year prospective study. *J Bone Joint Surg Am* 1996;78:1677-1684.

41. Bottoni CR, Wilckens JH, De Berardino TM, et al: A prospective, randomized evaluation of arthroscopic stabilization versus nonoperative treatment in patients with acute, traumatic, first-time shoulder dislocations. *Am J Sports Med* 2002;30:576-580.

   Twenty-four young male active-duty military patients with first-time shoulder dislocations were randomized to receive either 4 weeks of immobilization or arthroscopic Bankart repair with a bioabsorbable tack. All patients then followed the same supervised rehabilitation program. Of 12 patients who were treated nonsurgically and available for follow-up, 9 (75%) experienced another dislocation and 6 of these eventually had open Bankart reconstruction. In the 9 surgically treated patients who were available for follow-up, only 1 (11%) experienced another dislocation. The authors concluded that early arthroscopic intervention appears to be suitable treatment in active, young men with primary shoulder dislocations.

42. Larrain MV, Botto GJ, Montenegro HJ, Mauas DM: Arthroscopic repair of acute traumatic anterior shoulder dislocation in young athletes. *Arthroscopy* 2001;17:373-377.

43. Bono CM, Renard R, Levine RG, et al: Effect of displacement of fractures of the greater tuberosity on the mechanics of the shoulder. *J Bone Joint Surg Br* 2001;83:1056-1062.

Chapter 17

Fractures of the Humerus

Andrew Green, MD

J. Spence Reid, MD

DuWayne A. Carlson, MD

Proximal Humerus Fractures

Introduction

Proximal humerus fractures are common and encompass a broad spectrum of injuries and local anatomic pathology. With the aging population and the associated increased prevalence of osteoporosis, dramatic increases in the number of these fractures are anticipated. Most proximal humerus fractures are nondisplaced or minimally displaced and can be successfully treated without surgery. Less commonly, surgical treatment is indicated for displaced fractures. Although nonsurgical treatment is usually straightforward, surgical treatment can be difficult, and the reported results are often unsatisfactory.

The ability to accurately classify proximal humerus fractures is important in selecting the appropriate treatment because a variety of factors including associated soft-tissue injuries (neurovascular and rotator cuff), preexisting shoulder abnormalities, and patient factors impact treatment outcome. The surgical treatment of proximal humerus fractures is being facilitated by an improved understanding of both normal and pathologic anatomy as well as by new developments in surgical implants and techniques. Moreover, important advances in the outcome evaluation of shoulder disorders are helping orthopaedic surgeons to recognize the impact of proximal humerus fractures on patients and to direct treatment selection.

Epidemiology

Fractures of the proximal humerus comprise 4% to 5% of all fractures. The incidence increases rapidly with age and these fractures occur twice as often in women as in men. Eighty-seven percent of fractures occur as a result of a fall from a standing height. A Finnish study reviewed the incidence of osteoporotic proximal humerus fractures from 1970 to 1998 and found a dramatic age-adjusted increase during the period of review.[1] A 300% increase in these fractures has been projected for the next 30 years. Another study prospectively investigated risk factors for sustaining a proximal humerus fracture in 6,900 elderly women and found that

bone fragility and risk of falling were independent risk factors.[2] Women with both a low bone mineral density and risk factors for falling were more than twice as likely to experience a fracture than women with either one risk factor or no risk factors. A large study of proximal humerus fractures found that approximately 50% of proximal humerus fractures were minimally displaced.[3] Two-part surgical neck fractures were the most common displaced fracture, with an incidence of 28%.

Classification

It has been recognized that most proximal humerus fractures occur along the physeal scars of the proximal humerus. Based on this early observation, Neer developed the four-part classification system that remains the most recognized and widely used standard for assessing proximal humerus fractures. He described six different variations of displaced proximal humerus fractures and defined displacement as 45° of angulation or 1 cm of displacement of a part. More recent articles suggest that greater tuberosity displacement of 5 mm or less can have a clinically significant impact. Considering that the greater tuberosity is on average 8 ± 3.2 mm below the top of the articular segment, even small amounts of greater tuberosity displacement can be problematic.

The AO/ASIF/Orthopaedic Trauma Association (OTA) Comprehensive Long Bone Classification system organizes proximal humerus fractures into three main groups and three additional subgroups based on fracture location, the presence of impaction, translation, angulation or comminution of the surgical neck, and the presence or absence of a dislocation. Type A fractures are unifocal and involve the greater tuberosity or surgical neck. Type B fractures are bifocal. Type C fractures include intra-articular anatomic neck fractures and head splitting fractures. This classification system is less commonly referenced than the Neer system. In contrast to Neer's original classification, the AO/ASIF/OTA Comprehensive Long Bone Classification system clearly identifies a valgus impacted anatomic neck fracture as distinct from other four-part fractures. Patients with valgus impacted fractures, unlike those with true four-part fractures, can have partial preservation of the vascularity to the articular segment through the intact medial capsule and thus a lower incidence of osteonecrosis.

Unfortunately, all fracture classification systems have limited interobserver reliability. Several studies have demonstrated this to be true for proximal humerus fractures. Training with the Neer classification system significantly improved the interobserver reliability for classifying fractures with plain radiographs. Although CT has not been shown to improve the interobserver reliability of proximal humerus fracture classification, it is quite useful for the assessment of more specific details of fracture anatomy. Despite the apparent difficulties of fracture classification, these studies do not demonstrate that these systems are invalid. They remain clinically useful as they help clinicians to triage different injuries to appropriate treatment to achieve an optimal outcome. Neer addressed these concerns regarding the classification system by reaffirming that fracture classification and treatment were never intended to be made solely on the basis of radiographic evaluation.[4] For patients with complex injuries, the ultimate decision regarding classification and treatment may have to be deferred until the fracture and soft tissues are evaluated at the time of surgery.

Associated Injuries

Peripheral nerve injuries are commonly associated with proximal humerus fractures and can have a dramatic impact on the outcome of treatment. Nerve injuries that are detectable using electromyography occur in as many as 60% of patients and are more common with increasing age. The axillary nerve is the most commonly injured nerve in patients with a fracture of the proximal humerus. Axillary nerve injury often occurs in combination with other peripheral nerve injuries. Some of these combined injuries represent infraclavicular brachial plexus injuries. Unfortunately, recovery of associated nerve injuries is often incomplete.

Vascular injuries are a rare complication of proximal humerus fractures and fracture-dislocations. They usually involve the axillary artery, its branches, or the axillary vein. Vascular injuries most commonly occur in older patients who have fragile atherosclerotic vessels or in association with high-energy trauma and severe fracture displacement. An associated vascular injury must be treated as an emergency, and timely evaluation with arteriogram is imperative. It is possible to have a palpable distal pulse in the presence of a significant proximal vascular injury because of the extensive collateral blood supply around the shoulder.

Evaluation

A standardized approach to the evaluation of the injured shoulder should be used. This includes a detailed history that defines any comorbid conditions, preexisting shoulder problems, and the mechanism of injury. The social history is particularly important when the patient is elderly. Observation of patients should include assessment of their ambulatory and general physical condition. A stroke, seizure, or new medical condition such as syncope, should always be considered as a possible cause for a fall. Fracture-dislocation, especially posterior dislocation, may indicate new onset of a seizure disorder. Fracture through a metastatic lesion should also be considered in the older age group. If surgery is anticipated, a medical consultation should be considered. In a review of eight published series from 1974 to 1995, the death rate was 16% in patients with a mean age of 66 years who were followed for 3 years after surgery for proximal humerus fractures.

Good quality plain radiographs are essential for the diagnosis and classification of proximal humerus fractures. A true AP view of the glenohumeral joint with no glenohumeral overlap and an axillary lateral view are standard and should always be obtained. Important information including the diagnosis of a posterior dislocation may be missed if the axillary view is omitted. The axillary view can be accomplished with only a few degrees of shoulder abduction. Alternatively, a Velpeau view can be obtained in which the arm is held in internal rotation by the bandage and the patient leans backward with the x-ray beam directed superoinferiorly from the top of the shoulder onto a cassette located at the patient's elbow. Although the scapular Y-view can be difficult to interpret, it can demonstrate displacement of the posterior aspect of the greater tuberosity as well as surgical neck angulation. Additional AP views in internal and external rotation can provide more details about a fracture of the greater tuberosity as well as help to identify an occult surgical neck fracture.

Advanced imaging beyond plain radiographs should be considered when there is a question about the extent of fracture displacement and the choice of treatment is in question. In some patients, CT is required to further define the extent of tuberosity displacement. CT is particularly helpful to clarify head-splitting fractures and identifying posterior dislocations. Occasionally, standard axial CT may not clearly demonstrate the amount of fracture displacement in the vertical axis of the body. Coronal and three-dimensional reconstruction CT can be used to define the displacement of more complex proximal humerus fractures.

MRI is rarely indicated for routine evaluation of patients with proximal humerus fractures. However, if plain radiographs fail to demonstrate a fracture and the clinical course is not progressing satisfactorily, MRI is appropriate for diagnosing occult nondisplaced fractures, rotator cuff tearing, occult articular injury, or osteonecrosis.

Nonsurgical Treatment

Most proximal humerus fractures are either nondisplaced or minimally displaced and can be treated nonsurgically. Nonsurgical management of proximal humerus fractures should follow a defined protocol. Several authors and one meta-analysis suggest that a body bandage offers no advantage over simple sling immobilization. The timing of the initiation of shoulder motion remains controversial. One study found significantly better overall function and external rotation in those patients who started a supervised physical therapy program by day 14 compared with those whose therapy started after day 14.[5] In another study, the short-term results were better in patients starting shoulder motion by day 7, but there was no difference in outcome at 1 year between patients starting motion on day 7 versus day 21. Shoulder physiotherapy may be monitored by a physical therapist or self-directed in motivated, competent patients.

Rehabilitation decisions for individual patients need to be based on the specific clinical presentation and findings. When the fracture is impacted or stable, early range-of-motion exercises can be initiated. When the fracture is unstable, a period of immobilization is required. Most nondisplaced fractures are stable enough to begin range-of-motion exercises within 2 to 4 weeks after the injury. Early rehabilitation with shoulder range-of-motion exercises is associated with decreased pain and improved functional outcome.

Some fracture-dislocations can be reduced closed and then treated nonsurgically. A two-part anterior fracture-dislocation with displacement of the greater tuberosity is the most common type of fracture-dislocation. Most of these injuries reduce anatomically with closed reduction. Great care should be taken whenever a fracture-dislocation is reduced closed to avoid iatrogenic displacement. When any difficulty is encountered or there is concern about causing iatrogenic displacement, reduction should be performed with the patient under anesthesia or general or interscalene nerve block.

The amount of fracture displacement that is acceptable is controversial and depends on several factors. In addition to the specific type of fracture, the patient's premorbid functional status and outcome goals are important considerations. Despite the Neer criteria for displacement, most authors agree that the shoulder has very little tolerance for greater tuberosity displacement. Displacement of greater than 5 mm can result in substantial dysfunction. More recently, it was suggested that fractures with 3 mm of displacement should be reduced in athletes and laborers who are involved in activity that requires the arms to be raised over the head.[6]

Lesser tuberosity fractures are rare. Medial displacement of the lesser tuberosity can cause internal rotation weakness, block internal rotation, or result in subcoracoid impingement. Surgical neck angulation is usually directed apex anterolaterally. This angulation limits shoulder elevation and can result in subacromial impingement.

In some patients, comorbid factors render nonsurgical treatment the most appropriate option despite substantial displacement. One study suggested that nonsurgical management should be extended to include displaced medially translated two-part fractures and impacted valgus fractures in the elderly.[7,8]

Surgical Treatment

Surgical treatment is indicated for patients with displaced proximal humerus fractures and fracture-dislocations. There are numerous techniques available to treat these injuries, none of which are solely applicable or ideal for any specific or all fracture types.

Closed Reduction and Percutaneous Fixation

Some fractures can be adequately treated with closed reduction and percutaneous pinning. This technique is less invasive than open reduction and internal fixation and thus has the advantages of avoiding surgical trauma to the more superficial soft tissues, such as the deltoid muscle. Consequently, there is less scarring as well as minimal disruption of deeper soft tissues and a theoretically lower rate of osteonecrosis. Nevertheless, this type of fixation tends to be less stable than open reduction and internal fixation and requires hardware removal if pins are used. In addition, this technique does not allow for management of associated rotator cuff tearing or other intra-articular pathology that may impact the outcome of treatment. This technique is most easily applied to two-part surgical neck fractures, but it can also be used for more complex three- and four-part fractures. Terminally threaded pins provide superior fixation. More unstable and comminuted fractures and more severe osteopenia can compromise this technique. The initiation of shoulder motion is delayed because the fixation is not as secure. The best results have been reported with closed reduction and percutaneous pinning of two-part surgical neck fractures (Figure 1).

Careful pin placement is necessary to avoid iatrogenic neurovascular injury. A study of 10 cadavers investigated the safe location for percutaneous pins.[9] Lateral pins were located a mean distance of 3 mm from the anterior branch of the axillary nerve, and 20% of the lateral pins penetrated the humeral head cartilage. Anterior pins placed the cephalic vein and long head of the biceps at risk. The tip of the greater tuberosity pin was located 6 mm from the axillary nerve and 7 mm from the posterior humeral circumflex artery. Several authors have modified this technique by inserting cannulated screws over the percutaneously placed Kirschner wires, which eliminates the risk of pin sepsis, may increase

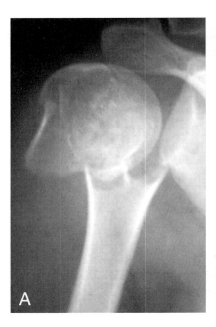 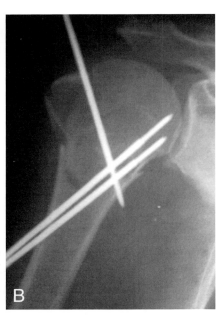

Figure 1 Plain radiographs of a displaced (angulated) two-part surgical neck fracture **(A)** that was treated with closed reduction and percutaneous pinning **(B)**.

fracture stability, and also may eliminate the need for hardware removal.

Open Reduction and Internal Fixation

The indications for open reduction and internal fixation of displaced proximal humerus fractures are controversial. The effect of residual fracture displacement on the outcome of treatment is difficult to determine. The outcome of surgical treatment depends on many factors in addition to the quality of the reduction of the fracture. The impact of osteopenic bone on the ability to obtain hardware purchase cannot be underestimated. Early studies recommended open reduction and internal fixation for two- and three-part fractures and prosthetic humeral head replacement for four-part fractures. Increasing experience with both techniques and critical outcome assessment has led to reconsideration of open reduction and internal fixation for the treatment of more complex displaced proximal humerus fractures.

The surgical approach depends on the specific fracture. Most fractures, including surgical neck, three-part, and four-part fractures, are treated via a deltopectoral approach. Greater tuberosity fractures can be treated via either a superior deltoid-splitting approach (similar to open rotator cuff repair) or a deltopectoral approach. Either approach can be used for treating valgus impacted fractures.

Many different internal fixation techniques are available. These include interosseous suture or wire, pins, screws, plates and screws, and rigid or flexible intramedullary rods. No single technique can be used exclusively for any specific fracture pattern. Comminution and osteopenia affect the stability or rigidity of any fixation technique; however, good bone is the exception, and techniques that achieve both interfragmentary and axial

stability without excessive soft-tissue dissection are preferred.

The security of screw fixation is often compromised because there is poor purchase in the humeral head. The best screw fixation can be achieved in the central aspect of the articular segment close to the subchondral bone where the cancellous bone is the thickest. Screw fixation of the greater tuberosity can fail because although the screw may have purchase in the humeral head articular segment, the fragile tuberosity may displace around the screw. Plate and screw fixation is best reserved for younger patients with good bone quality (Figure 2). When suture fixation is used the sutures can be placed through the bone or around the tuberosity fragments at the rotator cuff insertion. The latter is usually stronger and the preferred technique.

Metaphyseal comminution is particularly problematic. When there is comminution at the medial aspect of the surgical neck or proximal shaft area, it is difficult to maintain humeral length and the position of the articular segment. Varus malunion is a common sequela of comminution at the medial aspect of the surgical neck. Intramedullary fixation and fixed-angle plate and screw devices (blade and locking plates) can improve the stability of fixation. Conventional plate and screw fixation is prone to failure in this situation. In all patients with metaphyseal comminution, extraneous dissection should be avoided to preserve the vascularity to the articular segment.

Fixed-angle plate fixation has obvious advantages over traditional plate and screw techniques, particularly in patients with osteopenic bone. Blade plates and locking screw-plates have been recently introduced for treating proximal humerus fractures. The mode of failure of a

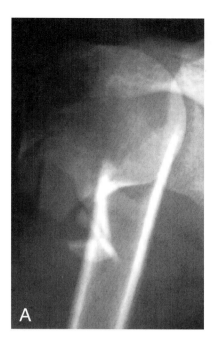
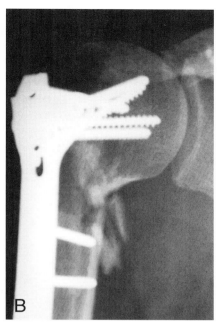

Figure 2 A, Preoperative plain radiograph of a displaced two-part surgical neck fracture in a 48-year-old woman. **B,** Postoperative plain radiograph of the same patient shows that nearly anatomic positioning was achieved with open reduction and internal fixation with a modified AO small fragment cloverleaf plate.

locking screw plate differs from that of a standard plate in that the entire construct has to fail as a unit instead of sequential screw pullout in the standard plate (Figure 3).

Recent biomechanical studies have evaluated the strength and stability of a variety of fixation techniques. In one study, antegrade locked intramedullary rodding was found to be superior to multiple pin fixation for the treatment of three-part greater tuberosity fractures.[10] Another study demonstrated that the addition of an intramedullary rod to a tension band construct significantly improved the fixation strength.[11] Tension band wiring supplemented with intramedullary fixation or Schanz pins was shown to be superior to tension band wiring alone for fixation of two-part surgical neck fractures.[5] Another biomechanical evaluation found tension band wiring in combination with Ender nails in a three-part fracture model to have less torsional and bending stiffness than either plate or locked intramedullary nail fixation.[12] Overall, the quality of the bone of the proximal humerus has been shown to have a significant effect upon the strength of all fracture fixation constructs.

Articular segment fractures are problematic because of the risk of arthritis resulting from articular incongruity as well as humeral head collapse secondary to osteonecrosis. Some simple articular fractures can be reduced and fixed internally. The articular reduction can be palpated through the rotator cuff interval and visualized with arthroscopic or fluoroscopic imaging. Displaced articular comminution is difficult to reduce without direct fracture exposure. Most fractures with significant articular comminution are treated with prosthetic replacement.

Valgus impacted four-part fractures are recognized as a distinct variation of four-part fractures. There appears to be a lower risk of osteonecrosis in patients with this type of fracture because the medial capsular vessels may remain intact. Thus, these fractures can be treated with open reduction and internal fixation (Figure 4). Limited soft-tissue dissection is required to achieve reduction. After the articular segment is reduced, the metaphyseal void can be filled with either autogenous or synthetic bone graft material.

Open reduction of true four-part fractures is controversial because of a high incidence of osteonecrosis. Achieving an anatomic reduction is critical when performing open reduction and internal fixation. A recent study of open reduction and internal fixation of three- and four-part fractures and fracture-dislocations found that osteonecrosis occurred in 5 of 11 three-part fractures and 8 of 9 four-part fractures.[13] Fracture-dislocation was also statistically associated with osteonecrosis. Although many of the patients with osteonecrosis had satisfactory outcomes, there were limitations of shoulder motion, and five of the eight patients with poor results had osteonecrosis. When there is osteonecrosis in the presence of an anatomic reduction, the clinical outcome is typically better.

Humeral head replacement is recommended for most four-part fractures and fracture-dislocations. In addition, humeral head replacement for some three-part fractures has been advocated, especially for those occurring in elderly patients with comminution and poor bone quality (Figure 5). Recent advances in implant design include modular humeral components. Modularity has several advantages, including improved ability to reconstruct the variable anatomy of the proximal humerus as well as facilitate revision from humeral head replacement to total shoulder replacement. Recognition of the impor-

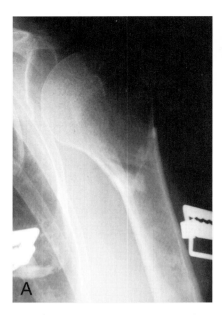
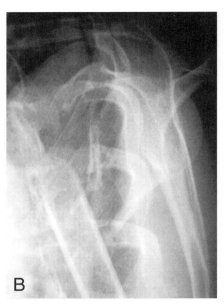
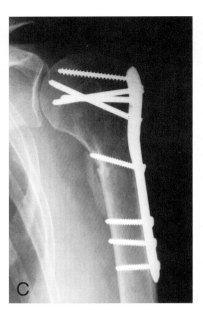

Figure 3 Preoperative true AP **(A)** and scapular Y-view **(B)** radiographs demonstrate a 100% displaced fracture of the surgical neck of the proximal humerus. **C,** Anatomic reduction and internal fixation was achieved using a locking proximal humeral plate.

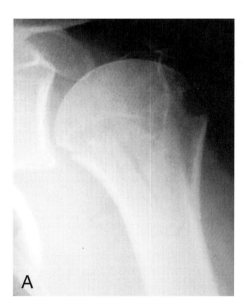
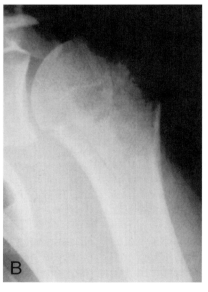

Figure 4 True AP radiographs of a patient with a valgus impacted proximal humerus fracture. **A,** Preoperative radiograph demonstrates the valgus position of the articular segment, which is impacted between the tuberosities. **B,** Postoperative radiograph demonstrates anatomic repositioning of the articular segment after open reduction and minimal internal fixation with heavy sutures.

tance of fixation and healing of the tuberosities has led to the development of new techniques that include circumferential suture fixation of the tuberosities around the humeral component (Figure 6). Although the functional outcomes of humeral head replacement for acute fracture remain variable, there is high patient satisfaction.

Complications

In addition to associated injuries, complications or poor results are not uncommon after proximal humerus fractures. Poor results after nonsurgical treatment are most commonly related to shoulder stiffness and limited mo-

tion or the consequences of displacement of the greater tuberosity. Even small amounts of superior displacement of the greater tuberosity can cause subacromial impingement. In fact, subacromial scarring without displacement can be sufficient to cause impingement. Surgical neck angulation and malunion are also relatively common. The typical angulation is apex anterolateral, and there is usually an associated loss of shoulder elevation and abduction (Figure 7). In addition, capsular contracture can occur and limit motion. Shoulder stiffness is best avoided by initiating passive motion exercises early in the rehabilitation process.

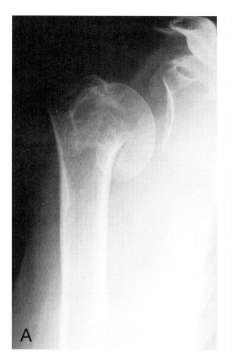
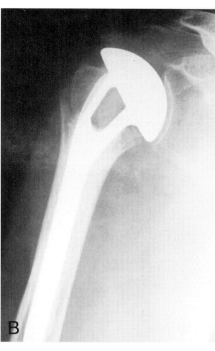

Figure 5 A, True AP radiograph of a three-part proximal humerus fracture in a 70-year-old woman. At the time of surgery an intra-articular head-splitting fracture was noted. **B,** Postoperative radiograph of the same patient after successful treatment with a humeral head replacement.

Although osteonecrosis is more common after four-part fractures, it can also occur after surgical treatment of less complex fractures. In contrast, osteonecrosis is rare after nondisplaced fractures or nonsurgical treatment of two- or three-part fractures. Posttraumatic arthritis usually occurs after articular segment fractures or malunions.

Late Posttraumatic Reconstruction

Late reconstruction after failed closed or open treatment is difficult. Although the results of late shoulder arthroplasty tend to be worse than the results of shoulder replacement for glenohumeral osteoarthritis, there is a high degree of patient satisfaction. The results of late reconstruction appear to correlate with the ability to correct the problems encountered at surgery, including malunion, nonunion, stiffness, and arthritis. The need for greater tuberosity osteotomy also correlates with the outcome. The outcome is better when reconstructive arthroplasty can be performed without tuberosity osteotomy.

Outcomes

There has been substantial recent interest in the evaluation of the outcome of various shoulder disorders. Most studies have focused on the treatment of atraumatic disorders. There is no outcome measure that is specifically designed to evaluate the outcome of shoulder fractures.

The outcome of nonsurgical treatment of nondisplaced proximal humerus fractures is often limited. The results of some studies comparing the nonsurgical and surgical treatment of more complex fractures in elderly patients suggest that in certain populations there may be little benefit to surgical treatment. In an older population, 40 patients with three-part fractures were randomized to undergo closed treatment or tension band internal fixation. Maximal function was achieved at 1 year.[14] The authors concluded that although surgery resulted in a better radiographic appearance, surgical treatment resulted in more complications and no significant improvement in overall patient outcome compared with nonsurgical treatment.

Several recent studies reported variable outcomes after surgical treatment of more severe proximal humerus fractures. It is difficult to determine why some studies report better outcomes than others, although varying patient populations, surgeon skill, and observer bias undoubtedly have an effect. The studies that use modern outcome assessments tend to report poorer outcomes for open reduction and internal fixation of more complex fractures, especially four-part fractures. Additionally, the selection of an optimal treatment plan is unfortunately not aided by a review of the orthopaedic literature. A meta-analysis of 24 reports spanning 30 years has been conducted, and the authors concluded that the published literature is inadequate for evidence-based decision making with regard to the treatment of complex proximal humerus fractures.[15]

Humeral Shaft Fractures

Epidemiology

Humeral shaft fractures account for approximately 3% of fractures. There is a bimodal age distribution of frac-

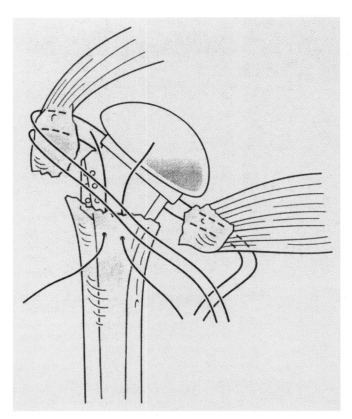

Figure 6 Diagram of circumferential suture fixation for tuberosity repair in humeral head replacement. *(Reproduced with permission from Browner B, Jupiter J, Levine A, Trafton P (eds): Skeletal Trauma: Basic Science, Management, and Reconstruction, ed 3. Philadelphia, PA, WB Saunders, 2003.)*

ture occurrence, with peaks of incidence occurring in the third decade of life for males and the seventh decade of life for females. However, approximately 60% of these fractures occur in individuals older than 50 years. The most common fractures occur in the middle third of the humerus and are of a simple fracture pattern (AO type A). In a tertiary referral center, 60% of patients with humeral shaft fractures were between the ages of 16 and 35 years, and most of the fractures were the result of high-energy mechanisms (43% caused by motor vehicle accidents and 17% caused by gunshot wounds).

Nonsurgical Management

Most humeral shaft fractures are best managed with functional bracing. In a report of 922 patients, of which 620 were available for follow-up, initial splinting or above-elbow casting followed by humeral fracture bracing resulted in a closed fracture nonunion rate of less than 2% and an open fracture nonunion rate of 6%.[16] Eighty-seven percent of fractures healed in less than 16° of varus, and 81% healed in less than 16° of anterior angulation. Overall, 98% of patients exhibited less than 25° of angulation in both planes, and the same percentage had shoulder limitation of 25° or less at brace re-

moval. Other studies confirmed these results, reporting nonunion rates of 1.2% to 8.9%, acceptable alignment, and excellent or good results in 69% to 95% of patients. Similar results have been achieved with immediate fracture brace application (Figure 8). However, one study reported loss of 5° to 40° of external rotation in 38% of patients treated with functional bracing secondary to malrotation of the humerus (as noted using CT) and/or soft-tissue contracture.[17] The authors of this report concluded that earlier application of the fracture brace (within 8 to 14 days after injury) may resolve humeral malrotation, whereas others recommend immediate fracture brace application.[18]

There is no consensus on what constitutes acceptable alignment of the humerus. In part, the amount of angulation that is clinically acceptable is related to the patient's size and body habitus. Shortening of 3 cm, 20° angulation in the sagittal plane, and 30° varus/valgus angulation in the average size patient is generally accepted as satisfactory. However, in slim patients, this amount of angulation may result in an unacceptable cosmetic result.

Contraindications for functional bracing included massive soft-tissue injury, bone loss, multiple injuries, lack of cooperation from the patient, or inability to obtain or maintain acceptable alignment. Methods of nonsurgical care other than fracture bracing have fallen out of favor because of shoulder and elbow stiffness resulting from lack of early joint mobilization.

Surgical Care

Although many diaphyseal humerus fractures are amenable to nonsurgical treatment, several indications for surgical intervention have been described in the literature (Table 1). Most of these surgical indications are relative, and the validity of some as surgical indications may be questioned. Absolute indications include fractures associated with a vascular injury, ipsilateral forearm fractures, and severe soft-tissue trauma.

One study reported outcome determinants for 7,687 patients with humeral shaft fractures.[19] Nonsurgical treatment failed in 2.5% of patients, with 7% of those with multiple trauma undergoing subsequent surgical intervention. Open fractures had a 12% infection rate in patients without fixation and 10.8% in those with internal fixation. Infection was associated with preexisting comorbid conditions, open fractures, and multiple trauma (not surgical intervention). Nonunions were associated with surgeon inexperience.

Plating

Plate and screw fixation for humeral shaft fractures has been the preferred treatment for many surgical indications. Union rates have been high (95% to 100%), with good shoulder and elbow function also reported. Infection rates have been low (0 to 4%, with most deep

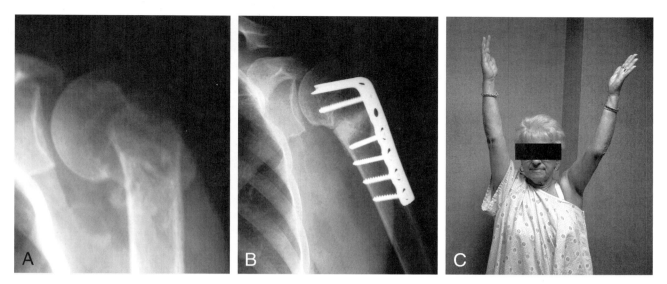

Figure 7 A, Preoperative plain radiograph of a patient who presented with pain and limited shoulder motion after a neck fracture demonstrates a varus malunion. **B,** Postoperative plain radiograph demonstrates that the malunion was successfully treated with an osteotomy and internal fixation with an angled blade plate. **C,** Photograph shows postoperative active forward elevation.

infections occurring in open fractures), and associated iatrogenic radial nerve palsies have been infrequent (0 to 4%, most of which are transient). The fixation failure rate has been 0 to 5%, with inadequate surgical technique (short plate syndrome) being responsible for most instances (Figure 9).

The main disadvantages of plate fixation that have been reported include the need for extensile exposure, risk of radial nerve injury, poor fixation in osteopenic bone, soft-tissue stripping leading to devascularization, stress shielding, and refracture after hardware removal. Concerns have also been raised that revisions (to treat infection, nonunion, or symptomatic hardware) through a scarred soft-tissue bed can lead to iatrogenic radial nerve injury, especially when the plate is placed under the nerve. One study addressed this concern by recommending transposition of the radial nerve through the fracture, thereby making a subsequent surgical exposure possible without encountering the radial nerve and the risk of injury.[20] Radial nerve transposition is a relatively new technique and further investigation is needed.

The introduction of fixed-angle screws has changed some of the thinking regarding the treatment of diaphyseal and metaphyseal fractures. A biomechanical study of Schuhli nuts, the first fixed-angle screw device that is anchored through a standard compression plate, revealed that the device had the greatest advantage over conventional screw fixation when there was a defect on the near cortex. It was also noted that there was less stress to the bone under the plate. In another report, the Schuhli nut was found to be useful in the treatment of difficult nonunions because the surgeons were able to place screws where cortical defects exist, improve purchase in osteoporotic bone, and create a fixed-angle de-

vice.[21] Union was achieved in these difficult nonunions during the index procedure in 41 of 44 patients.

Recently introduced locking plates are considered to be the next generation of fixed-angle implants because they provide theoretic advantages in fracture fixation, particularly for fractures and nonunions with comminution, bone loss, and osteopenia. Some locking plates allow for placement of either a fixed-angle locking screw or a standard cortical screw in each screw hole. The locking plate is not compressed against the bone, making it function much like an internal fixator. Therefore, devascularization and stress shielding of the bone beneath the plate are minimized. Biomechanically, the addition of one locking screw to a plating construct has been shown to increase the axial stability by 50% on each side of the fracture in an osteopenic bone model. With the same axial loading done in a hard cortical bone model, the differences in stability have been shown to be less. One study reported that in an osteopenic model AP bending, mediolateral bending, and torsional stability were similar for the limited-contact dynamic compression plate and the locking compression plate.[22] The average energy to failure was significantly greater in the locking compression plate. Because the axial stability of locked plating constructs appears to be improved, there is more of an onus on the orthopaedic surgeon to avoid gaps across the fracture site (avoiding stability in distraction) to prevent nonunions. Additional work needs to be done to determine when these locking plates are indicated over the currently available plating techniques.

Weight bearing on a plated humerus for a patient with multiple trauma has been a concern for orthopaedic trauma surgeons. In a study of 83 plated humerus frac-

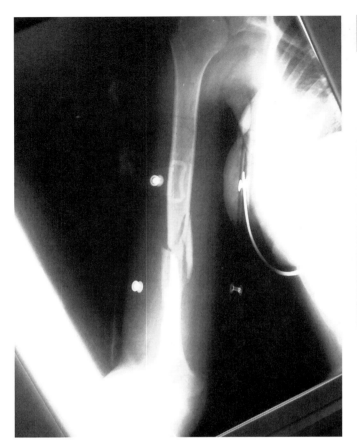

Figure 8 Radiograph of a patient with a comminuted humeral shaft fracture that shows evidence of healing in a fracture brace.

TABLE 1 | Indications for Surgical Treatment of Humeral Shaft Fractures

Vascular injury
Severe soft-tissue injury precluding bracing (such as burns)
Open fractures
Floating elbow
Pathologic fracture
Multiple trauma
Concomitant head injury
Inability to obtain or maintain reduction
Bilateral humeral shaft fractures
Shaft fracture with extension into joint
Segmental or severely comminuted fracture
Radial nerve injury during closed reduction
Distraction of bone fragments
Ipsilateral brachial plexus injury
Morbid obesity
Uncooperative or unreliable patient

tures separated into groups in which the humerus was used either in weight bearing (52%), no weight bearing (40%), or transfer weight bearing (8%), it was found that immediate weight bearing did not have an effect on union or malunion rates.[18] The patients did use a platform on their walker or crutch to decrease (at least theoretically) the moment arm of the forces exerted across the plate.

Immediate plate fixation of open humerus fractures has been a concern because it involves further stripping of soft tissues in an already compromised and contaminated wound bed. In a study of 53 open humeral shaft fractures, 46 were followed to fracture healing without problems with infection, further surgery to achieve union, or iatrogenic radial nerve palsies.[23] The authors concluded that immediate plate osteosynthesis is the treatment of choice for open humeral shaft fractures after thorough and aggressive débridement.

The question of how much fixation is sufficient for fractures is especially pertinent for the humeral shaft because most failures are reportedly secondary to inadequate fixation. In a biomechanical study that assessed the strength of plate fixation in relation to the number and spacing of bone screws, it was found that torsional stability is related to the absolute number of screws on either side of the fracture.[24] The authors reported that stability in bending depends on wide spacing of screws rather than on the absolute number of screws. Thus, long plates with screws placed close to and far away from the fracture site will most effectively improve stability. Although this logic can be extended to locking plates as well, biomechanical studies are needed to confirm whether this is true.

Intramedullary Rods

Interest has been increasing in the use of intramedullary rods to treat humeral shaft fractures because of successes seen using intramedullary rods to treat fractures of the lower extremities. Intramedullary rodding is less invasive, less devascularizing, and more load-sharing than plating.

In the first reported series of using intramedullary rods to treat humeral fractures, flexible intramedullary rods were used. When data from multiple flexible intramedullary rodding studies were combined, nonunions were found in 3% of patients, radial nerve palsy in 1%, and infections in 1% (all open fractures).[25] Shoulder deficits were reported in 3 of 32 patients whose fractures were treated with antegrade flexible rods, and elbow deficits were reported in 3 of 24 of those whose fractures were treated with retrograde flexible rods. Limitations of the flexible rods include lack of rotational control, inability to maintain axial stability in the presence of comminution, tendency for nail migration (backout), and need for postoperative bracing.

The introduction of locking intramedullary rods expanded the indications for treating humeral shaft fractures with intramedullary fixation. However, early reports on locked intramedullary nailing were fraught with

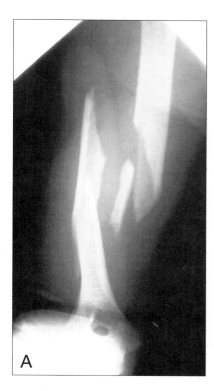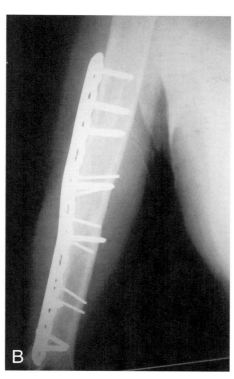

Figure 9 A, Preoperative radiograph of a comminuted and displaced humeral shaft fracture and complete radial and median nerve palsy in a 20-year-old man. **B,** Postoperative radiograph of the same patient after plating; median and radial nerve had eventual full recovery.

high nonunion rates (up to 33%) and frequent shoulder pain (27% to 100% of fractures treated with antegrade nailings). Follow-up studies have confirmed these relatively high rates of nonunion and shoulder pain, although a few authors report complication rates that are similar to those seen after plating. In particular, the incidence of shoulder pain is reduced when retrograde or anterior acromial approaches to nailing are used rather than a lateral deltoid-splitting incision (Figure 10).

Shoulder Pain Persistent shoulder pain has been reported to occur after antegrade intramedullary nailing of humeral shaft fractures, possibly because of the rotator cuff entry point. Anterior and straight lateral starting points have been described. The anterior starting point uses the anatomic interval between the anterior and middle third of the deltoid, with a starting point more centrally placed on the rotator cuff tendon. This starting point is thought to give a linear approach to the humeral canal if a straight nail is used, which may result in fewer problems with healing of the rotator cuff incision. Unfortunately, this approach to humeral shaft rodding most commonly results in violation of the superolateral articular surface, which may be why it takes up to 6 months for optimization of motion and function after nailing with this approach. Shoulder function was found to be good or excellent in 90% to 100% of humeral shaft fractures treated with the anterior approach. No known studies report a high percent of shoulder pain with the anterior approach.

The straight lateral starting point leads to splitting of the deltoid, an incision in the area near the insertion of

the rotator cuff (the avascular portion), and may lead to a starting point that is not in line with the humeral shaft canal. In a cadaver antegrade humeral shaft rod evaluation, an anterior approach resulted in a small incision in the midportion of the rotator cuff tendon that was aligned with the humeral canal. Clinical results from many studies using the lateral acromial approach have reported suboptimal shoulder function. Several authors, however, have reported shoulder problems in 17% of patients (or less) when using the lateral entry point. Unfortunately, not all such articles in the literature state which rod insertion approach was used. Nonetheless, a definite increase in shoulder pain has been reported to occur if the antegrade nail is left prominent with either approach.

Another factor affecting shoulder pain and starting point is the variability in the proximal humeral geometry (Figure 11). With increasing offset of the humeral head, there is a larger area of articular surface injury with the anterior approach. Unfortunately, this variable has not been addressed and may be difficult to reliably quantify unless reproducible, standard plain radiographic views are obtained.

Although shoulder pain decreases with the use of retrograde humeral nailing, some shoulder pain still occurs. This may be because of injury to proximally directed branches of the axillary nerve during proximal locking. However, one prospective randomized study of antegrade versus retrograde rodding shows no differences in shoulder pain between these two approaches.

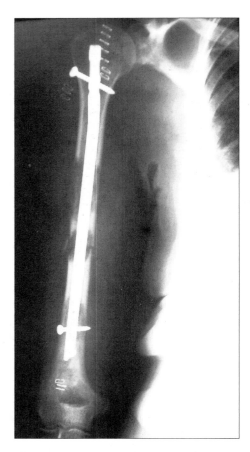

Figure 10 Radiograph showing a pathologic humerus fracture stabilized by an intramedullary rod.

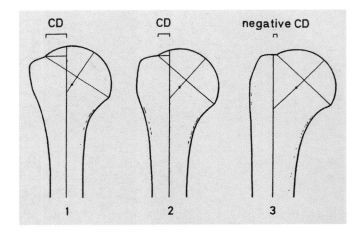

Figure 11 Illustration showing variations that can be noted in proximal humeral geometry that lead to variations in optimal humeral rod placement. *(Reproduced with permission from Hertel R, Knothe U, Ballmer FT: Geometry of the proximal humerus and implications for prosthetic design. J Shoulder Elbow Surg 2002;11:331-338.)*

Nonunions There are many causes of nonunions after humeral shaft nailing. The humerus is not normally a weight-bearing bone, which leads to a lack of natural fracture compressive forces with use. The slight anterior curvature and narrowing of the terminal centimeters of the distal humeral canal has led many orthopaedic surgeons to leave the humeral shaft fracture distracted as the intramedullary nail is impacted into this narrowed region. Fracture distraction has been correlated with nonunions in nailed humeral shaft fractures. One study found that the nonunion rate was lower in multiple trauma patients who needed to bear weight on the humerus with the intramedullary rod than those who had isolated injuries that did not require upper extremity weight bearing.

One popular intramedullary rodding system has reduced torsional stability in the first 25° to 30° of biomechanical testing. The rigidity to torsional load is similar to that of other nail designs, but the initial rotational play is significantly higher because of the nail design itself. The nail design has a single proximal screw and a single large, oval, distal interlocking screw hole. Nails with two proximal and distal locking screws did not exhibit this initial play with torsional testing. Because torsional stresses are significant in the humerus, this torsional shear may account for some nonunions when the less stable nail design is used.

Iatrogenic fractures have also been implicated as a cause for nonunion. Fracture extension or entry portal fractures can lead to implant and subsequently fracture instability, which in turn can lead ultimately to nonunion. The stability of the fracture based on insertion from proximal or distal entry sites has been studied as well. In a cadaver study, it was noted that intramedullary rodding from the short to the long segment resulted in improved fracture site stability. Fractures occurring at the isthmus were not reported to be significantly more stable with antegrade or retrograde insertion.

It has been reported that reaming of the humeral canal does not appear to affect union rates.[26,27] Reaming of the canal does, however, affect the ease of rod insertion and therefore the likelihood of iatrogenic fracture. Because iatrogenic fractures affect stability and possibly the union rate, reaming may affect union indirectly. Also, reaming may prevent jamming of the nail in the distal fragment (with antegrade insertion), decreasing the likelihood of persistent fracture gapping and nonunion. Disadvantages of reaming include potential thermal injury with aggressive reaming and injury to the endosteal blood supply. If used, limited reaming is preferred because complications can and do result with overreaming of the humeral canal.

Other Complications Associated With Humeral Shaft Nailing Iatrogenic supracondylar fractures and fracture site extensions commonly occur with the use of retrograde nails because the starting point is in dense cortical bone, and any variation from the ideal starting point and rod placement orientation can result in cracking of the supracondylar or fracture site cortex with rod insertion. Instability of the rod may result in nonunion of the fracture and iatrogenic fracture. In a cadaver study, it was noted that the alignment of the distal humerus in 14 of 20 cadavers led to an ideal starting point for rod placement at the superior rim of the olecranon fossa (Figure 12). In 6 of 20 cadavers, the ideal starting point remained in the distal metaphysis. In a separate cadaveric study, it was found that the intramedullary canal did extend to the olecranon fossa in all cadaveric specimens studied.[28] Although proximal entry point fractures during antegrade nailing are less common, they occur more commonly if the lateral starting point is used. It has been suggested that humeral nails should not be inserted with mallet impaction, but should instead be inserted only by hand to avoid iatrogenic fractures. If the nail is not inserted easily, some authors recommended further reaming to allow for easy placement.

Delayed fractures involving the distal humeral shaft entry point have also been problematic, as have fractures through distal locking screw holes. In a biomechanical study, it was found that the entry portal made in the distal humerus for insertion of a retrograde rod decreased the ultimate energy to failure in torsion to 18% of the intact specimen. However, another study found the decrease in bone strength to be only 11.1%. It is necessary to make a generous entry portal to decrease the risk of iatrogenic fractures; unfortunately this decreases the resistance to later injury and may affect the orthopaedic surgeon's decision to allow early upper extremity weight bearing.

Radial nerve palsy resulting from reaming of the humeral canal is also a concern. If a patient has no preoperative radial nerve palsy, holding an anatomic closed reduction during reaming and rod placement as well as pushing the motionless reamer through areas of severe comminution may protect the nerve. A fracture gap during the closed reduction likely indicates the presence of interposed tissue, with the nerve as a possible source, in which instance limited open reduction with nerve exploration may limit nerve injury. If the radial nerve is not functioning preoperatively, radial nerve exploration is indicated before fixation (whether intramedullary rodding or plating is planned). MRI or ultrasonography may be used for preoperative imaging of the radial nerve if there is concern about nerve entrapment.

Complications associated with the placement of locking screws are rare, but they can occur with the use of proximal and distal locking screws. Proximal locking with anterior to posterior placement of screws can injure the axillary nerve and even the axillary artery and vein if the screws are left prominent or if plunging is done with drilling of the posterior cortex. This risk is increased if the screws are placed with the shoulder maximally internally rotated. In lateral to medial proximal locking, there is a risk of injuring the axillary nerve or its branches, especially with the more distal of the two proximal holes. The anterior to posterior placement of distal locking screws can injure the lateral antebrachial cutaneous

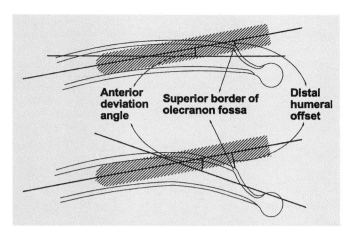

Figure 12 Illustration showing retrograde humeral nailing starting points based on the distal humeral anatomic variations. *(Reproduced with permission from Lin J, Hou SM, Inoue N, Chao EY, Hang YS: Anatomic considerations of locked humeral nailing. Clin Orthop 1999;368:247-254.)*

nerve, median nerve, or brachial artery. Lateral to medial screw placement can injure the radial nerve and posterior antebrachial cutaneous nerve. Dissection for anterior to posterior distal screw placement should be performed lateral to the biceps tendon. Incisions used for all distal interlocking screws should allow for placement of screws under direct vision, not percutaneously.

Another disadvantage of intramedullary nailing is that if revision is needed for any reason, the recovery of the nail will violate the rotator cuff again, which results in the increased risk of additional shoulder pain.

Overall, the results of treating humeral shaft fractures with intramedullary nails are not as consistently successful when compared with plating. The disparity in results using intramedullary rodding to treat humeral shaft fractures involves many variables, many of which are not documented in the literature. These variables include starting points for insertion of antegrade rods, the type of proximal humeral anatomy, static or dynamic locking of the rod, whether reaming is done, amount of fracture gap, and experience of the surgeon with humeral shaft rodding. The authors of articles that report good results with intramedullary rodding of humeral fractures often have published previous articles on humeral shaft rodding. Subsequent studies from the same authors usually show improved results as fine details that improve intraoperative and postoperative results are learned and incorporated with experience. Therefore, it may be concluded that one of the more important variables is surgeon experience.

Intramedullary Rods Versus Plates
Biomechanical comparisons of intramedullary rods and plates in axial loading found that under physiologic loading there was little difference between the two forms of fixation. When stressed to failure, the applied loads were 50% higher with intramedullary rods than plates, which

TABLE 2 | Comparative Studies for Plating and Nailing Humeral Shaft Fractures

Authors (Type of Study)	Treatment	No. of Patients	No. of Nonunion/ Malunion	No. of Infections	Radial Nerve Palsy	No. of Problems with Shoulder/Elbow	Additional Surgery	Iatrogenic Fractures
Chapman et al[29] (Prospective)	Plates	46	3/2	3 (deep)	1 (transient)	0/4	na	0
	Nails	38 (all antegrade)	2/1	0	2 (transient)	6/0	na	0
McCormack et al[30] (Prospective)	Plates	22	1/0	0	0	0/0	1	1
	Nails	21 (13 antegrade, 18 retrograde)	2/0	1	3 (2 transient)	4/0	7	2
Bolano et al[31] (Prospective)	Plates	14	1/NA	NA	NA	1/NA	NA	NA
	Nails	14	4/na	NA	NA	6/NA	NA	NA
Wagner et al[32] (Retrospective)	Plates	17	0/0	0	1 (transient)	0/0	0	0
	Nails	19 (all antegrade)	1/0	1 (superficial)	0	8/0	4	0
Meekers and Broos[33] (Retrospective)	Plates	80	0/0	0	4 (transient)	0/0	3	0
	Nails	81 (8 antegrade, 72 retrograde)	12/0	0	4 (3 transient)	2/9	18	4*
Linn[34] (Retrospective)	Plates	25	1/0	1	1 (transient)	0/0	9	0
	Nails	48 (15 antegrade, 33 retrograde)	0/1	0	0	1/3	22	1
Total	Plates	204	6/2	4	7 (transient)	1/4	13	1
	Nails	221	21/2	2	9 (7 transient)	21/12	51	7

*Three of these were changed to plate fixation because of comminution
NA = not applicable

is statistically significant. In other biomechanical studies, bending stiffness was reported to be greater with intramedullary nails, and torsional stiffness varied between studies with regard to plated or solid nail stabilized specimens.

Six studies have assessed the results of treatment with plating or interlocking intramedullary rods[29-34] (Table 2). Three of these were prospective randomized studies, and three were retrospective studies. Four of the studies recommended the use of plates instead of rods because of the increased complication rates associated with intramedullary rodding procedures. One article reported that both plates and rods provided reliable methods of fracture stabilization, and one article recommended rodding over plating.

Although significant improvements in the results of using intramedullary rods to treat humeral shaft fractures have been achieved, plating continues to give overall better results when considering nonunions, revision rates, and shoulder function. Intramedullary rods, however, are more beneficial than plating for patients with pathologic or impending fractures. Selected patients with severe comminution or segmental humeral shaft fractures and certain patients with multiple trauma may be best served with intramedullary rodding. Experience may broaden indications.

External Fixation

External fixation is not commonly used to treat humeral shaft fractures because of frequently associated complications. Generally accepted indications for external fixation of humeral shaft fractures include (1) massive soft-tissue injury, (2) bone injuries precluding the use of either plates or intramedullary rods, and (3) its use as a temporizing measure until another form of fixation can be implemented. Good results have been reported in a wider range of indications.

Radial Nerve Injury

Radial nerve injury is the most worrisome part of humeral shaft fracture treatment. Recovery rates for primary (fracture-related) nerve injuries are high (up to 92% of patients). The results of nerve decompression and repair are good (84.5% to 100%). Additional nerve injury may occur if early exploration is performed in closed fractures that do not require surgical intervention. For these reasons, it is recommended that primary nerve injuries be observed for the first 3 to 4 months. If no evidence of recovery is seen clinically or electromyographically, surgical intervention typically occurs within 6 months of injury. The exception to this treatment algorithm is open humeral shaft fractures because the incidence of radial nerve transection is higher with these injuries. This treatment algorithm has been challenged because not all radial nerves recover and observing primary nerve injuries for the first 3 to 4 months prolongs impairment. Additionally, the encasement of the radial nerve in callus can inhibit recovery or at least make the dissection for the repair difficult.

For secondary radial nerve palsies (those found after first examination of the patient), surgical intervention has classically been recommended. It is assumed that the nerve is either stretched or between the fracture fragments, either of which can delay nerve regeneration. However, it has been noted that secondary nerve palsies may recover without early decompression.

When the integrity of the radial nerve is not known (in patients who are intubated or sedated or those with closed head injuries) or when there is a high likelihood of radial nerve injury because of fracture pattern, somatosensory evoked potentials with continuous electromyography has been used to monitor radial nerve injury. One study found that changes identified during this type of monitoring altered treatment in 3 of 13 intramedullary rodding procedures.[35] No iatrogenic radial neuropathies were identified. Additional studies are necessary to confirm the usefulness of this technique because it results in not only increased costs, but also increased operating room time.

Ultrasound has been used successfully in the diagnosis of radial nerve entrapment, stretching, or transection. One report found that ultrasound provided accurate information regarding tenting, entrapment, and transection of the radial nerve. In nerves that were found to be contused using ultrasound, nerve recovery occurred at 6 months without the need for surgical intervention. This modality has promise for differentiating between contusion and surgical lesion, which can lead to earlier treatment and nerve recovery for patients with surgical lesions. The authors mentioned that high-quality ultrasonography equipment is needed and that there is a learning curve for ultrasonographers and radiologists.

During the surgical treatment of patients with humeral shaft fractures, it is important to initiate the care of the radial nerve as soon as the patient is anesthetized. The unsupported apex posterior angulation or "sag" of the fractured humerus stretches the radial nerve along with the rest of the posterior soft tissues. With the lateral intermuscular septum tethering the nerve, this slight stretching may result in a transient radial nerve palsy.

Nonunion

Humeral shaft nonunions often impair function, especially in the older population who already have functional challenges. Although good results have been reported using several methods of treating humeral shaft nonunions, the gold standard for treatment continues to be compression plate fixation. Bone grafting is typically included during compression plate fixation unless there is a hypertrophic nonunion. Union rates have been high (88% to 100%), and functional results have been good (76% to 90% good or excellent results).

Humeral shaft nonunions are commonly associated with disuse osteopenia and often with osteoporosis, which can make it difficult to gain stability using classic compression plating techniques. Adjuvant materials historically used for improving plating stability include polymethylmethacrylate, intramedullary fibula placement, and intramedullary plates. In a cadaveric study that compared pull-out strength with the use of Schuhli nut–augmented compression plates, standard compression plates, and compression plates augmented with polymethylmethacrylate, no significant difference was found between the Schuhli nut–augmented and the polymethylmethacrylate-augmented compression plates. A significant difference in pull-out strength, however, was found between these two methods of improving plating stability and compression plates. Schuhli nuts (and now the locking plates) have the benefit of not having the potential adverse effect on bone healing that polymethylmethacrylate has, especially when it extrudes between fracture fragments.

A study of 27 patients who received locking compression plates for the treatment of delayed unions and nonunions of the humeral shaft found that all 27 patients went on to achieve final union.[36] Two of these patients required a secondary bone grafting to achieve union. One fracture occurred above the plate, but no loss of fixation was reported in any of the patients.

The management of nonunion after humeral nailing is more difficult. The usual situation with postnailing nonunions is significant bone loss resulting from the windshield wiper effect. Subsequent intramedullary nailing has the potential to only compound this problem further. Exchange rodding for postnailing nonunions has not produced favorable results. When the nonunion site is taken down, stabilized with a humeral rod, and bone grafted, results are improved.

High union rates have been reported using both Ilizarov and unilateral external fixation in nonunion of the humeral shaft. For most orthopaedic surgeons, however, the routine use of these techniques should be limited to unusual circumstances (patients with infected nonunions or those with a compromised soft-tissue envelope).

Summary

A pain-free functional shoulder is the goal of treatment of a proximal humerus fracture. The optimal method of achieving this goal continues to be both a challenge and a controversy. The first hurdle is the correct classification of the fracture. Good quality radiographs are a must and may need to be augmented with advanced diagnostic imaging. In addition to minimally displaced proximal humerus fractures, certain valgus impacted fractures and two-part fractures may have good results when treated nonsurgically, particularly in the low-demand patient population. The results of surgical treatment of two-part proximal humerus fractures are generally very good. Surgical treatment of three-part proximal humerus fractures usually involves open reduction and internal fixation. Some four-part proximal humerus fractures, especially those occurring in younger patients, can be treated with open reduction and internal fixation. Humeral head replacement is reserved for some three-part and most four-part proximal humerus fractures and fracture-dislocations in older patients.

Most humeral shaft fractures can be treated nonsurgically with functional bracing. For most surgical indications, plating will give the most reliable results with the least likely need for later surgical intervention. As techniques and implants continue to improve, the results of plating, intramedullary rodding, and external fixation will improve the treatment of humeral shaft fractures.

Annotated References

1. Kannus P, Palvanen M, Niemi S, Parkkari J, Jarvinen M, Vuori I: Osteoporotic fractures of the proximal humerus in elderly Finnish persons: Sharp increase in 1970-1998 and alarming projections for the new millennium. *Acta Orthop Scand* 2000;71:465-470.

2. Lee SH, Dargent-Molina P, Breart G: Risk factors for fractures of the proximal humerus: Results from the EPIDOS prospective study. *J Bone Miner Res* 2002;17:817-825.

3. Court-Brown CM, Garg A, McQueen MM: The epidemiology of proximal humeral fractures. *Acta Orthop Scand* 2001;72:365-371.

4. Neer CS II: Four-segment classification of proximal humeral fractures: Purpose and reliable use. *J Shoulder Elbow Surg* 2002;11:389-400.

   This article provides an overview of the history of the Neer classification and its use in guiding treatment of proximal humerus fractures. The problem of intraobserver reliability and interobserver reproducibility of this classification system is addressed and the author notes that this classification system was never intended to rely only on the radiographs to assign a fracture type. Rather, it was assumed that the intraoperative findings would be an adjunct to confirm the fracture classification. The validity of the four-part system remains intact in that each category has an identifiable natural history, prognosis, and treatment requirement. The author reviews and updates his treatment recommendations for each fracture classification.

5. Koval KJ, Gallagher MA, Marsicano JG, Cuomo F, McShinawy A, Zuckerman JD: Functional outcome after minimally displaced fractures of the proximal part of the humerus. *J Bone Joint Surg Am* 1997;79:203-207.

6. Park TS, Choi IY, Kim YH, Park MR, Shon JH, Kim SI: A new suggestion for the treatment of minimally displaced fractures of the greater tuberosity of the proximal humerus. *Bull Hosp Jt Dis* 1997;56:171-176.

7. Court-Brown CM, Cattermole H, McQueen MM: Impacted valgus fractures (B1.1) of the proximal humerus: The results of non-operative treatment. *J Bone Joint Surg Br* 2002;84:504-508.

   This article describes a common type of proximal humerus fracture that occurs in elderly patients. It is unique to the AO classification and is distinct from the three-part fracture in the Neer classification in that the humeral head component is not rotated. The authors retrospectively evaluated 125 patients treated without surgery. At 1-year follow-up, good or excellent results were documented in 80.6% of patients. The outcome depended on the age of the patient and displacement of the fracture. The authors suggested that this common fracture does not require surgical treatment.

8. Court-Brown CM, Garg A, McQueen MM: The translated two-part fracture of the proximal humerus: Epidemiology and outcome in the older patient. *J Bone Joint Surg Br* 2001;83:799-804.

9. Rowles DJ, McGrory JE: Percutaneous pinning of the proximal part of the humerus: An anatomic study. *J Bone Joint Surg Am* 2001;83:1685-1699.

10. Wheeler DL, Colville MR: Biomechanical comparison of intramedullary and percutaneous pin fixation for proximal humeral fracture fixation. *J Orthop Trauma* 1997;11:363-367.

11. Beredjiklian PK, Iannotti JP, Norris TR, Williams GR: Operative treatment of malunion of a fracture of the proximal aspect of the humerus. *J Bone Joint Surg Am* 1998;80:1484-1497.

12. Ruch DS, Glisson RR, Marr AW, Russell GB, Nunley JA: Fixation of three-part proximal humeral fractures: a biomechanical evaluation. *J Orthop Trauma* 2000;14:36-40.

13. Wijgman AJ, Roolker W, Patt TW, Raaymakers EL, Marti RK: Open reduction and internal fixation of three and four-part fractures of the proximal part of the humerus. *J Bone Joint Surg Am* 2002;84-A:1919-1925.

The authors of this article evaluated intermediate- and long-term results for 60 patients with three- or four-part proximal humerus fractures. The fractures were fixed with either T plate or cerclage wires. At an average follow-up of 10 years, 87% of patients had good or excellent results and 13% had a poor result. Twenty-two patients (37%) developed osteonecrosis, seven of whom had a three-part fracture-dislocation, eight of whom had a four-part fracture-dislocation, and seven of whom had a fracture without dislocation. Overall, in the subgroup of patients with osteonecrosis, 9% had excellent results, 68% had good results, and 23% had poor results using the Constant score as the outcome measure. The clinical importance of this study is the recognition that the presence of osteonecrosis does not preclude a satisfactory outcome. Therefore, internal fixation of even a four-part fracture-dislocation in a relatively young patient is warranted.

14. Zyto K, Ahrengart L, Sperber A, Tornkvist H: Treatment of displaced proximal fractures in elderly patients. *J Bone Joint Surg Br* 1997;79:412-417.

15. Misra A, Kapur R, Maffulli N: Complex proximal humeral fractures in adults: A systematic review of management. *Injury* 2001;32:363-372.

16. Sarmiento A, Zagorski JB, Zych GA, Latta LL, Capps CA: Functional bracing for the treatment of fractures of the humeral diaphysis. *J Bone Joint Surg Am* 2000;82:478-486.

In this study, 620 of 922 patients with humeral shaft fractures (465 with closed fractures and 155 with open fractures) were followed to union. The authors reported that 87% of fractures healed in < 16° varus and 81% healed in < 16° anterior angulation. Nonunions were noted in 16 patients (3%), and 98% had limitation of 25° or less at time of brace removal.

17. Fjalestad T, Stromsoe K, Salvesen P, Rostad B: Functional results of braced humeral diaphyseal fractures: Why do 38% lose external rotation of the shoulder? *Arch Orthop Trauma Surg* 2000;120:281-285.

The authors of this study reported that functional bracing of 67 fractures resulted in an 8.9% nonunion rate and a 38% loss of external rotation from bony and/or soft-tissue contracture. They concluded that earlier placement of patients into a functional brace would improve rotational problems.

18. Tingstad EM, Wolinsky PR, Shyr Y, Johnson KD: Effect of immediate weightbearing on plated fractures of the humeral shaft. *J Trauma* 2000;49:278-280.

In this study, 83 humeral shaft fractures were treated with plates and full weight bearing (52%), transfer weight bearing (8%), or no weight bearing (40%). The authors reported that 94% of fractures went on to union. There were two nonunions in the non–weight-bearing group and three nonunions in the full weight-bearing group. Additionally, primary radial nerve palsies were noted in 34% of patients, and one transient iatrogenic radial nerve palsy was reported. The authors recommend bone grafting if patients have more than 50% cortical comminution.

19. Kreder HJ, Stephen DJG, Schemitsch EH, McKee MD, Williams JI, Yun J: A population review of 7687 humerus fractures in adults: Determinants of outcome, in *Final Program of the Orthopaedic Trauma Association Annual Meeting, October 11-13, 2002, Toronto, Ontario.* Rosemont, IL, Orthopaedic Trauma Association, 2002. Available at: http://www.hwbf.org/ota/am/ota02/otapo/OTP02091.htm. Accessed April 13, 2005.

20. Olarte CM, Darowish M, Ziran BH: Radial nerve transposition during humeral fracture fixation: Indications, technique, and results, in *Final Program of the Orthopaedic Trauma Association Annual Meeting, October 11-13, 2002, Toronto, Ontario.* Rosemont, IL, Orthopaedic Trauma Association, 2002. Available at: http://www.hwbf.org/ota/am/ota02/otapo/OTP02086.htm. Accessed December 14, 2004.

For patients with humeral fractures that were at high-risk for nonunion or revision surgery, the authors performed a radial nerve transposition through the fracture site to avoid injuring the nerve if revision surgery were necessary. Twelve transpositions were done with no iatrogenic nerve palsies reported. Of the three patients who had primary radial nerve palsies, two recovered completely and one had slight weakness.

21. Kassab SS, Mast JW, Mayo KA: Patients treated for nonunions with plate and screw fixation and adjunctive locking nuts. *Clin Orthop* 1998;347:86-92.

22. Hak DJ: Comparison of the AO locking plate with the standard limited-contact dynamic compression plate (LC-DCP) for fixation of osteoporotic humeral shaft fractures, in *Final Program of the Orthopaedic Trauma Association Annual Meeting, October 9-11, 2003, Salt Lake City, UT*. Rosemont, IL, Orthopaedic Trauma Association, 2003. Available at: http://www.hwbf.org/ota/am/ota03/otapo/OTP03013.htm. Accessed December 14, 2004.

23. Connolly S, Nair R, McKee MD, Waddell JP, Schemitsch EH: Immediate plate osteosynthesis of open fractures of the humeral shaft, in *Final Program of the Orthopaedic Trauma Association Annual Meeting, October 22-24, 1999, Charlotte, NC*. Rosemont, IL, Orthopaedic Trauma Association, 1999. Available at: http://www.hwbf.org/ota/am/ota99/otapo/OTP99012.htm. Accessed December 14, 2004.

24. Tornkvist H, Hearn TC, Schatzker J: The strength of plate fixation in relation to the number and spacing of bone screws. *J Orthop Trauma* 1996;10:204-208.

25. Gregory PR, Sanders RW: Compression plating versus intramedullary fixation of humeral shaft fractures. *J Am Acad Orthop Surg* 1997;5:215-223.

26. Achecar F, Whittle AP: Unreamed vs reamed interlocking nailing of humeral shaft fractures, in *Final Program of the Orthopaedic Trauma Association Annual Meeting, October 17-19, 1997, Louisville, KY*. Rosemont, IL, Orthopaedic Trauma Association, 1997. Available at: http://www.hwbf.org/ota/am/ota97/otapa/OTA97506.htm. Accessed December 14, 2004.

27. Blum J, Runkel M, Rommens PM: Clinical experience with three different retrograde interlocking nailing systems for humeral shaft fractures, in *Final Program of the Orthopaedic Trauma Association Annual Meeting, October 17-19, 1997, Louisville, KY*. Rosemont, IL, Orthopaedic Trauma Association, 1997. Available at: http://www.hwbf.org/ota/am/ota97/otapa/OTA97505.htm. Accessed December 14, 2004.

28. Bono CM, Levine R, Sabatino C, Tornetta P III: Dimensional analysis of the olecranon fossa in relation to retrograde humeral nail insertion, in *Final Program of the Orthopaedic Trauma Association Annual Meeting, October 12-14, 2000, San Antonio, TX*. Rosemont, IL, Orthopaedic Trauma Association, 2000. Available at: http://www.hwbf.org/ota/am/ota00/otapo/OTP00047.htm. Accessed December 14, 2004.

29. Chapman JR, Henley MB, Agel J, Benca PJ: Randomized prospective study of humeral shaft fracture fixation: Intramedullary nails versus plates. *J Orthop Trauma* 2000;14:162-166.

30. McCormack RG, Brien D, Buckley RE, McKee MD, Powell J, Schemitsch EH: Fixation of fractures of the shaft of the humerus by dynamic compression plate or intramedullary nail. *J Bone Joint Surg Br* 2000;82:336-339.

31. Bolano LE, Iaquitno JA, Vasicek V: Operative treatment of humerus shaft fractures: A prospective randomized study comparing intramedullary nailing with dynamic compression plating, in *Final Program of the Annual Meeting of the American Academy of Orthopaedic Surgeons, Orlando, FL, 1995*. Rosemont, IL, American Academy of Orthopaedic Surgeons, 1995.

32. Wagner MS, Patterson BM, Wilber JH, Sontich JK: Comparison of outcomes for humeral diaphysis fractures treated with either closed intramedullary nailing or open reduction: Internal fixation using a dynamic compression plate in the multiple trauma patient, in *Final Program of the Annual Meeting of the Orthopaedic Trauma Association, Orlando, FL, 1995*. Rosemont, IL, Orthopaedic Trauma Association, 1995.

33. Meekers FS, Broos PL: Operative treatment of humeral shaft fractures: The Leuven experience. *Acta Orthop Belg* 2002;68:462-470.

34. Lin J: Treatment of humeral shaft fractures with humeral locked nail and comparison with plate fixation. *J Trauma* 1998;44:859-864.

35. Mills WJ, Chapman JR, Robinson LR, Slimp JC: Somatosensory evoked potential monitoring during closed humeral nailing: A preliminary report. *J Orthop Trauma* 2000;14:167-170.

36. Ring DC, Kloen P, Kadzielski JJ, Helfet DL, Jupiter JB: Locking compression plates used for delayed unions and nonunions of the diaphyseal humerus, in *Final Program of the Orthopaedic Trauma Association Annual Meeting, October 11-13, 2002, Toronto, Ontario*. Rosemont, IL, Orthopaedic Trauma Association, 2002. Available at: http://www.hwbf.org/ota/am/ota02/otapo/OTP02095.htm. Accessed April 13, 2005.
    Twenty-seven patients (average age, 69 years) with humeral shaft delayed or nonunions were treated with locked compression plating with either bone grafting or demineralized bone application. There was no loss of fixation, but two patients required secondary bone grafting.

Chapter 18

Fractures of the Elbow

Michael D. McKee, MD, FRCSC

William M. Ricci, MD

Fractures of the Distal Humerus

The elbow is a unique mix of stability and motion of three separate articulations: the ulnohumeral, radiocapitellar, and proximal radioulnar joints. Given the intricate anatomic relationship between the distal humerus and proximal radius and ulna, disruption of the intra-articular anatomy has significant effects on motion and function.[1] Despite advances in surgical techniques and implants, reconstruction of the distal humerus remains a challenging problem and complications such as nonunion or malunion, posttraumatic osteoarthritis, and ulnar neuropathy are distressingly common. Intra-articular comminution from high-energy trauma in young patients or osteoporotic bone in older patients exacerbates technical difficulties. Open soft-tissue wounds, neurovascular damage, anterior osteochondral shearing fractures, metaphyseal comminution, and associated ipsilateral injuries add complexity to the treatment of these patients. Although it may not be possible to restore the elbow to "normal," advances in implant design, surgical approach, and postoperative rehabilitation help to optimize outcome. There is increasing use of primary elbow arthroplasty for the treatment of fractures in elderly patients with severe intra-articular comminution.[2-4]

Classification

Previous classification schemes of distal humerus fractures have been descriptive and based on the columnar/condylar concept, with terms such as supracondylar, transcondylar, condylar, and bicondylar. More recently, the classification scheme of the Orthopaedic Trauma Association (OTA) has been adopted.[5] Type A fractures are extra-articular, type B fractures are intra-articular but involve only a single column or condyle (a portion of the joint is still contiguous with the shaft), and complete articular or type C fractures are intra-articular fractures in which no portion of the joint remains contiguous with the shaft. Type C fractures are typically most difficult to treat, and they have a high associated complication rate. Each category of fracture is subclassified depending on the degree and location of fracture comminution.

To be effective, a classification scheme should be reliable, help guide treatment, and be able to predict outcome. It has been shown that the OTA/AO classification scheme had substantial agreement with regard to fracture type (A, B, and C), but it was not as reliable with regard to subtype classification.[6] No scheme has yet been related to treatment or outcome.

Surgical Indications

Despite the technical difficulties associated with surgical repair of these fractures, open reduction and internal fixation remains the standard of care for most, if not all, intra-articular fractures of the distal humerus in adult patients. Nonsurgical treatment is reserved for extra-articular fractures with minimal displacement. In adults, cast immobilization of periarticular or intra-articular fractures about the elbow is fraught with complications, including stiffness, loss of reduction, and delayed union or nonunion. In older patients with dementia or those in whom medical comorbidities are contraindications to surgery, the so-called "bag of bones" technique may be reasonable because it provides a minimal level of function with mild to moderate pain that is clinically acceptable. This technique involves a brief period (2 weeks) of splinting at elbow flexion of 90° followed by institution of range-of-motion exercises to restore elbow function. The goal is a stable, minimally painful pseudarthrosis with a functional range of motion.

Surgical Approach

The successful treatment of these injuries depends on adequate exposure. Although a medial or lateral approach can provide reasonable exposure of a single column, neither approach compares favorably with the view of the articular surface that is obtained from the posterior approach. It has been said that the front door to the elbow is from the back. Thus, a posterior surgical approach is optimal for the treatment of intra-articular fractures of the distal humerus that require surgical fixation. Because the extensor mechanism is interposed between the surgeon and the fracture, in this approach either an olecranon osteotomy or split/peel of the triceps muscle and tendon is required.

Although olecranon osteotomy has been considered the standard method of dealing with the extensor mechanism, it does have drawbacks (such as delayed union or nonunion of the osteotomy, prominent hardware, and increased surgical time). If an osteotomy is used, complications can be minimized by using Kirschner wires (K-wires) that engage the anterior cortex distally, are impacted well into the tip of the olecranon, and are secured with braided cable with two tensioning loops. Other techniques that provide sufficient exposure for the fixation of these injuries include triceps splitting or peeling approaches. Previous concerns that these soft-tissue procedures had a negative effect on extension strength (from weakened reattachment, direct muscle injury with resultant fibrosis, and injury to intra-muscular nerve branches) seem unfounded; studies of objective muscle strength testing following surgical repair of distal humeral fractures have shown no difference in elbow extension strength between the osteotomy and triceps split groups.[1,7]

In patients with open intra-articular distal humerus fractures, the humeral shaft often protrudes posteriorly as the condyles fracture, injuring the triceps muscle-tendon and exiting through the posterior skin (Figure 1). This defect can be easily incorporated into a triceps-splitting approach, thus avoiding the additional morbidity resulting from an olecranon osteotomy. A recent study of open distal humeral fractures suggested that this technique improved elbow scores and resulted in a modest (11°) increase in flexion-extension compared with an osteotomy.[7] Similarly, if an olecranon fracture is present, then this can be incorporated into the approach to facilitate exposure.

Techniques

The most technically challenging aspect of the surgical repair of a comminuted distal humerus fracture is intra-articular comminution, often with absolute bone loss or cartilaginous defect. The standard surgical approach is to reassemble the articular fragments first with a combination of lag screws or K-wires and then to fix this assembly to the metaphysis. However, if there is one large fragment of joint surface that can be anatomically reduced to either medial or lateral columns, this can be used to an advantage in patients with severe articular comminution by fixing this fragment anatomically; the other articular fragments can then be assembled to it. Maintenance of the dimensions of the trochlea is critical; trochlear narrowing will not allow the ulna to seat properly. This can be avoided by inserting screws used for this fixation in a nonlag fashion. One advantage of using the triceps-splitting or peeling approach is that the proximal ulna remains intact and can be used as a bony template

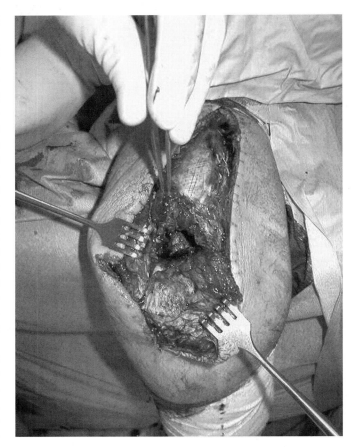

Figure 1 Intraoperative photograph of triceps muscle defect following an open distal humeral fracture in which the shaft protruded posteriorly, creating a posterior skin wound. This defect was débrided and incorporated into a triceps splitting approach. *(Reproduced with permission from McKee MD, Jupiter JB: Trauma to the adult elbow and fractures of the distal humerus, in Browner B, Jupiter JB, Levine A, Trafton P (eds): Skeletal Trauma. Philadelphia, PA, WB Saunders, 2001, vol 2, p 1446.)*

against which the trochlear reduction can be judged and resultant range of motion checked.

Small osteochondral fragments may be stabilized with Herbert screws countersunk through the articular surface perpendicular to the fracture line.[8] The head of the screw is inserted flush with the level of the subchondral bone to maximize purchase and avoid prominence in the event of cartilage loss. Alternative fixation options include minifragment 2.0- or 2.7-mm screws countersunk through the articular surface or small-diameter threaded wires that can be cut off flush with the cartilage surface.

One study reported on 21 patients with purely "articular" fractures of the distal humerus (defined as a fracture at or distal to the olecranon fossa) and identified five main articular fragments[8] (Figure 2). The authors pointed out that standard classification schemes did not recognize this pattern of injury, and they described techniques effective in their repair that depended primarily on Herbert screws for fixation of the joint fragments. They reported a mean arc of flexion-extension of 96°, and 16 of 21 patients had a good or excellent result according to the Mayo Elbow Performance index; how-

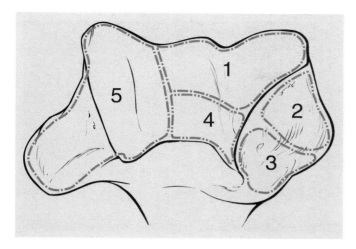

Figure 2 Schematic representation of the articular surface of the distal humerus showing the constituent parts of the articular fracture. 1 = Capitellum and lateral portion of the trochlea, 2 = Lateral epicondyle, 3 = Lateral epicondyle (posterior metaphyseal portion), 4 = Posterior aspect of the trochlea, 5 = Medial aspect of the trochlea and medial epicondyle.

ever, 10 patients required reoperation, mostly for stiffness.

Plate fixation of both medial and lateral columns is the mechanically optimal way to reestablish stability of the distal humerus in patients with bicondylar fractures (Figure 3). The ideal shape, orientation, and configuration of the plates have been the topics of many biomechanical and clinical studies, and some controversy exists.[9] Orthogonal plates (placed at 90° to each other, such as directly medially and posterolaterally) are superior to two plates placed directly posteriorly on the medial and lateral columns (in the plane of motion of the joint). There is some evidence that plates placed directly opposite each other (directly medially and laterally) are also biomechanically effective. Also, 3.5-mm compression plates or anatomic, precontoured plates designed specifically for the distal humerus are preferable to one third tubular or 3.5-mm pelvic reconstruction plates. These weaker plates have a higher failure rate, especially when there is metaphyseal comminution in the supracondylar area (Figure 4). Precontoured plates may be advantageous; when placed directly on a column they can be used to reestablish the normal profile of the distal humerus by enabling fracture reduction to the plate. This is useful when severe comminution makes reestablishing the column difficult. Also, in patients in whom distal screw purchase is poor because of comminution or osteoporosis, these plates can be contoured to "cradle" the distal fragments against a similarly applied plate on the opposite column, augmenting stability. Longer (60- or 70-mm) screws passed across to the opposite column will also improve fracture construct stability through a triangulation effect. Precontoured locking plates with fixed-angle screws are now available and may provide improved fixation in patients with comminuted fractures

and/or osteoporotic bone, but clinical results with these implants are not yet available.

Extensive metaphyseal comminution can complicate the anatomic reduction of the reassembled joint to the shaft. In this situation, deliberate shortening to gain better intrinsic stability and bony contact may be performed. However, this may compromise the depth and contour of the coronoid and olecranon fossae, possibly limiting full flexion and extension. Direct visual inspection during an arc of flexion-extension and trimming the tip of the olecranon or coronoid or deepening the corresponding fossa with a burr can eliminate this problem. It is also important to leave these fossae free of any fixation devices that may impede motion. Intraoperative radiographs should be obtained at the conclusion of the procedure for every patient.

In elderly patients, the combination of articular comminution and osteoporosis may make stable fixation unattainable. There are several series that describe good to excellent results following semiconstrained total elbow arthroplasty in this setting.[2-4] Because prosthesis longevity is a concern, this option is reserved for older patients, and the decision to proceed will depend on the surgeon's experience with fracture fixation and arthroplasty. It is important to use a semiconstrained device because there is no intrinsic condylar stability or anatomy; it is also important to preserve the proximal ulna (important for ulnar component stability) by using a triceps-splitting or peel approach. Excision of the fractured condyles creates a "working space" distally that facilitates component insertion without detaching the triceps in some patients. This decreases surgical time and triceps-related complications and enhances rapid restoration of elbow strength and motion, especially extension.

Postoperative Management

The goal of surgical repair of distal humerus fractures is to gain sufficient stability to allow early motion of the injured elbow. Prolonged immobilization following surgical repair typically results in unacceptable stiffness. In one study, immobilization for greater than 3 weeks postoperatively caused disabling stiffness.[10] A standard postoperative regimen for these injuries includes the application of a well-padded posterior slab splint (with the elbow at 90°) in the operating room with postoperative elevation of the arm. The splint is removed at 24 to 48 hours postoperatively in patients with isolated injuries, and active physiotherapy is initiated. The splint may be left on longer in patients with severe soft-tissue damage or in those with multiple injuries. Patients are encouraged to take responsibility for an active home exercise program monitored by a physiotherapist. For the typical posterior approach, resisted extension is avoided for the first 6 weeks to protect the extensor mechanism.

Patients without the anticipated slow, steady improvement in range of motion can be managed with

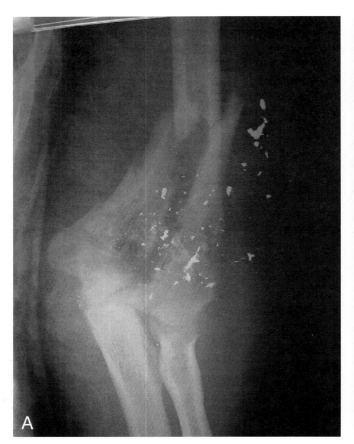
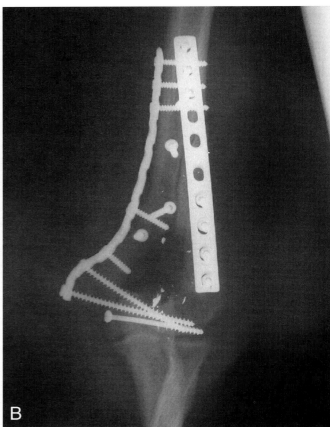

Figure 3 A, Preoperative AP radiograph of a comminuted, intra-articular distal humeral fracture caused by a gunshot wound. Fragments of bullet can be seen in the soft tissues; by their appearance and the anterior entry and posterior exit wounds, a significant defect in the triceps muscle was expected. The patient had a complete radial nerve palsy. The triceps defect was incorporated in the surgical approach, and a triceps split was performed. **B,** Postoperative AP radiograph shows rigid fixation with two plates that allowed early postoperative motion and enhanced the functional result. The radial nerve was explored and found to be contused but intact. At 1-year follow-up, the fracture had healed, the patient had a 115° arc of flexion-extension, and the radial nerve had recovered fully. *(Figure 3A reproduced with permission from McKee MD, Jupiter JB: Trauma to the adult elbow and fractures of the distal humerus, in Browner B, Jupiter JB, Levine A, Trafton P (eds): Skeletal Trauma: Basic Science, Management, and Reconstruction, ed 3. Philadelphia, PA, WB Saunders, 2003, vol 2, p 1460.)*

turnbuckle and nighttime extension splinting and flexion strapping. Prophylaxis for heterotopic bone is not routinely used.

Outcome

Although there is a wide range of reported results following this severe injury, a review of articles describing outcomes following the surgical repair of intra-articular distal humerus fractures using modern techniques and implants reveals that the average patient can expect a relatively pain-free, functional 105° arc of motion.[1,5,7-9] Forearm rotation is rarely affected unless there are concomitant, ipsilateral forearm or wrist injuries. Strength is also decreased; one recent report found that the measured strength of elbow flexion of the injured arm was only 74% of the normal side, whereas extension strength ranged from 71% to 76% (depending on elbow position).[1] In terms of patient-oriented outcome, the mean Disabilities of the Arm, Shoulder, and Hand (DASH) score was 20 (0= "perfect" and 100= "complete disability"), indicating mild residual impairment.

Common complications following surgical intervention for displaced intra-articular fractures of the distal humerus include fixation failure, nonunion, stiffness, elbow weakness, and ulnar neuropathy. Despite the complexity of fracture fixation and long surgical times, infection is relatively rare (especially in patients with closed fractures).

Elbow Dislocations and Fracture-Dislocations

Dislocation of the elbow joint (one of most stable articulations in the body) is second to shoulder dislocation as the most common dislocation of the upper extremity. Elbow dislocations have a high incidence of associated fracture. The injuries are classified as simple (no associated fracture) or complex (associated with fracture).[11] Simple dislocations can typically be managed with early mobilization after closed reduction, which is associated with a low risk of redislocation and generally good results. With closed reduction alone, the risk of recurrent

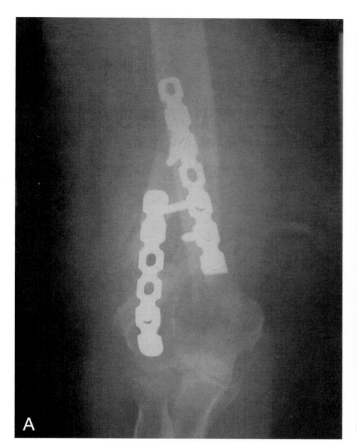
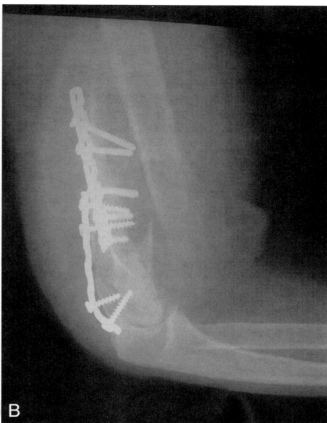

Figure 4 AP **(A)** and lateral **(B)** radiographs showing fixation failure after surgical repair of a distal humerus fracture. The posterior placement of both plates and lack of screw purchase proximal to the fracture contributed to the displacement at the fracture site.

instability or nonconcentric reduction is much higher in patients with complex dislocations (those with associated intra-articular fractures). Posterior elbow dislocations associated with a radial head fracture and coronoid fracture (the "terrible triad of the elbow") are very difficult to manage because of conflicting aims of ensuring elbow stability while maintaining early range of motion. Improved recognition of injury patterns, a better understanding of patterns of soft-tissue disruption, better fixation devices, and superior prosthetic implants have led to a more aggressive surgical approach to many of these injuries, with improved functional results[9,12-16] (Figure 5). However, surgical procedures for repair and reconstruction of the injured elbow are technically demanding and require careful planning because of the proximity of neurovascular structures.

Isolated Dislocations

Most acute elbow dislocations are posterior or posterolateral in direction, and closed reduction usually restores sufficient stability of the elbow to allow early motion. Stability can be evaluated with the forearm in supination and the elbow extended, which tends to be the most unstable position. Most of these injuries are quite stable after a brief period (7 to 10 days) in a splint with the elbow at 90° to allow for swelling and pain to subside. Early range of motion is indicated; immobilization for more than 3 weeks is associated with loss of motion, a flexion contracture, and a higher incidence of poor results. Long-term assessment of 52 patients at a mean 24-year follow-up revealed generally good results, with 50% of patients having no residual symptoms and no evidence of instability clinically, although 19 patients had some restriction of motion.[17]

Although both the medial and lateral collateral ligaments are usually disrupted in patients with simple elbow dislocations, routine surgical repair does not seem to offer any advantages. One prospective randomized study found essentially no difference in outcome between patients who had closed reduction and early motion and those who underwent open ligament repair.[18] However, there are isolated instances in which surgical intervention is indicated because of the inability to obtain or maintain a satisfactory closed reduction. It is thought that this is related to injury of the "secondary restraints" of the elbow such as the flexor-pronator mass and the common extensor origin, soft-tissue interposition, or entrapment of an unrecognized chondral or osteochondral fragment

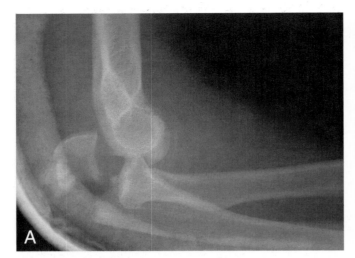 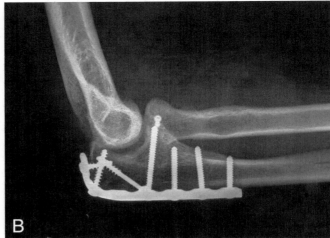

Figure 5 A, Preoperative lateral radiograph of an elbow dislocation associated with olecranon and radial head fractures in a 17-year-old boy. **B,** Postoperative lateral radiograph obtained after open reduction and internal fixation of the radial head fragment with a single countersunk Herbert screw, plate fixation of the ulna, and repair of the lateral collateral ligament through drill holes in the lateral column shows that a concentric reduction of both the radiocapitellar and ulnohumeral joints was achieved. This method provided sufficient stability to initiate immediate motion and enhanced the functional result.

in the joint. In this setting, CT can be helpful in excluding any occult bony pathology, and inability to obtain or maintain a concentric reduction is an indication for surgical intervention directed toward the specific pathology involved.

Anterior or "divergent" dislocations in which the radial head and ulna diverge are rare and typically result from high-energy trauma. Patients with these injuries typically have a much higher incidence of associated open wounds, neurovascular injury, fracture, and recurrent instability. Correspondingly, to achieve the principles of a concentric reduction and early motion, these injuries are much more likely to require early surgical repair.

Associated Radial Head Fracture

Radial head fractures associated with elbow dislocations are complex injuries. Radial head fractures were classified by Mason into three types, and a fourth type (type IV) was defined as fracture of the radial head with dislocation of the ulnohumeral joint. The treatment of a Mason type IV fracture is challenging; the goal is to restore sufficient joint stability that allows early motion yet maintains concentric reduction. Thus, these injuries usually require surgical repair. Because the lateral and medial ligaments are usually disrupted, preservation of the radial head (as an important secondary stabilizer of the elbow to valgus stress and posterior translation) is of paramount importance. Excision alone of the radial head can lead to valgus deformity, posterior subluxation, or even frank redislocation, and it should not be performed in patients with an associated elbow dislocation.

The radial head fracture is fixed with small, minifragment screws or Herbert screws that are inserted into the

nonarticular "safe zone" of the radial head and/or neck, which does not articulate with the proximal ulna.[19] This zone is identified as the perimeter between longitudinal lines drawn through the radial styloid and Lister's tubercle. If the fracture is irreparable, then metallic radial head replacement is the treatment of choice. What constitutes an irreparable fracture varies with the injury and the experience of the treating surgeon. One study found that 13 of 14 patients with more than three articular fragments had an unsatisfactory result following open reduction and internal fixation.[20] Additionally, simple two- or three-fragment fractures associated with an elbow dislocation had a significantly higher incidence of unsatisfactory outcome than isolated fractures. This suggests that open reduction and internal fixation of the radial head should be reserved only for patients with the simplest fracture patterns in the setting of associated elbow dislocation.

A reasonable alternative to repair of the radial head in patients with these difficult injuries is radial head replacement. One series described 25 patients with radial head fractures treated with metal radial head replacement; 23 had associated fractures or ligamentous injuries around the elbow. Although patients noted mild to moderate residual disability with a mean Mayo Elbow Performance score of 80, only three had "poor" results.[21] These results are superior to those described after internal fixation in similar patients.[9] A variety of metallic modular or bipolar radial heads are now available. Radial head replacement with silicone rubber arthroplasty is associated with a high incidence of clinical and radiologic complications because it has a low modulus of elasticity and offers little compressive resistance.[22] The complications of fragmentation and silicone-associated synovitis often necessitate late implant removal, and it is not indicated for radial head replacement in the patients with acute radial head fracture. Results with a bipolar or "floating" semiconstrained radial head that anchors in the radial shaft with a cemented intramedullary stem have been reported.[23] All patients had good or excellent results, there were no revisions, and no radiographic changes suggestive of cartilaginous erosion were seen in the capitellum. In another prospective study, 11 floating radial head prostheses were inserted at a mean of 4 days after injury in patients with irreparable radial head fractures.[24] Four patients also required internal fixation of associated fractures. At a mean follow-up 32 months, 8 of 11 patients had good to excellent results. Pain relief was good. Both these series emphasized the importance of reestablishing radiocapitellar stability in patients with complex elbow injuries.

Associated Coronoid Fractures

The coronoid process is important both as an anterior buttress of the greater sigmoid notch of the olecranon and the insertion of the anterior portion of medial collateral ligament and the middle part of the anterior capsule of the elbow. The coronoid process is vital to the stability of the ulnohumeral joint. Coronoid fractures typically result from an elbow dislocation or subluxation, and fracture of a large fragment of the coronoid will compromise the medial collateral ligament and disrupt the sigmoid notch, exacerbating elbow instability. Investigators have stressed the importance of fixation of large coronoid process fractures.[9,12,25,26]

Coronoid fractures have been classified into three types by Regan and Morrey: type I is a fracture of the tip of the coronoid process, type II is a fracture that involves 50% or less of the coronoid process, and type III is a fracture that involves more than 50% of the coronoid process. Although usually too small to fix, type I fractures are significant in that they alert the treating surgeon to the probability that the patient has had an episode of elbow instability.[27] The fixation of displaced type II and type III fractures helps to restore elbow stability and allows early motion. Larger fragments can be fixed with 3.0-, 3.5-, or 4.0-mm cannulated screws through the dorsal aspect of the ulna and directed to the coronoid process. When instability persists and the coronoid fracture is too small or too comminuted to repair, a cerclage wire or No. 5 nonabsorbable suture material placed around the fragments and attached anterior capsule and then brought through drill holes through the proximal ulna can help restore stability. Similarly, reattachment of the brachialis muscle and anterior capsule in chronically unstable elbows helps to restore elbow stability. There are few reports in the literature regarding the treatment or outcome of isolated coronoid fractures, and information

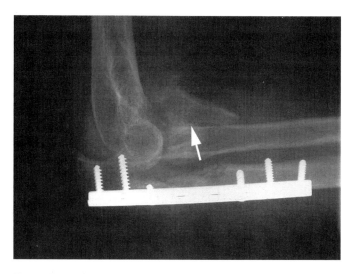

Figure 6 Radiograph showing technical errors in the management of a patient with a complex proximal ulna and radial head fracture. Note that the coronoid fracture fragment was not fixed (*arrow*), the radial head was excised and not reconstructed, and the elbow rapidly subluxated posteriorly. When ligamentous disruption exists, the radial head and coronoid provide a critical buttress against posterior subluxation.

must be gleaned from other larger series on elbow fractures and fracture-dislocations.

The long subcutaneous border of the ulna makes it vulnerable to direct trauma that can result in comminuted fractures of the proximal ulna. The mechanism of injury can include a direct blow to the ulna or a fall on the outstretched hand with the elbow in flexion. Higher-energy trauma can be associated with radial head fractures and dislocations of the elbow. Complex proximal ulnar fractures usually contain a significant coronoid fragment, which is critical to stability of the elbow for the reasons noted above. The coronoid fracture fragment is typically triangularly shaped and usually involves 50% to 100% of the coronoid process. When repairing these injuries, it is important to recreate the anterior buttress of the greater sigmoid notch of the proximal ulna. Thus, it is important to fix the coronoid fragment, typically with lag screws from the distal ulnar fragment, before reducing the primary ulnar fracture line (Figure 6). Once the main proximal-distal fragment fracture line is reduced, visualization (and repair) of the coronoid fragment becomes difficult. Tension band wiring of this type of comminuted fracture is contraindicated, and fixation of the proximal ulnar fracture should be performed with a small fragment compression plate contoured to project proximally around the tip of the olecranon (Figure 7). This configuration enhances stability through the buttress effect of the plate, which is useful when poor bone quality or comminution make screw purchase suboptimal.

The "Terrible Triad of the Elbow"

The "terrible triad of the elbow" consists of an elbow dislocation with concomitant radial head and coronoid

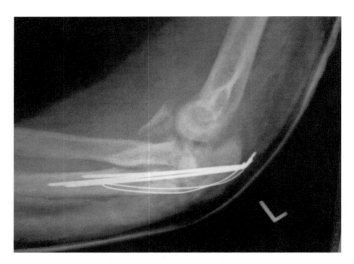

Figure 7 Radiograph showing early, recurrent posterior subluxation of the elbow in a 42-year-old patient after attempted fixation of a proximal ulnar fracture using a tension band technique. Note that the coronoid fragment has not been stabilized and that the associated fracture of the radial head has not been addressed. Tension band wiring is contraindicated in patients with complex proximal ulnar fractures, especially those that have associated elbow instability. It cannot reliably hold comminuted fragments and is unable to withstand the increased bending and rotational forces seen in this situation.

fractures. Poor outcomes have been reported for patients with this type of injury, especially when compared with patients with simple elbow dislocations caused by early recurrent instability of the elbow, stiffness, and arthrosis. There are few published reports that specifically assess this entity, and most information available is found in larger series of elbow injuries that contain small subsets of patients with this injury complex. In one series exclusively studying this injury, poor results, including early recurrent instability, stiffness, and loss of nonconcentric reduction, were noted in 7 of 11 elbows.[9,15] There was radiographic evidence of arthrosis of the ulnohumeral joint in 7 of 10 patients who retained their native elbow.

It is difficult to obtain and/or maintain concentric closed reduction of these injuries even with cast application, and prolonged immobilization leads to unacceptable levels of stiffness and dysfunction. However, improved understanding of the mechanism of elbow injuries and the primary and secondary constraints to stability in conjunction with better methods of surgical repair have led to a more aggressive surgical approach. Stability is achieved surgically through open reduction and internal fixation of coronoid fractures and/or repair of the anterior capsule, repair or replacement of the radial head, and repair of the lateral ligament complex. A recent study showed that the lateral collateral ligament complex is invariably injured in patients with this injury and that the most common pattern of injury was avulsion from the posterolateral aspect of the distal humerus, which typically leaves a characteristic "bare spot" on the bone.[28]

Chronic elbow instability is common following this injury and results from loss of soft-tissue constraints (especially the lateral collateral ligament complex), bony defect, or articular malalignment. Elbow reconstruction with an articulated fixator is an effective treatment in such situations. Good results were seen in 16 patients with posttraumatic elbow instability who were treated with a hinged external fixator for an average of 6 weeks.[29] Another series reported success in six of seven patients with unstable fracture-dislocation of the elbow treated with the Mayo hinged external fixator (mean arc of flexion/extension = 88°).[30] In both of these series, patients who had originally experienced a "terrible triad of the elbow" injury predominated.

These injuries are difficult to treat. Even with optimal care, stiffness, recurrent instability, and the need for secondary intervention can occur. However, it appears that successful treatment of elbow dislocations with associated radial head and coronoid fractures can be achieved using a standard surgical protocol that allows early motion and enhances functional results.

The Monteggia Lesion

Fracture of the proximal ulna with dislocation of the radial head was first described in 1814, and these injuries have been classified into four types according to the direction of the displacement of the radial head: anterior, posterior, lateral, and any direction with radial shaft fracture. Type I fractures (anterior radial head dislocation) are more common in children. Most adult patients with Monteggia injuries had posterior dislocations (Bado type II). This injury is typically seen in middle-aged adults and results from a fall on the outstretched hand with the elbow flexed and pronated. In adult patients with this type of injury, there is a high incidence of associated radial head fractures and triangular or quadrangular coronoid fragments as part of the ulnar fracture and a high complication rate (Figure 8).

Bado type II injuries have been subclassified based on the location of the ulnar fracture: fractures at the level of the coronoid process are type A, fractures just distal to the coronoid are type B, fractures through the diaphysis of the ulna are type C, and complex fractures that may involve the entire proximal one third to one half of the ulna are type D.[31,32] Coronoid process involvement can be associated with radial head fractures, and this combination of injuries can result in complete disruption of the osseous contributions to the stability of the elbow. Neurovascular injuries, including injury to the posterior interosseous, anterior interosseous, and ulnar nerves, have been reported.

Open reduction and internal fixation of the ulna with closed reduction of the radial head is the treatment of choice for Monteggia injuries in adults. The ulnar fracture is fixed with a 3.5-mm compression plate through a posterior approach; after stabilization, the elbow and proximal radioulnar joint should be assessed both clinically and radiographically. Ulnar fracture malreduction

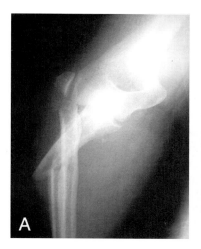
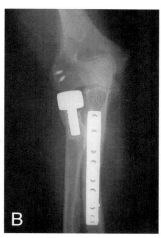
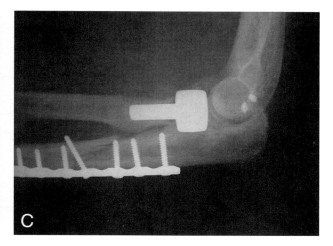

Figure 8 A, Preoperative radiograph showing a Monteggia-variant injury that occurred after the patient fell. Note that there is an angulated fracture of the proximal ulna with a comminuted posterolateral fracture-dislocation of the radial head. Postoperative AP **(B)** and lateral **(C)** radiographs of the same patient after open reduction and internal fixation of the ulnar shaft; radial head replacement with a modular, metallic prosthesis; and repair of the lateral collateral ligament with suture anchors in the lateral column.

can result in residual subluxation or dislocation of the radiocapitellar joint. If the radial head remains malreduced despite anatomic reduction of the ulnar fracture, then intra-articular interposition from the annular ligament, a torn joint capsule, or the presence of an osteochondral fragment should be suspected, in which instance an open reduction of the joint is indicated. This can be performed either through a Boyd approach (reflecting the anconeus from the radial side of the proximal ulna) or a separate lateral incision.

Olecranon Fractures

Anatomic restoration of the fractured articular surface of the olecranon with internal fixation that allows for early elbow range of motion can be accomplished with a variety of techniques. Complications related to loose or painful hardware are more common than complications related to healing. In general, good or excellent results should be expected after proper treatment of most olecranon fractures.

Classification

Several classification systems have been described for olecranon fractures; however, none are universally accepted. Colton's classification is perhaps the most widely used: type 1 fractures are avulsion fractures, type 2A through type 2D fractures are oblique fractures with increasing complexity, type 3 fractures are associated with a dislocation, and type 4 fractures are atypical high-energy multifragmented fractures. Classification systems by the AO/ASIF, the Mayo Clinic, and Schatzker are also useful and often cited.

Nonsurgical Treatment

Patients with fractures with less than 1 to 2 mm of displacement can often be treated nonsurgically. Immo-

bilization with the elbow flexed 60° to 90° for 7 to 10 days is typically followed by a program of gentle active range-of-motion exercises. Weight bearing and resistive elbow extension are limited for 6 to 8 weeks. Then a gradual increase in activity, weight bearing, and resistive exercises are allowed. Good results should be expected.

Surgical Treatment
Tension Band
Displaced olecranon fractures should be treated surgically. Tension band fixation is generally recommended for fractures that are both proximal to the coronoid process and not at risk of compressing the olecranon fossa. A tension band construct is advantageous because it theoretically converts dorsal distraction forces to compression at the fracture site on the articular surface. This theory has been recently challenged by a biomechanical analysis of cyclic loading of olecranon fixation constructs in which conversion of posterior tensile forces to articular compressive forces was not demonstrated.[33] If the articular surface is comminuted and unstable, then narrowing of the sigmoid notch can occur. In patients with dorsal comminution, there is risk of widening of the sigmoid notch. In such patients, other methods of fixation that provided neutralization should be used.

Clinical and biomechanical studies support a modified AO tension band technique for stable displaced olecranon fractures to maximize fixation strength and to minimize the risk of hardware-related complications[34,35] (Figure 9). Migration of K-wires and prominent or painful hardware are the most common complications and have been reported in up to 71% of patients.[35,36] Backing out of K-wires is three times more likely if the wires are passed down the intramedullary canal of the ulna rather than across the anterior cortex. The pullout strength and resistance to tensile force of transcortical wire placement

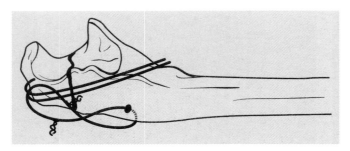

Figure 9 Schematic representation of the tension band fixation of a stable transverse olecranon fracture. (Adapted from Boyer MI, Galatz LM, Borrelli JJ, Axelrod TS, Ricci WM: Intra-articular fractures of the upper extremity: New concepts in surgical treatment. Instr Course Lect 2003;52:591-605.)

are significantly greater than for intramedullary K-wire placement. Two longitudinal splits in the triceps tendon should be made such that the bent K-wires can be impacted into the tip of the olecranon and deep to the tendon. These longitudinal splits should be closed with suture. The combination of engaging the anterior cortex at the distal tip of the K-wire, impaction of the K-wire into the tip of the olecranon, and closure of the triceps over the K-wire minimizes risk of hardware-related complications. The figure-of-8 tension band is secured proximally around these K-wires deep to the triceps to avoid strangulation of the tendon and distally through a drill hole in the ulna. This hole should be volar enough to avoid being unicortical, to minimize risk of pathologic fracture at this site, and to minimize risk of distraction of the articular surface. The tension band should be in a figure-of-8 configuration; either a monofilament stainless steel wire or a braided cable should be used, not a braided suture material. In biomechanical studies, braided cable has been shown to allow less fracture displacement than stainless steel wire.[37] No. 5 Ethibond suture (Ethicon, Somerville, NJ) is much less stiff and thus sustains longer displacements at equivalent loads when compared with 18-gauge wire; therefore, it is not suitable for the rigid fixation required for olecranon tension band fixation. The figure-of-8 band should have two tensioning loops to produce symmetric force at the fracture site, and the knots should be positioned to minimize hardware prominence.

Intramedullary Screw Fixation

Intramedullary screw fixation with large diameter screws must be used with caution. This method has a higher rate of fixation failure than tension band fixation. The threads of these large screws can tightly engage the intramedullary cortex, creating increased torque that can be mistaken for fracture compression leading to inadequate fixation. Conversely, when the threads are placed in a relatively large canal, poor purchase in the distal fragment can also lead to inadequate compression. Recent data, however, suggest that a properly placed 7.3-mm

partially threaded intramedullary lag screw combined with tension band wiring offers improved biomechanical fixation under conditions of cyclic loading compared with traditional K-wire and tension band constructs.[33]

Plate Fixation

Good results have been reported for both stable and comminuted olecranon fractures using plate fixation.[38] For comminuted olecranon fractures, compression techniques such as tension band wiring risk narrowing the greater sigmoid notch, are biomechanically less stable than plate fixation, and should be used with caution. Iliac crest bone graft should be considered if tension band fixation is chosen for these fractures. Also, fixation of oblique fractures that extend distal to the coronoid process is more stable with plates than with tension bands. Small screws and/or bioabsorbable pins can be used to anatomically reduce and stabilize comminuted articular fragments. Supplemental bone graft can be used to support depressed articular fragments. The choice of plate fixation depends on the quality of the bone and the location of the fracture. In general, the use of one third tubular hook-plates should be reserved for very proximal fractures. These thin plates are at risk for fatigue failure when used for more distal fractures. Reconstruction plates are of intermediate strength, are relatively easy to contour, and can be used in most patients requiring neutralization plates for olecranon fracture. Dynamic compression plates are difficult to contour, are the most prominent, have the highest risk of hardware-related pain, and should be reserved for patients with more distal fractures that involve the ulnar shaft. Plates are most commonly placed on either the dorsal or lateral aspect of the proximal ulna. The obliquity and comminution of the fracture can help dictate the most appropriate location. Dorsal plating may be advantageous for oblique fractures for which such plate position provides a buttress effect and allows lag screw fixation through the plate. Lateral plate position has been shown to be as biomechanically strong as dorsal placement for comminuted fractures. This plate position is less prominent and may reduce associated implant-related pain.

Excision

Excision of the tip of the olecranon with triceps tendon advancement can be successfully used for the treatment of nonreconstructible proximal olecranon fractures, especially in elderly patients or those with low functional demands. When the comminuted fragments are removed, the triceps tendon is advanced into the fracture bed of the distal fragment. Reattachment should be close to the articular surface (Figure 10). Resection of more than 50% of the olecranon should be avoided to minimize the risk of instability.

Postoperative Management

The goal of fracture fixation is early range of motion to minimize elbow joint contracture. Postoperative immo-

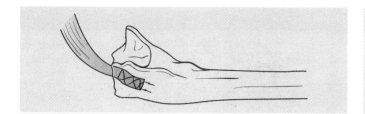

Figure 10 Schematic representation of triceps advancement. *(Adapted from Boyer MI, Galatz LM, Borrelli JJ, Axelrod TS, Ricci WM: Intra-articular fractures of the upper extremity: New concepts in surgical treatment. Instr Course Lect 2003;52:591-605.)*

bilization for short periods (no more than 7 days) can be used for comfort and for protection of the soft tissues. Thereafter, active range of motion is initiated with no weight bearing. After 6 to 8 weeks, depending on the stability of the fracture, gradual progression toward weight bearing and resistive exercises and strengthening can be initiated.

Radial Head Fractures

Many factors must be considered when treating patients with radial head fractures. First, the fracture pattern and its reconstructibility must be clearly defined. Then the presence of any associated dislocation, ligament disruption, and/or periarticular fractures must be identified. Patient-specific characteristics such as age, handedness, functional demands, and expectations can also influence treatment decisions. Finally, the surgeon's resources and technical ability with surgical management must be sufficient before undertaking surgical reconstruction of a complex radial head fracture and/or elbow dislocation.

Classification

According to the original Mason classification of radial head fractures, type I fractures are nondisplaced, type II fractures are partial articular with displacement, and type III fractures are comminuted fractures involving the entire head of the radius (Figure 11). Comminuted partial articular fractures are often described as Mason type III fractures, but they should be classified as Mason type II fractures. Fractures with associated ligamentous injury or other associated fractures are often referred to as Mason type IV injuries. These represent a complex and diverse group of injuries for which treatment is determined both by the fracture pattern of the radial head and by the associated injuries.

Nonsurgical Treatment

Patients with nondisplaced (Mason type I) fractures should be treated nonsurgically. Range of motion is initiated within 7 days of the injury as pain allows. Weight bearing is protected for approximately 6 weeks. Activity and weight bearing can then be advanced as tolerated. Good results should be expected; however, displacement

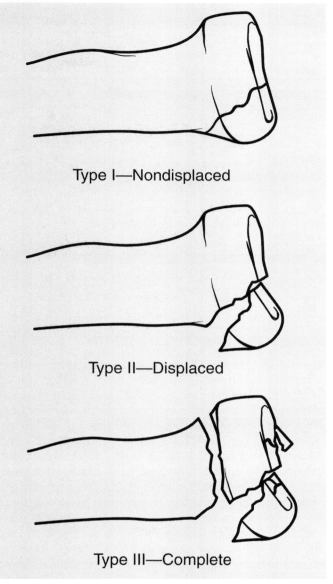

Type I—Nondisplaced

Type II—Displaced

Type III—Complete

Figure 11 Schematic representation of the Mason classification of radial head fractures. Type IV (fracture-dislocation) is not shown. *(Adapted from Boyer MI, Galatz LM, Borrelli JJ, Axelrod TS, Ricci WM: Intra-articular fractures of the upper extremity: New concepts in surgical treatment. Instr Course Lect 2003;52:591-605.)*

with loss of motion and symptomatic nonunion can occur. Nonsurgical management can be recommended for patients with simple displaced (Mason type II) fractures if two conditions are met: fracture fixation is not required for elbow stability and there is no significant barrier to elbow motion (at least 20° to 120° of flexion and 70° of each pronation and supination should be achieved). When these conditions are met, nonsurgical management is similar to that for nondisplaced fractures. Published results of nonsurgical treatment of Mason type II fractures are marginal. One study reported good range of motion but functional results were graded good or excellent in only 44% of the patients[39] (Table 1). Commi-

TABLE 1 | Treatment Outcomes for Patients With Mason Type Fractures

Author(s)	Mason Type	Treatment	No. of Patients	Follow-up (months)	Range of Motion (degrees*)				Good/ Excellent Results
					Elbow Flexion	Elbow Extension	Forearm Pronation	Forearm Supination	
Leppilahti and Jalovaara[45†]	II	Excision	6	60	135	-15	77	75	48%
	III		17						
Ikeda and Oka[44]	II	Excision	4	132	131	-9	85	85	
	III		11	116	132	-17	77	81	
Moro et al[21]	III	Titanium radial head replacement	10	40	140	-5	78	66	40%
	IV		15	39	140	-10	78	70	87%
Sanchez-Sotelo et al[46]	IV	Excision	10	55	140	-8	86	84	90%
Popovic et al[24]	IV	Floating radial head replacement	11	32	130	-20	-14	-16	73%
Ring et al[20]	II	Open reduction and internal fixation	30	58	130	-11	72	72	93%
	III		26	44‡	129	-18	67	59	46%

*All values are to the nearest degree, with negative values representing motion loss compared with normal and positive values representing limit of motion in the direction described
†Results for patients with Mason type II and III fractures could not be distinguished ‡Excludes 10 patients who underwent subsequent radial head excision
(Adapted from Boyer MI, Galatz LM, Borrelli JJ, Axelrod TS, Ricci WM: Intra-articular fractures of the upper extremity: New concepts in surgical treatment. *Instr Course Lect* 2003;52:591-605.)

nuted radial head (Mason type III) fractures without associated ligamentous injury or other fracture can be treated nonsurgically or by radial head excision or replacement. The elbow must be stable to consider nonsurgical management. If results of nonsurgical management are poor, late excision can be considered. This treatment algorithm assumes that initial nonsurgical management is better than surgical management and that delayed excision has good results. Neither of these assumptions has been proven true. One study reviewed 21 cases of late radial head excision (1 month to 20 years after injury) with an average follow-up of 15 years.[40] Pain improved in 76% of the patients; however, 73% remained symptomatic. Better results have been achieved using other treatment algorithms, including open reduction and internal fixation, radial head replacement, and acute excision.[20]

Surgical Treatment
Open Reduction Internal Fixation
Surgical treatment is indicated for patients with Mason type II fractures when the radial head is required for elbow stability and/or there is a block to satisfactory elbow motion caused by the fracture. Surgical options include open reduction with internal fixation or partial radial head excision. Miniature lag screws, screws with differential pitch, and/or bioabsorbable pins can be used when the fracture does not involve the radial neck; otherwise, the use of small plates is indicated. Several studies have shown good results with the use of open reduction and internal fixation to treat Mason type II fractures. One such study found better results in patients treated with open reduction and internal fixation than those treated nonsurgically.[39] The authors reported that elbow and forearm motion were excellent, and 90% of patients had good or excellent results. Another study also reported excellent elbow and forearm motion, and 100% of patients had good or excellent clinical ratings after undergoing open reduction and internal fixation to treat Mason type II fractures.[41] Another more recent study found that the results of open reduction and internal fixation in the treatment of Mason type II fractures were less predictable when patients had more than a single simple fragment, particularly when associated with a complex elbow or forearm injury pattern.[20] Open reduction and internal fixation used to treat comminuted radial head fractures was not as successful. One study found significantly worse results for open reduction and internal fixation of Mason type III fractures than similar treatment of Mason type II fractures.[42] Another study found that open reduction and internal fixation of Mason type III fractures is much less likely to be successful when patients have more than three articular fragments.[20]

Excision
Partial excision of the radial head can be considered for Mason type II fractures when the fragments are relatively small and elbow stability is preserved after excision. The advantages of early complete radial head excision for patients with comminuted fractures are good pain relief and range of motion. The disadvantages include potential for radial shortening leading to wrist pain and/or arthritis and decreased forearm strength. Excision

also causes altered load transfer at the ulnohumeral joint that can lead to elbow arthritis. At an average 16-year follow-up after undergoing radial head excision, one study reported a 100% incidence of radiographic arthrosis, but this apparently did not affect functional scores.[43] Two more recent studies each found similar results at medium- to long-term follow-up of patients who underwent radial head excision for isolated fractures.[44,45] Elbow and forearm range of motion were good, but most patients had radial shortening, elbow pain, and elbow arthritis. Symptoms and arthritis at the wrist were variable. One study reviewed early results of radial head excision for the treatment of patients with elbow fracture-dislocation with unsalvageable radial head fracture.[46] Although range of motion was excellent and 90% of patients had good or excellent results, radial shortening at the wrist averaged 1.6 mm and was symptomatic in two patients who each had more than 4 mm of shortening. Eighty percent had radiographic evidence of elbow arthritis and 40% had elbow pain. These studies indicate that although range of motion can be quite good after radial head excision, patients may have persistent elbow and wrist pain. Therefore, radial head excision for Mason type III fractures should be reserved for elderly patients with relatively low functional demands.

Radial Head Replacement

Radial head replacement for Mason type III fractures provides stability, prevents radial shortening, and provides appropriate load transfer at the elbow. Biomechanical studies indicate that the radial head provides less than 30% of the resistance to valgus stress and is a secondary stabilizer when the medial collateral ligament is intact. However, following disruption of the medial collateral ligament or the interosseous membrane, the radial head becomes a main stabilizer to valgus stress[41] and longitudinal compressive forces, respectively. In medial collateral ligament–deficient elbows, both monoblock and bipolar metal radial head implants provide improved valgus stability that approaches that of an intact radial head. Therefore, preservation of the radial head is desired whenever possible; otherwise, radial head replacement is indicated. The major concerns with radial head replacement are capitellar arthritis and implant-related complications. Implanted materials were initially silicone, but better results have been accomplished with metal implants. Biomechanical studies show silicone implants are incapable of transferring physiologic loads across the radial capitellar joint. Clinical results support these laboratory data by showing a high incidence of elbow arthritis and radial shortening after silicone arthroplasty. One study found good range of motion with 70% of patients having good or excellent results after silicone radial head replacement.[22] However, 56% of patients had elbow arthritis, and radial shortening averaged 2.0 mm.

Monoblock metal radial head implants provide more physiologic load transfer and therefore theoretically protect against radial shortening and ulnohumeral joint arthritis. Results for metal radial head replacement for Mason type III fractures are difficult to discern from results for Mason type IV fractures because patients with associated fractures or ligament deficiencies are not distinguished from those without associated injuries in most reports.

Metal radial head replacement has been reported to result in a similar range of motion, better clinical scores, decreased radial shortening, and decreased elbow arthritis compared with excision or silicone arthroplasty. In one report of 25 patients who underwent metal radial head replacement, motion at the elbow was reported as excellent, forearm motion was good, and 68% of patients were graded as having good or excellent results.[21] Only 21% had elbow arthritis, no patient had radial shortening, and no implants required removal despite 17 patients having evidence of periprosthetic lucency. Another study reviewed 31 patients who received vitallium radial head implants.[47] Two patients required implant removal for painful loosening and only one of the remaining patients had radial shortening (2 mm). In 7 patients, there was evidence of nonprogressive radiolucent lines surrounding the prosthesis. A more recent study reviewed a new floating radial head implant for patients with radial head fractures associated with elbow dislocation.[24] The floating radial head design theoretically provides better articulation with the capitellum at varying degrees of elbow flexion, and 73% of patients had good or excellent results. There was no radial shortening, no elbow arthritis, and no patients required revision. These results are similar or worse than those achieved using solid metal radial head implants for patients with Mason type IV injuries (Table 1). Potential problems with floating implants include mechanical failure, debris formation, and osteolysis. It is yet to be determined which metallic implant material is ideal for the treatment of these injuries, and whether floating radial head implants will offer improved long-term results remains unknown. Radial head replacement appears to be the best option for the treatment of Mason type III fractures. The goal of postoperative management after radial head replacement is to optimize motion. A short period of immobilization (< 7 days) can be used for comfort. Active range of motion with protected weight bearing for 6 weeks is typically followed by a progressive increase in activities. Prolonged protection from heavy weight bearing should be considered after radial head replacement.

Surgical Approach

Access to the radial head is usually best accomplished through a lateral Kocher approach. To avoid disruption of the lateral collateral ligament, dissection posterior to the midcapitellum should be avoided. A lateral safe zone of 110° has been described.[19] In this safe zone, screws placed through the lateral articular surface will not impinge at the radioulnar articulation. Associated proximal ulnar and radial head fractures can be approached either with one or two incisions. Radial head replacement and open reduction and internal fixation of the proximal ulna can usually be accomplished through one posterior lateral incision. When open reduction and internal fixation of the radial head or neck is indicated, two incisions may be required.

Annotated References

1. McKee MD, Wilson TL, Winston L, Schemitsch EH, Richards RR: Functional outcome following surgical treatment of intra-articular distal humeral fractures through a posterior approach. *J Bone Joint Surg Am* 2000;82:1701-1707.

   Using objectively measured strength testing and patient-oriented outcome measures, this article defined functional outcome following the treatment of these injuries with a modern surgical approach. Mean flexion strength was 74% of normal, mean extension strength was 74% to 76% of normal, mean range of motion was 25° to 133°, and the mean DASH Outcome Measure score was 20.

2. Frankle MA, Herscovici D, Dipasquale TG, Vasey MB, Sanders RW: A comparison of open reduction and internal fixation and primary total elbow arthroplasty in the treatment of intraarticular distal humeral fractures in women older than age 65. *J Orthop Trauma* 2003;17(7):473-480.

   The authors found that 4 of 12 elderly patients who underwent fixation of comminuted intra-articular distal humeral fractures required conversion to total elbow arthroplasty, whereas those treated with primary arthroplasty had superior outcome, shorter hospital stay, and no revisions.

3. Gambirasio R, Riand N, Stern R, Hoffmeyer P: Total elbow replacement for complex fractures of the distal humerus: An option for the elderly patient. *J Bone Joint Surg Br* 2001;83:974-978.

   Ten elderly patients who underwent primary total elbow arthroplasty for fracture had a mean Mayo Elbow Performance score of 94 and a mean arc of flexion-extension of 102°, with a negligible complication rate.

4. Garcia JA, Mykula R, Stanley D: Complex fractures of the distal humerus in the elderly. *J Bone Joint Surg Br* 2002;84:812-816.

   This series reports a mean Mayo Elbow Performance score of 93, a mean arc of flexion-extension of 101°, and no reoperations in 16 elderly patients who underwent total elbow arthroplasty for treatment of a complex distal humeral fracture.

5. Fracture and dislocation compendium: Orthopaedic Trauma Association Committee for Coding and Classification. *J Orthop Trauma* 1996;10(suppl 1):1-154.

6. Wainwright AM, Williams JR, Carr AJ: Interobserver and intraobserver variation in classification systems for fractures of the distal humerus. *J Bone Joint Surg Br* 1999;82:636-642.

7. McKee MD, Kim J, Kebaish K, Stephen DJG, Kreder HJ, Schemitsch EH: Functional outcome after open supracondylar fractures of the humerus. *J Bone Joint Surg Br* 2000;82:646-651.

   This study compared a triceps-splitting approach and an olecranon osteotomy approach in the treatment of 25 patients with open, intra-articular distal humeral fractures, most of whom had a posterior wound. A modest 11° improvement in flexion-extension range and higher elbow scores were found in the triceps-splitting group.

8. Ring D, Jupiter JB, Gulotta L: Articular fractures of the distal part of the humerus. *J Bone Joint Surg Am* 2003;85:232-238.

   For patients with fractures entirely at or distal to the olecranon fossa, most reported good results with surgical treatment (16 of 21 reported good or excellent results, with a mean arc of motion of 96°); however, the authors noted that the surgical procedure was technically difficult and 10 patients required reoperation.

9. McKee MD, Jupiter JB: Trauma to the adult elbow and fractures of the distal humerus, in Browner B, Jupiter JB, Levine A, Trafton P (eds): *Skeletal Trauma*. Philadelphia, PA, WB Saunders, 2001, vol 2, pp 1455-1522.

10. Wadell JP, Hatch J, Richards RR: Supracondylar fractures of the humerus: Results of surgical treatment. *J Trauma* 1988;28:1615-1621.

11. Hildebrand KA, Patterson SD, King GJ: Acute elbow dislocations: Simple and complex. *Orthop Clin North Am* 1999;30(1):63-79.

12. Cook RE, McKee MD: Techniques to tame the terrible triad: Unstable fracture dislocations of the elbow. *Oper Tech in Orthop* 2003;13(2):130-137.

   The authors of this article outline a standard surgical approach to treating patients with these devastating injuries with an emphasis on technique.

13. Frankle MA, Koval KJ, Sanders RW, Zuckerman JD: Radial head fractures with dislocations treated by immediate stabilization and early motion. *J Shoulder Elbow Surg* 1999;8:355-356.

14. Ring D, Jupiter JB: Fracture dislocation of the elbow: Current concepts review. *J Bone Joint Surg Am* 1998;80(14):566-580.

15. Ring D, Jupiter JB, Zilberfarb J: Posterior dislocation of the elbow with fractures of the radial head and coronoid. *J Bone Joint Surg Am* 2002;84-A:547-551.

   The authors of this study reported that excision of a fractured radial head, when associated with posterior elbow dislocation and coronoid fracture (the terrible triad), resulted in redislocation in 100% of patients. Unsatisfactory results occurred on 7 of 11 patients. The four patients with satisfactory results had retention of the radial head, and two of these also had repair of the lateral collateral ligament.

16. Schmeling GJ: Elbow and forearm: Adult trauma, in Koval KJ (ed): *Orthopaedic Knowledge Update 7.* Rosemont, IL, American Academy of Orthopaedic Surgeons, 2002, pp 307-316.

17. Josefsson PO, Johnell O, Gentz CF: Long-term sequelae of simple dislocation of the elbow. *J Bone Joint Surg Am* 1984;66:927-930.

18. Josefsson PO, Gentz CF, Johnell O, Wendeberg B: Surgical versus nonsurgical treatment of ligamentous injuries following dislocation of the elbow joint: A prospective randomized study. *J Bone Joint Surg Am* 1987;69:605-608.

19. Smith GR, Hotchkiss RN: Radial head and neck fractures: Anatomic guidelines for proper placement of internal fixation. *J Shoulder Elbow Surg* 1996;5: 113-117.

20. Ring D, Quintero J, Jupiter JB: Open reduction and internal fixation of fractures of the radial head. *J Bone Joint Surg Am* 2002;84:1811-1815.

   In this retrospective review of 56 patients who underwent open reduction and internal fixation of a radial head fracture, the authors found that for those with Mason type II fractures (N = 30), all 15 with noncomminuted fractures had satisfactory results and 4 of 15 with comminuted fractures had unsatisfactory results. All four patients with unsatisfactory results had associated fracture-dislocations. For those patients with Mason type III fractures (N = 26), 13 of 14 with more than three fragments had unsatisfactory results.

21. Moro JK, Werier J, MacDermid JC, Patterson SD, King GJ: Arthroplasty with a metal radial head for unreconstructible fractures of the radial head. *J Bone Joint Surg Am* 2001;83:1201-1211.

   In this study, 25 patients with comminuted, unreconstructible radial head fractures were treated with radial head replacement. At an average follow-up of 39 months, the authors reported that patients had a mild to moderate impairment of physical capability of the elbow and wrist. The authors concluded that this is a safe and effective treatment option in this patient group.

22. Carn RM, Medige J, Curtain D, Koenig A: Silicone rubber replacement of the severely fractured radial head. *Clin Orthop* 1986;209:259-269.

23. Judet T, Garreau de Loubresse C, Piriou P, Charnley G: A floating prosthesis for radial head fractures. *J Bone Joint Surg Br* 1996;78:244-250.

24. Popovic N, Gillet PH, Rodriguez A, Lemaire R: Fracture of the radial head associated with elbow dislocation: Results of treatment using a floating radial head prosthesis. *J Orthop Trauma* 2000;14:171-177.

   This article described the use of a new articulating bipolar type of prosthesis in the treatment of patients with unstable fracture-dislocations of the elbow associated with radial head fractures. At a mean of 32-month follow-up, the authors reported that four patients had excellent results, four had good results, two had fair results, and one had poor results.

25. O'Driscoll SW, Jupiter JB, Cohen MS, Ring D, McKee MD: Difficult elbow fractures: Pearls and pitfalls. *Instr Course Lect* 2003;52:113-134.

26. Pugh DM, Wild LM, Schemitsch EH, King GJ, McKee MD: Standard surgical protocol to treat elbow dislocations with radial head and coronoid fractures. *J Bone Joint Surg Am* 2004;86-A:1122-1130.

   This article describes superior results (mean Mayo Elbow Performance score, 88) with the use of a standard protocol (surgical stabilization and immediate motion) in the treatment of 36 consecutive patients with the terrible triad of the elbow.

27. Terada N, Yamada H, Seki T, Utabe T, Takayama S: The importance of reducing small fractures of the coronoid process in the treatment of unstable elbow dislocation: A case report. *J Shoulder Elbow Surg* 2000;9(4):344-347.

   The authors of this case report emphasize the significance of the coronoid fracture and the importance of fixation in the setting of elbow dislocation.

28. McKee MD, Schemitsch EH, Sala MJ, O'Driscoll SW: The pathoanatomy of lateral ligamentous disruption in complex elbow instability. *J Shoulder Elbow Surg* 2003;12:391-396.

   This study analyzed the soft-tissue injury patterns on the lateral aspect of the elbow in 62 consecutive patients with elbow dislocation or fracture-dislocation that required surgical repair. Avulsion of the lateral collateral ligament and avulsion of the posterior capsule from the posterolateral humerus were the most commonly associated soft-tissue and concomitant ruptures of the common extensor origin (41 patients). The authors reported that ulnar-based pathology was rare.

29. McKee MD, Bowden SH, King GJ, et al: Management of recurrent, complex instability of the elbow with a hinged external fixator. *J Bone Joint Surg Br* 1998;80(6):1031-1037.

30. Cobb TK, Morrey BF: Use of distraction arthroplasty in unstable fracture dislocations of the elbow. *Clin Orthop* 1995;312:201-210.

31. Ring D, Jupiter JB, Simpson NS: Monteggia fractures in adults. *J Bone Joint Surg Am* 1998;80(12): 1733-1744.

32. Ring D, Jupiter JB: Proximal ulnar fractures and fractures-dislocations, in Norris TR (ed): *Orthopaedic Knowledge Update Shoulder and Elbow 2*. Rosemont, IL, American Academy of Orthopaedic Surgeons, 2002, pp 369-377.

33. Hutchinson DT, Horwitz DS, Ha G, Thomas CW, Bachus KN: Cyclic loading of olecranon fracture fixation constructs. *J Bone Joint Surg Am* 2003;85: 831-837.

    In this cadaveric study evaluating cyclic loading of transverse olecranon fracture fixation constructs, a 7.3-mm cancellous screw either with or without associated tension band was shown to have nearly five times greater stability than K-wire techniques.

34. Finsen V, Lingaas PS, Storro S: AO tension-band osteosynthesis of displaced olecranon fractures. *Orthopedics* 2000;23:1069-1072.

35. Mullett JH, Shannon F, Noel J, Lawlor G, Lee TC, O'Rourke SK: K-Wire position in tension band wiring of the olecranon: A comparison of two techniques. *Injury* 2000;31:427-431.

    The authors of this study compared tension band technique with K-wires passed down the long axis of the ulna and K-wires passed across the anterior cortex. Patients with K-wires passed down the long axis had a three time higher rate of radiographic evidence of wires backing out. Forty two percent of patients with K-wires passed down the long axis required hardware removal compared with only 11% of those in the transcortical group. Transcortical wires were reported to have twice the maximum pullout strength.

36. Romero JM, Miran A, Jensen CH: Complications and re-operation rate after tension-band wiring of olecranon fractures. *J Orthop Sci* 2000;5:318-320.

    In this retrospective review of 55 patients treated for a displaced olecranon fracture with tension brand technique, the authors reported an overall revision rate of 72%, with the main reason for removal of hardware being pain (61% of patients).

37. Harrell RM, Tong J, Weinhold PS, Dahners LE: Comparison of the mechanical properties of different tension band materials and suture techniques. *J Orthop Trauma* 2003;17:119-122.

    The authors of this study reported that stainless steel wire had a significantly higher load to failure and approximately 20 times greater stiffness than 5-mm woven polyester tape and either one or two loops of No. 5 braided polyester suture. The authors concluded that neither woven polyester tape nor braided polyester suture materials were suitable for rigid tension band fixation.

38. Bailey CS, MacDermid J, Patterson SD, King GJ: Outcome of plate fixation of olecranon fractures. *J Orthop Trauma* 2001;15:542-548.

    In this study, 25 patients underwent plate fixation for the treatment of displaced olecranon fractures; although none of these patients had any difference in motion or strength, they did have reduced supination compared with their uninjured sides. The mean DASH Outcome Measure score was near normal and the Medical Outcome Study Short Form-36 scores showed no difference compared with that of the average American population. Twenty percent of patients required plate removal. The authors recommended plate fixation as an alternative for the treatment of displaced olecranon fractures.

39. Khalfayan EE, Culp RW, Alexander AH: Mason type II radial head fractures: Operative versus nonoperative treatment. *J Orthop Trauma* 1992;6:283-289.

40. Broberg MA, Morrey BF: Results of delayed excision of the radial head after fracture. *J Bone Joint Surg Am* 1986;68:669-674.

41. King GJ, Zarzour ZD, Rath DA, Dunning CE, Patterson SD, Johnson JA: Metallic radial head arthroplasty improves valgus stability of the elbow. *Clin Orthop* 1999;368:114-125.

42. King GJW, Evans DC, Kellam JF: Open reduction and internal fixation of radial head fractures. *J Orthop Trauma* 1991;5(1):21-28.

43. Goldberg I, Peylan J, Yosipovitch Z: Late results of excision of the radial head for an isolated closed fracture. *J Bone Joint Surg Am* 1986;68:675-679.

44. Ikeda M, Oka Y: Function after early radial head resection for fracture: A retrospective evaluation of

15 patients followed for 3-18 years. *Acta Orthop Scand* 2000;71:191-194.

45. Leppilahti J, Jalovaara P: Early excision of the radial head for fracture. *Int Orthop* 2000;24:160-162.

46. Sanchez-Sotelo J, Romanillos O, Garay EG: Results of acute excision of the radial head in elbow radial head fracture-dislocations. *J Orthop Trauma* 2000; 14(5):354-355.

47. Knight DJ, Rymaszewski LA, Amis AA, Miller JH: Primary replacement of the fractured radial head with a metal prosthesis. *J Bone Joint Surg Br* 1993; 75:572-576.

Chapter 19

Fractures of the Forearm and Distal Radius

Gregory J. Schmeling, MD

Gregory Rafijah, MD

Daniel Zinar, MD

Forearm Fractures

The function of the upper extremity is to position the hand in space. The forearm axis includes the wrist, forearm, and elbow. The unique contribution of the forearm to the function of hand positioning is supination and pronation. The forearm axis should be considered as a single joint complex. Injury to any of the components of the forearm axis will have an impact on function. When developing a treatment plan for patients with forearm fractures, the impact of each component of the injury on the function of other parts of the forearm axis should be considered. In addition, when an injury to one component of the forearm axis is identified, injury to other components should be ruled out.

Of the nearly 1.5 million hand and forearm fractures identified in 1998, almost 650,000 were fractures of the radius and/or ulna.[1] Forearm fractures, therefore, result in significant health care costs. The most common mechanisms of injury include falls, being struck by another person or object, and motor vehicle accidents. Although it was reported that most of these fractures occurred in individuals between the ages of 5 to 14 years and in those older than 65 years, approximately 110,000 fractures occurred in individuals between the ages of 18 and 64 years. Even though the period of temporary disability may be relatively short for patients with forearm fractures, it may have a significant financial impact on individuals with limited resources. Any significant permanent disability in the population of working individuals also represents a significant cost to society.

Fracture prevention in the aging population helps maintain independence and function. Risk factors have been identified in one study that assessed fractures of the forearm and wrist in elderly men and women.[2] Femoral neck bone mineral density, height loss, and calcium intake were reported to be independent predictors for fracture in men. Femoral neck bone mineral density, height loss, and history of falls were reported to be independent predictors for fracture in women. Strategies to prevent forearm and wrist fractures in elderly men and women should focus on these risk factors.

Classification

Multiple classification systems exist for fractures or injuries to the forearm axis. Criteria that are most often used include location, pattern, displacement, wrist or elbow involvement, comminution or bone loss, and soft-tissue envelope. The Orthopaedic Trauma Association attempted to standardize fracture classifications by developing a fracture and dislocation compendium. This system is complex and may have a high level of interobserver variability. Intraobserver consistency makes it useful for individual research and outcome assessment.

To understand injuries and plan treatment, it is useful to classify them as either simple or complex injuries of the forearm axis. The forearm axis has both bone and soft-tissue components. Simple injuries are single forearm axis component injuries (isolated ulnar fractures, isolated radial fractures, and fractures of both the ulna and radius). Complex injuries represent injury to multiple components of the forearm axis (Galeazzi fracture-dislocations, Monteggia fracture-dislocations, and the Essex-Lopresti fracture-dislocation).

Interosseous Membrane

The interosseous membrane plays a pivotal role in forearm stability and couples the motion of the distal radioulnar joint (DRUJ) and the proximal radioulnar joint (PRUJ). The interosseous membrane is divided into the proximal, middle, and distal thirds. The middle third is the strongest and has been described as the most significant contributor to longitudinal stability of the forearm.

Anatomically, there are three main fiber groups (descending) on the volar side and two main fiber groups (ascending) on the dorsal side[3] (Figure 1). The two main groups are the intermediate descending fibers on the volar surface and the proximal ascending bundle. Both bundles attach to the radius at the interosseous tubercle (8.5 cm from the elbow) and to the ulna.[3] The central third of the interosseous membrane is made up of the proximal ascending bundle and intermediate descending fibers. The proximal ascending bundle provides most of the resistance to distal migration of the radius when the

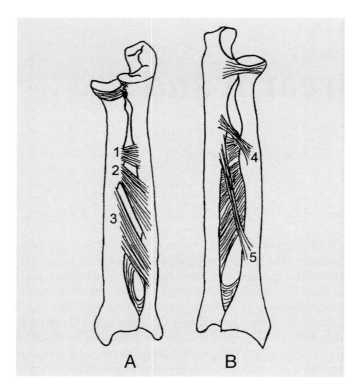

Figure 1 Anterior **(A)** and posterior **(B)** aspects of the interosseous membrane. 1 = Proximal descending fibers, 2 = Intermediate descending fibers, 3 = Distal descending fibers, 4 = Proximal ascending bundle, and 5 = Distal ascending bundle. *(Reproduced with permission from Poitevin LA, Valente S: La membrana interossea y la estabilidad longitudinal del antebrazo. Rev AAOT 1999;64:220-228.)*

DRUJ and PRUJ are resected. The intermediate descending fibers provides most of the resistance to proximal migration of the radius when the DRUJ and PRUJ are resected.[3] The other fiber groups contribute radius migration resistance as well but not nearly as much as the proximal ascending bundle and intermediate descending fibers.

The proximal ascending bundle and intermediate descending fibers converge and attach to the radius at the interosseous tubercle. They allow the ulna to resist longitudinal stress and transmit loads from one bone to the other.[3] Because longitudinal stress is resisted by all of the ligaments, injury to the proximal ascending bundle or intermediate descending fibers alone may not result in significant migration. The transmission of load from the wrist to the elbow by way of the forearm is complex and depends on wrist anatomy, position of the forearm, and soft-tissue links between the radius and ulna.[4] The interosseous membrane plays a significant role in force transmission when the elbow is in varus but plays an insignificant role in force transmission when the elbow is in valgus.

Clinical suspicion of an interosseous membrane injury should be high when a patient reports pain at the DRUJ or midforearm associated with a radial head injury. This diagnosis can be confirmed with ultrasound or MRI.[5] Both diagnostic imaging modalities have demon-

strated a high degree of sensitivity, specificity, accuracy, and positive and negative predictive value for this type of injury.[5] Studies have described a clinical test based on a cadaveric model to assess the integrity of the interosseous membrane.[6] To perform this test, the radius is pulled proximally. If greater than 3 mm of instability is present, the interosseous membrane is injured; if there is greater than 6 mm of instability, both the interosseous membrane and triangular fibrocartilage are injured. Optimal treatment of complex forearm axis injuries requires a complete understanding of the injury. If the interosseous membrane injury is not fully appreciated, significant long-term problems may occur.

Indications for Open Reduction and Internal Fixation
The treatment goal for forearm axis injuries is to restore the anatomy to provide early return to function. Because the forearm must be thought of as a joint, most injuries in adult patients are treated with open anatomic reduction, internal fixation, and early motion.

Isolated Ulnar Fractures
Isolated ulnar fractures often are defensive injuries. Functional bracing has been recommended for isolated ulnar fractures that are stable. Stable fractures have been defined as those with less than 50% of displacement. The model used to arrive at this definition was a distal third fracture of the ulna with the central third of the interosseous membrane intact. The authors of a systematic review[7] that identified 1,876 patients in 33 published series concluded that fractures with minimal displacement are best treated with a short arm cast, displaced or unstable fractures are best treated with compression plating, and fractures with 25% to 50% of displacement or angulated 10° to 15° are unstable. Others studies have reported the presence of significant rotational instability of the ulna in patients with midshaft osteotomies.[8] These authors concluded that treatment should not be based on displacement alone because rotational instability may persist. An evidence-based medicine review concluded that there was insufficient evidence to conclude which method of treatment was best for isolated fractures of the ulna in adult patients.[9]

Nondisplaced, isolated ulnar fractures around the junction of the middle third and distal third may be treated with a short arm cast for 2 to 4 weeks followed by bracing until union occurs. Displaced, unstable isolated fractures are treated with open reduction and internal fixation, with progression to motion when the postoperative pain decreases. As the fracture approaches the joint on either end of the ulna, less displacement is better tolerated and open reduction and internal fixation is recommended.

Isolated Radial Shaft Fractures
Isolated radial shaft fractures are uncommon. DRUJ integrity should be evaluated to exclude the Galeazzi

injury. Most isolated radial shaft fractures are treated with open reduction and internal fixation because the radius rotates around the ulna and casting the adult arm above the elbow is associated with significant morbidity.

Fractures of the Radius and Ulna

Fractures of both the radius and ulna in adult patients are best treated with open reduction and internal fixation unless significant medical contraindications exist. The bone stability that contributes to the forearm axis should be restored and permit early return to function.

Galeazzi Fracture

Galeazzi fractures, fractures of the radius, most commonly occur at the junction of the middle and distal thirds associated with injury to the DRUJ and the interosseous membrane. Open reduction and internal fixation is almost always indicated for this type of injury. After open reduction and internal fixation, the forearm is supinated and the DRUJ is assessed for stability. Unstable joints are reduced and pinned. In one study, 38 patients with Galeazzi fractures were reviewed and the DRUJ was found to be unstable in 55% of patients when the radial fracture was less than 7.5 cm from the midarticular surface of the radius; the DRUJ was unstable in only 6% of patients when the radial fracture was farther away than 7.5 cm.[10] The authors recommended using the location of the radial fracture as an aid in making the diagnosis of an unstable DRUJ. One recent case report described the extensor carpi ulnaris as a block to the reduction of the DRUJ associated with a Galeazzi fracture.[11] If the DRUJ does not reduce after anatomic reduction and fixation of the radius, exploration of the joint may be required.

Monteggia Fractures

Monteggia fractures are proximal ulnar fractures associated with a dislocation of the radial head. Posterior dislocation of the radial head most commonly occurs in adults. Treatment involves fracture reduction and internal fixation first. The radial head usually relocates and is stable. The radial head does not reduce frequently because of a nonanatomic reduction of the ulna. If the ulna is anatomic and the radial head does not reduce, an open reduction of the joint is required.[12]

Monteggia equivalent injuries are proximal ulnar fractures associated with a fracture of the radial head. When a patient with a Monteggia equivalent injury also has a comminuted radial head fracture, there is no consensus on whether reduction and internal fixation of the comminuted radial head fracture should be done or the entire radial head replaced.[12] If an interosseous membrane injury is also suspected, replacing the radial head to increase radiocapitellar contact and ulnohumeral stability is warranted. The complication rate is high for patients who undergo treatment for Monteggia equivalent injuries.[12,13]

The Role of Bone Grafting

Acute bone grafting has been advocated in the past for the treatment of forearm fractures when more than 30% of the circumference is comminuted. This recommendation was based on the assumption that because the rate of union for comminuted, grafted fractures was the same as the rate for noncomminuted, nongrafted fractures the addition of bone graft increased the rate of union for comminuted fractures. It was also assumed that the rate of union for comminuted fractures would be less than the rate of union for noncomminuted fractures. One study, however, concluded that the union rate for patients with comminuted, nongrafted fractures was the same as that for patients with noncomminuted, nongrafted fractures.[14] Thirty percent comminution of the shaft of the forearm bone, therefore, should no longer be used as an indication for acute bone grafting. Current biologic plating techniques are able to overcome the negative influence of the comminution.

Bone grafting has a role in the treatment of forearm fractures with segmental bone loss or severe open fractures with poor local biology. After soft-tissue reconstruction, short segmental defects can be reconstructed with tricortical iliac crest autograft[15] or fibular allograft.

Fixation Techniques
Plating

Plate fixation for the treatment of forearm fractures has been around for some time and has gone through many iterations. Noncompression plates gave way to anatomic reduction and compression plating. Large (4.5-mm) plates and thin neutralization plates are no longer recommended because of the risk of fracture occurring on hardware removal and loss of fixation, respectively. Open reduction and internal fixation with small (3.5-mm) compression plates became the subsequent treatment of choice and gave way to techniques such as bridge plating that preserve biology rather than restore mechanics. The concept of biologic fixation was then developed.

In an attempt to preserve biology without sacrificing mechanical stability, the AO/ASIF developed the point contact fixator, a noncompression plate with screws that are threaded into the plate. Unicortical screw fixation holds the plate to the bone. The plate is placed on the bone without disturbing the fracture blood supply and is not contoured to the bone. Several authors have reported union rates ranging from 92% to 100% using this technique.[16-18] Infection rates range from 0 to 1% of patients,[16,17] and refracture after plate removal is approximately 5%,[17] which is as good as or better than rates reported for compression plating techniques using biologic fixation.[16]

The locking compression plating systems evolved from the point contact fixator.[19] Unicortical fixation can be achieved with locking screws, but compression is also possible with the plate design. The preservation of the biology allows early fracture healing via callus formation. The implant provides mechanical stability for early mobilization and return to function. Prospective comparisons with traditional biologic fixation methods are lacking to date, but the method appears promising.

Intramedullary Fixation

Intramedullary nailing is not meant to replace compression plating in the treatment of forearm fractures. It is an internal splint only, and supplemental bracing or casting often is required. Intramedullary nailing can be considered an alternative to plating pathologic or impending pathologic fractures,[20] segmental fractures, comminuted gunshot fractures, refractures that occur after plate removal, fractures at either end of a plate, or fractures in athletes who participate in contact sports. This technique should not be used if insertion of the intramedullary nail crosses a growth plate or in patients with small diameter canals (< 3 mm), fractures < 3 cm from the end of the bone, preexisting deformity, corrective osteotomies, and nonunions.

Intramedullary nailing has found greater application in pediatric orthopaedics. One study used intramedullary Kirschner wire fixation in 57 patients younger than 14 years and showed that alignment was maintained and no adverse growth plate events occurred.[21] Another study reported similar results in 31 patients.[22] The authors of another study concluded that intramedullary fixation with Kirschner wires or flexible titanium intramedullary rods is ideal for the treatment of transverse fractures of the forearm in children and adolescents.[23] Cast immobilization is required because rigid fixation is not achieved.

External Fixation

Forearm shaft fractures rarely require external fixation. Compression plating in the treatment of open forearm fractures, which is not associated with increased complications, remains the treatment of choice. External fixation of forearm fractures, however, can be complicated by pin tract infection, nerve injury, and a high rate of nonunion when compared with compression plating. External fixation may have a role as a temporizing measure in the treatment of open forearm fractures in underresuscitated multiple trauma patients or in those with severely contaminated open fractures.

Outcomes

Supination and pronation, based on the rotation of the radius around the ulna, are unique functions of the forearm. Malunion of a forearm fracture alters the position of one bone relative to the other, thereby altering the arc of motion. Loss of motion in the supination-pronation arc is one criterion used to define outcome.

In a study in which a cadaveric model was used to assess the effect of rotational malunion of the radius on the supination-pronation arc of motion, a significant loss of supination was noted to occur with > 30° of pronation deformity of the radius and a significant loss of pronation occurred with > 30° of supination deformity.[24] The amount of rotational loss in the opposite direction was comparable whether the rotational deformity was supination or pronation. It can therefore be concluded that the forearm axis tolerates up to 30° of rotational deformity of the radius without significant loss of motion. In the clinical situation, however, deformities do not occur in isolation. Deformity in other planes may be synergistic and result in greater amounts of motion loss.

Rotational malunion of the ulna was evaluated in a cadaver study and the authors concluded that rotational malunion of the ulna did not lead to loss in the arc of supination and pronation.[25] Rotational deformity in one direction increased the motion in the opposite direction. Rotational deformity of the ulna changes the location of the arc of rotation of the forearm. Correction of a rotational deformity of the ulna should not increase the arc of motion, only the position of the arc in space. Correction of a significant rotation deformity of the radius, however, could be expected to increase the arc of rotation.

Another cadaver study assessed the effect of rotational malunion of the ulna, radius, or ulna and radius on forearm rotation.[26] The authors found that supination deformity of the ulna had little effect on rotation, supination deformity of the radius produced a significant reduction in forearm rotation, and a pronation deformity of either the radius or ulna produced a moderate reduction in rotation. A rotational deformity of both the radius and ulna in the same direction produced a pattern similar to that caused by an isolated radial deformity. A rotational deformity of both the radius and the ulna in the opposite direction produced the greatest loss of forearm rotation.

Computer models have also been developed to determine the effect of deformity on the rotation of the forearm.[27,28] It has been reported that computer modeling may be useful in preoperative planning for deformity correction in the forearm because it can help predict the result based on the amount of correction.

Early mobilization may also affect outcome. One study reported that immobilization for more than 2 weeks had a significant impact on strength and endurance of patients with forearm fractures that were treated with open reduction and internal fixation.[29] Goal-oriented exercises were reported to have improved patient strength and endurance over the period of the study. At 8 weeks postoperatively, patients with goal-oriented exercises were stronger and had better endurance than control subjects.

The outcome measures used in the published literature typically rely on union rate and the physician's interpretation of the patient's outcome based on range of

TABLE 1 | Outcome Measures Used to Assess Forearm Fractures

Functional Result	Criteria
Excellent	Union, < 10° flexion-extension loss, < 25° pronation-supination loss
Satisfactory	Union, < 20° flexion-extension loss, < 50° pronation-supination loss
Unsatisfactory	Union, > 30° flexion-extension loss, > 50° pronation-supination loss
Failure	Nonunion

(Adapted with permission from Anderson LD, Sisk TD, Tooms RE, Park WI III: Compression-plate fixation in acute diaphyseal fractures of the radius and ulna. *J Bone Joint Surg Am* 1975;57:287-297.)

TABLE 2 | Forearm Fracture Outcomes by Treatment Type

Treatment		Union	Satisfactory or Better
Compression plate	Ulna, radius, or both bones	88% to 98%	80% to 92%
Intramedullary nailing	Ulna, radius, or both bones	94% to 100%	70% to 78%
Compression plate	Monteggia	90% to 100%	83% to 86%
Compression plate	Galeazzi	94% to 100%	92% to 100%

motion and union (Table 1). Union rates are high for forearm fractures treated with all methods of fixation and for simple and complex forearm axis injuries. Outcomes are poorer for patients with forearm fractures treated with intramedullary fixation techniques and even worse for those with Monteggia equivalent injuries and open fractures with significant soft-tissue injury (Table 2).

Complications

Complications associated with forearm fractures include infection, nerve injury, compartment syndrome, malunion, nonunion, synostosis (union of normally distinct bones) or heterotopic ossification, and refracture after plate removal.

Infection

The infection rate ranges from 0.8% to 7% of patients with forearm fractures.[17,18] For those with open fractures, the infection rate ranges from 1.2% to 20%. Superficial infections usually respond to treatment with antibiotics. Deep infections require surgical irrigation and débridement and treatment with intravenous antibiotics. In most patients, the hardware can be maintained. Patients with osteomyelitis, however, may require seg-

mental resection of the diaphysis and soft-tissue and bone reconstruction.

Nerve Injury

Nerve injury associated with forearm fractures is most often related to excessive swelling or retraction during surgical exposure. Most of these injuries do not represent an anatomic disruption and therefore recover with time. Transection of the median nerve by diaphyseal forearm fracture has been reported. The superficial radial nerve is at risk for a traction injury during surgical exposure of the middle and distal thirds of the radius. The posterior interosseous nerve is at risk during exposure of the proximal third of the radius. When a volar approach is used, the arm should be kept in supination. When a dorsal or posterolateral approach is used, the arm should be kept in pronation. With the forearm fully pronated, a safe zone extending from the edge of the proximal radial articular surface from 40 mm (minimum) to 60 mm (maximum) and from 44 to 60 mm has been reported.[30] Supination reduced this safe zone to as little as 22 mm (mean, 33 mm).

Compartment Syndrome

Compartment syndrome is a rare complication in patients with forearm fractures. One study that reviewed the etiology of compartment syndrome in 164 patients treated over an 8-year period, which represented an average annual incidence of 0.7 and 7.3 per 100,000 in women and men, respectively, found that compartment syndrome was associated with a distal radial fracture in 16 patients and a forearm fracture in 13 patients.[31] The incidence of compartment syndrome was 0.25% for distal radial fractures and 3% for forearm fractures. Another study reported a much higher incidence of compartment syndrome (7%) associated with proximal ulnar fractures caused by a low-velocity gunshot wound in five patients and high-energy blunt trauma in one patient.[32] If a high incidence of suspicion for compartment syndrome is maintained and physicians are prepared to perform rapid release of compartments to prevent muscle neurosis, then the sequelae of compartment syndrome can be avoided.

Malunion

Malunion can have a profound effect on function. Although rotational malunion of either bone or malunion of the ulna may be better tolerated, loss of radial bow or change in its location can result in a significant risk for loss of forearm rotation.[24-28] A malunion that results in significant loss of forearm rotation is best treated with osteotomy, deformity correction, and compression plating.

Nonunion

Historically, the incidence of nonunion has ranged from 0 to 9% of patients.[17,18] With modern techniques, the nonunion rate ranges from 0 to 2%.[17,18] Infected nonunions are best treated with segmental resection of the infection and reconstruction of the soft tissues. Bone reconstruction should take place after antibiotic therapy. Noninfected nonunions are treated with débridement of the nonunion or bone grafting, revision compression plating, or both. The diagnosis of nonunion can be difficult. In patients with ulnar shaft fractures, ossification of the fracture often occurs slowly because of the greater percentage of cortical bone. In addition, primary bone healing without callous formation may occur in patients with rigid compression plating.

Synostosis or Heterotopic Ossification

The incidence of synostosis of the forearm is generally low (2%), but it is disabling because it reduces the arc of supination and pronation to 0°. The incidence of interosseous membrane heterotopic ossification is higher, but it does not always limit the arc of forearm rotation. Head injury, burns, genetic predisposition, severe soft-tissue injury, and the presence of bone fragments or bone graft on the interosseous membrane are risk factors for the development of synostosis.[33] The treatment of synostosis is resection, early motion, and recurrence prevention, which includes radiation therapy and anti-inflammatory medications.[34] Factors related to poor outcome of forearm synostosis treatment include fracture location (proximal and distal fractures have poorer outcomes than midshaft fractures) and size, severity of the initial injury, and timing of the resection.[34] One study reported excellent results for the resection of proximal radioulnar synostosis within 6 to 12 months after injury using a meticulous technique, fat interposition, and no recurrence prophylaxis.[34] Whether these results are applicable to patients with middle or distal synostosis is unknown. Another study reported excellent results for resection of forearm synostosis within 4 months of injury, using postoperative radiation therapy and indomethacin for recurrence prophylaxis.[35] With adequate recurrence prophylaxis, resection of synostosis should be considered sooner rather than later because a better outcome may be achieved. Restoration of good forearm rotation has also been reported using resection of a 1-cm portion of the radial shaft distal to treat nonoperable proximal radioulnar synostosis.[33]

Refracture After Plate Removal

The incidence of refracture after plate removal has been reported to range from 3% to 17% of patients.[17-29] Refracture can occur either through the old fracture or through screw holes. Refractures associated with the old fracture line are a result of premature removal of the implant. Refracture through a screw hole is often a result of the stress concentration effect of the screw hole. Refracture after plate removal is most often associated with the use of 4.5-mm plates and screws, but it can occur with smaller implants. Although routine forearm plate removal is not recommended, indications for removal include hardware pain and participation in physical activities that place significant stress on the forearm (such as military service and athletic activity). To reduce the risk of refracture, plates should not be removed until complete bone remodeling is demonstrated on radiographs. Even though bone mineral density does not return for 21 months after injury, plates can be removed sooner if remodeling is complete. After implant removal, patients are restricted to nonphysical activities for 8 to 12 weeks. Refracture after implant removal is most often treated with repeated compression plating, but intramedullary nailing or cast immobilization has also been recommended.

Distal Radial Fractures

Fifteen percent to 20% of all fractures involve the distal radius, and up to 50% of these are intra-articular fractures.[36] Colles, who first described this clinical entity in 1814 without the benefit of radiography, reported that although all such fractures healed without any disability, deformity usually persisted throughout life. Much has been learned since then, and distal radial fracture treatment has been revolutionized in the past 20 years. Better understanding of distal radial fractures and refinements in fixation techniques continue to improve treatment results.

Most distal radial fractures are the result of a fall, with a bimodal age distribution that mostly affects children and the elderly. In a prospective cohort of Caucasian women followed in a 10-year study (average patient age at the time of fracture, 76 years) 73% of the fractures were extra-articular and occurred after a fall.[37] A decline in bone mineral density was associated with a fracture.

The advent of high-speed transportation and recreation has increased the incidence of complicated fractures. High-energy injuries often disrupt the articular surface of the distal radius and typically occur in young, active individuals who place heavy demands on their wrists. Because near-anatomic reconstruction of these fractures is required for a good outcome in this patient population, efforts have been made to better understand these fractures and improve treatment options.

Classification

Most clinicians refer to distal radial fractures in terms of eponyms. Although descriptions such as Colles fracture, Barton fracture, or die-punch fracture are used regularly, they provide little information about the fracture personality or assist in the selection of treatment options. Classification systems have been developed as a clinical aid and research comparison tool. To be useful, a classification system should be simple, clinically relevant, guide treatment, and be reproducible enough for meaningful research. Numerous classification systems exist for fractures of the distal radius, but none of these are univer-

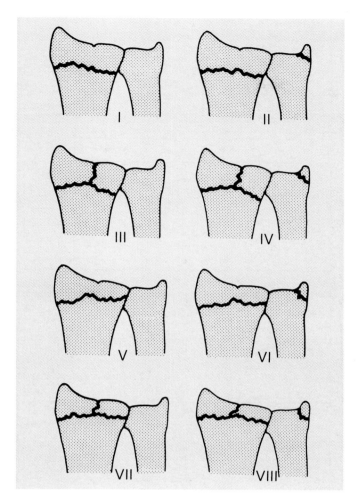

Figure 2 Frykman classification of distal radius fractures. Types I, III, V, and VI do not have an associated fracture of the distal ulna. Fractures III through VIII are intra-articular fractures. Higher classification fractures have poorer prognoses. *(Reproduced with permission from Fernandez DL, Palmer AK: Fractures of the distal radius, in Green DP, Hotchkiss RN, Pederson WC (eds): Green's Operative Hand Surgery, ed 4. New York, NY, Churchill Livingstone, 1999, p 935.)*

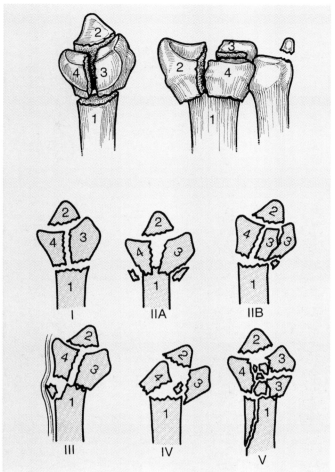

Figure 3 Melone classification of distal radius fractures. The four major fragments are (1) the radial shaft, (2) the radial styloid region, (3) the dorsal medial facet, and (4) the volar medial facet. The major fragment of this four-part fracture is the medial facet (fragments 3 and 4). Types I through IV represent increasingly comminuted fractures, with type V being an extremely comminuted, unstable fracture without large identifiable facet fragments. *(Reproduced with permission from Fernandez DL, Palmer AK: Fractures of the distal radius, in Green DP, Hotchkiss RN, Pederson WC (eds): Green's Operative Hand Surgery, ed 4. New York, NY, Churchill Livingstone, 1999, p 936.)*

sally accepted in the orthopaedic community. The Frykman classification system is commonly used, and it differentiates between intra-articular and extra-articular fractures with and without ulnar styloid fractures (Figure 2). The Frykman system, however, does not help guide treatment and has limited interobserver reliability. Intra-articular fractures of the distal radius follow a consistent pattern.[38,39] The joint surface often fractures along fault lines into a radial styloid fragment and lunate facet fragment that often splits coronally into a volar medial and a dorsomedial fragment (Figure 3).

Distal radial fractures have also been defined in terms of parts.[38-40] A part extends to the radial or ulnar joint surface, is displaced more than 1 to 2 mm, and can be surgically manipulated and potentially stabilized. Fractures are described as two-, three-, or four-part injuries, and the major patterns include the radial styloid, radial shaft, and palmar and dorsal fragments of the lunate facet.

The AO/ASIF classification system divides fractures into three major groups. Type A fractures are extra-articular, type B fractures are simple articular, and type C fractures are complex articular (Figure 4). These groups are subdivided such that there are 144 possibilities, making the AO/ASIF system rather cumbersome for clinical use. Studies have shown limited interobserver and intraobserver reliability with the Frykman, Melone, and standard AO/ASIF classification systems.[41]

The Fernandez classification system is based on mechanism of injury and is designed to be clinically useful (Figures 5 and 6 and Tables 3 and 4). According to this system, injuries are described as bending fractures (type I), articular shear fractures (type II), compression fractures (type III), fracture-dislocations (type IV), or combined mechanisms (type V). This classification sys-

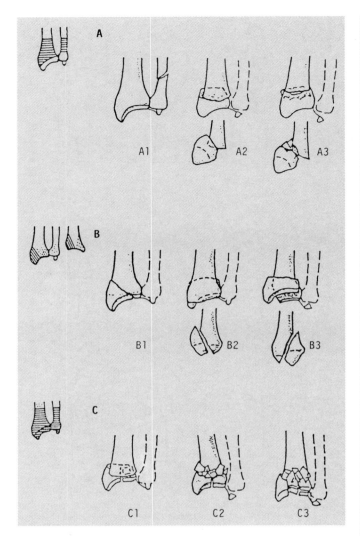

Figure 4 The comprehensive classification of fractures (AO). **A,** Extra-articular: fractures affect neither the articular surface of the radiocarpal nor the radioulnar joins. A1, extra-articular fracture of the ulna with the radius intact; A2, extra-articular fracture of the radius, simple and impacted; A3, extra-articular fracture of the radius, multifragmentary. **B,** Partial articular: fracture affects a portion of the articular surface, but the continuity of the metaphysis and epiphysis is intact. B1, partial articular fracture of the radius, sagittal; B2, partial articular fracture of the radius, dorsal rim (Barton); B3, partial articular fracture of the radius, volar rim (reverse Barton, Goyrand-Smith II). **C,** Complete articular: fracture affects the joint surfaces (radioulnar and/or radiocarpal) and the metaphyseal area. C1, complete articular fracture of the radius, articular simple and metaphyseal simple; C2, complete articular fracture of the radius, articular simple and metaphyseal multifragmentary; C3, complete articular fracture of the radius, multifragmentary. *(Reproduced with permission from Müller ME, Nazarian S, Koch P, Schatzker (eds): The Comprehensive Classification of Long Bones. New York, NY, Springer-Verlag, 1990.)*

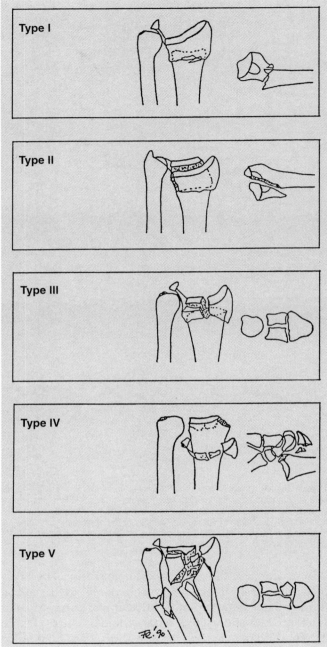

Figure 5 Fernandez classification of distal radius fractures (fracture types in adults based on the mechanism of injury). *(Reproduced with permission from Fernandez DL, Palmer AK: Fractures of the distal radius, in Green DP, Hotchkiss RN, Pederson WC (eds): Green's Operative Hand Surgery, ed 4. New York, NY, Churchill Livingstone, 1999, p 940.)*

tem helps surgeons select treatment options and identify unstable fracture patterns.

Type I fractures result from bending forces that usually create an extra-articular fracture of the distal radial metaphysis. The fracture can be displaced dorsally or volarly; volarly displaced fractures are quite unstable.

Type II fractures are shearing injuries of the joint surface. The resulting shear fracture can involve either the volar or dorsal lip or radial styloid. These are usually

unstable injuries resulting from fracture line obliquity, and carpal subluxation usually occurs. Most articular shear fractures require internal fixation.

Type III fractures are compression injuries of the articular surface that usually result from an axial load to the wrist. These die-punch injuries result in joint surface disruption and depression and usually follow the pattern of joint surface comminution described by Melone and

TABLE 3 | Fernandez Classification of Distal Radius Fractures

Fracture Types (Adults) Based on the Mechanism of Injury	Children Fracture Equivalent	Stability/Instability (High risk of secondary displacement after initial adequate reduction)	Displacement Pattern	Number of Fragments	Associated Lesions (Carpal ligament, fractures, median, ulnar nerve, tendons, ipsilateral fracture upper extremity, compartment syndrome)	Recommended Treatment
Type 1: Bending fracture of the metaphysis	Distal forearm fracture Salter II	Stable Unstable	Nondisplaced Dorsal (Colles) Volar (Smith) Proximal Combined	Always two main fragments plus Varying degree of metaphyseal comminution (instability)	Uncommon	Conservative (stable fractures) Percutaneous pinning (extrafocal or intrafocal) External fixation (exceptionally bone graft)
Type II: Shearing fracture of the joint surface	Salter IV	Unstable	Dorsal (Barton) Radial (Chauffeur) Volar (revised Barton) Combined	Two-part Three-part Comminuted	Less common	Open reduction Screw-plate fixation
Type III: Compression fracture of the joint surface	Salter III, IV, V	Stable Unstable	Nondisplaced Dorsal Radial Volar Proximal Combined	Two-part Three-part Four-part Comminuted	Common	Conservative Closed, limited, arthroscopically assisted or extensile open reduction Percutaneous pins External fixation Internal fixation Plate, bone graft
Type IV: Avulsion fractures, radiocarpal fracture dislocation	Very rare	Unstable	Dorsal Radial Volar Proximal Combined	Two-part (radial styloid, ulnar styloid) Three-part (volar, dorsal margin) Comminuted	Frequent	Closed or open reduction Pin or screw fixation Tension wiring
Type V : Combined fractures (I-IV) high-velocity injury	Very rare	Unstable	Dorsal Radial Volar Proximal Combined	Comminuted and/ or bone loss (frequently intra-articular, open, seldom extra-articular)	Always present	Combined method

(Reproduced with permission from Fernandez DL, Palmer AK: Fractures of the distal radius, in Green DP, Hotchkiss RN, Pederson WC (eds): *Green's Operative Hand Surgery*, ed 4. New York, NY, Churchill Livingstone, 1999, p 940.)

others. Open reduction is usually required to disimpact the articular fragments.

Type IV injuries are rare and are usually the result of high-energy trauma. The fracture-dislocation of the wrist occurs when the major ligamentous supports of the wrist are avulsed with the accompanying radial and ulnar styloids. There is usually significant and sometimes dramatic fracture displacement. Surgical repair of the avulsed styloids usually restores stability, but volar capsular and intercarpal ligament injuries may also need to be addressed.

Type V injuries are the result of a combination of mechanisms. Usually the result of high-energy trauma, these are the most severe and unstable fractures. A combination of surgical techniques and exposures may be required to restore alignment and stability.

Diagnostic Evaluation

No classification system or treatment algorithm can be used without accurate diagnostic studies. High-quality prereduction and postreduction radiographs are essential. Projections should be taken in AP, lateral, and oblique views. Several studies recommend using the lateral tilt or lunate facet view as an additional lateral projection.[42] The tilted lateral view of the distal radius is obtained with the wrist elevated 20° from the perpendicular. This projection neutralizes the 20° inclination of the radial styloid and effectively eliminates the radiographic overlap of the radial styloid. Improved assessment of the articular surface, especially the lunate fossa, is noted with this view. It is helpful for assessing both reduction and application of internal fixation. One study reported findings of tilted lateral radiographs obtained for seven cadaver wrists.[42] Lunate facet fractures were created and AP, lateral, and 22° tilted lateral radiographs were obtained. Because a statistically significant improvement in measurement accuracy was noted, routine use of the tilted lateral wrist view was recommended to evaluate intra-articular fractures of the distal radius (especially of the lunate facet).

Digital radiography is becoming increasingly common, and many surgeons are concerned about how this new diagnostic technology compares with standard radiography. One study compared digital radiography to standard radiography with regard to ability to measure specific elements of a fractured distal radius.[43] The use of digital software improved interobserver reliability significantly with regard to measurement of radial length, palmar tilt, and articular step-off. These findings suggest that digital radiography is at least equivalent to plain radiography in regard to the ability to measure important fracture parameters.

Evaluation of complicated intra-articular fractures may benefit from diagnostic scanning in addition to plain radiography. CT has been shown to improve measurement of articular incongruity and angulation and improve interobserver reproducibility.[44] CT also helps in the assessment of comminution and formulation of treatment plans. MRI has also been used to assess distal radial fractures. One study noted that MRI provided good evaluation of osseous injuries and can also detect occult soft-tissue injuries.[45]

Outcomes

Restoration of anatomic alignment is the best predictor of a good outcome in young, active patients with distal radial fractures. Good long-term results can be expected when healing occurs with a smooth joint surface, neutral radial length, neutral volar tilt, at least 5° of radial inclination, and a stable DRUJ. Residual articular surface incongruity may be the most important factor that affects long-term results. In a study of 40 young patients with

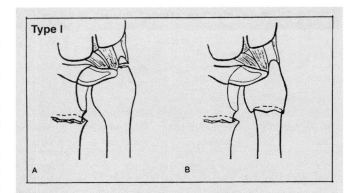

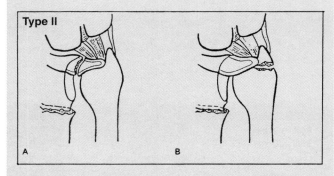

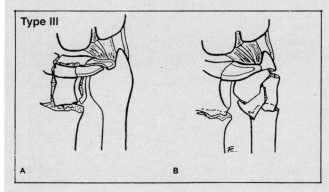

Figure 6 Fernandez classification of associated distal radioulnar joint lesions. *(Reproduced with permission from Fernandez DL, Palmer AK: Fractures of the distal radius, in Green DP, Hotchkiss RN, Pederson WC (eds): Green's Operative Hand Surgery, ed 4. New York, NY, Churchill Livingstone, 1999, p 941.)*

distal radial fractures, 65% were reported as having radiographic evidence of posttraumatic arthrosis at 6.7 years; 91% of the patients with articular incongruity developed radiographic evidence of arthritis and 11% of patients with a smooth articular surface developed arthritis.[46] Step-offs of the articular surface of 2 mm or more predict a poor outcome, and some authors note that even a 1-mm step-off can affect the overall result.[36,46-48]

Loss of radial length and volar tilt has been shown to influence outcome, whereas restoration of radial inclination is less influential on the final functional result. Shortening causes distortion of the triangular fibrocartilage complex (TFCC) and significantly alters load distribution

TABLE 4 | Fernandez Classification of Associated Distal Radioulnar Joint Lesions

	Pathoanatomy of the Lesion	Joint Surface Involvement	Prognosis	Recommended Treatment
Type I: Stable (Following reduction of the radius, the distal radioulnar joint is congruous and stable)	A: Fracture tip ulnar styloid B: Stable fracture ulnar neck	None	Good	A + B: Functional aftertreatment Encourage early pronation-supination exercises Note: Extra-articular unstable fractures of the ulna at the metaphyseal level or distal shaft require stable plate fixation
Type II: Unstable (Subluxation or dislocation of the ulnar head present)	A: Tear of triangular fibrocartilage complex and/or palmar and dorsal capsular ligaments B: Avulsion fracture base of the ulnar styloid	None	Chronic instability Painful limitation of supination if left unreduced Possible late arthritic changes	A: Closed treatment (Reduce subluxation, sugar tong splint in 45° supination 4 to 6 weeks) A + B: Surgical treatment (Repair triangular fibrocartilage complex or fix ulnar styloid with tension band wiring; immobilize wrist and elbow in supination [cast] or transfix ulna/radius with Kirschner wire and forearm cast)
Type III: Potentially Unstable (Subluxation possible)	A: Intra-articular fracture of the sigmoid notch B: Intra-articular fracture of the ulnar head	Present	Dorsal subluxation possible together with dorsally displaced die punch or dorsoulnar fragment Risk of early degenerative changes and severe limitation of forearm rotation if left unreduced	A: Anatomic reduction of palmar and dorsal sigmoid notch fragments; if residual subluxation tendency present, immobilize as in type II injury B: Functional aftertreatment to enhance remodeling of ulnar head If distal radioulnar joint remains painful, partial ulnar resection, Darrach or Sauvé-Kapandji procedure at a later date

(Reproduced with permission from Fernandez DL, Palmer AK: Fractures of the distal radius, in Green DP, Hotchkiss RN, Pederson WC (eds): *Green's Operative Hand Surgery*, ed 4. New York, NY, Churchill Livingstone, 1999, p 941.)

within the carpus and DRUJ. Radial shortening also results in pain from ulnar impaction, weakness of grip, and loss of forearm rotation. Along with loss of radial inclination, shortening often produces the unsightly cosmetic deformity associated with neglected fractures of the distal radius. Studies have shown that restoration of radial length correlates with improved outcome, especially in patients with extra-articular fractures.[47,49]

Increased dorsal tilt alters force distribution within the carpus that can lead to pain and degeneration of the wrist. As little as 10° of dorsal tilt can result in dorsal intercalated segment instability posture and dorsal subluxation of the carpus. In a clinical study of 13 patients with dorsally angulated malunions of the distal radius, all had dorsal intercalated segment instability posture and persistent pain.[50] Both pain and deformity were relieved by corrective osteotomy of the distal radius. Dorsal angulation was also found to be deleterious in a biomechanical cadaver study.[51] Increased dorsal tilt significantly affected wrist motion and carpal alignment. Adaptive dorsal intercalated segment instability posture of the midcarpal joint and dorsal subluxation of the radiocarpal joint were observed.

Severity of injury plays a role in overall outcome. Outcome and complication rates were reviewed in a study of 18 patients with open fractures of the distal radius.[52] Patients with type III open fractures had worse outcomes and more complications than patients with type I and type II injuries.

Patients with low functional demands may achieve good outcomes even with significant deformity of the distal radius. A study of 25 low-demand elderly patients who were treated nonsurgically revealed a wide variety of final radiographic outcomes, including 24% of patients whose outcomes were classified as poor.[53] Functional results, however, were generally good to excellent (88%). The authors noted that radiographic and functional outcomes did not correlate in this age group. Although more than half of the patients had obvious cosmetic deformities, none claimed to be unhappy about their clinical appearance. These findings suggest that patients in this age group with low functional demands can expect good results with nonsurgical management. However, the authors noted that activity level is a more important criterion than age and recommended surgical treatment of active patients older than 60 years with severely displaced intra-articular fractures of the distal radius.

Associated Injuries

A wide variety of associated injuries may complicate distal radial fracture treatment and final outcome. Injuries to the median nerve, intercarpal ligaments, carpal bones, and DRUJ have been reported extensively.[36,54-58] Arthroscopic studies have identified a high degree of associated injuries, including injuries to the TFCC and scapholunate ligament. In one such study, 68% of 60 patients had a significant intercarpal injury at the time of arthroscopy.[55] Another study used arthroscopy to assist in open reduction and internal fixation of distal radial fractures; a 54% rate of TFCC tears and an 18% rate of scapholunate injuries were noted.[58] The TFCC tears were all peripheral. The authors recommended acute repair of the associated soft-tissue injuries and reported only good to excellent results in their series. These findings suggest that these associated injuries may have a significant effect on the overall outcome of distal radial fractures.

Complications

Several complications have been associated with distal radial fractures.[59] In a study assessing such complications, 250 patients were prospectively evaluated for complications related to treatment. Patients and physicians completed questionnaires at 6-month follow-up. The physicians reported a complication rate of 27%, whereas the patients reported a complication rate of 21%.[60]

Malunion is the most common complication associated with fractures of the distal radius, and it can have a significant effect on wrist and DRUJ function. Surgical procedures to correct malunion include corrective osteotomy of the distal radius and shortening or resection of the distal ulna. Although simple articular malunions can be corrected with osteotomy, complex articular surface malunions may be best treated with total or partial wrist fusion. Nonunion is a rare complication of distal radial fractures, and it is usually related to injury severity, smoking, infection, and iatrogenic overdistraction by internal or external fixation. Nonunion of a distal radial fracture can be difficult to treat. If at least 2 cm of bone remains in the distal fragment, then open reduction and bone grafting may be performed; otherwise, total wrist fusion may be required to obtain a stable union.

Tendon ruptures can follow distal radial fractures treated surgically and nonsurgically. Common causes include attrition on hardware or bone fragments. Ruptures of the extensor pollicis longus tendon can occur even after nondisplaced distal radial fracture.[61] The communicating fracture hematoma can result in an ischemic injury to the tendon as it passes through the third dorsal extensor compartment. Patients who report crepitus and pain with thumb motion should be carefully evaluated for third dorsal compartment release to prevent tendon rupture. Extensor pollicis longus tendon rupture can be successfully reconstructed with transfer of the extensor indicis proprius tendon.

Median nerve injury is common following distal radial fracture, and a complete neurologic examination should be performed on presentation and at regular intervals. Most nerve injuries will respond to closed reduction and observation, but in some patients numbness may persist. Patients with significant median neuropathy that does not improve after reduction should undergo carpal tunnel release.

Complex regional pain syndromes can occur during the treatment of distal radial fractures. Associated causes include excessive prolonged traction, immobilization in extreme positions (for example, in a cotton-loader position cast), untreated carpal tunnel syndrome, and injuries to the superficial radial nerve from percutaneous hardware. The symptoms can include severe pain and swelling without an obvious clinical cause. Early recognition of a complex regional pain syndrome and early intervention is essential to avoid a disastrous final result. Hand therapy, sympathetic blockade, and correction of nerve entrapment are the cornerstones of treatment.

The DRUJ must be carefully evaluated for stability in patients with distal radial fractures. In a retrospective study of 166 distal radial fractures, 14 patients had instability of the DRUJ. All of the patients with complications related to DRUJ instability had fractures of the ulnar styloid.[57] Instability was most likely when associated with fracture at the base of the ulnar styloid. Other studies have reported, however, the presence of DRUJ instability without fracture of the ulnar styloid. Supination splinting allows the distal ulna to seek a stable position and allow for satisfactory healing in most patients. Patients with persistent DRUJ instability should be considered for repair of an avulsed ulnar styloid or the TFCC. A prospective study used arthroscopy to determine whether peripheral TFCC tears in 51 young patients with distal radial fractures resulted in DRUJ instability and noted that the TFCC was injured in 43 patients, 11 of whom had complete peripheral tears.[56] At 1-year follow-up, 10 of these 11 patients had chronic DRUJ instability. All of the patients with DRUJ instability had poor outcomes as assessed using Gartland-Werley wrist scores.

Treatment

Many factors must be considered when creating a treatment plan for patients with fractures of the distal radius. Surgeons must carefully assess each fracture for degree of displacement, comminution, fracture pattern, osteopenia, and the presence of soft-tissue injuries. Each patient also must be assessed for level of health, daily functional demands, and activity level.

Nonsurgical Management

Most fractures of the distal radius can be successfully managed without surgical intervention. Minimally displaced fractures that have stable metaphyseal support can be treated nonsurgically. Immobilization of the wrist with a properly molded cast or splint until fracture union occurs usually provides good results. Regular follow-up ensures that the fracture maintains radiographic alignment and that the patient is properly caring for the limb.

Displaced or angulated fractures of the distal radius should be evaluated for reduction. Reduction is recommended if there is significant fracture displacement, articular displacement greater than 1 to 2 mm, angulation greater than 20°, shortening of more than 3 mm, and acute median nerve compression.

Fresh distal radial fractures can be reduced in a cast room setting with a hematoma block. Alternatively, reduction can be performed under conscious sedation. Hematoma blocks are effective when performed within 24 to 48 hours of the injury. Ten to 15 mL of 0.5% plain lidocaine is aseptically injected directly into the fracture site. Excellent anesthesia can be obtained in patients with a fresh fracture, but patients with fractures more than 48 hours old will likely require regional or general anesthesia for successful closed reduction. The technique of closed reduction first requires longitudinal traction to disimpact bony fragments and stretch the shortened soft tissues. Several minutes of traction may be required, and the use of finger traps can be quite helpful. A pronated position of the forearm will assist in reduction of the dorsally displaced fracture. Palmar translation of the distal fragment will restore volar tilt.

After reduction, a well-molded double sugar-tong splint is applied. Although there is no consensus regarding the best position for immobilization, gentle pronation, wrist flexion, and ulnar deviation is generally recommended. Extreme positioning of the wrist in flexion

and ulnar deviation (in a cotton-loader position cast, for example) should be avoided in all patients.

Radiographs obtained after reduction should be evaluated for fracture alignment and splint molding. An acceptable reduction will have less than 2 mm of articular incongruity, neutral volar tilt, and restoration of radial length. The patient should be instructed to keep the hand elevated, and digital motion should be prescribed. The fracture reduction should be monitored on a weekly basis to ensure maintenance of acceptable alignment. Loss of fracture position is by definition a sign of instability, and if it occurs, the patient should be evaluated for remanipulation and surgical stabilization.

Indications for Surgery

Unstable fractures of the distal radius require surgical intervention to maintain fracture reduction. Fractures with severe fracture displacement, extensive comminution, or loss of fracture reduction are at risk. In addition, articular shear fractures and joint compression injuries usually require open reduction and internal fixation to restore articular incongruity.

Percutaneous Pinning

There are many advocates of closed reduction and percutaneous pinning, and many unstable distal radial fractures can be successfully treated with this technique. An image intensifier is used to help place Kirschner wires of 0.045 to 0.062 inches in diameter into the radial styloid after closed reduction. Dorsally placed wires can further enhance stability, but care must be taken to avoid extensor tendon injury. The pins are protected with an appropriate cast until fracture union occurs, and then they are removed. Physical therapy, if needed, is usually begun at this time.

Percutaneous pinning may not be appropriate for all patients. Fractures complicated by osteopenia and comminution may not offer adequate support and if unrecognized can lead to fixation failure and subsequent malunion. Additional risks include pin tract infections, injury to branches of the superficial radial nerve, and complex regional pain syndromes.

The Kapandji technique of distal radius pinning is an effective alternative to standard interfocal pinning. Intrafocal Kirschner wires are inserted into the fracture site and used as a lever to reduce the fracture. The pin is then drilled into the opposite cortex, providing a buttress to fracture reduction. Pins can be inserted radially and dorsally to reduce radial inclination and volar tilt, respectively. Intrafocal pins alone are effective if only one cortex is comminuted. Augmentation of intrafocal pinning with external fixation is recommended when two or more cortices are comminuted or if significant osteopenia is present.

External Fixation

There are many who advocate use of external fixation in the treatment of distal radial fractures. Improved understanding of the potential complications of external fixation has allowed evolution of the technique, and external fixation still has its place in the treatment of distal radial fractures. Excessive traction and fixation in extreme positions of wrist position, however, can lead to severe hand and wrist dysfunction. Pin tract infections, radial nerve injury, and complex regional pain syndromes can also complicate external fixation of the wrist.

External fixation can effectively overcome deforming muscle forces and maintain radial length, even in fractures with severe metaphyseal comminution. The device can provide excellent force neutralization to protect internal fixation or it can be used to reduce fresh fractures by traction ligamentotaxis. Distraction can often reduce major fragments, but it will not elevate impacted articular fragments. Multiplanar ligamentotaxis can be used with fixation devices that allow the surgeon to "dial in" the reduction as needed.

Several studies suggest that additional Kirschner wire fixation greatly improves the stability of an external fixation construct. One such study created unstable distal radial fracture models in seven cadaver wrists.[62] The fractures were stabilized with four different types of external fixators, and the stability of each construct was tested before and after supplemental Kirschner wire fixation. The data showed that Kirschner wire supplementation greatly improved overall stability of the fracture models. No difference between the four different types of fixators was found.

Attention to detail is required to prevent complications with external fixation. Pins should be placed through ample incisions to prevent injury to the superficial radial nerve. Although extreme positioning of the wrist may be required to obtain fracture reduction, the fixator should allow the wrist to seek a neutral position for immobilization. Traction should not be excessive, and the lunate should be distracted only approximately 1 mm from its fossa in the radius. If the traction is appropriate, full supple passive finger motion will be possible at the end of the procedure.

The standard technique for external fixation of the radius uses two pins in the index metacarpal and two more pins in the radial shaft. Some studies suggest that additional pins in the distal fragment of the radius will gain control of the distal fragment and improve fracture stability.[62,63] A prospective study assessed the use of a fifth pin in the distal radial fragment and reported better radiographic and functional results at final follow-up using this technique.[63] There has also been interest in the use of nonbridging external fixators to treat these fractures. These fixators use pins in the distal fragment to avoid some of the complications of carpal distraction and potentially allow for early wrist range of motion. Good outcomes with this technique have been reported.[64,65]

Open Reduction and Internal Fixation

There have been many reports favoring open reduction and internal fixation of distal radial fractures.[36,66-71] Low-profile implants designed for the distal radius have improved the ability of surgeons to stabilize small but important fracture fragments. Buttress plating of articular shear fractures has long been the accepted practice, but mini-implants have expanded the application of open reduction and internal fixation in the treatment of distal radial fractures. Locking internal fixation and fragment-specific fixation devices are additional recent developments.[70,71]

Volar Versus Dorsal Plate Application

No consensus exists regarding whether plates should be applied on the volar or dorsal surface of the radius. Advocates of volar plating cite several advantages over dorsal plating.[71] The volar surface has more space available for internal fixation than the dorsal surface, and the pronator quadratus muscle provides additional protection of volar hardware. Problems with tendon adhesions and ruptures have been reported more frequently with dorsally placed fixation than with volar fixation.[71] Advocates of volar fixation also note the importance of restoring the substantial volar cortex. The dorsal cortex is thin and offers little intrinsic support, but the thick volar cortex can offer significant support when directly restored by open reduction and internal fixation.

Disadvantages of the volar approach include difficulty in performing an articular reduction. Arthrotomy of the important volar wrist capsular ligaments should be avoided, and reduction is usually accomplished indirectly with fluoroscopic assistance. Alternatively, arthroscopy or a dorsal arthrotomy can be performed to allow direct visualization and reduction of the articular surface.

Approach to the volar surface of the radius is most commonly performed from the radial side through the flexor carpi radialis tendon sheath. Elevation of the pronator quadratus provides excellent visualization of the volar surface, except for the most volar-ulnar corner. If the key to the fracture includes reduction of the palmar-medial corner, then an ulnar side approach that releases the carpal tunnel can be used with superb visualization.

The dorsal approach to the distal radius is best performed through the third dorsal extensor compartment. After release of the extensor pollicis longus tendon, the wrist and digital extensor tendons are elevated without disruption of their sheaths. Dorsal plate fixation allows for direct buttressing of dorsal rim fractures and dorsally angulated metaphyseal fractures. Arthrotomy of the dorsal wrist capsule provides excellent visualization of the articular surface. Tendon dysfunction and ruptures have been reported to occur frequently with dorsally placed hardware.[71]

The best construct for internal fixation of the distal radius has yet to be identified. In a cadaver biome-

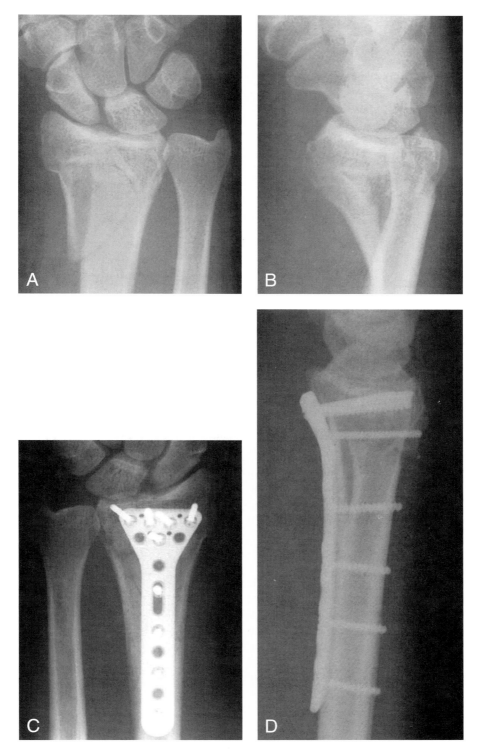

Figure 7 **A** through **D**, Radiographs showing a distal radius fracture treated with open reduction and internal fixation with volar locking plate.

chanical study, the strength and stiffness of dorsally applied hardware was evaluated.[67] The study compared three constructs: a 3.5-mm AO T-plate, two dorsally placed 2.0-mm plates, and the dorsal locking pi plate. The two dorsally placed 2.0-mm plates construct was reported to be the strongest construct tested in this study. In a prospective clinical study, 73 dorsally displaced and unstable distal radial fractures were treated with open reduction and internal fixation using a low-profile plate designed for dorsal application to the distal radius.[66] Satisfactory reduction was achieved in 93% of fractures and maintained in 88%; 95% of

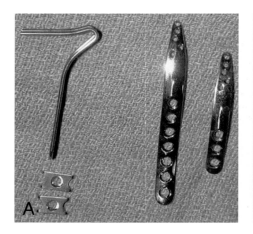
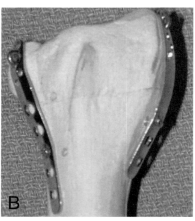
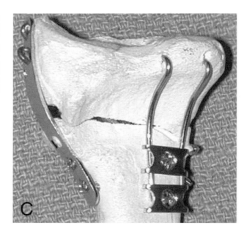

Figure 8 A, Photograph of fragment-specific devices for distal radius fixation. **B** and **C,** Photographs of fragment-specific devices applied to a bone model.

patients were judged to have a good or excellent outcome.

Arthroscopy has been used as an alternative method to obtain articular reduction of distal radial fractures and allow evaluation and treatment of associated soft-tissue injuries. In a study of 33 distal radial fractures treated with pins and external fixation, arthroscopy was used to facilitate reduction.[58] The authors reported good to excellent results in 100% of patients, with good maintenance of the distal radial articular surface. They also repaired peripheral tears of the TFCC in 54% of these patients.

Fragment-Specific Internal Fixation
Fragment-specific internal fixation is a novel concept in the treatment of distal radial fractures. The use of small, low-profile plates that are custom-designed for the radial styloid, dorsal ulnar corner, and volar lip of distal radial fractures has received some support in the literature[69,70] (Figure 7). The plates are placed orthogonally, and although small, provide reportedly strong fixation. In a biomechanical study of cadaver wrists, fragment-specific internal fixation was compared with static augmented external fixation in three- and four-part fracture models.[69] Fragment-specific internal fixation was found to exceed the strength of the augmented external fixation. Physiologic loading of the cadaver models suggested that this technique provides adequate strength for an early range of motion program. In a prospective clinical study of 20 distal radial fractures, fragment-specific internal fixation was used in a clinical setting.[70] Two-year follow-up revealed good to excellent results in all but two patients. The authors concluded that the technique is safe and strong enough to maintain alignment for initiation of an early range-of-motion program.

Locked Plating of Distal Radial Fractures
Locking internal fixation has received considerable interest in the treatment of distal radial fractures. Plates have been developed that allow for threaded pins and screws to lock into distally threaded holes. On engage-

ment, the fixation locks to the plate and essentially becomes a fixed-angle device. Locking internal fixation improves articular support and reduces the need for bone grafting. Locking devices are available for both volar and dorsal application. Locking fixation allows for potential volar plate fixation of dorsally displaced distal radial fractures by capturing the distal fragment with its fixed-angle pegs and screws (Figure 8). In one study, 29 consecutive patients with 31 dorsally displaced fractures were treated with a volar only approach and a locking plate designed for the volar surface of the distal radius.[71] The use of locking internal fixation provided enough stability to allow early range of motion and maintain anatomic alignment, even for dorsally displaced fractures. They reported 19 excellent and 12 good clinical results.

Annotated References

1. Chung KC, Spilson SV: The frequency and epidemiology of hand and forearm fractures in the United States. *J Hand Surg [Am]* 2001;26:908-915.

2. Nguyen TV: Center JR, Sambrook PN, Eisman JA: Risk factors for proximal humerus, forearm, and wrist fractures in elderly men and women: The Dubbo Osteoporosis Epidemiology Study. *Am J Epidemiol* 2001;153:587-595.

3. Poitevin LA: Anatomy and biomechanics of the interosseous membrane: Its importance in the longitudinal stability of the forearm. *Hand Clin* 2001;17:97-110.
   This anatomic and biomechanical cadaver study defines the interosseous membrane and its function. It points out the components of the interosseous membrane that are clinically significant for forearm stability.

4. Markolf KL, Lamey D, Yang S, Meals R, Hotchkiss RN: Radioulnar load-sharing in the forearm: A study in cadavera. *J Bone Joint Surg Am* 1998;80:879-888.

5. Fester EW, Murray PM, Sanders TG, Ingari JV, Leyendecker J, Leis HL: The efficacy of magnetic resonance imaging and ultrasound in detecting disruptions of the forearm interosseous membrane: A cadaver study. *J Hand Surg [Am]* 2002;27:418-424.

   The authors of this cadaver study examined the sensitivity and specificity of MRI and ultrasound when used to determine complete disruptions of the interosseous membrane. Both modalities were very sensitive and specific. Either modality may be used to assist in the diagnosis of forearm interosseous membrane injury.

6. Smith AM, Urbanosky LR, Castle JA, Rushing JT, Ruch DS: Radius pull test: Predictor of longitudinal forearm instability. *J Bone Joint Surg Am* 2002;84: 1970-1976.

7. Mackay D, Wood L, Rangan A: The treatment of isolated ulnar fractures in adults: A systematic review. *Injury* 2000;31:565-570.

8. Muellner T, Fuchs M, Kwasny O: Rotational instability and integrity of the interosseous membrane in cadaveric ulnar shaft fractures. *Arch Orthop Trauma Surg* 1998;118:53-56.

9. Handoll HH, Pearce PK: Interventions for isolated diaphyseal fractures of the ulna in adults. *Cochrane Database Syst Rev* 2004;2:CD000523.

   The authors evaluated randomized or quasirandomized trials of nonsurgical and surgical treatment of isolated ulnar fractures in adults. They concluded that there is insufficient evidence to determine the most appropriate method of treatment for isolated fractures of the ulna.

10. Rettig ME, Raskin KB: Galeazzi fracture-dislocation: A new treatment-oriented classification. *J Hand Surg [Am]* 2001;26:228-235.

11. Budgen A, Lim P, Templeton P, Irwin LR: Irreducible Galeazzi injury. *Arch Orthop Trauma Surg* 1998; 118:176-178.

12. Ring D, Jupiter JB, Simpson NS: Monteggia fractures in adults. *J Bone Joint Surg Am* 1998;80:1733-1744.

13. Biyani A, Olscamp AJ, Ebraheim NA: Complications in the management of complex Monteggia-equivalent fractures in adults. *Am J Orthop* 2000;29: 115-118.

14. Wright RR, Schmeling GJ, Schwab JP: The necessity of acute bone grafting in diaphyseal forearm fractures: A retrospective review. *J Orthop Trauma* 1997;11:288-294.

   The authors report the results of a retrospective review of 183 forearm bone fractures in 137 patients. The union rate of comminuted nongrafted forearm fractures was the same as the union rate for noncomminuted, nongrafted forearm fractures. Comminution alone may no longer be an indication for acute bone grafting of forearm fractures.

15. Barbieri CH, Mazzer N, Mazer MR: Use of a delayed cortical bone graft to treat diaphyseal defects in the forearm. *Int Orthop* 1999;23:295-301.

16. Fernandez Dell'Oca AA: Tepic S, Frigg R, Meisser A, Haas N, Perren SM: Treating forearm fractures using an internal fixator: A prospective study. *Clin Orthop* 2001;389:196-205.

17. Haas N, Hauke C, Schutz M, Kaab M, Perren SM: Treatment of diaphyseal fractures of the forearm using the Point Contact Fixator (PC-Fix): Results of 387 fractures of a prospective multicentric study (PC-Fix II). *Injury* 2001;32(suppl 2):B51-B62.

18. Hertel R, Eijer H, Meisser A, Hauke C, Perren SM: Biomechanical and biological considerations relating to the clinical use of the Point Contact-Fixator: Evaluation of the device handling test in the treatment of diaphyseal fractures of the radius and/or ulna. *Injury* 2001;32(suppl 2):B10-B14.

19. Frigg R: Locking compression plate (LCP): An osteosynthesis plate based on the dynamic compression plate and the Point Contact Fixator (PC-Fix). *Injury* 2001;32(suppl 2):63-66.

20. Martin WN, Field J, Kulkarni M: Intramedullary nailing of pathological forearm fractures. *Injury* 2002;33:530-532.

21. Yung SH, Lam CY, Choi KY, Ng KW, Maffulli N, Cheng JC: Percutaneous intramedullary Kirschner wiring for displaced diaphyseal forearm fractures in children. *J Bone Joint Surg Br* 1998;80:91-94.

22. Kucukkaya M, Kabukcuoglu Y, Tezer M, Eren T, Kuzgun U: The application of open intramedullary fixation in the treatment of pediatric radial and ulnar fractures. *J Orthop Trauma* 2002;16:340-344.

23. Flynn JM: Pediatric forearm fractures: Decision making, surgical techniques, and complications. *Instr Course Lect* 2002;51:355-360.

24. Kasten P, Krefft M, Hesselbach J, Weinberg AM: How does torsional deformity of the radial shaft influence the rotation of the forearm? A biomechanical study. *J Orthop Trauma* 2003;17:57-60.

The authors performed a biomechanical analysis of the effects of isolated torsional radial malunion on forearm motion and report that more than 30° of rotational malunion will result in significant loss of supination or pronation. They conclude that supination deformity causes loss of pronation and vice versa.

25. Tynan MC, Fornalski S, McMahon PJ, Utkan A, Green SA, Lee TQ: The effects of ulnar axial malalignment on supination and pronation. *J Bone Joint Surg Am* 2000;82:1726-1731.

26. Dumont CE, Thalmann R, Macy JC: The effect of rotational malunion of the radius and ulna on supination and pronation: An experimental investigation. *J Bone Joint Surg Br* 2002;84:1070-1074.

27. Kasten P, Krefft M, Hesselbach J, Weinberg AM: Computer simulation of forearm rotation in angular deformities: A new therapeutic approach. *Injury* 2002;33:807-813.

28. Yasutomi T, Nakatsuchi Y, Koike H, Uchiyama S: Mechanism of limitation of pronation/supination of the forearm in geometric models of deformities of the forearm bones. *Clin Biomech (Bristol, Avon)* 2002;17:456-463.

29. Solanki PV, Mulgaonkar KP, Rao SA: Effect of early mobilisation on grip strength, pinch strength, and work of hand muscles in cases of closed diaphyseal fracture radius-ulna treated with dynamic compression plating. *J Postgrad Med* 2000;46:84-87.

30. Diliberti T, Botte MJ, Abrams RA: Anatomical considerations regarding the posterior interosseous nerve during posterolateral approaches to the proximal part of the radius. *J Bone Joint Surg Am* 2000; 82:809-813.

31. McQueen MM, Gaston P, Court-Brown CM: Acute compartment syndrome: Who is at risk? *J Bone Joint Surg Br* 2000;82:200-203.

32. Ghobrial TF, Eglseder WA Jr, Bleckner SA: Proximal ulna shaft fractures and associated compartment syndromes. *Am J Orthop* 2001;30:703-707.

33. Kamineni S, Maritz NG, Morrey BF: Proximal radial resection for posttraumatic radioulnar synostosis: A new technique to improve forearm rotation. *J Bone Joint Surg Am* 2002;84:745-751.

The authors report the results in seven patients of resection of 1 cm of proximal radius to treat proximal radioulnar synostosis. The method is recommended for patients with a proximal radioulnar synostosis that is too extensive for discrete resection, involves the articular surface, or is associated with an anatomic deformity. Although this procedure was not free of complications, the average functional score improved from 57 to 81.

34. Jupiter JB, Ring D: Operative treatment of posttraumatic proximal radioulnar synostosis. *J Bone Joint Surg Am* 1998;80:248-257.

35. Beingessner DM, Patterson SD, King GJW: Early excision of heterotopic bone in the forearm. *J Hand Surg [Am]* 2000;25:483-488.

36. Simic PM, Weiland AJ: Fractures of the distal aspect of the radius: Changes in treatment over the past two decades. *Instr Course Lect* 2003;52:185-195.

This instructional course lecture provides an excellent review of the current state of distal radial fracture management.

37. Vogt MT, Cauley JA, Tomaino MM, Stone K, Williams JR, Herndon JH: A 10-year follow-up study of descriptive characteristics and risk factors: The study of osteoporotic fractures. *J Am Geriatr Soc* 2002;50: 97-103.

Caucasian women 65 years and older were enrolled as cohorts in this 10-year prospective study. The incidence of fractures was 7.3 per 1,000 person-years. Seventy three percent of fractures were extra-articular and occurred after a fall. The average age at time of fracture was 76 years, and a decline in bone mineral density was associated with a fracture.

38. Melone CP: Articular fractures of the distal radius. *Orthop Clin North Am* 1984;15:217-236.

39. Jupiter JB, Fernandez DL: Comparative classification for fractures of the distal end of the radius. *J Hand Surg [Am]* 1997;22:563-571.

40. Cohen MS, McMurty RY, Jupiter JB: Fractures of the distal radius, in Browner B, Jupiter J, Levine A, Trafton P (eds): *Skeletal Trauma*, ed 2. Philadelphia, PA, WB Saunders, 1992.

41. Andersen DJ, Blair WF, Steyers CM Jr, Adams BD, el-Khoui GY, Brandser EA: Classification of distal radius fractures: An analysis of inter-observer reliability and intra-observer reproducibility. *J Hand Surg [Am]* 1996;21:574-582.

42. Lundy DW, Quisling SG, Lourie GM, Feiner CM, Lins RE: Tilted lateral radiographs in the evaluation of

of distal radius fractures. *J Hand Surg [Am]* 1999;24: 249-256.

43. Bozentka DJ, Beredjiklian PK, Westawski D, Steinberg DR: Digital radiographs in the assessment of distal radius fracture parameters. *Clin Orthop* 2002; 397:409-413.

In this study, digital radiographs were compared with plain radiographs to assess the ability of each to measure specific elements of a fractured distal radius. The use of digital radiography improved interobserver reliability significantly with regard to measurement of radial length, palmar tilt, and articular step-off. The findings suggest that digital radiography is at least equivalent to plain radiography in its ability to measure important fracture parameters.

44. Katz MA, Beredjiklian PK, Bozentka DJ, Steinberg DR: Computed tomography scanning of intra-articular distal radius fractures: Does it influence treatment? *J Hand Surg [Am]* 2001;26:415-421.

In this study, four hand surgeons reviewed radiographs of 15 intra-articular fractures of the distal radius. The results were reassessed after evaluation of CT scans of the fractures. Improved intra-observer and interobserver agreement was noted after review of the CT scans. The scans aided in the measurement of gaps, step-offs, and comminution and helped with the development of treatment plans.

45. Spence LD, Savenor A, Nwachuku I, Tilsley J, Eustace S: MRI of fractures of the distal radius: Comparison with conventional radiographs. *Skeletal Radiol* 1998;27:244-249.

46. Knirk JL, Jupiter JB: Intra-articular fractures of the distal end of the radius in young adults. *J Bone Joint Surg Am* 1986;68:647-659.

47. Trumble TE, Schmitt SR, Vedder NB: Factors affecting functional outcome of displaced intra-articular distal radius fractures. *J Hand Surg [Am]* 1994;19: 325-340.

48. Wagner WF, Tencer AF, Kiser P, Trumble T: Effects of intra-articular depression on wrist joint contact characteristics. *J Hand Surg [Am]* 1996;21:554-560.

49. Trumble TE, Wagner W, Hanel DP, Vedder NB, Gilbert M: Intrafocal (Kapandji) pinning of distal radius fractures with and with out external fixation. *J Hand Surg [Am]* 1998;23:381-394.

50. Taleisnik J, Watson HK: Midcarpal instability caused by malunited fractures of the distal radius. *J Hand Surg [Am]* 1984;9:350-357.

51. Park MJ, Cooney WP, Hahn ME, Looi KP, An KN: The effects of dorsally angulated distal radius fractures on carpal kinematics. *J Hand Surg [Am]* 2002; 27:223-232.

This biomechanical cadaver study evaluated carpal kinematics in dorsally angulated distal radial fracture models. Significant effects on carpal motion and carpal alignment were noted. This included dorsal intercalated segment instability deformity and dorsal carpal subluxation.

52. Rozental TD, Beredjiklian PK, Steinberg DR, Bozentka DJ: Open fractures of the distal radius. *J Hand Surg [Am]* 2002;27:77-85.

The authors of this study assessed 18 patients with open fractures of the distal radius. Using the Gustilo and Anderson classification system, nine type I fractures (50%), three type II fractures (17%), and six type III fractures (34%) were noted. Patients were evaluated for outcome using the Disabilities of the Arm, Shoulder, and Hand Questionnaire; complication rate and the number of surgical procedures were also assessed. The authors reported that patients with type I fractures had a similar complication rate and prognosis as those with type II fractures, but patients with type III fractures had many more complications and poorer overall outcomes.

53. Young BT, Rayan GM: Outcome following nonoperative treatment of displaced distal radius fractures in low demand patients older than 60 years. *J Hand Surg [Am]* 2000;25:19-28.

In this retrospective review of 25 low-demand patients with distal radial fractures (average age, 72 years), the authors reported a wide variety of final radiographic outcomes, 24% of which were identified as poor. Functional results, however, were generally good to excellent (88% of patients). The authors noted that radiographic and functional outcomes do not correlate in this age group. More than half of the patients had an obvious cosmetic deformity, but none claimed to be unhappy about their clinical appearance. The authors concluded that patients in this age group with low functional demands can expect good result with nonsurgical management, and they recommended surgical intervention for active patients older than 60 years with severely displaced intra-articular fractures of the distal radius.

54. Richards RS, Bennett JD, Roth JH, Milne K: Arthroscopic intra-articular soft tissue injuries associated with distal radial fractures. *J Hand Surg [Am]* 1997;22:772-776.

55. Geissler WB, Freeland AE, Savoie FH, McIntyre LW, Whipple TL: Intra-carpal soft tissue lesions associated with an intra-articular fracture of the distal end of the radius. *J Bone Joint Surg Am* 1996;78:357-365.

56. Lindau T, Adlercreutz C, Aspenberg P: Peripheral tears of the triangular fibrocartilage complex cause distal radioulnar joint instability after distal radial fractures. *J Hand Surg [Am]* 2000;25:464-468.

This prospective study was conducted to determine whether peripheral TFCC tears associated with distal radial fractures result in DRUJ instability. Fifty-one patients with distal radial fractures were evaluated arthroscopically. The TFCC was injured in 43 patients. One third of patients had an element of DRUJ instability that was associated with a TFCC tear. Fifty-four percent of patients also had an injury to the scapholunate ligament. Ten of 11 patients with complete peripheral TFCC tears had DRUJ instability 1-year after fracture. Patients with DRUJ instability had poor outcomes as assessed using Gartland-Werley wrist scores. The risk of instability was reported to be greatest in male patients younger than 60 years and female patients younger than 50 years.

57. May MM, Lawton JN, Blazar PE: Ulnar styloid fractures associated with distal radius fractures: Incidence and implications for distal radioulnar joint instability. *J Hand Surg [Am]* 2002;27:965-971.

This is a retrospective review of 166 distal radial fractures that were reviewed for an association between DRUJ instability and fractures of the ulnar styloid. All distal radial fractures that were complicated by DRUJ instability had a fracture of the ulnar styloid. More than one third of ulnar styloid fractures involved the base. Fractures at the base of the ulnar styloid were found to be especially at risk for instability.

58. Shih JT, Lee HM, Tan CM: Arthroscopically-assisted reduction of intra-articular fractures and soft tissue management of the distal radius. *Hand Surg* 2001;6:127-135.

The authors of this study treated 33 patients with distal radial fractures by using percutaneous pinning with or without external fixation after arthroscopically assisted reduction. The authors reported that 54% of patients had associated TFCC tears, and 18% had scapholunate tears. They also reported 100% good to excellent results with good maintenance of the distal radial articular surface. In all patients, the TFCC tears were peripheral. The authors recommended addressing soft-tissue injuries with repair.

59. Jupiter JB, Fernandez DL: Complications following distal radial fractures. *Instr Course Lect* 2002;51:203-219.

60. McKay SD, Macdermid JC, Roth JH, Richards JS: Assessment of complications of distal radius fractures and development of a complication checklist. *J Hand Surg [Am]* 2001;26:916-922.

In this study, 250 patients were prospectively evaluated for complications related to treatment of distal radial fractures. Questionnaires were completed by patients and physicians at 6-month follow-up. Physicians reported a complication rate of 27%, whereas patients reported a complication rate of 21%. Reflex sympathetic dystrophy was noted in 20% of patients. The authors also review complications associated with distal radial fracture treatment and provide a complication checklist for future research.

61. Skoff HD: Postfracture extensor pollicis longus tenosynovitis and tendon rupture: A scientific study and personal series. *Am J Orthop* 2003;32:245-247.

62. Wolfe SW, Austin G, Lorenze M, Swigart CR, Panjabi MM: A biomechanical comparison of different wrist external fixators with and without K-wire augmentation. *J Hand Surg [Am]* 1999;24:516-524.

63. Werber KD, Raeder F, Brauer RB, Weiss S: External fixation of distal radial fractures: Four compared with five pins. A randomized prospective study. *J Bone Joint Surg Am* 2003;85:660-666.

The authors of this prospective randomized study compared a standard four-pin fixator to a five-pin construct (the fifth pin is designed to capture the distal radial articular fragment). The authors concluded that the fifth pin improved control the distal radial fragment and that the five-pin fixator also achieved better final radiographic and functional results than the four-pin fixator.

64. McQueen MM, Simpson D: Use of Hoffman 2 compact external fixator in the treatment of re-displaced unstable distal radial fractures. *J Orthop Trauma* 1999;13:501-505.

65. McQueen MM: Redisplaced fractures of the distal radius: A randomised, prospective study of bridging vs nonbridging fixation. *J Bone Joint Surg Br* 1998;80:665-669.

66. Carter PR, Fredrick HA, Laseter GF: Open reduction and internal fixation of unstable distal radius fractures with a low profile plate: A multi-center study of 73 fractures. *J Hand Surg [Am]* 1998;23:300-307.

67. Peine R, Rikili DA, Hoffmann R, Duda G, Regazzoni P: Comparison of three different plating techniques for the dorsum of the distal radius: A biomechanical study. *J Hand Surg [Am]* 2000;25:29-33.

Cadavers were used in this biomechanical study to compare the strength and stiffness of the AO 3.5-mm T-plate, two dorsally placed 2.0-mm plates, and the dorsal pi plate. The two dorsally placed 2.0-mm plate construct was determined to be the strongest construct tested.

68. Jupiter JB, Ring DR, Weitzel PP: Surgical treatment of redisplaced fractures of the distal radius in pa-

tients older than 60 years. *J Hand Surg [Am]* 2002; 27:714-723.

The authors of this study assessed 20 patients with distal radial fractures who presented with displacement after closed reduction. Open reduction and internal fixation and early rehabilitation was performed in each patient. Results were judged as excellent in 7 patients, good in 11, and fair in 2.

69. Dodds SD, Cornelissen S, Jossan S, Wolfe SW: A biomechanical comparison of fragment-specific fixation and augmented external fixation for intra-articular distal radius fractures. *J Hand Surg [Am]* 2002;27:953-964.

This biomechanical study used cadaver wrists to compare the use of low-profile modular implants and static augmented external fixation. The low-profile fragment-specific fixation implants are custom designed to treat fractures of the volar lip, radial styloid, and dorsal-ulnar facet of the distal radius. Three- and four-part fractures were evaluated. The authors reported that fragment-specific fixation exceeded the strength of the augmented external fixation and that this implant system allows for free range of motion. Physiologic loading of the cadaver models suggested that the system provides adequate strength for the initiation of early range of motion.

70. Konrath GA, Bahler S: Open reduction and internal fixation of unstable distal radius fractures: Results

using Trimed fixation system. *J Orthop Trauma* 2002; 16:578-585.

The authors of this study used open reduction and internal fixation to treat patients with unstable distal radial fractures with fragment-specific fixation. They reported that the system was stable and had a safety profile comparable to other systems. Good to excellent results were achieved in all but two patients. The authors concluded that this system is safe and strong enough for early rehabilitation.

71. Orbay JL, Fernandez DL: Volar fixation for dorsally displaced fractures of the distal radius: A preliminary report. *J Hand Surg [Am]* 2002;27:205-215.

The authors of this study performed open reduction and internal fixation on 29 consecutive patients with 31 dorsally displaced distal radial fractures. A volar approach was used in each patient, with a locking fixed-angle plate designed for the volar surface of the radius. The authors reported that the volar approach allowed accurate reduction of the more substantial volar cortex and improved stability. Volar plate application reduced the soft-tissue problems associated with dorsal plates. The use of locking internal fixation provided enough stability to allow early range of motion and maintain anatomic alignment, even for patients with dorsally displaced fractures. The enhanced stability decreased the need for bone graft. Excellent results were reported in 19 patients and 12 had good clinical results.

Chapter 20

Injuries to the Hand and Carpus

Joseph F. Slade III, MD

David Ring, MD

Phalanx Fractures

It is tempting to consider open reduction and internal fixation for the treatment of isolated, closed, spiral, or long oblique phalanx fractures, but pinning is usually preferred for its simplicity, safety, and limitation of trauma to the gliding tendon structures in the hand. In a randomized trial of pinning versus open screw fixation, there were no significant differences in recovery rate, pain scores, alignment, motion, or grip strength.[1] Although this research did not observe the diminished results typically associated with open treatment, it did not demonstrate any advantage to using screws.

Unstable fractures of the proximal phalanx are common. One of the most popular treatment methods is transarticular pinning (Eaton-Belsky technique) in which a Kirschner wire is drilled across the metacarpal head and metacarpophalangeal joint into the intramedullary space of the proximal phalanx. A recent report of this technique observed good results overall in 12 patients (average total active motion of 265°), but the technique is not without complications.[2] One patient had a substantial flexion contracture, one had flexor tendon adhesions, and one had significant rotational deformity.

Fracture-Dislocations of the Proximal Interphalangeal Joint

Fracture-dislocations of the proximal interphalangeal joint can be challenging to treat effectively. The key element of treatment is restoration and maintenance of joint alignment. In a retrospective review of the long-term follow-up of injuries treated with closed reduction and transarticular pinning of the proximal interphalangeal joint without an attempt to reduce the associated fracture of the middle phalanx base, an average of 85° of motion was observed.[3]

With the use of intraosseous Kirschner wires and dental rubber bands, a simplified external fixator to treat fracture-dislocations or pilon-type fractures of the proximal interphalangeal joint was developed.[4] This external fixator spans the proximal interphalangeal joint and provides continuous traction throughout a full range of mo-

tion of the joint (Figure 1). If closed fracture reduction restores articular congruity and spanning external fixation maintains an anatomic joint relationship, then active motion can be initiated immediately after surgery.

Open reduction and internal fixation has been less successful in the treatment of fracture-dislocations of the proximal interphalangeal joint, but it is sometimes necessary for very large fractures of the middle phalanx base. Similarly, if a large portion of the articular surface is injured, volar plate arthroplasty is an option. A study comparing open reduction and internal fixation with volar plate arthroplasty found early redislocation in six patients; however, favorable results were achieved provided joint alignment was maintained.[5] Another option when the fracture is large or unsalvageable is to use an osteochondral graft from the hamate to reconstruct the volar aspect of the middle phalanx base. In a study of 13 patients, all of the grafts healed—two with dorsal subluxation of the joint—and an average 85° arc of motion was achieved with 80% grip strength.[6]

Mallet Fractures

The complications associated with surgical treatment of mallet fractures have reinforced the reasonable results observed for nonsurgical treatment. In one recent study, 24 of 59 patients with surgically treated mallet fractures (41%) had a complication, including dorsal skin necrosis, recurrent extension lag, permanent nail deformities, transient pin tract infections, or osteomyelitis.[7] The only indication for surgical treatment for which there is general consensus is subluxation of the distal interphalangeal joint, but some surgeons are concerned about large displaced fracture fragments.

Extension block pinning has proved useful, and this technique is expanding the indications for surgical treatment for some surgeons. In this technique, the distal phalanx is flexed and a wire is drilled into the middle phalanx head to support the mallet fragment in anatomic position. The phalanx is then extended, realigned, and pinned. One study reported good or excellent results in 78% of patients treated with this technique.[8] Another

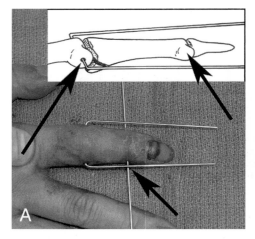
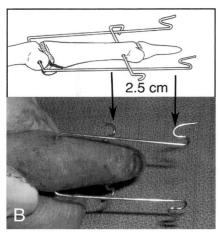
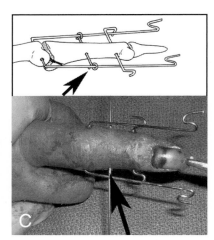

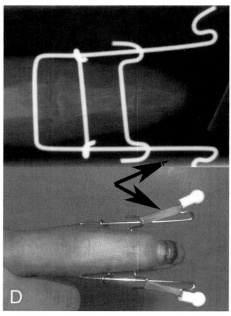
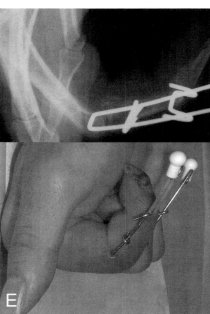

Figure 1 Schematic representations and photographs of a simplified external fixator created intraoperatively from Kirschner wires and dental bands that spans the proximal interphalangeal joint and provides continuous traction throughout a full range of motion of the joint. **A,** The dynamic distraction splint is assembled using three 0.045-in Kirschner wires placed parallel to each other and perpendicular to the lateral axis of the digit. The long arrow indicates the placement of the first 0.045-inch Kirschner wire as it is placed through the rotational center of the head of the proximal phalanx and is parallel to the joint surface. The short arrows indicate the placement of the second 0.045-inch Kirschner wire, which is also parallel to the joint surface of distal interphalangeal joint and the first Kirschner wire. **B,** The free ends of both wires are fashioned into hooks (*arrows*) for attachment of the dental loop rubber bands. The distance between the hooks is 2.5 cm. **C,** The final Kirschner wire is parallel to the other two and passes through the middle phalanx in the midaxial line. Its free ends are cut short and bent around the limbs of the first Kirschner wire. This middle pin (*arrows*) acts as a fulcrum to maintain congruent reduction through a full arc of motion. **D** and **E,** Dental loop rubber bands (*arrows*) are then placed between the two hooks in sufficient quantity (usually three per pair of hooks) to distract the joint and maintain its reduction throughout the full range of motion, and joint reduction through a complete arc of motion is confirmed with radiographic imaging.

study reported joint congruity in 17 of 18 patients, with an average 80° arc of motion.[9] In yet another study, open reduction and Kirschner wire fixation led to a 67° arc of motion with few complications in 33 patients.[10] It remains unclear whether these techniques are superior to those used for the nonsurgical treatment of mallet fractures without joint subluxation.

Metacarpal Fractures

Metacarpal Neck Fractures

The degree of acceptable angulation for small finger metacarpal neck fractures is still debated. An in vitro study investigating the effect of malalignment on the intrinsic hand musculature recommended 30° as the maximum acceptable angulation based on observations suggesting that greater angulation may limit grip strength and motion.[11] Conversely, two prospective randomized trials of reduction and splinting versus buddy taping or

symptomatic treatment found no differences in ultimate hand function—one group of authors concluded that splinting provided better early comfort, whereas the other group of authors concluded that splinting slowed recovery.[12,13] In another study that questioned the strict angular criteria for acceptable reduction, the interobserver and intraobserver reliability of both angular measurements and treatment recommendations were limited.[14]

Metacarpal Base Fractures

Articular fractures of the small finger metacarpal base can be complex and difficult to repair. Some surgeons favor open reduction and internal fixation for even minor amounts of articular surface incongruity or impaction, whereas others prefer nonsurgical treatment of most of these fractures. In a recent study, 10 of 25 patients who underwent surgical treatment for articular fractures of the small finger metacarpal base reported painful arthritis at an average follow-up of 3.3 years.[15] These results suggest that surgical treatment is often unsuccessful in preventing the rapid onset of arthritis, but it remains unclear how patients with similar fractures would fare with nonsurgical treatment and also whether the type or quality of surgical treatment influences the results.

Similar controversy exists in the treatment of thumb metacarpal base fractures. In a study comparing 32 patients with Bennett fractures that had adequate reduction and were treated with either closed reduction and pinning or open reduction and internal fixation, no clinical or radiographic differences were observed.[16]

Metacarpal Shaft Fractures

Treatment of diaphyseal fractures of the small finger metacarpal is straightforward. In a recent study of 25 patients treated with transverse pinning of a fifth metacarpal shaft fracture, excellent clinical and radiologic results were reported.[17] Another group of authors reported on the use of multiple intramedullary Kirschner wires inserted through a hole in the base of the metacarpal and buried permanently in the bone in 22 patients.[18] This study was unique in that the implants were intended to be permanent, and the authors did not immobilize the patients postoperatively. The overall results were good, but in two patients the wires bent at the fracture site and in another the wires migrated into the carpometacarpal joint and had to be removed.

Plate and Screw Fixation

Plate and screw fixation of metacarpal and phalanx fractures is usually reserved for combined injuries (fractures associated with soft-tissue injury), multiple fractures, and some complex articular injuries. Two studies have evaluated the complications of plate and screw fixation. One study of plate fixation in 157 patients with nonthumb metacarpal fractures found 15% of patients had delayed union or nonunion and 10% had stiffness—both more likely a reflection of the severity of the injuries selected for plate fixation rather than any shortcoming of the plates themselves.[19] Another investigation reached the same conclusion, with open wound and phalanx fractures being associated with stiffness after plate and screw fixation.[20]

Interest in the development of resorbable plates for use in the hand continues. As with other resorbable implants, the challenge continues to be balancing the strength of a plate with its resorbability without causing a substantial inflammatory response. A biomechanical study demonstrated strength comparable to 1.7- and 2.3-mm metal plates.[21] Another study demonstrated gradual loss of strength during 12 weeks of in vitro degradation, with adequate strength for in vivo loads maintained for 8 weeks.[22] It is still unclear whether

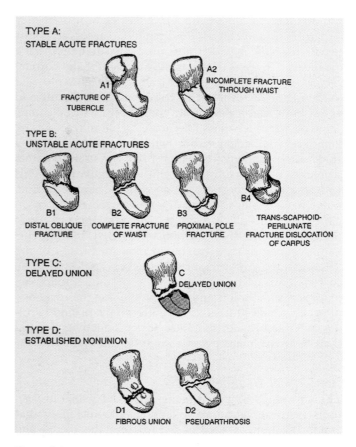

Figure 2 Schematic representation of the Herbert classification of scaphoid fractures. Note that type B scaphoid fractures are differentiated by the instability of those fracture patterns in the acute setting. *(Reproduced with permission from Green DP (ed):* Green's Operative Hand Surgery, *ed 4. New York, NY, Churchill Livingstone, 1999, p 815.)*

resorbable implants will have a major role in the treatment of hand injuries.

Scaphoid Fractures

Fractures of the scaphoid typically fall into two categories: displaced and nondisplaced. They have been further classified by anatomic location (proximal, waist, or distal) or by the stability of the fracture itself (Figure 2). Often not visible on initial radiographic views, these fractures challenge the diagnosing physician to use clinical presentation and physical examination combined with three-dimensional or follow-up imaging. The mechanism of injury usually involves a fall onto the radial side of an extended wrist. Physical examination typically demonstrates snuffbox and scaphoid tubercle tenderness as well as pain with longitudinal compression of the thumb.[23] Management of these injuries begins with short arm-thumb spica immobilization until definitive diagnosis and a treatment plan are made.

Diagnostic Imaging

Delayed diagnosis of a scaphoid fracture typically occurs when the fracture line is difficult to visualize on plain radiographs, including the navicular view. Emergency departments and clinics with immediate access to CT or live fluoroscopy may use these modalities to help reach a diagnosis. CT scans of the wrist with sagittal and coronal reconstructions continue to be a standard technique used to characterize scaphoid fractures and, importantly, to assess bony union during the course of fracture healing.

MRI accurately identifies acute scaphoid fractures by demonstrating inflammation within the scaphoid. In a study of 195 patients for whom MRI was used to detect scaphoid fractures or other occult wrist injury in patients with snuffbox tenderness but no visible evidence of fracture on plain films, occult fractures were found in 76 patients, 37 of which were scaphoid fractures.[24] Additionally, these authors demonstrated that 180 patients had a change in their treatment plan as a result of the MRI findings. Additional studies have found MRI to be cost-effective when compared with traditional follow-up physical examination and radiographs for the diagnosis of occult scaphoid fractures.[25,26] Certainly, promptly ruling out fracture can minimize lost productivity for patients who are unnecessarily immobilized in a cast.

Nonsurgical Treatment

The advantage of closed management of scaphoid fractures is preservation of a tenuous blood supply that enters the bone at its distal end from the dorsal and palmar branches of the radial artery. Additionally, the scaphoid has only ligamentous and capsular attachments, which make it susceptible to osteonecrosis when a fracture or iatrogenic soft-tissue injury occurs. Scaphoid fractures have been shown to heal well with casting, but debate continues as to whether long or short arm cast immobilization should be used. Biomechanical studies testing distal and proximal fracture fragment motion in short arm-thumb spica casts after a scaphoid waist osteotomy have demonstrated contradictory results with respect to interfragmentary motion.[27,28] A recent clinical study has shown that patients with stable scaphoid fractures managed in a short arm-thumb spica cast have a 90% union rate, but slower healing times than patients with a long arm-thumb spica cast that eliminates pronation and supination.[29,30]

Surgical Treatment

There is general agreement in the literature that the risk of nonunion is increased with displaced, unstable, and proximal pole fractures or even fractures for which the diagnosis has been delayed.[31] Consequently, reduction and surgical stabilization of these types of scaphoid fractures has been the standard of care. For nondisplaced scaphoid fractures, advancements in surgical fixation, specifically percutaneous and arthroscopically assisted techniques, offer patients distinct advantages to conservative management: healing rates are improved, func-

tional recovery is accelerated, and morbidity from prolonged casting is reduced.[32-35]

The use of a headless, variable-pitch threaded lag screw has changed the effectiveness of internal fixation for scaphoid fractures. Traditionally, these fractures are approached by open reduction either through dorsal or volar incisions.[36] Despite the risk of disrupting inherent ligamentous stability and jeopardizing the tenuous blood supply to scaphoid fracture fragments, open reduction and internal fixation has been shown to provide satisfactory healing and function at follow-up.[37-39]

Percutaneous reduction and fixation techniques with or without arthroscopic assistance have multiple theoretic advantages: preservation of blood supply, maintenance of inherent ligamentous stability, minimal iatrogenic soft-tissue injury, and early restoration of wrist motion. Recent studies have shown excellent results with respect to union, functional recovery, and return to work.[32,34,35,40-42] Two recent studies compared cast immobilization with internal fixation for the treatment of nondisplaced scaphoid fractures and demonstrated significantly improved time to union and time to return to work following internal fixation.[34,35]

Displaced and unstable fractures may also be treated with an open or arthroscopically assisted percutaneous technique. In the open approach, a reduction under direct visualization is performed. To use a minimally invasive approach, displaced fracture fragments may be reduced by manipulating percutaneously placed Kirschner wire joysticks driven into the proximal and distal pole fragments. Temporary fixation can then be maintained with a cannulated screw guidewire placed down the central axis of the scaphoid.[32,43] The importance of a centrally placed guidewire cannot be overstated. In a biomechanical study on cadaveric scaphoids, centrally placed scaphoid screws demonstrated greater stiffness and load to failure than eccentrically placed screws.[44] After fracture reduction and preliminary fixation have been obtained, wrist arthroscopy can be used to assess intra-articular congruency.[41,45,46] Finally, a headless variable-pitched cannulated screw can be placed percutaneously, which minimizes iatrogenic soft-tissue trauma (Figures 3 and 4).

Perilunate Injuries

Perilunate injuries consist of a spectrum of ligamentous and bony injuries that occur about the lunate. Historically, patient outcomes after these devastating dislocations or fracture-dislocations are satisfactory at best. Radiographic evidence of midcarpal or radiocarpal arthrosis and loss of carpal height are common findings at follow-up.[47,48] However, satisfactory pain relief and return to occupation can be achieved with current treatment methods.[49,50]

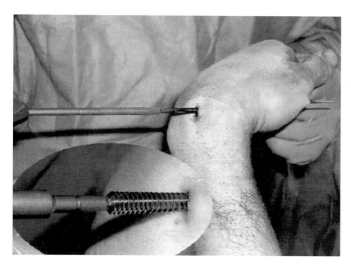

Figure 3 Photograph and inset showing the percutaneous placement of a scaphoid screw through a dorsal approach. *(Reproduced with permission from Slade JF III, Geissler WB, Gutow AP, Merrell GA: Percutaneous internal fixation of selected scaphoid nonunions with an arthroscopically assisted dorsal approach. J Bone Joint Surg Am 2003;85[suppl 4]:20-32.)*

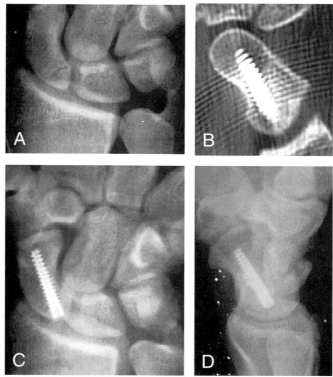

Figure 4 A, Preoperative radiograph of a patient with a proximal pole fracture who presented 50 days after injury. CT scan **(B)** and radiographs **(C** and **D)** obtained at 3-month postoperative follow-up after percutaneous placement of scaphoid screw fixation demonstrate that the fracture is healed. Cortical bridging is present on the CT scan. *(Reproduced by permission from Slade JF III, Gutow AP, Geissler WB: Percutaneous internal fixation of scaphoid fractures via an arthroscopically assisted dorsal approach. J Bone Joint Surg Am 2002;84[suppl 2]:21-36.)*

The traditional classification for these traumas to the wrist was introduced in a biomechanical study.[51] The energy of injury typically travels through the scapholunate interval (stage I) and past the lunocapitate articulation, disrupting the space of Poirier (stage II). Next, the lunotriquetral ligamentous complex is disrupted (stage III—dorsal perilunate dislocation), and finally the lunate dislocates from its fossa into the carpal tunnel volarly (stage IV—lunate dislocation) (Figure 5). If the energy of injury traverses through an individual bone rather than a ligamentous complex, then the resultant perilunate fracture is labeled with the prefix "trans" (for example, dorsal transscaphoid perilunate dislocation).

A multicenter, retrospective review of patients with perilunate injuries demonstrated that the initial diagnosis of these complex carpal injuries was missed in 25% of patients.[47] Initial radiographs of any dramatically swollen wrist secondary to a high-energy trauma require careful examination by an experienced radiologist or orthopaedist. The authors showed that perilunate fracture-dislocations were twice as common as perilunate dislocations. Also, open injuries and delayed treatment negatively affected clinical outcomes, but the specific type of perilunate injury tended not to affect final results.

Once the diagnosis has been made and a careful neurovascular examination has been performed, the dislocation or fracture-dislocation must be urgently reduced. When performed with adequate muscle relaxation (using either axillary nerve block or general anesthesia), re-creation of the mechanism of injury followed by axial traction across the wrist using a wrist traction tower or weights will reduce most of these inju-

ries. Fluoroscopic inspection of the reduction in multiple planes and with stress views allows for critical assessment of the injury and accurate diagnosis of carpal disruptions. Examination should include visualization and evaluation of the distal radius and ulna, carpal height, Gilula's arcs, carpal interosseous spaces, scapholunate and radiolunate angles, and the rotatory positions within the proximal carpal row.

Open reduction and internal fixation for these injuries has been advocated,[52] and it has been described as providing better results than closed reduction alone—without internal fixation.[48,50,53] With direct visualization of fracture reduction and fixation or ligamentous repair, authors have reported satisfactory patient outcomes but limited functional results.[48,49] One study used a combined dorsal and volar approach and found suboptimal outcomes despite fracture reduction and restoration of radiolunate and scapholunate angles.[52] The authors reported changes in mean revised carpal height ratio (from 1.59 to 1.49), mean scapholunate angle (from 44° to 58°), and mean radiolunate angle (from −10° to 6°). In addition, grip strength and range of motion in all planes were significantly less than those of the uninjured contralateral wrist.

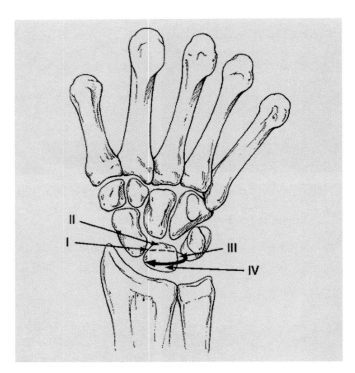

Figure 5 Schematic representation of the progressive stages of perilunate instability as classified by Mayfield. Stage I represents scapholunate ligament disruption; stage II, dislocation of the capitate (dorsally); stage III, lunotriquetral ligament disruption; and stage IV, complete dislocation of the lunate (volarly). *(Reproduced from Bednar JM, Osterman AL: Carpal instability: Evaluation and treatment.* J Am Acad Orthop Surg *1993;1:13.)*

Using a pure dorsal approach to treat all dorsal transscaphoid perilunate fracture-dislocations, another group of investigators demonstrated encouraging results at a mean 8-year follow-up.[48] These authors performed closed reduction of the fracture-dislocations with axial traction, then performed an open anatomic reduction and internal fixation. Internal fixation consisted of screw or Kirschner wire fixation for scaphoid fractures, Kirschner wire fixation for lunotriquetral and scapholunate ligament tears, and pinning of the reduced radiolunate relationship. At final follow-up, the authors found satisfactory maintenance of scapholunate and radiolunate angles, and Mayo wrist scores were comparable to those in previously published reviews.

Open reduction and internal fixation has many distinct advantages in the management of these injuries, such as reduction of dislocated or fractured bones that have buttonholed through supporting ligamentous structures and wrist capsule or direct ligamentous repair of interosseous and capsular ligament disruptions. A volar lunate dislocation (Mayfield stage IV) certainly should be treated with open reduction. Although open reduction and internal fixation is the current standard of care for perilunate injuries, an open approach to dorsal perilunate injuries increases the total soft-tissue injury of the affected wrist, resulting in a well-healed but functionally stiff wrist.

In an attempt to maximize postoperative wrist function, minimally invasive methods are becoming increasing popular for difficult and complex injuries to the wrist joint. For example, if an anatomic reduction of a perilunate fracture-dislocation cannot be obtained by traction and manipulation, fractures and dislocations may be reduced with the assistance of percutaneously placed Kirschner wire joysticks. After closed reduction, carpal fractures can be fixed with variable-pitched headless cannulated screws using minimally invasive techniques, and ligamentous disruptions can be stabilized with percutaneously placed Kirschner wires.[54] Whether reduction is open or closed, stable bony fixation with minimal soft-tissue disruption typically provides the best possible functional results.

Annotated References

1. Horton TC, Hatton M, Davis TR: A prospective randomized controlled study of fixation of long oblique and spiral shaft fractures of the proximal phalanx: Closed reduction and percutaneous Kirschner wiring versus open reduction and lag screw fixation. *J Hand Surg [Br]* 2003;28:5-9.

   This randomized trial of closed reduction and percutaneous Kirschner wire fixation (15 patients) versus open reduction and screw fixation of a spiral or long oblique fracture of the proximal phalanx (13 patients) showed no significant differences in recovery rate, pain scores, alignment, motion, or grip strength.

2. Hornbach EE, Cohen MS: Closed reduction and percutaneous pinning of fractures of the proximal phalanx. *J Hand Surg [Br]* 2001;26:45-49.

   Among 12 patients with unstable extra-articular fractures of the proximal phalanx that were treated with transarticular intramedullary Kirschner wires, an average total active motion of 265° was achieved with one significant proximal interphalangeal joint flexion contracture, one flexor tendon adhesion, and one significant rotational deformity.

3. Newington DP, Davis TR, Barton NJ: The treatment of dorsal fracture-dislocation of the proximal interphalangeal joint by closed reduction and Kirschner wire fixation: A 16-year follow up. *J Hand Surg [Br]* 2001;26:537-540.

   An average of 85° of proximal interphalangeal joint motion with an average 8° flexion contracture with mild but not severe degenerative changes was observed an average of 16 years after Kirschner wire fixation of 11 unstable dorsal fracture-dislocations of finger proximal interphalangeal joints without attempt to reduce the fracture of the base of the middle phalanx.

4. Slade JF, Baxamusa TH, Wolfe SW: External fixation of proximal interphalangeal joint fracture dislocations. *Atlas Hand Clin* 2000;5:1-29.

This is a detailed review discussing the treatment of complex fractures and fracture-dislocations of the proximal interphalangeal joint. This report also demonstrates the clinical advantages and step-by-step application of a straightforward proximal interphalangeal joint external fixator for the treatment of unstable fracture-dislocations.

5. Deitch MA, Kiefhaber TR, Comisar BR, Stern PJ: Dorsal fracture dislocations of the proximal interphalangeal joint: Surgical complications and long-term results. *J Hand Surg [Am]* 1999;24:914-923.

6. Williams RM, Kiefhaber TR, Sommerkamp TG, Stern PJ: Treatment of unstable dorsal proximal interphalangeal fracture/dislocations using a hemi-hamate autograft. *J Hand Surg [Am]* 2003;28:856-865.

   Among 13 patients with a hemi-hamate autograft for the treatment of an unstable dorsal proximal interphalangeal fracture-dislocation, an average 85° arc of proximal interphalangeal motion and 80% grip was achieved. Two patients had recurrent dorsal subluxation, but all of the grafts healed.

7. King HJ, Shin SJ, Kang ES: Complications of operative treatment for mallet fractures of the distal phalanx. *J Hand Surg [Br]* 2001;26:28-31.

   In this study, 24 of 59 surgically treated mallet fractures (41%) developed a postoperative complication, including dorsal skin necrosis, recurrent extension lag, permanent nail deformities, transient pin track infections, and osteomyelitis.

8. Pegoli L, Toh S, Arai K, Fukuda A, Nishikawa S, Vallejo IG: The Ishiguro extension block technique for the treatment of mallet finger fracture: Indications and clinical results. *J Hand Surg [Br]* 2003;28:15-17.

   In this study, 65 consecutive patients with a mallet fracture of the distal phalanx with either a large bone fragment, palmar subluxation, or substantial joint incongruity were treated with extension block Kirschner wire fixation. The authors reported good or excellent results (using the Crawford rating system) in 78% of patients.

9. Tetik C, Gudemez E: Modification of the extension block Kirschner wire technique for mallet fractures. *Clin Orthop* 2002;404:284-290.

   Extension block Kirschner wiring of 18 mallet fractures achieved a healed, congruous joint surface in 17 patients, with an average 81° of flexion and a 1.6° extensor lag.

10. Takami H, Takahashi S, Ando M: Operative treatment of mallet finger due to intra-articular fracture of the distal phalanx. *Arch Orthop Trauma Surg* 2000;120:9-13.

Open reduction and Kirschner wire fixation of 33 mallet fractures (13 with distal interphalangeal joint subluxation) achieved an average loss of extension of 4° and an average flexion of 67°, with few complications and degenerative changes in only 6 patients.

11. Ali A, Hamman J, Mass DP: The biomechanical effects of angulated boxer's fractures. *J Hand Surg [Am]* 1999;24:835-844.

12. Harding IJ, Parry D, Barrington RL: The use of a moulded metacarpal brace versus neighbour strapping for fractures of the little finger metacarpal neck. *J Hand Surg [Br]* 2001;26:261-263.

    In this prospective, randomized comparison of buddy taping and splinting in 65 patients with fifth metacarpal neck fractures, the authors found equally good final results, but patients were more comfortable during treatment with a brace.

13. Kuokkanen HO, Mulari-Keranen SK, Niskanen RO, Haapala JK, Korkala OL: Treatment of subcapital fractures of the fifth metacarpal bone: A prospective randomised comparison between functional treatment and reposition and splinting. *Scand J Plast Reconstr Surg Hand Surg* 1999;33:315-317.

14. Leung YL, Beredjiklian PK, Monaghan BA, Bozentka DJ: Radiographic assessment of small finger metacarpal neck fractures. *J Hand Surg [Am]* 2002;27:443-448.

    Serial evaluation of 96 radiographs of small finger metacarpal neck fractures by three observers demonstrated limited agreement on the measured angulation of the fracture and the treatment recommendation between observers and by the same observer 6 weeks later.

15. Papaloizos MY, Le Moine P, Prues-Latour V, Borisch N: Della Santa DR: Proximal fractures of the fifth metacarpal: a retrospective analysis of 25 operated cases. *J Hand Surg [Br]* 2000;25:253-257.

    Among 25 patients who underwent surgical treatment of fractures of the fifth metacarpal, 10 developed painful degenerative arthritis at an average of 3.3 years after surgery.

16. Lutz M, Sailer R, Zimmermann R, Gabl M, Ulmer H, Pechlaner S: Closed reduction transarticular Kirschner wire fixation versus open reduction internal fixation in the treatment of Bennett's fracture dislocation. *J Hand Surg [Br]* 2003;28:142-147.

    This comparison of 32 patients with adequately reduced Bennett fractures that were evaluated an average of 7 years after undergoing either closed reduction and pinning or open reduction an internal fixation demonstrated no clinical or radiographic differences between these two groups.

17. Galanakis I, Aligizakis A, Katonis P, Papadoko-stakis G, Stergiopoulos K, Hadjipavlou A: Treatment of closed unstable metacarpal fractures using percutaneous transverse fixation with Kirschner wires. *J Trauma* 2003;55:509-513.

In this study, 25 patients with fifth metacarpal fractures were treated with manipulative reduction and Kirschner wire fixation with excellent radiographic and functional results.

18. Faraj AA, Davis TR: Percutaneous intramedullary fixation of metacarpal shaft fractures. *J Hand Surg [Br]* 1999;24:76-79.

19. Fusetti C, Meyer H, Borisch N, Stern R, Santa DD, Papaloizos M: Complications of plate fixation in metacarpal fractures. *J Trauma* 2002;52:535-539.

Among 157 patients with extra-articular fractures of nonthumb metacarpals that were treated with plate and screw fixation, 12 patients (15%) had delayed union or nonunion, 8 (10%) had stiffness, 7 (8%) had plate loosening or breakage, and 1 (< 1%) had a deep infection.

20. Page SM, Stern PJ: Complications and range of motion following plate fixation of metacarpal and phalangeal fractures. *J Hand Surg [Am]* 1998;23:827-832.

21. Waris E, Ashammakhi N, Happonen H, et al: Bioabsorbable miniplating versus metallic fixation for metacarpal fractures. *Clin Orthop* 2003;410:310-319.

The authors of this study performed mechanical testing on human metacarpals and reported that bioabsorbable plates have stability comparable to 1.7- and 2.3-mm plates.

22. Bozic KJ, Perez LE, Wilson DR, Fitzgibbons PG, Jupiter JB: Mechanical testing of bioresorbable implants for use in metacarpal fracture fixation. *J Hand Surg [Am]* 2001;26:755-761.

The authors of this study reported that bioresorbable plates gradually lost bending strength and stiffness during 12 weeks of in vitro degradation. The plates appear to retain adequate strength for physiologic loads for about 8 weeks.

23. Parvizi J, Wayman J, Kelly P, Moran CG: Combining the clinical signs improves diagnosis of scaphoid fractures: A prospective study with follow-up. *J Hand Surg [Br]* 1998;23:324-327.

24. Brydie A, Raby N: Early MRI in the management of clinical scaphoid fracture. *Br J Radiol* 2003;76:296-300.

In this study, 195 patients with snuffbox tenderness and no evidence of scaphoid fracture on plain films were prospectively assessed with MRI of the wrist. The authors reported identifying 37 scaphoid fractures, 28 distal radius fractures, and 9 other carpal fractures. The management of 92% of the patients was changed because of the MRI results.

25. Dorsay TA, Major NM, Helms CA: Cost-effectiveness of immediate MR imaging versus traditional follow-up for revealing radiographically occult scaphoid fractures. *AJR Am J Roentgenol* 2001;177:1257-1263.

The authors of this study compared the cost of scaphoid fracture screening done with MRI of the wrist and the total charges of a traditional protocol of follow-up examinations and radiographs. The study revealed MRI costs of $770 and traditional follow-up costs of $677; therefore, the authors concluded that MRI screening of patients with suspected scaphoid fractures is fiscally reasonable.

26. Saxena P, McDonald R, Gull S, Hyder N: Diagnostic scanning for suspected scaphoid fractures: An economic evaluation based on cost-minimisation models. *Injury* 2003;34:503-511.

This study compared five different imaging screening protocols for patients with clinical signs but no radiographic evidence of scaphoid fracture. Early MRI was shown to be cost-competitive and was seen as an opportunity to minimize costs of clinic visits, cast changes, and repeat radiographs.

27. Kaneshiro SA, Failla JM, Tashman S: Scaphoid fracture displacement with forearm rotation in a short-arm thumb spica cast. *J Hand Surg [Am]* 1999;24:984-991.

28. McAdams TR, Spisak S, Beaulieu CF, Ladd AL: The effect of pronation and supination on the minimally displaced scaphoid fracture. *Clin Orthop* 2003;411:255-259.

CT was used to track interfragmentary motion in cadaveric wrists with scaphoid osteotomies while pronated and supinated. The authors reported that total motion between fragments in wrists immobilized in short arm thumb spica casts averaged 0.2 mm.

29. Hambidge JE, Desai VV, Schranz PJ, Compson JP, Davis TR, Barton NJ: Acute fractures of the scaphoid: Treatment by cast immobilisation with the wrist in flexion or extension? *J Bone Joint Surg Br* 1999;81:91-92.

30. Gellman H, Caputo RJ, Carter V, Aboulafia A, McKay M: Comparison of short and long thumb-spica casts for non-displaced fractures of the carpal scaphoid. *J Bone Joint Surg Am* 1989;71:354-357.

31. Trumble TE: Management of scaphoid nonunions. *J Am Acad Orthop Surg* 2003;11:380-391.

This is a concise review of the diagnosis and treatment of scaphoid nonunions.

32. Slade JF III, Gutow AP, Geissler WB: Percutaneous internal fixation of scaphoid fractures via an arthroscopically assisted dorsal approach. *J Bone Joint Surg Am* 2002;84(suppl 2):21-36.

    This is an instructional review and step-by-step guide for a novel, minimally invasive approach to internal fixation of scaphoid fractures using arthroscopically assisted fracture reduction and percutaneous fixation.

33. Saeden B, Tornkvist H, Ponzer S, Hoglund M: Fracture of the carpal scaphoid: A prospective, randomised 12-year follow-up comparing operative and conservative treatment. *J Bone Joint Surg Br* 2001;83:230-234.

    In this retrospective comparison of the long-term results of open reduction and internal fixation versus short arm thumb spica casting for treating acute scaphoid fractures, the authors reported an earlier return to function in the surgically managed group of patients.

34. Adolfsson L, Lindau T, Arner M: Acutrak screw fixation versus cast immobilisation for undisplaced scaphoid waist fractures. *J Hand Surg [Br]* 2001;26:192-195.

    The authors of this prospective, randomized trial of percutaneously placed screw fixation compared with short arm thumb spica casting for the treatment of acute, nondisplaced scaphoid waist fractures reported better range of motion at 16 weeks in patients with fixed fractures. The early mobilization of the surgically managed group did not impact fracture healing.

35. Bond CD, Shin AY, McBride MT, Dao KD: Percutaneous screw fixation or cast immobilization for nondisplaced scaphoid fractures. *J Bone Joint Surg Am* 2001;83:483-488.

    In this study of patients with acute nondisplaced scaphoid fractures who were randomized to be treated with either percutaneous screw fixation or cast immobilization, the authors reported faster time to healing and quicker return to work in patients in the percutaneous screw fixation group.

36. Polsky MB, Kozin SH, Porter ST, Thoder JJ: Scaphoid fractures: Dorsal versus volar approach. *Orthopedics* 2002;25:817-819.

    In a comparison of using volar and dorsal approaches during open reduction and internal fixation for the treatment of scaphoid fractures, the authors reported no differences between the two groups with respect to wrist range of motion, grip strength, or pain level.

37. Rettig ME, Kozin SH, Cooney WP: Open reduction and internal fixation of acute displaced scaphoid waist fractures. *J Hand Surg [Am]* 2001;26:271-276.

    The authors of this study reported that 14 consecutive patients with displaced scaphoid fractures that were treated using open reduction and internal fixation with bone grafting for comminution had return of function, wrist range of motion, and radiographic evidence of union with preservation of scaphoid alignment and height.

38. Rettig ME, Raskin KB: Retrograde compression screw fixation of acute proximal pole scaphoid fractures. *J Hand Surg [Am]* 1999;24:1206-1210.

39. Trumble TE, Gilbert M, Murray LW, Smith J, Rafijah G, McCallister WV: Displaced scaphoid fractures treated with open reduction and internal fixation with a cannulated screw. *J Bone Joint Surg Am* 2000;82:633-641.

    The authors of this study retrospectively reviewed scaphoid fractures that were treated with open reduction and internal fixation with the Herbert-Whipple screw and open reduction and internal fixation with an AO/ASIF 3.5-mm cannulated screw. They reported no difference in healing rates, time to union, or functional results between these two groups of patients.

40. Slade JF III, Jaskwhich D: Percutaneous fixation of scaphoid fractures. *Hand Clin* 2001;17:553-574.

    The approach for percutaneous screw fixation from the dorsal aspect of the proximal scaphoid pole is described and its potential benefits, such as central guidewire placement and avoidance of volar ligament injury, are discussed.

41. Slade JF III, Grauer JN, Mahoney JD: Arthroscopic reduction and percutaneous fixation of scaphoid fractures with a novel dorsal technique. *Orthop Clin North Am* 2001;32:247-261.

    This clinical review of scaphoid fractures treated surgically with arthroscopically assisted fracture reduction and percutaneous screw fixation demonstrated excellent patient outcomes with regards to fracture union, wrist range of motion, and patient satisfaction.

42. Yip HS, Wu WC, Chang RY, So TY: Percutaneous cannulated screw fixation of acute scaphoid waist fracture. *J Hand Surg [Br]* 2002;27:42-46.

    These authors describe the technique and report the 2-year follow-up results of 49 patients with scaphoid fractures who were treated with percutaneous screw fixation from the volar aspect of the scaphoid tubercle. There was a 100% union rate, and patients had excellent functional results.

43. Slade JF III, Geissler WB, Gutow AP, Merrell GA: Percutaneous internal fixation of selected scaphoid nonunions with an arthroscopically assisted dorsal approach. *J Bone Joint Surg Am* 2003;85(suppl 4):20-32.

A novel technique for the percutaneous management of scaphoid nonunions is presented in this article. The authors report the results of arthroscopically assisted closed reduction and percutaneous screw fixation used to treat 15 patients with painful fibrous unions or nonunions without sclerosis. The average time from initial injury was 10.6 months. Although bone grafting was not performed in these patients, all the fibrous unions and nonunions healed with evidence of cortical bridging on CT scans. Modified Mayo wrist scores revealed 12 excellent and 3 good patient outcomes.

44. McCallister WV, Knight J, Kaliappan R, Trumble TE: Central placement of the screw in simulated fractures of the scaphoid waist: A biomechanical study. *J Bone Joint Surg Am* 2003;85:72-77.

45. Geissler WB, Hammit MD: Arthroscopic aided fixation of scaphoid fractures. *Hand Clin* 2001;17:575-588.

    This article provides a thorough description of the technique of scaphoid fracture reduction under arthroscopic visualization.

46. Toh S, Nagao A, Harata S: Severely displaced scaphoid fracture treated by arthroscopic assisted reduction and osteosynthesis. *J Orthop Trauma* 2000;14:299-302.

    These authors present a case report of the successful minimally invasive treatment of a displaced scaphoid fracture.

47. Herzberg G, Comtet JJ, Linscheid RL, Amadio PC, Cooney WP, Stalder J: Perilunate dislocations and fracture-dislocations: A multicenter study. *J Hand Surg [Am]* 1993;18:768-779.

48. Herzberg G, Forissier D: Acute dorsal transscaphoid perilunate fracture-dislocations: Medium-term results. *J Hand Surg [Br]* 2002;27(6):498-502.

    The authors of this article treated 11 of 14 patients with transscaphoid perilunate fracture-dislocations with open reduction through a dorsal approach and obtained satisfactory results. Volar ligamentous injuries were not reconstructed, but the dorsal capsule was repaired.

49. Sotereanos DG, Mitsionis GJ, Giannakopoulos PN, Tomaino MM, Herndon JH: Perilunate dislocation and fracture dislocation: A critical analysis of the volar-dorsal approach. *J Hand Surg [Am]* 1997;22:49-56.

50. Melone CP Jr, Murphy MS, Raskin KB: Perilunate injuries: Repair by dual dorsal and volar approaches. *Hand Clin* 2000;16:439-448.

    The authors of this article present a concise review of the two-incision approach to treating perilunate injuries and contend that for active individuals precise repair of all injured structures can provide a satisfactory functional outcome that had not been achieved with closed reduction.

51. Mayfield JK, Johnson RP, Kilcoyne RK: Carpal dislocations: Pathomechanics and progressive perilunar instability. *J Hand Surg [Am]* 1980;5:226-241.

52. Hildebrand KA, Ross DC, Patterson SD, Roth JH, MacDermid JC, King GJ: Dorsal perilunate dislocations and fracture-dislocations: Questionnaire, clinical, and radiographic evaluation. *J Hand Surg [Am]* 2000;25:1069-1079.

    In this series of 23 patients with perilunate injuries, the authors advocate a combined volar and dorsal approach for reduction, fixation, and ligamentous repair. They reported that 73% of patients returned to their prior occupations, and that average flexion and extension arc and grip strength were 57% and 73% of the uninjured side, respectively.

53. Apergis E, Maris J, Theodoratos G, Pavlakis D, Antoniou N: Perilunate dislocations and fracture-dislocations: Closed and early open reduction compared in 28 cases. *Acta Orthop Scand Suppl* 1997;275:55-59.

54. Soejima O, Iida H, Naito M: Transscaphoid-transtriquetral perilunate fracture dislocation: Report of a case and review of the literature. *Arch Orthop Trauma Surg* 2003;123:305-307.

    This case report and literature review details experience in the management of these rare perilunate injuries.

Section 4

Axial Skeleton— Including Spine and Pelvis

Section Editors:
Jens R. Chapman, MD
Michael D. Stover, MD

Chapter 21

Pelvic Fractures: Evaluation and Acute Management

Peter J. O'Brien, MD, FRCSC

Kyle F. Dickson, MD

Introduction

Low-energy fractures of the pelvis are common injuries. Major disruptions of the pelvic ring that are associated with life-threatening hemorrhage, however, are not commonly seen in general orthopaedic practice. High-energy pelvic fractures often occur in conjunction with multiple injuries. Patients with these devastating injuries need emergent, well-coordinated, multidisciplinary assessment and treatment and are best managed in trauma referral hospitals. This chapter reviews the basic concepts of pelvic ring injury in terms of mechanism of injury and classification, the initial evaluation of patients with pelvic ring injuries, and the protocols for emergent resuscitation and treatment. Definitive treatment and expected outcomes of pelvic ring fractures are covered in chapter 22.

Anatomy and Stability of the Pelvis

The osseous and soft-tissue anatomy of the pelvis is complex. Surgeons caring for patients with pelvic fractures must be familiar with the intricacies of pelvic anatomy.

Treating physicians must be knowledgeable about the anatomy of the soft-tissue structures within the pelvis because these structures are at risk of injury when a pelvic ring fracture occurs. Injuries to major blood vessels (the internal iliac artery and its branches, the median sacral artery and the pelvic veins), neurologic tissue (lumbosacral plexus and the cauda equina), the lower gastrointestinal tract, and the lower genitourinary tract (particularly the urinary bladder and the male urethra) are frequently associated with pelvic ring injuries.

From a functional standpoint, the pelvis should be considered to be a ring structure. The ring is composed of three bones (the sacrum and the two innominate bones) and the ligamentous structures that bind them together. The pelvic ligaments that are essential for maintaining stability of the pelvic ring include the posterior ligaments, anterior ligaments, and pelvic floor ligaments. The major posterior ligaments are the anterior sacroiliac, interosseous sacroiliac, and posterior sacroil-

iac ligaments along with the iliolumbar and lateral lumbosacral ligaments. The anterior ligamentous complex is called the symphysis pubis, and the major structures of the pelvic floor are the sacrospinous and sacrotuberous ligaments.

Stability is the major anatomic feature of the pelvis and depends on the integrity of the bony and ligamentous structures. A failure of the pelvic ring (fracture or ligament disruption) at one site only will not render the pelvis unstable. When the ring is disrupted in two places, however, instability is present; therefore, unstable pelvic ring injuries always have injuries in at least two parts of the ring—an anterior and a posterior lesion.

Mechanism of Injury

High-energy pelvic ring fractures are frequently associated with significant injuries to other regions of the body. They generally occur as a result of motor vehicle collisions, industrial machinery crushes, or falls from a height.[1] The major forces that act on the pelvis to produce injury are anteroposterior compression (external rotation of the hemipelvis), lateral compression (internal rotation of the hemipelvis), vertical shear, or a combination of these forces. The fracture pattern can help orthopaedic surgeons determine the direction and magnitude of the injuring force. This information is useful in predicting the spectrum of associated injuries to other organ systems.[2,3] Knowing the mechanism of injury and the force vectors that have produced the pelvic injury are also essential for planning treatment of the pelvic injury.

Initial Evaluation and the Role of the Orthopaedic Surgeon

A team approach is necessary for the simultaneous assessment and resuscitation of patients with a pelvic fracture. In addition to nursing and paramedical personnel, the team should include a trauma-trained general surgeon, orthopaedic surgeon, interventional radiologist, and when appropriate, an intensivist, urologist, and neurosurgeon. The protocols developed by the Advanced Trauma Life Support program should be followed. Most multiple trauma patients with pelvic fracture who do not survive die from head injury, chest injury, or abdominal injury.[4] Nevertheless, ongoing blood loss from the pelvic injury can be a significant contributor to a poor outcome, and there are some situations in which pelvic bleeding is the major contributing factor in the death of a patient. In particular, patients with unstable pelvic fracture patterns tend to have significant pelvic bleeding.[2] Active participation by an orthopaedic surgeon in the initial assessment and management of patients with pelvic fractures can lead to improved rates of patient survival.[5]

The conscious trauma patient will give a history that is invaluable in the initial assessment of the pelvic injury and associated injuries. However, many patients with serious pelvic injuries are intubated or unconscious and are therefore unable to provide any history. A thorough physical examination, identification of associated injuries, and careful review of the diagnostic imaging studies are required for successful management.

Physical examination of the pelvis starts with inspection of the integument. Open wounds must be carefully inspected for size, location, and contamination. Degloving injuries, contusions, ecchymosis, and crush injuries to the soft tissue all are important aspects of the assessment. The patient will need to be log rolled to examine the posterior soft tissues. Deformity of the pelvis or lower extremities may be obvious on inspection and may be indicative of pelvic injury. Tenderness to palpation is also a sign of underlying pelvic ring injury. The entire anterior and posterior pelvis must be carefully palpated to elicit tenderness. Clinical examination can reliably detect or rule out significant pelvic fracture in patients with blunt trauma who are alert.[6-8] Provocative physical examination of the pelvis assists the surgeon in determining mechanical instability if plain radiographs show no evidence of definite instability. Rotational instability is evaluated by placing the hands on each iliac crest at the level of the anterior-superior iliac spine and gently trying to open and close the pelvis. The pelvis should move as a unit. Movement of one side of the pelvis in respect to the other side indicates rotational instability. Once a mechanically unstable pelvis is identified via examination, repeated manipulation of the pelvis should be avoided to minimize the possible dislodgement of clot and the subsequent worsening of hemodynamic instability. Physical examination to determine pelvic instability is often best performed in the operating room after the patient has been anesthetized.

The search for associated injuries to the intrapelvic structures begins with a carefully conducted neurologic and vascular assessment of the lower extremities and the perianal region. Pelvic fractures are frequently associated with neurologic injury, particularly lumbosacral plexus injuries. Neurologic deficits in the lower extremities can involve any of the nerve roots from L2 to S4, with L5 and S1 nerve root injuries being the most com-

mon. Bowel or bladder incontinence and sexual dysfunction are often long-term sequelae of high-energy pelvic ring injuries and need to be identified during the initial assessment. Patients with fractures that involve the central portion of the sacrum (zone III) are at high risk of having severe bowel and/or bladder dysfunction.

The skin and soft tissues need to be carefully examined for injury. Open fractures require accurate early diagnosis for appropriate management. Perineal lacerations and vaginal or rectal injuries are life-threatening and require early diagnosis for successful treatment. Therefore, all patients with significant pelvic injuries require a rectal examination and, when appropriate, a vaginal examination. Closed degloving injuries are commonly associated with high-energy pelvic injuries. The subcutaneous tissue is sheared away from the underlying fascia. The large hematoma and necrotic adipose tissue that are present can lead to infection in over one third of patients. Débridement and closure over drains may be necessary.[9]

Genitourinary injuries are commonly associated with pelvic fractures. Scrotal swelling, blood at the urethral meatus, a displaced prostate, or inability to easily pass a Foley catheter are all classic signs of urethral injury and require assessment with retrograde urethrogram. Hematuria may be a sign of bladder rupture. Bladder ruptures are usually extraperitoneal, but they can be intraperitoneal. The diagnosis is confirmed by cystogram.[10] Urethral and bladder injuries require treatment by a skilled urology team, which frequently works in conjunction with those who provide definitive orthopaedic care.

Radiographic evaluation of pelvic injuries starts with the AP view, which is generally a standard part of the assessment of patients with multiple trauma. Pelvic injuries are then further evaluated with inlet and outlet pelvic views and lateral lumbosacral views. The AP pelvic view provides information about the location, pattern, and displacement of the fracture. The inlet view clearly demonstrates the direction and displacement of the injury and provides an excellent view of posterior injuries. The outlet view demonstrates sagittal plane deformities and sacral fracture patterns. The lateral view of the sacrum best demonstrates displacement and rotation of transverse components of H-pattern sacral fractures (Figures 1 and 2).

Axial CT is a routine part of the imaging of pelvic ring injuries. CT is more accurate in determining the presence, exact location, and pattern of pelvic injuries than are plain radiographs.[11] Sagittal and coronal reformat images and three-dimensional reconstructions may be useful in assessing patients with complex injury patterns. CT can also be used to estimate the size of pelvic hematomas, can predict the need for transfusion, and can help identify which patients may benefit from pelvic angiography.[12] Contrast-enhanced CT may also be used for the same purposes[13-15] (Figure 3).

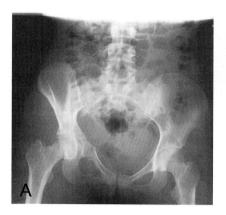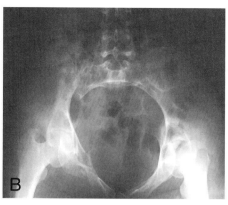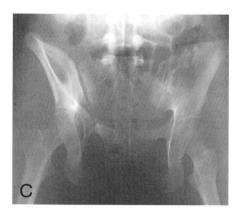

Figure 1 AP **(A)**, inlet **(B)**, and outlet **(C)** views of a patient with a type II lateral compression injury.

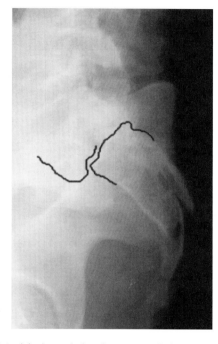

Figure 2 Lateral lumbosacral view demonstrates displacement in the transverse component of an H-type sacral fracture.

ries and has important implications for definitive management. The classification systems based on stability are also important for planning definitive treatment. In general, pelvic ring fractures are considered to be stable, rotationally unstable, or rotationally and vertically unstable. Some fractures will have one type of instability in one hemipelvis and another type on the other side. The classification system based on the mechanism of injury is useful in the acute phase of treatment to predict blood loss and associated injuries. Type III anteroposterior compression injuries are generally associated with greater blood loss and transfusion requirements than are type III lateral compression injuries. Type I and type II lateral compression injuries are usually caused by lateral impact and have a 50% incidence of head injury associated with them. Type III lateral compression injuries are generally caused by rollover mechanisms, are not typically associated with head injury, but they are associated with a high risk of bowel injury and lower extremity fracture. Vertical shear injuries are associated with a high risk of hypovolemic shock (63%) and mortality (25%).[16]

Radiographic signs of pelvic instability include more than 5 mm of displacement of the posterior sacroiliac complex, the presence of a posterior fracture gap (as opposed to impaction), and the presence of an avulsion fracture of the ischial spine, ischial tuberosity, sacrum, or the transverse process of the fifth lumbar vertebra.

Classification of pelvic ring fractures can be based on the anatomic location of the injuries (using the Letournel classification system), stability (using the Bucholz, Tile, or Orthopaedic Trauma Association classification systems), or mechanism of injury (using the Young and Burgess classification system) (Figure 4). Each classification system has important features and they should be used together. The anatomic classification system describes the exact location of the bone and ligament inju-

Protocols for Emergent Treatment and Resuscitation

The initial management of the hemodynamically unstable patient with a pelvic fracture should follow Advanced Trauma Life Support protocols, which emphasize simultaneous assessment and resuscitation. The ABCs (airway, breathing, and circulation) of the primary survey for the assessment of immediately life-threatening injuries are well known. Initial treatment includes, when appropriate, intubation, ventilation, chest tube insertion, aggressive fluid resuscitation, and avoidance or management of hypothermia and coagulopathy. In conjunction with a careful secondary survey, all associated injuries (head, chest, abdomen, spine, integument, and extremities) should be identified.

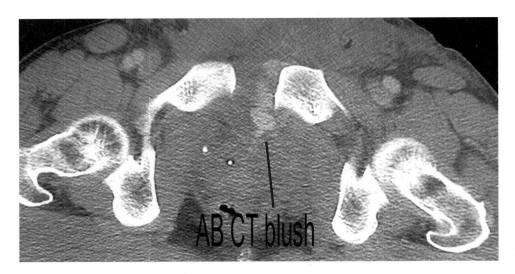

Figure 3 Contrast blush seen on a pelvic CT scan provides an indication for angiography.

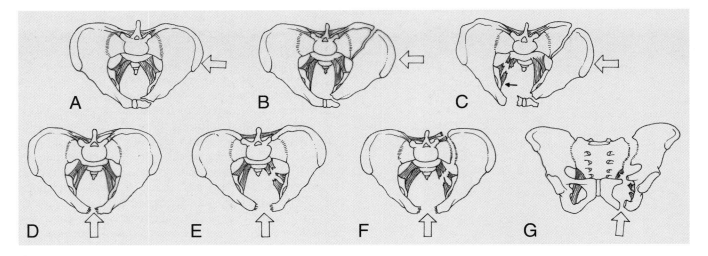

Figure 4 The Young and Burgess classification of pelvic injuries. The arrows indicate the direction of the force causing the injury. **A** through **C** represent lateral compression injuries. Type I is a stable injury that includes rami fractures. Further displacement results in a type II injury with hemipelvic instability usually from a fracture-dislocation posteriorly. If the force continues across the body, a type III injury with an opening of the contralateral pelvic occurs. **D** through **F** depict the increasing injury to the ligaments of the pelvis with anteroposterior compression injuries. A type I injury is stable with only the symphysis disrupted. As the force and displacement increases, the sacrospinous and sacrotuberous ligaments rupture and allow rotational instability, a type II injury. Last, the posterior sacroiliac ligaments fail, creating a completely unstable hemipelvis, a type III injury. **G** shows a vertical shear injury, which ruptures the pelvis anteriorly and posteriorly. *(Reproduced from Beaty JH (ed): Orthopaedic Knowledge Update 6. Rosemont, IL, American Academy of Orthopaedic Surgeons, 1998, pp 427-439.)*

Orthopaedic intervention is required for patients in whom bleeding from the pelvic fracture is contributing to ongoing hypotension. Lateral compression fracture patterns are not associated with major pelvic hemorrhage, whereas anterior-posterior compression and vertical shear patterns can be. The acute resuscitation of the patient must include a strategy to rapidly stabilize the unstable pelvis (anterior-posterior or vertical shear patterns). Pelvic stabilization will reduce pelvic bleeding and can provide some pain relief. Some of the techniques available to provide emergent stabilization of the unstable pelvic fracture include traction, military antishock trousers, vacuum beanbags, sheets,[1,17,18] binders,[18] and external fixators. Angiographic embolization and surgical packing of the pelvis may also be needed to control bleeding in the pelvis.[19]

Most pelvic blood loss is caused by bleeding cancellous bone surfaces and disrupted pelvic veins. Some form of early pelvic fracture stabilization may assist in controlling this type of hemorrhage by reducing motion and allowing clots to stabilize. It is unlikely that these techniques control hemorrhage by reducing pelvic volume and thereby allowing tamponade.[20]

Pneumatic antishock garments have been used in the past as a form of temporary pelvic stabilization that could be applied in the field. Problems with decreased ventilatory capacity, lower extremity compartment syndrome, and difficulty with hypotension on

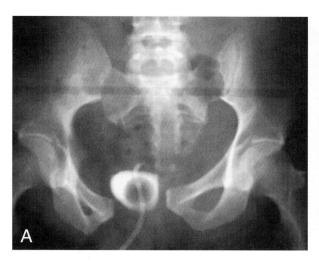 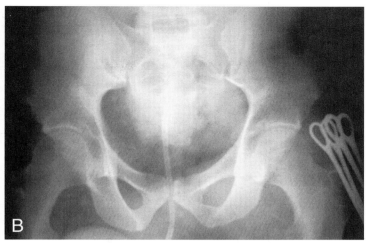

Figure 5 Radiographs of a patient with an unstable pelvic fracture without **(A)** and with **(B)** a circumferential sheet wrap; note that the circumferential sheet wrap resulted in temporary fracture reduction and stabilization.

removal of the devices has led most centers to discontinue their use.

A simple alternative that can be applied in the field or in the emergency department is a pelvic binder or a circumferential sheet. Circumferential wrapping with a sheet is a readily available and inexpensive technique. A sheet or towel is wrapped snugly around the pelvis and is then clamped or knotted. The sheet can be positioned at the hips if access to the abdomen is needed[21] (Figure 5).

Temporary pelvic ring stabilization can be effectively achieved using an external skeletal fixator. Although some controversy exists about its use in the treatment of patients with acute pelvic fractures, several studies have documented decreased mortality rates in patients with pelvic fractures that were treated with external fixation.[21-27] Frames are typically used as a temporary fixation device for resuscitation, but they occasionally can be left in place as definitive or supplemental fixation. An external fixator can be emergently applied either in the emergency department or in the operating room. A standard anterior external fixator with pins in the iliac crest and configured as a one-bar, two-bar, or trapezoidal frame works well to stabilize the pelvis in patients with open book (type II anteroposterior compression) fracture patterns. Pins can be inserted rapidly and accurately. Fluoroscopic guidance may facilitate pin placement between the iliac crest cortical tables.[28] In patients with fracture patterns that have complete posterior pelvic instability, an anterior frame may worsen the posterior pelvic reduction. An alternative to the simple anterior frame in that situation is the C-shaped pelvic clamp. Use of the C clamp is contraindicated if the posterior fracture of the ilium is anterior to the sacroiliac joint, and it should be used with caution if there is comminution of the sacrum. These devices apply a posterior compression force and can be applied percutaneously. There are several significant potential complications associated with

the use of the C clamp, and the surgeon using such a device must be fully aware of the correct technique. External fixation devices should be applied before emergency laparotomy when possible and can be turned down to allow access to the abdomen for laparotomy.

Persistent arterial bleeding in the pelvis can be a cause of ongoing hypotension and may be amenable to angiographic embolization. There is controversy as to whether hemodynamically unstable patients should undergo pelvic stabilization with external fixation before angiography.[15,29-31] In many centers, external fixation is applied to the pelvis for hemodynamically unstable patients and if the patients remain hypotensive, angiographic arterial embolization is performed. The rationale for this approach is that only a small percentage of patients with pelvic fractures (10%) have pelvic bleeding from arteries that are amenable to embolization. Other centers, however, proceed to angiography before any pelvic fracture fixation and have demonstrated good outcomes.[31] In most patients, branches of the internal iliac artery are identified and embolized directly. Success rates of over 90% in controlling pelvic arterial bleeding have been reported.[32]

Surgical exploration and ligation of bleeding sites is not an effective technique to control hemorrhage in pelvic trauma. There is evidence that surgical packing of the pelvis, however, may be effective for controlling blood loss in hypotensive patients. In this technique, the retroperitoneal space is packed with surgical sponges. The packing is changed or removed in 24 to 48 hours. Patients who are candidates for this type of management are those who remain in "extremis" despite fluid resuscitation and emergency external fixation. The technique has been used in some European centers, but it has not gained wide acceptance in North America. The rationale for pelvic packing is that bleeding from the venous plexus can be controlled by packing, arterial bleeding

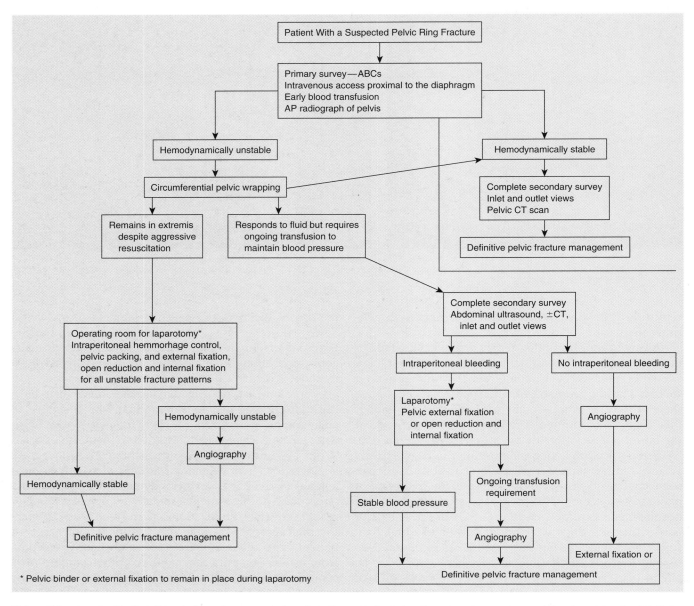

Figure 6 Sample protocol for the initial evaluation and management of a patient with a pelvic ring fracture. The various steps remain somewhat controversial, and each institution will need to develop its own protocol depending on resources and facilities. The protocol should be developed collaboratively by trauma surgeons, orthopaedic surgeons, and interventional radiologists.

can also be controlled with packing, and complex pelvic injuries are often combined with intraperitoneal lesions that require laparotomy[33] (Figure 6).

Open Fractures

Open fractures of the pelvis require additional treatment considerations. Open pelvic fractures have been associated with high mortality rates. Early death often results from uncontrolled hemorrhage, and late mortality can be caused by overwhelming sepsis. The principles of open fracture care that are used to treat open fractures elsewhere in the body should be applied, including prophylactic antibiotic therapy, tetanus pro-

phylaxis, emergent wound débridement and irrigation, early skeletal stabilization, and delayed wound coverage. Additionally, patients with open pelvic fractures are at risk of exsanguination, and packing of the wound may be necessary.

When the open wound is in the perineum, there is a high risk of fecal contamination that can lead to major wound infection and uncontrolled sepsis. Patients with open pelvic fractures and perineal wounds generally have been managed with fecal diversion via a transverse colostomy and rectal stump washout. There has been some controversy as to which patients require fecal diversion; however, it is generally accepted that colostomy

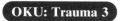

should be used for patients with extensive open perineal or open posterior pelvic wounds.[1,34-36]

Patients with a rectal tear have a serious form of open pelvic fracture. Rectal tears must be recognized early and managed with diverting colostomy. Vaginal lacerations associated with pelvic fractures also are open fractures and require débridement and repair.

Biomechanics of External and Internal Fixation

Most commonly, external fixation is used only as a temporary measure in the acute management of patients with unstable pelvic ring injuries. Anterior pelvic external fixation frames can provide enough stability to be used as definitive fixation for some rotationally unstable pelvic ring injuries.[37] However, no external fixation system provides enough stability to allow mobilization of patients with vertically unstable pelvic fractures.[38,39] Although a combination of external fixation and internal fixation will provide improved biomechanical stability, the strongest constructs for vertically unstable fracture patterns are a combination of anterior and posterior internal fixation.

Summary

The evaluation and acute management of patients with a high-energy pelvic fracture require a multidisciplinary approach. The orthopaedic surgeon must have an understanding of the complex pelvic anatomy, injury patterns, and associated injuries. Resuscitation and initial evaluation are critical steps that require input from the orthopaedist. Protocols for emergent treatment must include plans for simple, rapid, and effective pelvic stabilization in the appropriate circumstances. Effective assessment and treatment of pelvic ring fractures in the acute phase will improve the outcomes for patients with these serious injuries.

Annotated References

1. Routt ML, Nork SE, Mills WJ: Treatment of complex fractures: High-energy pelvic ring disruptions. *Orthop Clin North Am* 2002;33:59-72.

2. Eastridge BJ, Starr A, Minei JP, O'Keefe GE: The importance of fracture pattern in guiding therapeutic decision-making in patients with hemorrhagic shock and pelvic ring disruptions. *J Trauma* 2002;53:446-451.

   In this study, 86 patients with pelvic fracture who had laparotomy and/or angiography were reviewed retrospectively. In those patients with a stable pelvic fracture pattern, the cause of hypotension was intra-abdominal injury in 85% and the mortality rate was 25%. In those patients with an unstable pelvic fracture pattern, 59% had arterial pelvic bleeding and the mortality was 52%.

3. Dalal SA, Burgess AR, Siegel JH, et al: Pelvic fracture in multiple trauma: Classification by mechanism is key to pattern of organ injury, resuscitative requirements, and outcome. *J Trauma* 1989;29:981-1002.

4. Ankarath S, Giannoudis PV, Barlow I, Bellamy MC, Matthews SJ, Smith RM: Injury patterns associated with mortality following motorcycle crashes. *Injury* 2002;33:473-477.

5. Biffi WL, Smith WR, Moore EE, Gonzalez RJ, Morgan SJ, Hennessey T: Evolution of a multidisciplinary clinical pathway for the management of unstable patients with pelvic fractures. *Ann Surg* 2001;233:843-850.

6. Gonzalez RP, Fried PQ, Bukhalo M: The utility of clinical examination in screening for pelvic fractures in blunt trauma. *J Am Coll Surg* 2002;194:121-125.

7. Duane TM, Tan BB, Golay D, Cole FJ, Weireter LJ, Brit LD: Blunt trauma and the role of routine pelvic radiographs: A prospective analysis. *J Trauma* 2002;53:463-468.

8. McCormick JP, Morgan SJ, Smith WR: Clinical effectiveness of the physical examination in diagnosis of posterior pelvic ring injuries. *J Orthop Trauma* 2003;17:257-261.

   In this study, 66 patients were prospectively evaluated for pelvic fracture with physical examination and CT. The authors reported that 49 had evidence of posterior pelvic ring injury on their CT scans and that 48 of those 49 (98%) had posterior pelvic tenderness on physical examination.

9. Hak DJ, Olson SA, Matta JM: Diagnosis and management of closed internal degloving injuries associated with pelvic and acetabular fractures: The Morel-Lavallee lesion. *J Trauma* 1997;42:1046-1051.

10. Morey AF, Iverson AJ, Swan A, et al: Bladder rupture after blunt trauma: Guidelines for diagnostic imaging. *J Trauma* 2001;51:683-686.

11. Guillamondegui OD, Pryor JP, Gracias VH, Gupta R, Reilly PM, Schwab CW: Pelvic radiography in blunt trauma resuscitation: A diminishing role. *J Trauma* 2002;53:1043-1047.

12. Blackmore CC, Jurkovich GJ, Linnau KF, Cummings P, Hoffer EK, Rvara FP: Assessment of volume of hemorrhage and outcome from pelvic fracture. *Arch Surg* 2003;138:504-508.

13. Pereira SJ, O'Brien DP, Luchette FA, et al: Dynamic helical computed tomography scan accurately de-

tects hemorrhage in patients with pelvic fracture. *Surgery* 2000;128:678-685.

14. Stephen DJ, Kreder HJ, Day AC, et al: Early detection of arterial bleeding in acute pelvic trauma. *J Trauma* 1999;47:638-642.

15. Miller PR, Moore PS, Mansell E, Meredith JW, Chang MC: External fixation or arteriogram in bleeding pelvic fracture: Initial therapy guided by markers of arterial hemorrhage. *J Trauma* 2003;54: 437-443.

    In this retrospective review, 35 patients with pelvic ring fractures had hypotension attributed to the pelvic injury. Three of four stable patients who had a contrast blush seen on CT scans had arterial bleeding on angiography; 19 of 26 (73%) unstable patients who did not respond to initial resuscitation had arterial bleeding on angiography. The authors reported that delay in angiography for external fixation in patients not responding to initial resuscitation would have delayed embolization in the presence of arterial bleeding in 7 of 16 patients (44%).

16. Whitbeck MG Jr, Zwally HJ II, Burgess AR: Innominosacral dissociation: Mechanism of injury as a predictor of resuscitation requirements, morbidity, and mortality. *J Orthop Trauma* 1997;11:82-88.

17. Routt ML Jr, Falicov A, Woodhouse E, Schildhauer TA: Technical trick: Circumferential pelvic antishock sheeting. A temporary resuscitation aid. *J Orthop Trauma* 2002;16:45-48.

18. Bottlang M, Simpson T, Sigg J, Krieg JC, Madey SM, Long WB: Noninvasive reduction of open-book pelvic fractures by circumferential compression. *J Orthop Trauma* 2002;16:367-373.

19. Grimm MR, Vrahas MS, Thomas KA: Pressure-volume characteristics of the intact and disrupted pelvic retroperitoneum. *J Trauma* 1998;44:454-459.

20. Kregor PJ, Routt ML Jr: Unstable pelvic ring disruptions in unstable patients. *Injury* 1999;30(suppl 2):B19-B28.

21. Edeiken-Monroe BS, Browner BC, Jackson H: The role of standard roentgenograms in the evaluation of instability of pelvic ring disruption. *Clin Orthop* 1989;240:63-76.

22. Reimer BL, Butterfield SL, Diamond DL, et al: Acute mortality associated with injuries to the pelvic ring: The role of early patient mobilization and external fixation. *J Trauma* 1993;35:671-677.

23. Moreno C, Moore EE, Rosenberger A, et al: Hemorrhage associated with major pelvic fracture: A multi-specialty challenge. *J Trauma* 1986;26:987-994.

24. Gyling SF, Ward RE, Holcroft JW, Bray TJ, Champman MW: Immediate external fixation of unstable pelvic fractures. *Am J Surg* 1985;150:721-724.

25. Flint L, Babikian G, Anders M, Rodriguez J, Seligson DL: Definitive control of mortality from severe pelvic fracture. *Ann Surg* 1990;211:703-707.

26. Cryer HM, Miller FB, Evers BM, Rouben LR, Seligson DL: Pelvic fracture classification: Correlation with hemorrhage. *J Trauma* 1988;28:973-980.

27. Edwards CC, Meier PJ, Browner BD, et al: Results treating 50 unstable pelvic injuries using primary external fixation. *Orthop Trans* 1985;9:434.

28. Tucker MC, Nork SE, Simonian PT, Routt ML Jr: Simple anterior pelvic external fixation. *J Trauma* 2000;49:989-994.

    In this study, 41 patients with unstable pelvic ring fractures had a single-pin anterior pelvic external fixator applied. Fluoroscopic outlet-obturator oblique views were used for pin insertion. The authors reported that 94% of the pins were completely contained between the iliac cortical tables and that the initial pelvic reduction was maintained in 93% of patients until the frame was removed.

29. Cook RE, Keating JF, Gillespie I: The role of angiography in the management of haemorrhage from major fractures of the pelvis. *J Bone Joint Surg Br* 2002;84:178-182.

    In this study, 23 patients with unstable pelvic ring fractures had angiography for uncontrolled hypotension. Fracture morphology (classification as anteroposterior compression, lateral compression, or vertical shear injuries) was not a reliable guide to identifying associated vascular injury. Although the number of patients assessed in this study was small, the authors concluded that pelvic skeletal stabilization and laparotomy (when indicated) should be performed before angiography.

30. Starr AJ, Griffin DR, Reinert CM, et al: Pelvic ring disruptions: Prediction of associated injuries, transfusion requirement, pelvic arteriography, complications, and mortality. *J Orthop Trauma* 2002;16:553-561.

    This review of database information of 325 patients with closed pelvic fractures revealed that shock on admission and the Revised Trauma Score were useful predictors of mortality, transfusion requirement, and Abbreviated Injury Scores.

31. Gruen GS, Leit ME, Gruen RJ, Peitzman AB: The acute management of hemodynamically unstable multiple trauma patients with pelvic ring fractures. *J Trauma* 1994;36:706-713.

32. Velmahos GC, Toutouzas KG, Vassiliu P, et al: A prospective study on the safety and efficacy of angiographic embolization for pelvic and visceral injuries. *J Trauma* 2002;53:303-308.

33. Ertel W, Keel M, Eid K, Platz A, Trentz O: Control of severe hemorrhage using C-clamp and pelvic packing in multiply injured patients with pelvic ring disruption. *J Orthop Trauma* 2001;15:468-474.

   In this study, 14 multiply injured patients with pelvic ring disruption and hemorrhagic shock were treated with C-clamp stabilization followed by laparotomy and pelvic packing. Three patients died acutely of hemorrhage and one died later of multiple organ failure. The authors concluded that pelvic packing and C-clamp fixation are effective in controlling severe hemorrhage.

34. Brenneman FD, Katyal D, Boulanger BR, et al: Long-term outcomes in open pelvic fractures. *J Trauma* 1997;42:773-777.

35. Pell M, Flynn WJ Jr, Seibel RW: Is colostomy always necessary in the treatment of open pelvic fractures? *J Trauma* 1998;45:371-373.

36. Woods RK, O'Keefe G, Rhee P, et al: Open pelvic fracture and fecal diversion. *Arch Surg* 1998;133:281-286.

37. Bellabarba C, Ricci WM, Bolhofner BR: Distraction external fixation in lateral compression pelvic fractures. *J Orthop Trauma* 2000;14:475-482.

38. Ponson KJ, Hoek van Dijke GA, Joosse PMS, Snijders CJ: Improvement of external fixator performance in Type C pelvic ring injuries by plating of the pubic symphysis: An experimental study on 12 external fixators. *J Trauma* 2002;53:907-913.

39. Ponsen KJ, Hoek van Dijke GA, Joosse P, Snijders CJ: External fixators for pelvic fractures: Comparison of the stiffness of current systems. *Acta Orthop Scand* 2003;74:165-171.

Chapter 22

Pelvic Fractures: Definitive Treatment and Expected Outcomes

M.L. Routt Jr, MD

Carol Copeland, MD

Definitive Radiographic Evidence of Injury

Plain pelvic radiographs can demonstrate evidence of pelvic ring disruptions. An AP plain radiograph should be obtained for patients who report pelvic pain or who have experienced multiple trauma and intubated patients who are unable to cooperate with examination. Recent studies emphasize that the screening AP pelvic film may not be indicated for minimally injured, alert patients without specific complaints.[1] When abnormalities are noted on the initial image, biplanar plain pelvic radiographs further define the injury and displacements. These inlet and outlet pelvic radiographs define symphyseal, pubic ramus, iliac, sacroiliac, and sacral injuries as well as combinations thereof. When a paradoxical inlet appearance of the upper sacral region is noted on an AP pelvic image, a transverse sacral fracture may be present. The addition of lateral sacral radiographs will help to define these unusual transverse sacral fractures as well as their displacements and deformities.[2] Soft-tissue air densities remote from the bowel may be noted on plain pelvic films. Such a finding heralds an open skin wound, bowel perforation, or subcutaneous emphysema caused by a chest wall injury (Figure 1).

Screening AP pelvic radiographs may be confusing for several reasons. It is important to know exactly how the radiograph was obtained. If the patient is encircled in a snug circumferential pelvic wrap such as a sheet or binder, initial pelvic displacements and deformities may be missed. The circumferential pelvic wrap often reduces pelvic deformities, and the clinician must be aware of this[3] (Figure 2). Morbid obesity and poor bone quality may limit evaluation of the screening pelvic image. Previously administered contrast agents may also obstruct visualization of injured areas.

Routine two-dimensional pelvic CT scans refine the clinician's understanding of the pelvic injury. These contiguous axial images include the entire pelvis and soft-tissue envelope from iliac crest to ischium and progress in 5-mm increments. The routine pelvic CT scan further delineates the posterior pelvic ring, acetabular areas, and soft-tissue structures (Figure 3). Contrast-enhanced CT scans may be used to identify associated genitourinary, vascular, and visceral injuries. Pelvic CT scans are especially helpful and sensitive in pediatric patients with pelvic ring injuries.[4] For the most complex pelvic injuries, three-dimensional pelvic CT scans may aid in understanding the injury. High-quality three-dimensional pelvic CT scans require additional axial images for processing; therefore, additional patient radiation exposure and scanner time is also required. For these reasons, these studies are reserved for the most difficult or confusing pelvic injuries (Figure 4). Significant pelvic soft-tissue injuries such as open wounds and closed degloving injuries are readily identified on the pelvic CT scan.

Pelvic angiography is indicated for those patients with pelvic ring disruptions and hemodynamic instability that is resistant to routine resuscitative measures. Pelvic arterial injuries can be embolized (Figure 5). Dynamic fluoroscopy done at the time of pelvic angiography is also helpful in imaging of pelvic injury. The fluoroscope can be positioned in a variety of positions without moving the injured patient.[5]

Anatomic-Mechanical Classification of Pelvic Injury

The anatomic-mechanical pelvic classification scheme identifies the specific sites of pelvic injury, displacements, and deformities.[6] It also considers the pelvic instability noted on physical examination. This classification system, as with all others, is dependent on a thorough radiographic assessment that includes pelvic plain radiographs and CT. Injuries are described according to specific anatomic sites. The associated displacements are quantified on the radiographs. Anatomic classification does not require memorization of various pelvic classification schemes, but necessitates an understanding of pelvic osseous anatomy and obvious radiographic displacement patterns. Using the anatomic method, injury details are factored into the treatment decision-making process along with the instability noted on physical examination. Surgical exposures, reduction maneuvers, clamp applications, and implant locations and sequenc-

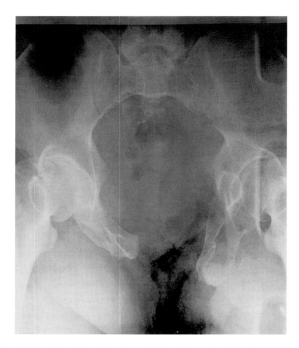

Figure 1 An inlet pelvic plain radiograph of an adult male patient who was injured in a motorcycle accident demonstrates the various pelvic ring injuries and associated deformities. Soft-tissue air densities are caused by the open perineal traumatic wound.

ing are planned preoperatively to ensure surgical effectiveness. The anatomic pelvic injury classification also takes into consideration associated soft-tissue injuries.

Most clinicians prefer more detailed injury descriptions provided by the anatomic mechanical classification rather than the abbreviations provided by other classifications because they are easy to communicate and remember in guiding treatment.

Nonsurgical Treatment
Nonsurgical treatment methods include bed rest, circumferential wrapping, skeletal traction, pelvic slings, and spica casting. These techniques are selected less commonly as surgical experience, intraoperative fluoroscopy, and pelvic fixation techniques have advanced. Nonsurgical treatment of unstable injuries is indicated in patients whose overall medical condition prevents safe surgical intervention. Nonsurgical treatment requires serial radiographic evaluations to ensure that the reduction is maintained during healing. For nonunions, electrical stimulation is a nonsurgical option.[7]

Injury-Specific Indications for Surgical Treatment
Instability
Because most unstable pelvic ring injuries have numerous sites of instability because of the ringed structure, confusion may arise regarding certain fixation principles. Over time, fixation of pelvic ring injuries has evolved.

Clinical series have evaluated surgical timing, surgical exposures, quality of reduction, and fixation techniques, as well as outcomes and complications.[8-33] Biomechanical laboratory evaluations have tested a variety of surgical devices and demonstrated that stable fixation of each site contributes to overall ring stability.[34,35]

Deformity
Certain pelvic traumatic injuries such as the overlapping or locked symphysis pubis as well as displaced pubic ramus fractures that intrude into the vagina or bladder or those that cause flow disturbances of the iliac vessels require surgical intervention. Certain displaced iliac fractures put patients at increased risk for skin necrosis and warrant surgical management. Displaced posterior pelvic ring injuries require reduction and fixation to avoid pelvic malunion and nonunion that have been associated with consistently poor outcomes.[7] Surgical intervention is indicated for open pelvic fractures. The traumatic wound is thoroughly débrided and then irrigated. Open wound management is advocated for most traumatic pelvic open wounds. Traumatic pelvic ring instability in association with direct rectal injuries or perineal wounds that involve the rectum warrant fecal diversion using an end (no loop) colostomy. Perineal traumatic open wounds that spare the rectum may not need diversion and are treated with open wound management.[30] In patients with concomitant pelvic ring disruptions and spinal fractures, pelvic fixation may be indicated if wear associated with the spinal orthotic device involves the injured pelvic ring. Similarly, pelvic stabilization should be strongly considered in patients with concurrent spinal cord and pelvic ring injuries.

Anterior Pelvic Ring Injuries
Anterior pelvic ring injuries include symphysis pubis disruptions, pubic rami fractures, and certain associated acetabular fractures. Disruptions of the symphysis pubis can result from a variety of mechanisms, with variable resultant deformities. The deformities can include external-internal rotation, flexion-extension, and cephalad-caudad translation, depending on the associated posterior ring injury. The degree of symphyseal disruption has been categorized in multiple classification schemes in an attempt to determine the degree of posterior pelvic ring injury and instability.[6]

Surgical treatment has been advocated when the symphyseal diastasis exceeds 2.5 cm. This clinical recommendation is based on experimental evidence that indicates at least involvement of the anterior sacroiliac ligaments in association with symphyseal distraction. This rule may not be applicable to children or adults of small stature. Furthermore, such absolute parameters fail to take into account variable radiographic technique and magnification, the effect of temporizing stabilization of the pelvis,

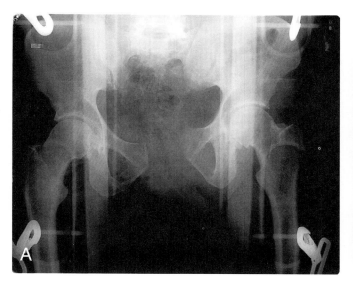

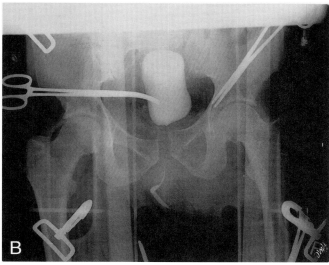

Figure 2 **A,** A plain radiograph demonstrates a pelvic ring injury that includes a distraction injury of the symphysis pubis in a patient who was hemodynamically unstable at the scene of the accident and on presentation to the emergency department. **B,** An AP pelvic film obtained after a circumferential pelvic sheet was snugly applied and secured with clamps reveals that symphyseal closure was achieved. The patient's vital signs and hematocrit level normalized after circumferential pelvic sheet application. An anterior pelvic external fixator was applied using the circumferential pelvic sheet to maintain the reduction by cutting holes in the sheet in the areas of iliac crest pin insertions. After frame application, the sheet was loosened and removed. Definitive pelvic reduction and fixation was carried out after the patient was stabilized and evaluated.

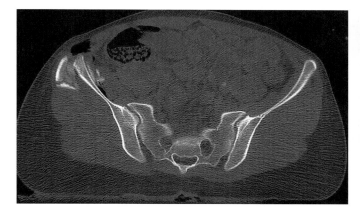

Figure 3 A pelvic CT axial scan demonstrates the presence of an open and comminuted right iliac crest fracture. Air densities within the local soft tissues and beneath the iliacus muscle reveal the open wound status.

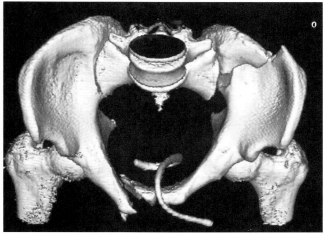

Figure 4 Three dimensional pelvic CT scan, which is used to further understand complex injury patterns, demonstrates a left iliac fracture with ipsilateral sacroiliac joint disruption along with the right parasymphyseal pubic fracture. A suprapubic catheter was inserted initially to treat the patient's associated urethral disruption.

or that static radiographic images may underestimate symphyseal displacement at the time of injury. This rule also does not consider the "locked" symphysis disruption. If the CT scan shows evidence of any widening of the anterior sacroiliac joint, significant rotational displacement at the time of injury can be inferred. Anterior pelvic ring treatment is directed according to the patient's medical history, physical examination findings, radiographic findings, associated injuries, and other variables.

Anterior pelvic external fixation is a treatment option for nonobese patients with minor symphyseal disruptions or rami fractures and incomplete rotational posterior pelvic instability. Supplemental posterior pelvic internal fixation is indicated for patients with unstable injuries.[35]

The fixation clamps are loosened 6 to 8 weeks after injury, and pelvic stability is evaluated. AP inlet and outlet pelvic radiographs assess healing. If the symphysis pubis is not tender to palpation and the radiographs demonstrate reduction maintenance, the iliac pins are removed in the clinic.

Symphysis Pubis Disruptions
Open reduction and internal fixation is recommended for complete symphyseal disruptions in association with posterior pelvic injuries. A Pfannenstiel exposure centered

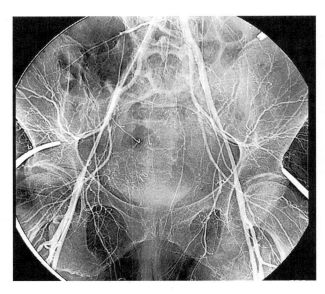

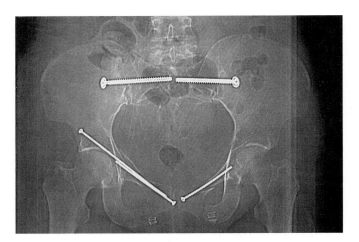

Figure 6 This AP pelvic plain radiograph reveals bilateral anterior and posterior pelvic ring injuries in a patient who was crushed by a horse. The patient underwent pelvic stabilization using percutaneous fixation at each site of instability.

Figure 5 A pelvic arteriogram helps identify and control arterial bleeding sites in hemodynamically unstable patients with pelvic ring injuries who do not respond to volume resuscitation, thermoregulation, and pelvic volume reduction.

slightly above the pubic tubercles allows symphyseal access for reduction and plate fixation. In both distraction and "locked" injuries, the reduction is adjusted to perfection before fixation. A uniplanar plate construct is used when the posterior pelvic ring is not significantly disrupted. Two-holed dynamic compression plates manifest early incomplete fixation failure when the individual screws are noted to separate radiographically on the outlet pelvic image. These two-holed dynamic compression plates also permit symphyseal flexion-extension and rotation. Laparoscopic repair techniques are currently being investigated for use in the management of symphyseal injuries.[36] A single contoured six-holed 3.5-mm pelvic reconstruction plate using two or three screws on each side of the symphyseal disruption is recommended. In patients with posterior pelvic ring instability, either multiplanar symphyseal plating techniques or, more preferably, posterior ring stabilization is recommended.[35] Multiplanar symphyseal plate constructs have demonstrated improved stability in laboratory experiments; however, the plate separation necessary to achieve these mechanical advantages is not always possible clinically without significant soft-tissue stripping. Modified perpendicular plate designs were not found to be biomechanically superior to conventional uniplanar plates.[37] Malleable pelvic reconstruction plates may demonstrate evidence of fatigue fracture on follow-up radiographs without clinical correlation.

Pubic Rami Fractures

Fractures occur at different locations along the pubic ramus (parasymphyseal, midramus, and pubic root) and may also occur in association with symphyseal disrup-

tions. Pubic root fractures may involve the anterior acetabular articular area. Inferior pubic rami fractures occur similarly adjacent to the caudal aspect of the pubic body and at the transition of the ramus into the ischial tuberosity. Segmental inferior ramus fractures are common. Pubic rami fractures are associated with local visceral injuries, such as bladder and urethral disruptions. Vaginal impingement may result from a displaced, malrotated inferior pubic ramus fracture. Retropubic anastomotic communications between the inferior epigastric (or external iliac) and obturator vascular systems, known as the corona mortis, may be disrupted because of the superior pubic ramus fracture and cause unexplained hemorrhage.[38]

Pubic rami fractures may be managed differently depending on the pattern of pelvic instability. Nonsurgical management is the rule if the posterior pelvic ring is sufficiently stabilized. Anterior stabilization is preferable for rotationally unstable injuries or to supplement posterior fixation in patients with more complex injury patterns. A simple anterior pelvic external fixation device can be used. Unstable and displaced parasymphyseal pubic fractures can be approached using a Pfannenstiel exposure with plate fixation performed similar to that for symphysis pubis disruptions. Unstable and displaced pubic root fractures are more laterally located; if fixation is necessary, open reduction may require either an extended Pfannenstiel (Stoppa) or ilioinguinal exposure to facilitate plate fixation. Retrograde medullary superior pubic rami screws provide an alternative fixation technique to internal fixation and may not require the exposure necessary for open reduction and plate fixation; additionally, this technique has been shown to provide biomechanical stability comparable to plate fixation[35] (Figure 6).

Inferior pubic rami fractures that produce vaginal impingement should be treated surgically. Using a Pfannenstiel exposure, the malrotated segmental inferior ramus fracture can either be excised or reduced and stabilized with a medullary screw. For malunited inferior rami fractures or delayed presentations, a direct medial surgical exposure is used to excise the impinging ramus.

Anterior pelvic injuries are often associated with inguinal soft-tissue traumatic disruptions. During the surgical exposure, the inguinal soft tissue should be explored after the local hematoma is removed. The reduction and fixation can often be performed using the deep traumatic interval. Similarly, this defect should be repaired after fixation to prevent subsequent hernia formation.

Associated Acetabular Fractures

Pelvic ring injuries infrequently occur in association with acetabular fractures. Open reduction and internal fixation of the displaced acetabular fracture is typically the first treatment option for such patients when clinical status allows. Even minor malreductions of pelvic ring injuries make accurate acetabular reduction difficult. Therefore, in hemodynamically stable patients, anatomic acetabular reduction and fixation is achieved followed by treatment of the pelvic ring instabilities (during the same anesthetic session when possible). Early management decisions regarding the pelvic ring disruption should be carefully considered in these patients. In conjunction with general and urologic surgeons, the physician should carefully place incisions for early treatment of associated injuries or for resuscitation from a pelvic injury in consideration of future surgical exposures for the pelvis or acetabulum. For example, low-midline laparotomy wounds or contaminated anterior external fixation pin sites may complicate a planned ilioinguinal acetabular surgical exposure.

Iliac Fractures

Iliac fractures occur in a variety of patterns. Nondisplaced, stable iliac fractures are treated conservatively. Iliac fractures may result from donor bone graft harvesting adjacent to the anterior-superior iliac spine. Other more comminuted iliac fractures are the result of high-energy direct forces applied to the iliac crest. Severe local flank contusions are associated with this type of iliac fracture. The adjacent skin may be abraded, or open iliac traumatic wounds may be present. In such patients, the buttock and flank may be ecchymotic and swollen. Careful evaluation for intra-abdominal pathology should be performed.[23,33] Displaced fractures into the greater sciatic notch may involve the superior gluteal artery with associated hemorrhagic complication. For fractures that are displaced into the greater sciatic notch, a preoperative arteriogram delays surgical management, but is advocated to ensure the superior gluteal artery patency. Embolization is indicated preoperatively when the supe-

rior gluteal artery is disrupted, even in the hemodynamically stable patient.[33]

The indications for surgical fixation of iliac fractures include displaced or unstable iliac fractures associated with open wounds; severely displaced or comminuted iliac fractures; patients with unstable iliac fractures that compromise adequate pulmonary function because of pain, bowel entrapment, or herniation within the iliac fracture; or iliac/flank skin compromise caused by fracture displacement.

Routine anterior pelvic external fixation is contraindicated for iliac fractures. Displaced and comminuted iliac fractures are best treated with open reduction and stable internal fixation. Open reduction of an iliac fracture is best performed using an internal iliac exposure. The skin incision usually parallels the iliac crest; however, when local skin abrasions are present, the incision may be modified to avoid them. Traumatic open wounds are usually directly over the iliac crest. Open wound margins are sharply débrided, and then extended to allow reduction and internal fixation. When soft-tissue degloving injuries are encountered, the tissues should be adequately débrided. Dissection and retraction near the anterior-superior iliac spine should avoid lateral femoral cutaneous nerve injury. Direct access to the internal iliac surfaces is accomplished after subperiosteal elevation of the iliacus muscle. Lag screws between the iliac tables may be used to secure the reductions and are supported using pelvic reconstruction plates.[33] Patients with associated bowel injuries should be treated during the same anesthetic session.

Sacroiliac Joint Injuries

Disruptions of the sacroiliac joint may be associated with complete or incomplete disruption of the posterior ligamentous complex, resulting in global or rotational instability of the posterior ring.[6] Unstable, displaced sacroiliac joint disruptions should be reduced and stabilized. Internal fixation of the posterior pelvis is used for those injuries traditionally classified as vertically unstable or in which all the ligamentous structures of the sacroiliac joint have been disrupted. Stabilization of the sacroiliac joint from a posterior surgical approach has been evaluated. Tension band wiring, lag screw fixation, and plate fixation have all been shown to be complicated by posterior wound problems in early clinical series, but the incidence of such complications has diminished as surgical experience and techniques have advanced.[39] Sacroiliac joint disruptions can also be accessed using the anterior iliac surgical exposure. With the patient supine, the iliac exposure can be combined with a Pfannenstiel exposure to address the anterior pelvic and sacroiliac injuries simultaneously. Sacroiliac joint injuries are stabilized using anterior plates that span the joint or iliosacral screws. Both techniques have been associated with injury to the fifth lumbar and upper sacral nerve roots. Recent

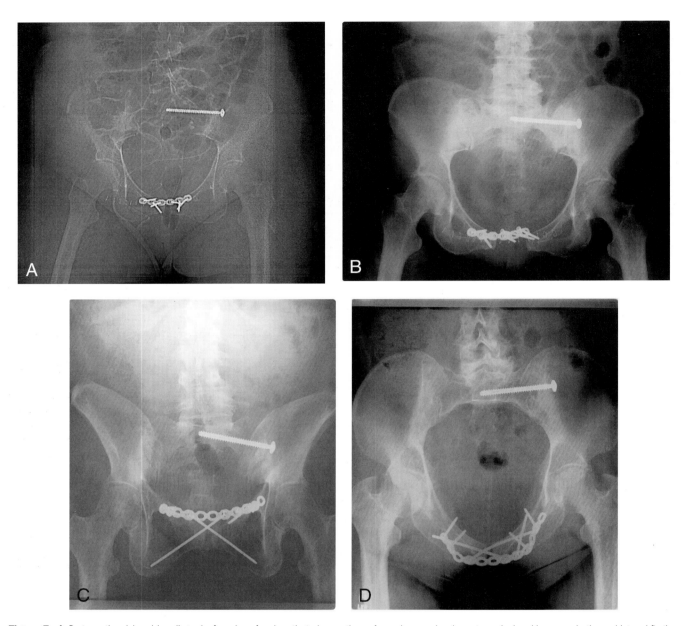

Figure 7 **A,** Postoperative plain pelvic radiograph of an obese female patient who was thrown from a horse and underwent symphysis pubis open reduction and internal fixation; left sacroiliac joint disruption was treated with percutaneous iliosacral screw fixation. The patient noted pelvic pain during bed exercises with the physical therapist and a plain radiograph **(B)** demonstrated pelvic fixation failure anteriorly. **C** and **D,** These biplanar plain pelvic radiographs show that revision of the symphyseal reduction was done with transsymphyseal screws and a more peripheral fixation construct. The patient healed uneventfully thereafter.

data suggest that the most stable construct may be a combination of plate and iliosacral screw fixation.[40]

Fracture-dislocations of the sacroiliac joint (crescent fractures) are combination disruptions of the posterior pelvic ring.[41] In patients with this type of injury, the anterior sacroiliac joint capsule and ligamentous structures are injured, producing distraction or compression through the articular surfaces depending on the application of load. As the disruptive force encounters the dense interosseous ligaments, either the iliac or sacral bone is fractured. When these traumatic events are caused by laterally applied loads, the iliac fracture is oblique and

the anterior sacral ala may be impacted. The crescent iliac fragment may also be unstable, having lost its ligamentous attachments to the sacrum, but this is a rare occurrence.

Unstable and displaced crescent injuries are treated surgically. In some patients, there is minimal displacement yet significant instability. If the fracture pattern allows, these injuries can be managed using percutaneously inserted iliosacral screws (Figure 7). Open reduction of crescent fractures is performed using either an anterior or posterior exposure, each of which has advantages. The sacroiliac joint can be accessed for débridement through either approach. The posterior exposure requires subperiosteal elevation of the hip abductors from the lateral ilium. Using the posterior exposure, the fracture is accurately reduced along the crescent fragment and secured with clamps. Stability is achieved using lag screws and plates through this posterior exposure. If the crescent fragment is initially unstable, iliosacral screw fixation is necessary to stabilize the innominate bone to the sacrum. The anterior approach can be useful, especially in the setting of compromised posterior soft tissues. Implant choice depends on the size of the intact posterior iliac crescent fracture fragment. Lag screws are placed from the internal iliac fossa into the crescent fragment and along the iliac crest. Plate fixation across the sacroiliac joint and/or iliosacral lag screws are used when possible.

Sacral Fractures

Many of the principles of sacroiliac joint disruptions apply to management of sacral fractures. Sacral fractures have been classified according to the area of injury. Alar, transforaminal, and central fracture patterns have been described to reflect associated neurologic injury rates. Transverse sacral fractures are not easily visualized on routine inlet and outlet plain pelvic radiographs. True lateral sacral radiographs are necessary to predictably identify these unusual injuries. Other level potential spinal injuries should be excluded in patients with sacral fractures, and detailed neurologic evaluations are documented.

Stabilization of the sacrum from a posterior approach has been evaluated clinically, and the biomechanical and clinical stabilities of various implants have been reported for the treatment of unstable sacral fractures.[35] Open reduction of sacral fractures is indicated in displaced and unstable patterns and when osseous debris within the nerve root tunnel correlates with specific nerve root symptoms and signs. A posterior exposure is used. Nerve decompression can be accomplished by fracture reduction and removal of bone if necessary. No clinical data are available to support the use of routine decompression after reduction. Internal fixation is used to secure the open reduction and protect the local nerve roots from further potential damage. Posterior tension plates, sacral bars, iliosacral screws, and other techniques have been recommended. All forms of compression fixation are used cautiously to avoid iatrogenic nerve root damage, especially in patients with transforaminal fracture patterns. Unstable sacral fractures treated shortly after injury (within 24 to 72 hours) may be amenable to closed reduction performed by external manipulation of the hemipelvis and stabilization using percutaneous iliosacral screws. Because the screws are placed percutaneously, the potential problem of soft-tissue infection complications are greatly diminished.

Pelvic ring disruptions are not common in children. These injuries are usually caused by high-energy traumatic events such as crush accidents. Plastic deformation can occur in the pelvic ring just as it can occur in the long bones of children, producing unusual injury patterns. Closed management using spica casting and traction has been advocated because of potential bone remodeling of deformities and inexperience with these injuries. Critical investigations of pediatric pelvic internal fixation are ongoing. In all pediatric pelvic ring disruptions, follow-up evaluations should include serial radiographic assessment of the developing triradiate cartilage.

Specific Surgical Indications

Open and/or Percutaneous Fixation

A variety of fixation techniques are available to manage unstable pelvic ring disruptions. These implants can be inserted either open and/or percutaneously. Percutaneous techniques are used to treat unstable pelvic injuries when displacement is minimal, or to treat pelvic injuries that can be reduced accurately using closed manipulative techniques, typically within the first 5 days after injury.[32] Percutaneous fixation includes the use of external fixation, iliosacral screws, medullary pubic ramus screws, and transiliac screws[42] (Figure 8). Open fixation techniques are selected when open reduction is necessary, intraoperative fluoroscopy is insufficient, or the injury pattern or local anatomy does not allow for safe percutaneous management.

Anterior Pelvic External Fixation

Routine anterior pelvic external fixation is a form of percutaneous fixation. Anterior pelvic external fixation can be used temporarily before internal fixation, as definitive fixation in some patients, or as an external support for internal fixation. The iliac crests must be intact for routine anterior pelvic external fixation to be successful. The pins are inserted between the iliac cortical tables, and the deformity is corrected using the pins to manipulate and then stabilize the reduction. This technique may result in elongated insertion incisions that interfere with subsequent surgical exposures. To avoid such problem wounds, the pelvic deformity can be manipulated and the reduction achieved initially using a circumferential pelvic wrap, such as a sheet or binder. With the pelvic reduction temporarily maintained, the iliac pins are inserted and the frame is applied. The anterior frame should be assembled to allow abdominal expansion and hip flexion to accommodate sitting. Single-pin anterior pelvic external fixation is effective, especially when used with posterior internal fixation. If bilateral single iliac crest pins are used, the insertion should be performed using fluoroscopy to accurately insert the pins between the iliac cortical tables for reliable long-term fixation.[43]

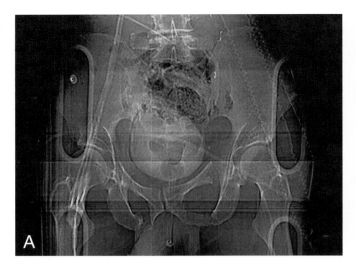
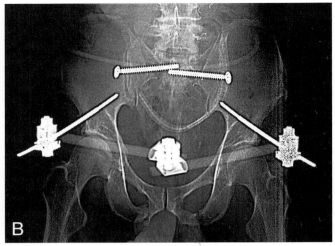

Figure 8 **A,** A preoperative pelvic CT scout image, which is often the best pelvic AP film, demonstrates bilateral sacroiliac injuries and bilateral pubic ramus fractures. The patient also had significant abdominal injuries. **B,** A postoperative plain pelvic radiograph demonstrates that the pelvic ring injuries were reduced and stabilized using an anterior pelvic external fixator and bilateral iliosacral screws.

Anterior inferior iliac pins have also been advocated for anterior pelvic external fixation frames.[42,44] These pins are directed from the anterior-inferior iliac spine into the supra-acetabular bone. These pins are more difficult to insert because of the anterior-inferior iliac spine depth, and the hip joint must be avoided. Anterior-inferior iliac spine pins also interfere with patient mobilization to the seated position because the pins obstruct hip flexion. Anterior-inferior iliac spine pins are especially useful when iliac crest comminution or flank soft-tissue injuries preclude use of routine iliac crest pins.

Percutaneous Techniques

Percutaneous techniques such as iliosacral screw fixation are attractive treatment options because soft-tissue dissection and blood loss are minimized. Posterior percutaneous techniques are associated with a low incidence of infections (0 in a series of 177 consecutive patients).[45] These techniques are demanding and require a conceptual understanding of the anatomy of the pelvis as well as the mandatory presence of a skilled technician to run the fluoroscopy unit. Fluoroscopy may not be possible because of intra-abdominal contrast or morbid obesity. As with all pelvic surgery, neurologic and vascular structures are at risk. Complications of percutaneous fixation after closed reduction include poor reductions, failures of fixation, misplaced screws, and neurologic injury.

Perioperative Protocol

Deep venous thrombosis prophylaxis begins when the patient is admitted to the hospital. Mechanical deep venous thrombosis prophylaxis includes sequential compression devices applied to the upper or lower extremities, including the feet, as the patient's other injuries allow. Preoperative chemical deep venous thrombosis prophylaxis may complicate surgical intervention. Short-duration agents or continuous infusions are selected for surgical patients preoperatively. Sequential compression devices are also used intraoperatively whenever possible. After surgery, sequential compression devices are used in conjunction with chemical prophylaxis. Special consideration is given to those patients with extensive surgical or trauma-related wounds. Early administration of chemical prophylactic agents may increase wound complication rates.

Postoperative Rehabilitation

Patients with stable fracture patterns can be mobilized soon after injury and may bear weight as allowed by comfort. Close radiographic follow-up is necessary to detect occult instability.[46] Postoperative rehabilitation protocols supervised by a licensed physical therapist serve both to mobilize patients and educate them regarding recommended physical activities and exercises. Depending on associated injuries, rehabilitation and daily activities are modified appropriately. For patients with unilateral pelvic injuries treated with stable fixation, the affected hemipelvis is protected with crutch-assisted ambulation and weight of limb weight-bearing restrictions. Abdominal, lumbar, and lower extremity isometric exercises begin the day after surgery. Active and passive hip and knee range-of-motion exercises provide comfort and mobility. Some patients can benefit from a hydrotherapy program after secure wound healing, which allows the patient to exercise with minimal weight bearing. During this early healing phase, ambulation in chest-deep water is also allowed. Assuming that uneventful healing occurs, activities are advanced 6 to 8 weeks after surgery. Light resistance, high repetition strengthening exercises, and progressive partial weight bearing can gradually restore function over the ensuing 6 weeks. Daily abdominal and lumbar strengthening and low-impact aerobic programs are advised thereafter. Patients with bilateral posterior pelvic injuries are restricted to bed or chair activities for the initial 6 or 8 weeks after surgery.

Complications

Vascular Injury

Hemorrhage from pelvic arterial injuries is most frequently seen in injuries associated with major ligamentous disruption. In particular, certain types of pelvic ring disruptions have been shown to be associated with higher blood loss, greater transfusion requirements, and higher rates of arterial embolization (Burgess and Young anteroposterior compression types II and III and lateral compression type III).[6] In a recent retrospective study of a strictly applied protocol for angiographic intervention in a population of 364 pelvic fracture patients, arterial embolization was found to be more necessary for the treatment of fractures associated with major ligamentous disruption.[47] Older age (median, 42 versus 29 years; $P = 0.028$) and higher pelvic girdle Abbreviated Injury Scale score (3 versus 2; $P = 0.015$) were the only other variables that were significantly different between the embolized and nonembolized groups. In this study, patients requiring arterial embolization were significantly older (median age, 55 years) in the subgroups of patients with or without major ligamentous disruption (27 and 30 patients; $P = 0.002$ and $P = 0.048$, respectively). This finding was corroborated in a study of pelvic fractures in the geriatric population. Patients older than 55 years with lateral compression type injuries were four times as likely to require blood transfusions than their younger counterparts.[8] Older patients appear to be the exception to the general rules of fracture pattern as a determinant of blood loss.

Deep Venous Thrombosis

The reported rate of clinically evident deep venous thrombosis after pelvic ring disruption is between 13% to 31%.[9,10,48] Pulmonary embolism has been reported in approximately 3% to 13% of patients. Fatal pulmonary embolism occurs in 2.5% to 2.7% of patients with pelvic ring disruption. Weighing the risks of hemorrhage with chemoprophylaxis against the risks of deep venous thrombosis is challenging in polytraumatized patients. Sequential compression devices are accepted as safe and are frequently used in this population. Accepting the risks of prophylactic placement of an inferior vena cava filter for unstable pelvic ring injuries may be appropriate in certain patients.[49] However, definition of the high-risk patient is difficult, and an appropriate screening tool for occult pelvic deep venous thrombosis has yet to be identified. Pelvic vein thromboses can be missed during screening of the lower extremities for deep venous

thrombosis. Ascending venography of the pelvis is considered the most reliable method of detecting pelvic thrombosis, but because the procedure is invasive it can result in associated morbidity. Contrast-enhanced CT and magnetic resonance venography were found to be unacceptable as screening tools for occult pelvic deep venous thrombosis because, followed by venography, each method had unacceptable false-positive rates in a prospective study of pelvic and acetabular fracture patients.[50]

Heterotopic Ossification

The incidence of clinically significant heterotopic ossification is approximately 8%.[10] Predictors for clinically significant heterotopic ossification are unknown. Associated local soft-tissue trauma, hypoxia, and systemic factors related to multiple and head injuries are thought to contribute to the development of heterotopic ossification. Routine radiation therapy or indomethacin prophylaxis is not generally used because patterns of heterotopic ossification are less predictable than those occurring after acetabular fractures.

Infection and Soft-Tissue Complications

The incidence of postoperative hematomas is 8% to 14% after open reduction and internal fixation of types B and C pelvic ring disruptions.[9,10,48,51] The incidence of deep infection requiring repeat surgical intervention ranges from 3% to 14% after open surgical procedures.[9,10,48] Deep infections have not been reported after percutaneous posterior fixation.[45,48] The presence of a large subcutaneous degloving injury with hematoma must be recognized because the risk of infection and skin necrosis increases dramatically in patients with these injuries. The treatment of the fracture with an associated degloving lesion is still controversial. Percutaneous techniques may minimize the risk of infection and skin injury associated with the opening of these injuries. Careful débridement and dead space management at the time of open fixation is recommended, especially if the wound is contiguous with the surgical exposure. Staged limited open débridement of the soft-tissue lesion may have a role in the management of these lesions.

Iliosacral Screw Misplacement

The complex three-dimensional structure of the sacrum creates multiple opportunities for misplacement. Attempting to use the lag function of the screw to diminish residual widening of the sacroiliac joint can lead to perforation of the anterior sacral cortex if the screw is placed from slightly posterolateral to anteromedial in the plane perpendicular to the sacroiliac joint. This is easily avoided by accounting for the anticipated compression when determining screw length. In one series, 13% of the screws were either protruding out of the anterior sacral cortex or into the S1 foramen.[48] Misplacement caused by surgeon error occurred in 2% of patients.[45] In this series, the fluoroscopic lateral view of the sacrum was found to be crucial for avoiding anterior penetration of the sacral cortex and the inlet view was found to be less reliable. Complications include screw misplacement, fixation failure, and neurovascular injury among others related to intraoperative fluoroscopy or navigation systems.

Reduction

After complete sacroiliac joint dislocation, displacement is generally in a posterior direction as seen on the inlet view, flexion is generally seen on the outlet view, and vertical translation is generally seen on the AP view.[45] Residual sacral displacement of greater than 10 mm significantly decreases the safe space available for screw placement and puts the neurovascular structures at risk.[46] Early closed manipulation and stabilization may be more successful than delayed closed manipulation and stabilization because it minimizes the effects of the formation of consolidated hematoma and muscle spasm. Intraoperative traction in a combined anterior and distal vector while the patient is in the supine position may help correct the deformities.

Malunion and Fixation Failure

Healing in a nonanatomic position can lead to gait disturbance and sitting abnormalities. Although the definition of malunion is somewhat arbitrary, it was defined in one study of a small group of patients with surgically treated vertically unstable fractures as displacement of greater than 1 cm in any plane or clinical limb-length discrepancy of greater than 2 cm.[48] The authors of this study found that malunion was present in 46% of patients. Additionally, malunion was more common in patients with fractures without anterior stabilization and in those with fractures through the sacrum than in patients with anterior stabilization or more than one point of fixation posteriorly; these differences, however, did not reach clinical significance.

A recent study reported on 63 patients with vertically unstable pelvic ring injuries treated with closed reduction and iliosacral screw fixation.[11] All fixation failures occurred in the presence of vertical sacral fractures; anterior fixation was present in each instance. Failure did not correlate with the absence of anterior fixation or the number or position of the screws. Patient noncompliance has been shown to contribute to loss of reduction in 1.7% to 13% of patients treated with percutaneous or open techniques for unstable fractures.[9,10,45,51] Careful medical management of delirium tremens and head injury-related spasticity, which commonly occur in the trauma patient population, must be undertaken to prevent premature weight bearing.

Current recommendations to avoid displacement and subsequent malunion or nonunion include accurate reduction, maximizing fixation, and careful evaluation of patients for compliance and to determine effective rehabilitation protocols. Open reduction of vertical sacral fractures and consideration of additional fixation methods have been suggested, but are also associated with complications.[39]

Nerve Injury

Nerve injury after pelvic ring disruption has a poorer prognosis than after acetabular fracture or other lower extremity injuries. Nerve injury is associated with adverse short-term effects, particularly on pain management, as well as adverse effects on rehabilitation and the long-term function of patients. The severity of the associated neurologic injury is likely related to the displacement and the severity of the posterior pelvic ring injury. Displaced lumbosacral fractures and sacroiliac joint disruptions are more commonly associated with nerve injuries than are iliac wing fractures. Motor deficits occur more commonly in Tile type C (33%) than Tile type B injuries.[9] It has been reported that vertically unstable fractures of the sacrum are associated with a 56% incidence of neurologic deficit.[48] Residual deficits at long-term follow-up were common in this study. Of eight patients with preoperative neurologic deficit and long-term clinical follow-up, no patient exhibited complete recovery from neurologic deficit. In another series of surgically treated Tile type B and C fractures, the incidence of neurologic dysfunction was 13.5%, and only 30% of these patients experienced full neurologic recovery.[10]

Functional Outcomes

The negative effects of pelvic fracture on function are well documented in the literature. Even with low-energy, stable, type A pelvic fractures in the geriatric population, 84% of patients require some form of additional community support.[12] A simple outcome measure for short-term function is the Functional Independence Measure, which scores for feeding, transfer mobility, locomotion, expression, and social interaction. Using this scale, one study reported that 88 children with pelvic fractures were found to be significantly impaired, and 80% of patients with unstable fractures and 52% of those with stable fractures were found to require assistance for transfer and locomotion.[13] A gross measure of outcome that is often reported is return to work status. The low rates of patients with unstable pelvic fractures who are able to return to their original employment (range, 46% to 63%) underscore the complexity and severity of these injuries.[9,14,48]

A validated disease-specific outcome tool can allow comparison between populations and treatment methods, but one has yet to be developed and validated for pelvic injuries. The Majeed scoring system is one of the earliest outcome tools specifically for pelvic injuries and has been modified.[15] A 7-point system has been developed based on radiologic result (displacement of the anterior and posterior ring at the time of healing), clinical result (pain and physical activity level), and social reintegration (professional activities).[9] Another group of authors developed the Iowa Pelvic Score, which consists of 20 questions concerning activities of daily living, and weighted questions concerning work history, pain, limp, a visual pain analog, and cosmesis.[17] The Iowa Pelvic Score has been shown to correlate well with the Medical Outcomes Study Short Form 36-Item Health Survey (SF-36) scores on all but the mental health scale.[16,17] It has not, however, been validated for reproducibility, and it has not been applied to normal populations. The Oswestry score, a validated score for low back pain that is used frequently by physiotherapists, has also been used to evaluate patients with pelvic fractures.[18,19]

In addition to a disease-specific pelvic outcome tool, many outcome studies use a generic outcome measure such as the SF-36 or the Sickness Impact Profile.[18-20] These generic outcome measures have been validated and are reproducible. Published age and gender normative data are available for comparison to the general population. For example, a consecutive series of Tile type B and type C fractures, all surgically treated by the same surgeon, reported SF-36 results in which the patients with pelvic fracture showed a 14% impairment on the physical component score and a 5% impairment on the mental outcome score when compared with the normal population. There was no significant difference between the patients with Tile type B and type C fractures.[20] As with other generic measures, the effects of associated injuries on outcome must be considered. It is important to note that no known prospective functional outcome studies comparing different treatment methods have yet been conducted.

The Role of the Injury and Anatomic Reduction

Anatomic reduction is believed to be correlated with a higher probability of a good clinical result. Posterior pelvic ring correction and limb-length discrepancy correction were correlated with clinical outcome as measured by the SF-36 in a series of surgically treated unstable Tile type B and type C fractures.[10] Several long-term outcome studies, however, suggest that clinical results after pelvic fracture are multifactorial, and the role of anatomic reduction is less clear. Severity of injury and displacement (which may in turn adversely affect a surgeon's ability to achieve anatomic results) have been shown to correlate with poorer functional results.[9,21,48] Even in patients with accurate posterior reduction of Tile type C fractures, 20% had fair clinical results, and pa-

tients with Tile type B fractures were significantly more likely to be pain free than those with Tile type C fractures (89% versus 30%).[9] Other factors including severity of injury, soft-tissue injuries, neurologic injuries, and posttraumatic degenerative disease of the sacroiliac joint were thought to contribute to these poorer outcomes. When patients with vertically displaced fractures treated with external fixation but no internal fixation were assessed, no correlation was found between residual vertical displacement and either SF-36 score or Iowa Pelvic Score. A limb-length discrepancy was perceived by 63% of patients, but this did not correlate with radiographic residual vertical displacement. The combination of perceived limp plus perceived limb-length discrepancy and cosmetic deformity correlated with the Iowa Pelvic Score and the scores on three of eight SF-36 scales, but it did not correlate with radiographic evidence of vertical displacement.[17]

The Role of Associated Injuries

Associated injuries have a significant effect on mortality in patients with pelvic ring disruption.[14,22,23,52] The mortality rate in patients with closed pelvic fractures (18%) was primarily related to closed head injuries and multiple organ failure. A significantly higher mortality rate (25%) was noted in patients with open pelvic fractures, and mortality was associated with pelvic hemorrhage in more than half of these patients.[14] One study found that hypotension and injury severity score were the only factors that correlated with mortality in a subgroup of patients requiring angiography.[52] The study population consisted of 38 patients undergoing angiography according to a strict protocol. Indications were transfusion requirements of 4 units in 24 hours, 6 units in 48 hours, unstable patients with negative or borderline peritoneal lavage, and intraoperative findings of large retroperitoneal hematoma during laparotomy. Thirty-five patients were found to have bleeding from an arterial source in the pelvis, and the remaining three patients had splenic embolizations performed. Patients presenting with hypotension were significantly more likely to die than those who were normotensive (44% versus 17%). The authors suggested that once bleeding from the pelvic ring has been controlled the ultimate outcome is related to associated injuries.

In addition to affecting mortality, associated injuries adversely impact long-term functional outcomes. One study analyzed 74 patients with unstable pelvic ring injuries treated with open reduction internal fixation. Forty-three patients had associated head, maxillofacial, pulmonary, abdominal, genitourinary, or orthopaedic injuries, most of which required surgical intervention. Patients with associated injuries scored significantly lower on all scales of the SF-36 than those without associated injuries.[10]

Comorbidities

One study found a positive direct correlation with medical comorbidities (arthritis, diabetes, obesity, cardiovascular disease) in the presence of pelvic fracture and low scores on the physical function scale of the SF-36.[24] The effect of medical comorbidities on outcome, as measured by multivariate regression analysis, was greater than that of fracture displacement or severity.

Open Fractures

Another study reviewed a cohort of 44 patients with open pelvic fractures (4% of all pelvic fractures).[14] Mortality was high (25%), and blood product requirements were significantly higher than those of the patients with closed fractures. All patients who did not undergo fecal diversion in the presence of perineal wounds developed intrapelvic septic complications. Most were treated with external fixation. Significant chronic disability was documented. Comparing these results to those from a previously reported population of patients with closed pelvic fractures, patients with open pelvic fractures were found to have significantly poorer scores on the physical and physical functioning subscales when compared with age- and gender-matched normative data.[14,24]

Pregnancy and Pelvic Fracture

Maternal mortality rates in pregnant trauma patients with pelvic fractures range from 4% to 28%.[25] In the same scenario, fetal mortality ranged from 35% to 80% when associated with pelvic trauma.[25,26,52] Direct trauma to the fetus, placenta, or uterus is more commonly the cause of death than maternal hemorrhage with hypotension and/or maternal death (56% versus 36%). The trimester at the time of pelvic fracture had no influence on fetal outcome.

The orthopaedic outcome of pelvic fracture treatment has rarely been investigated in patients with pelvic fractures during pregnancy. In one study, the presence of the pregnancy necessitated modification of pelvic fracture treatment in two of three patients with live fetuses, and acceptable orthopaedic outcomes were achieved in all patients.[53] Although pelvic or acetabular surgery before delivery is rare, no fetal deaths have been reported as a result of such surgery in the absence of maternal multisystem organ failure and death.[26,53]

Genitourinary Outcomes

Although primary injury of the genitourinary tract may be more common after Tile type B injuries, genitourinary complaints were more common in higher-energy, Tile type C injuries (25%), even in the absence of primary injury to the genitourinary tract.[9] In a group of female patients with pelvic fractures, also with no primary genitourinary trauma, 21% reported genitourinary complaints. These were more common in patients with unstable fracture patterns and in those with fractures with initial and residual displacement ≥5 mm. Fractures that were specifically displaced vertically or laterally and exposed the pelvic floor to tensile stresses were associated with a statistically significant increase in the rate of urinary complaints.[26] One study reported a 33% incidence of bladder or sexual dysfunction in patients with vertically displaced fractures, but this did not correlate with residual vertical displacement, Iowa Pelvic Scores, or SF-36 scores.[17] Dyspareunia has been reported to occur in approximately 5.5% to 19% of women with pelvic fractures.[9,26] Erectile deficiency has been reported to occur in 12.5% of men after undergoing surgical treatment of Tile type C fractures.[9]

The use of open treatment and the timing of treatment for anterior pelvic ring lesions in the presence of urologic injury remains controversial. Late attention to urethral repair has been recognized in the literature to be detrimental to long-term orthopaedic outcome. In one study of 23 patients with posterior urethral injuries associated with pelvic fractures, the urologic management of 8 patients (35%) was found to adversely impact the management of the pelvic fracture.[27] Delayed urethral repair and the use of suprapubic cystostomy was found to preclude early aggressive fixation of pelvic fractures in four patients, three of whom remained disabled because of pelvic pain. In contrast, none of the patients treated with acute endoscopic realignment remained disabled from the pelvic injury. In another study, an aggressive combined orthopaedic and urologic team approach was used for 23 patients with combined pelvic ring and genitourinary injuries.[51] The protocol included open reduction and internal fixation of anterior pelvic ring injuries with simultaneous repair of bladder and/or urethral repair using magnet-facilitated realignment techniques. The use of suprapubic cystostomy tubes was avoided. There were no early infections, and only one late infection (4.3%) occurred. A total of four fixation failures (17%) occurred, one of which was associated with late deep infection. Late urologic complications were frequent (30%). Male patients had stricture (44%) and impotence (17%). One female patient (20%) had incontinence, which resolved after a bladder suspension surgery.

Summary

Closed treatment with external fixation and surgical stabilization is useful in improving patient survival, relieving pain, and improving patient mobilization. Controversies remain regarding the relative roles of closed versus open techniques and the ultimate importance of perfect anatomic reduction. Prospective randomized studies with functional outcome data and the development of a pelvis specific validated outcome tools are necessary to answer these questions.

Annotated References

1. McCormick JP, Morgan SJ, Smith WR: Clinical effectiveness of the physical examination in diagnosis of posterior pelvic ring injuries. *J Orthop Trauma* 2003;17:257-261.

   The authors of this article report that physical examination, specifically palpation of the posterior pelvis, in patients with pelvic fractures can accurately detect injuries of the posterior ring.

2. Nork SE, Jones CB, Harding SP, Mirza SK, Routt ML Jr: Percutaneous stabilization of U-shaped sacral fractures using iliosacral screws: Technique and early results. *J Orthop Trauma* 2001;15:238-246.

   The authors report that U-shaped sacral fractures are rare and occur after significant spinal axial loading. A paradoxic inlet view of the upper sacrum on the AP plain pelvic radiograph is typically sufficient for diagnosis. Delayed diagnosis can be avoided by physicians having a high degree of clinical suspicion and obtaining early lateral sacral radiographs and pelvic CT scans. Surgical stabilization may assist in early mobilization of the patient from recumbency and prevents progressive deformity with associated nerve root injury. Although percutaneous fixation diminishes potential blood loss and surgical times, it still allows subsequent sacral decompression of the local neural elements using open techniques when necessary.

3. Routt ML Jr, Falicor A, Woodhouse E, Schildhauer TA: Circumferential pelvic anti-shock sheeting: A temporary resuscitation aid. *J Orthop Trauma* 2002; 16:45-48.

4. Guillamondegui OD, Mahboubi S, Stafford PW, Nance ML: The utility of the pelvic radiograph in the assessment of pediatric pelvic fractures. *J Trauma* 2003;55:236-239.

   The authors of this article discuss the usefulness of the pelvic radiograph in the assessment of pediatric pelvic fractures and report that pelvic radiographs lack the sensitivity of pelvic CT scans for detecting pelvic fractures in all anatomic areas evaluated. Pelvic CT scans also provide additional information regarding soft-tissue injury that is not available on most pelvic radiographs.

5. Patel NH, Hunter J, Weber TG, Routt ML Jr: Rotational imaging of complex acetabular fractures. *J Orthop Trauma* 1998;12:59-63.

6. Dalal SA, Burgess AR, Siegel JH: Pelvic fracture in multiple trauma: Classification by mechanism is key to pattern of organ injury, resuscitative requirements, and outcome. *J Trauma* 1989;29:981-1002.

7. Mears DC, Velyvis J: Surgical reconstruction of late pelvic post-traumatic nonunion and malalignment. *J Bone Joint Surg Br* 2003;85:21-30.

   For patients with a pelvic nonunion with local osteopenia and malalignment, stabilization of all three pelvic columns is recommended. The authors found that true pelvic (united) malunions were the most satisfactorily realigned and had the fewest complications. Patients with ununited and unstable malalignments, especially those with heterotopic bone, had the poorest corrections and the most neurologic complications. The authors suggest that local resection of a symptomatic bony prominence and fixation in situ of a posterior pelvic nonunion provides highly effective symptomatic relief with fewer complications. Despite this, many patients had persistent low back pain.

8. Henry SM, Pollak AN, Jones AL, Boswell S, Scalea TM: Pelvic fracture in geriatric patients: A distinct clinical entity. *J Trauma* 2002;53:15-20.

9. Pohlemann T, Gansslen A, Schellwald O, Culemann U, Tscherne H: Outcome after pelvic ring injuries. *Injury* 1996;27(suppl 2):B31-B38.

10. Korovessis P, Baikousis A, Stamatakis M, Katonis P: Medium- and long-term results of open reduction and internal fixation for unstable pelvic ring fractures. *Orthopedics* 2000;23:1165-1171.

11. Griffin DR, Starr AJ, Reinert CM, Jones AL, Whitlock S: Vertically unstable pelvic fractures fixed with percutaneous iliosacral screws: Does posterior injury pattern predict fixation failure? *J Orthop Trauma* 2003;17:399-405.

   In this retrospective study of 62 patients whose vertically unstable pelvic ring disruptions were treated using closed reduction and iliosacral screw fixation (anterior fixation was performed in all but six patients), four patients with vertical sacral fractures lost fixation within the first 3 weeks. Failure was not associated with anterior fixation or length, number, or position of iliosacral screws.

12. Morris RO, Sonibare A, Green DJ, Masud T: Closed pelvic fractures: Characteristics and outcomes in older patients admitted to medical and geriatric wards. *Postgrad Med J* 2000;76:646-650.

13. Upperman JS, Gardner M, Gaines B, Schall L, Ford HR: Early functional outcome in children with pelvic fractures. *J Pediatr Surg* 2000;35:1002-1005.

14. Brenneman FD, Katyal D, Boulanger BR, Tile M, Redelmeier DA: Long-term outcomes in open pelvic fractures. *J Trauma* 1997;42:773-777.

15. Majeed SA: External fixation of the injured pelvis: The functional outcome. *J Bone Joint Surg Br* 1990; 72:612-614.

16. Miranda MA, Riemer BL, Butterfield SL, Burke CJ III: Pelvic ring injuries: A long term functional outcome study. *Clin Orthop* 1996;329:152-159.

17. Nepola JV, Trenhaile SW, Miranda MA, Butterfield SL, Fredericks DC, Riemer BL: Vertical shear injuries: Is there a relationship between residual displacement and functional outcome? *J Trauma* 1999; 46:1024-1030.

18. Gruen GS, Leit ME, Gruen RJ, Garrison HG, Auble TE, Peitzman AB: Functional outcome of patients with unstable pelvic ring fractures stabilized with open reduction and internal fixation. *J Trauma* 1995; 39:838-845.

19. Fairbank JC, Couper J, Davies JB, et al: The Oswestry low back pain disability questionnaire. *Physiotherapy* 1980;66:271-273.

20. Oliver CW, Twaddle B, Agel J, Routt ML Jr: Outcome after pelvic ring fractures: Evaluation using the medical outcomes short form SF-36. *Injury* 1996;27: 635-641.

21. Lindahl J, Hirvensalo E, Bostman O, et al: Failure of reduction with an external fixator in the management of injuries of the pelvic ring: Long term evaluation of 110 patients. *J Bone Joint Surg Br* 1999;81: 955-962.

22. Ferrera PC, Hill DA: Good outcomes of open pelvic fractures. *Injury* 1999;30:187-190.

23. Demetriades D, Karaiskakis M, Toutouzas K, Alo K, Velmahos G, Chan L: Pelvic fractures: Epidemiology and predictors of associated abdominal injuries and outcomes. *J Am Coll Surg* 2002;195:1-10.

24. McCarthy ML, MacKenzie EJ, Bosse MJ, Copeland CE, Hash C, Burgess AR: Functional status following orthopaedic trauma in young women. *J Trauma* 1995;39:828-837.

25. Leggon RE, Wood GC, Indeck MC: Pelvic fractures in pregnancy: Factors influencing maternal and fetal outcomes. *J Trauma* 2002;53:796-804.

26. Copeland CE, Bosse MJ, McCarthy ML, et al: Effect of trauma and pelvic function on female genitourinary, sexual, and reproductive function. *J Orthop Trauma* 1997;11:73-81.

27. Mayher BE, Guyton JL, Gingrich JR: Impact of urethral injury management on the treatment and outcome of concurrent pelvic fractures. *Urology* 2001;57:439-442.

28. Connor GS, McGwin G Jr, MacLennan PA, Alonso JE, Rue LW III: Early versus delayed fixation of pelvic ring fractures. *Am Surg* 2003;69:1019-1023.

The authors of this article report that because pelvic ring fracture fixation within the first week of injury results in significantly reduced incidence of pulmonary complication, shorter hospital stays, and reduced cost of care regardless of injury severity, a coordinated team approach to ensure prompt resuscitation, stabilization, and surgical fixation can result in more optimal patient outcomes.

29. Kabak S, Halici M, Tuncel M, Avsarogullari L, Baktir A, Basturk M: Functional outcome of open reduction and internal fixation for completely unstable pelvic ring fractures (type C): A report of 40 cases. *J Orthop Trauma* 2003;17:555-562.

Morbidity and mortality rates are higher in patients with completely unstable pelvic ring injuries. Emergency department stabilization and reconstruction of the pelvic ring with optimal surgical techniques in these patients can reduce morbidity and mortality rates. The authors of this study report that anterior and posterior internal fixation results in satisfactory clinical and radiologic outcomes and conclude that the affective status of patients is an important aspect that should be considered during the entire course of patient care.

30. Woods RK, O'Keefe G, Rhee P, Routt ML Jr, Maier RV: Open pelvic fracture and fecal diversion. *Arch Surg* 1998;133:281-286.

31. Kutsy RL, Robinson LR, Routt ML Jr: Lumbosacral plexopathy in pelvic trauma. *Muscle Nerve* 2000;23: 1757-1760.

32. Routt ML Jr, Nork SE, Mills WJ: High-energy pelvic ring disruptions. *Orthop Clin North Am* 2002;33:59-72.

High-energy pelvic ring disruptions are associated with numerous primary organ system injuries. Early, accurate pelvic reduction and stable fixation optimize patient outcome. A variety of fixation techniques have been advocated. The authors report that a multispecialty team approach is advantageous when managing these patients and their pelvic injuries.

33. Switzer JA, Nork SE, Routt ML Jr: Comminuted fractures of the iliac wing. *J Orthop Trauma* 2000;14: 270-276.

Because comminuted iliac fractures occur in two distinct patterns and are associated with numerous local injuries that complicate management, the authors of this article suggest that management protocols include early open reduction and stable internal fixation. Traumatic open wounds should not be closed primarily. Primary closure with closed suction drainage is effective in the management of associated degloving injuries. Extension of the fracture into the greater sciatic notch warrants further evaluation with pelvic angiography.

34. Ponson KJ, Hoek van Dijke GA, Joosse P, Snijders CJ, Agnew SG: Improvement of external fixator performance in type C pelvic ring injuries by plating of the pubic symphysis: An experimental study on 12 external fixators. *J Trauma* 2002;53:907-912.

35. Simonian PT, Routt ML Jr: Biomechanics of pelvic fixation. *Orthop Clin North Am* 1997;28:351-367.

36. Zobrist R, Messmer P, Levin LS, Regazzoni P: Endoscopic-assisted, minimally invasive anterior pelvic ring stabilization: A new technique and case report. *J Orthop Trauma* 2002;16:515-519.

37. Leighton RK, Waddell JP, Bray TJ, et al: Biomechanical testing of new and old fixation devices for vertical shear fractures of the pelvis. *J Orthop Trauma* 1991;5:313-317.

38. Teague DC, Graney DO, Routt ML Jr: Retropubic vascular hazards of the ilioinguinal exposure: A cadaveric and clinical study. *J Orthop Trauma* 1996;10: 156-159.

39. Howlett A, Nork SE, Routt ML Jr: Perioperative complications after open posterior pelvic surgery, in *Proceedings: 2005 Annual Meeting.* Rosemont, IL, American Academy of Orthopaedic Surgeons, 2005, p 602.

40. Yinger K, Scalise J, Olson SA, Bay BK, Finkemeier CG: Biomechanical comparison of posterior pelvic ring fixation. *J Orthop Trauma* 2003;17:481-487.

41. Borrelli J Jr, Koval KS, Helfet DL: Operative stabilization of fracture dislocations of the sacroiliac joint. *Clin Orthop Relat Res* 1996;329:141-146.

42. Barei DP, Bellabarba C, Mills WJ, Routt ML Jr: Percutaneous management of unstable pelvic ring disruptions. *Injury* 2001;32(suppl 1):SA33-SA44.

    Because percutaneous pelvic fixation stabilizes pelvic ring disruptions without extensive pelvic dissection, anterior and posterior percutaneous pelvic fixation techniques allow for acute and definitive treatment. Successful percutaneous pelvic fixation techniques depend on accurate closed reduction, excellent intraoperative fluoroscopic imaging, and detailed preoperative planning. Early pelvic stability diminishes hemorrhage, provides patient comfort, and allows early patient mobilization from recumbency.

43. Tucker MC, Nork SE, Simonian PT, Routt ML Jr: Simple anterior pelvic external fixation. *J Trauma* 2000;49:989-994.

    The authors of this study report that simple anterior pelvic external fixation frames can be used as either temporary, definitive, or supplementary fixation, depending on the pelvic injury pattern. Fluoroscopic imaging was used to insert all of the fixation pins into the iliac crest between the iliac cortical tables to a depth of at least 5 cm. Each patient had closed manipulative reduction. Seventy-five of the 80 pins (94%) were completely contained between the iliac cortical tables, according to the CT scans. The initial pelvic closed reductions were maintained until the fixators were removed in 37 of 40 patients (93%). Only one deep pin-tract infection developed, mandating early frame removal and intravenous antibiotic therapy.

44. Bellabarba C, Stewart JD, Ricci WM, DiPasquale TG, Bolhofner BR: Midline sagittal sacral fractures in anterior-posterior compression pelvic ring injuries. *J Orthop Trauma* 2003;17:32-37.

45. Routt ML, Simonian PT, Mills WJ: Iliosacral screw fixation: Early complications of the percutaneous technique. *J Orthop Trauma* 1997;11:584-589.

46. Reilly MC, Bono CM, Lithouki B, Sirkin M, Behrens FF: The effect of sacral malreduction on the safe placement of iliosacral screws. *J Orthop Trauma* 2003;17:88-94.

47. Hamill J, Holden A, Paice R, Civil I: Pelvic fracture pattern predicts pelvic arterial haemorrhage. *Aust N Z J Surg* 2000;70:338-343.

48. Keating JF, Werier J, Blachut P, Broekhuyse H, Meek RN, O'Brien PJ: Early fixation of the vertically unstable pelvis: The role of iliosacral screw fixation of the posterior lesion. *J Orthop Trauma* 1999;13:107-113.

49. Webb LX, Rush PT, Fuller SB: Greenfield filter prophylaxis of pulmonary embolism in patients undergoing surgery for acetabular fracture. *J Orthop Trauma* 1992;6:139-145.

50. Stover MD, Morgan SJ, Bosse MJ, et al: Prospective comparison of contrast-enhanced computed tomography versus magnetic resonance venography in the detection of occult deep pelvic vein thrombosis in patients with pelvic and acetabular fractures. *J Orthop Trauma* 2002;16:613-621.

51. Routt ML, Simonian PT, Defalco AJ, Miller J, Clarke T: Internal fixation in pelvic fractures and primary repairs of associated genitourinary disruptions: A team approach. *J Trauma* 1996;40:784-790.

52. O'Neill PA, Riina J, Sclafani S, Tornetta P III: Angiographic findings in pelvic fractures. *Clin Orthop* 1996;329:60-67.

53. Pape HC, Pohlemann T, Gansslen A, Simon R, Koch C, Tscherne H: Pelvic fractures in pregnant multiple trauma patients. *J Orthop Trauma* 2000;14:238-244.

Chapter 23

Acetabular Fractures: Acute Evaluation

Michael J. Bellino, MD

Anatomic Considerations

The innominate bone is a complex structure that supports the acetabulum. A clear understanding of the anatomy of the acetabular region is needed to achieve successful reconstruction of the hip. The acetabulum can be described as a structure contained in the limbs of an inverted Y. The anterior limb of the Y is the anterior column or iliopubic segment, and the posterior limb is the posterior column or ilioischial segment. The arch between the limbs of the Y is the roof of the acetabulum (Figure 1). The columns are surgical divisions of the innominate bone that relate to differing aspects of surgical access.

The anterior column extends from the iliac crest to the symphysis pubis. It includes the gluteus medius tubercle, the anterior pillar, and the anterior halves of the acetabulum and cotyloid fossa. When viewed from the anteroposterior and medial lateral perspectives, the anterior column is concave. The anterior border of this segment is the anterior-superior iliac spine, the interspinous notch, and the anterior-inferior iliac spine. The posterior column extends from the sciatic buttress at the anterior and superior border of the greater sciatic notch to the ischiopubic ramus. The posterior border of the posterior column is the anterior border of the greater sciatic notch, the ischial spine, and the lesser sciatic notch.

Mechanisms of Injury

Fractures of the acetabulum result from forces directed through four points of the body—the foot with an extended knee; the knee, which is usually flexed; the greater trochanter; and the posterior aspect of the pelvis. An infinite variety of fracture patterns can result depending on the attitude of the extremity and the direction and magnitude of the force (Figure 2). The velocity of the force also plays a role in determining the fracture pattern in conjunction with the strain rate sensitivies of the involved tissues.[1]

Associated Injuries

Fractures of the acetabulum frequently occur as the result of high-energy trauma, which occurs with the highest prevalence in younger patient populations. Patients with fractures of the acetabulum (essentially fractures of the pelvic ring) are challenging to treat. Acetabular injuries frequently involve associated injuries to other systems, which must be treated promptly to avoid both early and late complications.[2]

In a study of 262 displaced acetabular fractures, there was at least one additional injury in 56% of patients.[3] Fifty-one fractures (19%) had an associated head injury; 20 fractures (8%) occurred with an abdominal injury, 40 fractures (18%) with a chest injury, 17 fractures (6%) with a genitourinary injury; 91 fractures (35%) with an injury involving an extremity, 11 fractures (4%) with an injury of the spine, and 33 fractures (13%) with a nerve palsy. Two or more associated injuries were found in 34 fractures (13%); 114 fractures (44%) were not associated with other injuries.

A Morel-Lavallé lesion is a soft-tissue internal degloving injury associated with pelvic and acetabular fractures. These lesions also may occur as a result of blunt trauma to the pelvis in the absence of a fracture. The blunt trauma imparts a sheer force that disrupts the

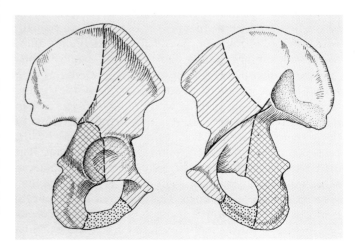

Figure 1 The external and internal aspects of the innominate bone showing the areas of the anterior column (hatched area), posterior column (cross-hatched area), and ischiopubic rami (speckled area). *(Reproduced with permission from Letournel E, Judet R (eds): Fractures of the Acetabulum, ed 2. Berlin, Germany, Springer-Verlag, 1993.)*

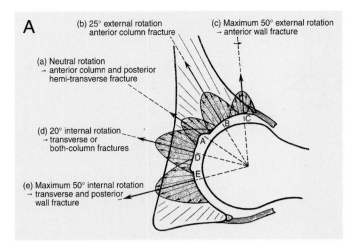

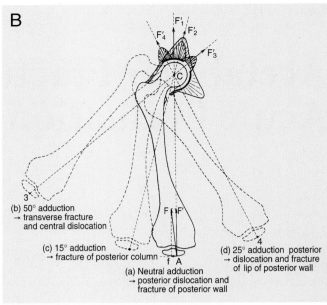

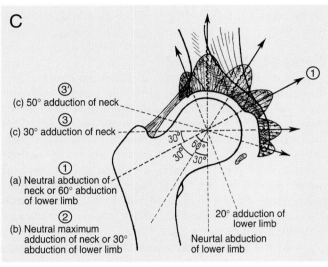

Figure 2 A, Coronal section through the hip joint showing types of fractures produced by varying degrees of hip rotation. **B,** Axial section through the hip joint showing the types of fractures produced by varying the degree of adduction. F = force applied at point A, F' = component of force transmitted to the acetabulum, C = center of rotation of femoral head. **C,** Coronal section through the hip joint showing types of fractures produced by varying degree of adduction. *(Reproduced with permission from Letournel E, Judet R (eds): Fractures of the Acetabulum, ed 2. Berlin, Germany, Springer-Verlag, 1993.)*

subcutaneous tissue from the deep fascia. The subcutaneous space that is created is filled with serosanguineous fluid and a variable amount of viable and necrotic adipose tissue. The incidence of Morel-Lavallé lesions is likely underreported. In one review, 8.3% of patients with acetabular fractures that resulted from blunt trauma to the trochanteric region had a Morel-Lavallé lesion.[1] Another retrospective review of 24 patients with a Morel-Lavallé lesion showed that 46% of the lesions were culture positive, most with *Staphylococcus epidermidis*. Three of these patients subsequently developed a deep bone infection.[4] The lesion is diagnosed by the presence of a soft-tissue swelling that is fluctuant. The area may be ecchymotic or have decreased cutaneous sensation. The lesion may occur anywhere from the lumbosacral region to the knee. The preferred treatment for a Morel-Lavallé lesion is incision and débridement, either before or during definitive fixation of the acetabular fracture (when the lesion is on the surgical side of the fracture). The wound is packed open. When granulation tissue appears, the wound may be considered for delayed primary closure. The incision must be placed in a loca-

tion that will not compromise the subsequent incision for definitive fixation of the acetabular fracture. Also, the incision must not create a large skin flap that could result in compromised blood flow to the skin edge.

A posterior hip dislocation associated with fracture of the acetabulum does not correlate with a poor prognosis.[1,3] In the study of 262 displaced acetabular fractures, 59 of 83 hips (71%) associated with a posterior dislocation showed good to excellent clinical outcomes compared with 109 of 140 hips (78%) that were not associated with a posterior hip dislocation.[3] It is generally accepted that an isolated posterior dislocation of the hip results in a high incidence of osteonecrosis of the femoral head. The reason that this risk is lower in fracture-dislocations is unknown. A posterior fracture-dislocation of the hip should be urgently reduced. The reduction may be performed in the emergency department after giving the patient a rapidly acting general anesthetic agent and should include appropriate airway monitoring. The procedure also may be done in the operating room. Reduction of the dislocation may be prevented by several factors including not providing the patient with adequate anesthesia or muscle relaxant, the presence of interposed soft tissue (such as capsule or external rotators), and the presence of interposed bony fragments (such as posterior wall or femoral head fragments). An associated femoral fracture, especially a proximal fracture, may complicate the reduction because it is difficult to obtain adequate leverage. A Schantz pin placed in the intertrochanteric region or in the anterior femoral neck may facilitate the reduction when the patient has a proximal femoral fracture. If the attempt at closed reduction fails, then open reduction must be performed.

Patients with a femoral head fracture that is associated with an acetabular fracture often have poor outcomes. Femoral head fractures can occur as a separate fragment (a Pipkin fracture) or an impaction of the femoral head. One study of 35 femoral head fractures showed overall good results in 47% of patients. Complications included 11 instances of osteonecrosis, 11 instances of traumatic arthritis, and 3 instances of hip infections.[5] There are numerous treatment options for patients with femoral head fractures that occur with acetabular fractures. Femoral head fractures, which are small and infrafoveal, typically occur in combination with a posterior wall fracture, and may be considered for incision. It is possible to perform the excision of the femoral head fragment through the Kocher-Langenbeck approach. If the femoral head fracture is large and infrafoveal, the posterior approach affords poor access for reduction and fixation and may jeopardize the blood supply to the fragment and to the femoral head. Under these circumstances, the femoral head fracture is best treated through the Smith-Petersen approach followed by subsequent reduction and fixation of the acetabular fracture through the Kocher-Langenbeck approach; alternatively, a trochanteric flip can be used in selected patients.[6] If the posterior acetabular fracture is being treated nonsurgically, the femoral head fracture can be treated through the Smith-Petersen approach.

Certain types of acetabular fractures may be associated with an impaction injury to the femoral head resulting in articular cartilage and subchondral bone injury. This injury may occur with a transverse or T-shaped fracture pattern in which the femoral head is displaced medially and the superior and lateral aspect of the femoral head impacts on the roughened fracture surface of the intact ilium. Alternatively, in a posterior wall fracture-dislocation, the femoral head may contact the bony fracture surfaces as it pushes the posterior wall fragment posteriorly. In the posteriorly dislocated position, femoral head damage may occur as the femoral head is impacted onto the retroacetabular surface. Either bony or articular injury to the femoral head is clearly the most predictive factor for poor outcome.[3] Older patients with damage involving more than 25% of the femoral head should be considered for total hip replacement. The younger patient with this type of injury is not an ideal candidate for total hip replacement and therefore should be considered for treatment with rotational osteotomy of the femur.[7]

A fracture of the femoral neck that occurs in combination with an acetabular fracture is rare. A displaced femoral neck fracture in a young patient is considered an orthopaedic emergency. When this combination of injuries occurs, priority is given to treatment of the femoral neck fracture. Both injuries should be treated with the approach that offers the best probability of a satisfactory reduction. The Smith-Petersen approach affords excellent exposure of the femoral neck and may be used concomitantly with the Kocher-Langenbeck approach. Alternatively, the Watson-Jones approach may be used; however, the incision for the Watson-Jones approach must be placed in a slightly more anterior location if the posterior approach is later to be used.[7]

Radiographic Evaluation

Radiographic assessment of the acetabulum includes AP and Judet (45° oblique) views of the pelvis (Figure 3). The AP view of the pelvis is obtained with the x-ray beam centered over the symphysis pubis (Figure 4). The Judet views include the obturator oblique and iliac oblique views. The iliac oblique view is obtained with the patient tilted 45°; the affected hip is adjacent to the x-ray cassette and the x-ray beam is centered over the affected hip (Figure 5). The obturator oblique view is obtained with the patient tilted 45°; the unaffected hip is adjacent to the x-ray cassette, and the x-ray beam is centered over the affected hip (Figure 6). The innominate bone viewed from cephalad to caudad has a superior iliac segment that is 90° perpendicular to the inferior ischiopubic section (Figure 7). When the x-ray beam is tangent to these surfaces of the innominate bone, each section is seen in profile. The iliac oblique view exposes the profile of the ilium, whereas the obturator oblique views expose the obturator foramen. The iliac oblique view essentially superimposes the anterior superior iliac spine with a view of the posterior superior iliac spine. On the obturator oblique view, the tip of the coccyx should be centered slightly above the femoral head. These views are obtained by rotating the patient 45° from side to side rather than tilting the beam of the x-rays. For an injured patient this is an uncomfortable maneuver; therefore, patients must be adequately premedicated before obtaining these views. It is imperative that the entire pelvis is visible on the radiograph.

There are six essential landmarks of the acetabulum that are evaluated on the AP radiograph (Figure 8). The radiographic landmarks are the posterior wall, the anterior wall, the roof of the acetabulum, the radiographic U or teardrop, the ilioischial line (the landmark of the posterior column), and the iliopectineal line (the landmark of the anterior column). Each landmark corre-

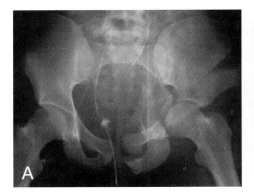 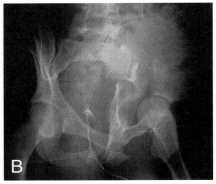 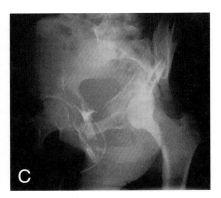

Figure 3 **A,** AP radiographic view of the pelvis. **B,** Iliac oblique radiographic view of the left hip. **C,** Obturator oblique radiographic view of the left hip.

sponds to a specific structure with the exception of the teardrop. The teardrop is a radiographic finding produced by the x-ray beam being tangent to the outer wall of the obturator canal, which forms the inner limb of the teardrop. The external limb of the teardrop is formed by the surface of the outer aspect of the acetabular fossa. The oblique views allow comparison between the injured side and the uninjured side.

The iliac oblique view is best suited to see the anterior wall as it lies unobstructed from the superimposed view of the posterior wall. The iliac oblique view also shows the unobstructed posterior border of the bone. The obturator oblique view best shows the anterior column and iliopectineal line, whereas the posterior wall is more apparent as it lies unobstructed from superimposition of the anterior wall. In addition, the bony structure of the obturator ring is clearly seen.

The two-dimensional CT scan is an essential part of the radiologic evaluation of fractures of the acetabulum. A CT scan can be used to detect impaction injury to the articular surfaces of the femoral head and acetabulum, as well as for identifying each articular loose fragment (Figures 9 and 10). The two-dimensional CT scan also is helpful in determining fracture planes, which are often difficult to determine accurately on the plain radiographs (Figure 11). Plain radiographs primarily have been used to assess the quality of reduction following surgery. A recent study has compared the use of plain radiographs with CT scans to assess articular fragment displacements in acetabular fractures.[8] Investigators retrospectively evaluated a series of CT scans and plain radiographs of patients with displaced acetabular fractures and also used a canine acetabulum fracture model. Plain radiographs showed poor sensitivity at detecting step deformity in fractures involving a single column. CT scans were superior in assessing step and gap displacement compared with plain radiographs in this model.[8]

The introduction of three-dimensional CT reconstruction of the pelvis has improved the understanding of the complex nature of fractures of the acetabulum (Figure 12). The three-dimensional image may be manipu-

lated to visualize fracture planes from different perspectives. The femur and sacrum may be subtracted from the innominate bone for an unobstructed view of the fracture (Figure 13). The three-dimensional CT reconstruction is particularly useful to verify the interpretation of the plain radiographs and CT scan, preoperative planning, and provides less experienced physicians with an acceptable level of correct diagnoses.

Classification

The Letournel classification system for acetabular fractures, based on the column concept of the anatomy of the acetabulum, was first presented by Letournel in 1961 and was based on a study of 75 cases.[9] The classification system has evolved since its inception and is the most widely accepted classification system for acetabular fractures in use today.[1]

The Letournel system can provide information that will assist in surgical treatment decisions. This system has been assessed for interobserver and intraobserver reliability and has been compared with the reliability of CT scans. In a recent study,[10] three different groups of reviewers with different levels of training were given AP and Judet radiographs randomly selected from an acetabular fracture database. These radiographs were then used to classify the fracture pattern using the Letournel system. The reviewers were later given CT scans to use in conjunction with the radiographs to classify the fractures. The Letournel acetabular fracture classification system was determined to have substantial reliability; the additional information provided by the CT scans did not appear to improve the reliability of the classification.

Acetabular fractures are divided into two main groups—elementary fractures and associated fractures. Elementary fractures involve a portion of a column or the column in its entirety (Figure 14). The transverse fracture is included in this group because of its simple form, despite the fact that it involves both the anterior and posterior columns. Elementary fractures are further divided into five forms including the posterior wall, pos-

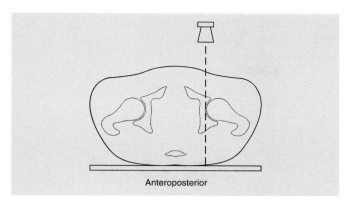

Figure 4 The AP view of the pelvis is obtained with the x-ray beam centered over the symphysis pubis.

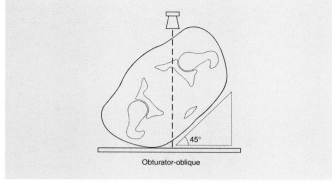

Figure 6 The obturator oblique view of the pelvis is obtained with the patient tilted 45°, the unaffected hip is adjacent to the x-ray cassette, and the x-ray beam is centered over the affected hip.

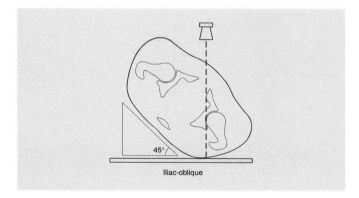

Figure 5 The iliac oblique view of the pelvis is obtained with the patient tilted 45°, the affected hip is adjacent to the x-ray cassette, and the x-ray beam is centered over the affected hip.

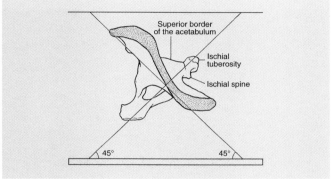

Figure 7 The innominate bone viewed from the cephalad to the caudad direction shows that the iliac segment and the ischiopubic segment are oriented orthogonally with respect to one another. *(Reproduced with permission from Letournel E, Judet R (eds): Fractures of the Acetabulum, ed 2. Berlin, Germany, Springer-Verlag, 1993.)*

terior column, interior wall, anterior column, and transverse (Figure 15).

Associated fracture patterns involve at least two of the elementary fracture patterns. The five associated fracture patterns are T-shaped, associated posterior column and posterior wall, associated transverse and posterior wall, associated anterior and posterior hemitransverse, and both-column fractures.

Simple Fracture Patterns

Fractures of the posterior wall typically involve the rim of the acetabulum, a portion of the retroacetabular surface, and a variable portion of the articular cartilage. Impaction of the articular cartilage is a common finding for this fracture pattern and should be diagnosed preoperatively using plain radiographs or a CT scan. Extended posterior wall fractures can involve the entire retroacetabular surface, and include a portion of the greater or lesser sciatic notch and/or the ischial tuberosity. The ilioischial line remains intact on the AP view. Posterior column fractures include only the ischial portion of the bone. The entire retroacetabular surface is displaced

with the posterior column. As the vertical line separating the anterior from the posterior column traverses inferiorly, it most commonly enters the obturator foramen. A fracture of the inferior pubic ramus is typically found. In some cases, the fracture line traverses just posterior to the obturator foramen, splitting the ischial tuberosity. The ilioischial line is typically displaced and disassociated from the teardrop. However, when a large portion of the quadrilateral surface remains intact with the posterior column, the teardrop and a portion of the pelvic brim will be displaced along with the posterior column.

Fractures of the anterior wall involve the central portion of the anterior column. The inferior pubic ramus is not fractured. The pelvic brim is displaced in its midportion. AP and obturator oblique radiographs show displacement of the iliopectineal line. The AP and iliac oblique radiographs show interruption of the anterior rim contour.

Anterior column fractures can occur anywhere from a very low to a very high level. Low-level fractures involve only the superior ramus and pubic portion of the acetabulum. High-level fractures can involve the entire

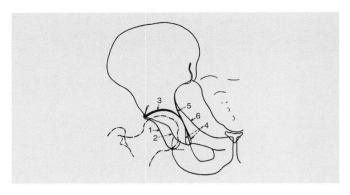

Figure 8 The six radiographic landmarks of the acetabulum. (1) Posterior wall. (2) Anterior wall. (3) Roof. (4) Radiographic U. (5) Ilioischial line. (6) Iliopectineal line. *(Adapted with permission from Letournel E, Judet R (eds): Fractures of the Acetabulum, ed 2. Berlin, Germany, Springer-Verlag, 1993.)*

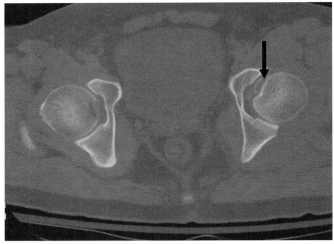

Figure 10 Axial two-dimensional tomography scan through the hip joints. The arrow points to an intra-articular osteochondral fragment of the left hip joint.

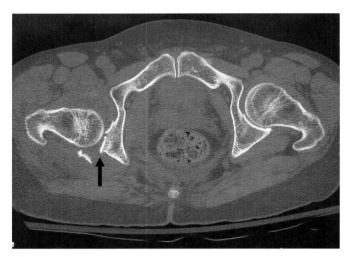

Figure 9 Axial two-dimensional tomography scan through the hip joint showing marginal impaction of the right posterior wall acetabulum fracture. The arrow points to the segment of articular cartilage and subchondral bone that is impacted.

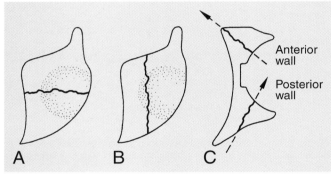

Figure 11 Fracture planes as seen with axial two-dimensional tomography scan. **A,** Plane of a both-column fracture. **B,** Plane of a transverse fracture. **C,** Plane of anterior and posterior wall fractures. *(Reproduced with permission from Letournel E, Judet R (eds): Fractures of the Acetabulum, ed 2. Berlin, Germany, Springer-Verlag, 1993.)*

anterior border of the innominate bone. The pelvic brim and iliopectineal line are displaced. Medial translation of the entire roof, or a portion of the roof, is typical of displacement of a high- or intermediate-level anterior column fracture. This type of displacement also can be seen with anterior column plus posterior hemitransverse, and both column fracture patterns.

Transverse fractures divide the innominate bone into two portions, with a horizontally displaced fracture line crossing the acetabulum at a variable level. The innominate bone is then divided into a superior part composed of the iliac wing and a portion of the roof of the acetabulum. The lower part of the bone, the ischiopubic segment, is composed of an intact obturator foramen with the anterior and posterior walls of the acetabulum. Letournel subdivided transverse fractures into the following groups: transtectal, the transverse fracture line crosses the superior acetabular articular surface; juxtatectal, the transverse fracture line crosses at the junction of the superior acetabular articular surface and superior cotyloid fossa; and infratectal, the transverse fracture line crosses through the cotyloid fossa.

Associated Fracture Patterns

The association of a posterior column and posterior wall fracture divides the posterior column into a larger posterior column component and an associated posterior wall component. The ilioischial line is typically displaced and disassociated from the teardrop.

The association of the transverse plus posterior wall fracture combines a normal transverse configuration with one or more separate posterior wall fragments. A fracture of the inferior pubic ramus does not typically occur.

The T-shaped fracture is similar to the transverse fracture except for the addition of a vertical split along the quadrilateral surface and acetabular fossa (the stem of the T), which divides the anterior from the posterior column. An associated fracture of the inferior pubic

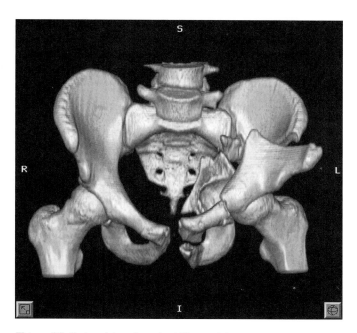

Figure 12 AP view of three-dimensional CT scan of the pelvis.

ramus is typically present. This vertical fracture line can enter the obturator foramen, or leave it intact, exiting through the ischium.

The anterior plus posterior hemitransverse fracture combines an anterior wall or anterior column fracture with a horizontal and horizontal transverse component, which traverses the posterior column at a low level. The distinction between the associated anterior column plus associated posterior hemitransverse and T-shaped patterns is often subtle. In the anterior plus posterior hemitransverse fracture, the anterior component is typically at a higher level and is more displaced than the posterior component.

It is important to realize that transverse, associated transverse plus posterior wall, T-shaped, and anterior plus posterior hemitransverse fractures all show involvement of the anterior and posterior columns of the acetabulum but are not both-column fractures. In these four fracture types, a portion of the articular surface remains in its normal position, attached to the intact portion of the ilium. The both-column fracture is therefore unique, with its division of all segments of articular cartilage from the ilium. The both-column fracture is associated with the "spur" sign—the fractured edge of the intact posterior iliac wing is seen prominently relative to the medially displaced articular segments on the obturator oblique radiographic view. This sign is pathognomonic of a both-column fracture.

As with all anatomic classification systems, there is some overlap between fracture types. If this system of classification was perfectly symmetric there would be more than 10 categories. The additional groups are incorporated into the 10 fracture types. Associated ante-

rior column and anterior wall fractures are included with anterior column fractures. Similarly, anterior wall plus posterior hemitransverse fractures are included with anterior column plus posterior hemitransverse fractures. Associated posterior column and anterior hemitransverse fractures are considered T-shaped fractures.

Emergent Treatment

Acetabular fractures are the result of high-energy mechanisms, which frequently result in injury to other body systems. The dramatic appearance of the pelvic radiograph must not divert attention from the possibility of life-threatening visceral injury. The resuscitation and primary survey of the patients should proceed simultaneously according to Advanced Trauma Life Support guidelines.[11] A detailed neurologic examination is performed to identify existing deficits. The pelvis, perineum, and surrounding integument are examined. The position of the lower extremities is examined to rule out the presence of a dislocated hip. A careful evaluation of the AP pelvic radiograph will identify most injuries to the hip and pelvis.

Open fractures of the acetabulum are uncommon. Contamination of the hip joint may occur with open pelvic fractures as a result of severe perineal and gluteal wounds, vaginal lacerations, or bowel injury. Bladder injuries occurring with a pelvic ring injury are repaired at the time of débridement and fixation. Urinary catheter drainage is preferable to suprapubic catheter drainage of the bladder. Surgical drains placed in the retropubic Retzius space will decrease the rate of infection. Bowel injury may require diversion. Coordination and planning with the trauma surgeon will help prevent compromise of subsequent approaches required for acetabular reconstruction.

In the past, the use of skeletal traction before surgical treatment of fractures of the acetabulum was not advocated by some surgeons. It was believed that traction was unnecessary because it would not maintain a perfect reduction and would not maintain the reduction of an unstable dislocation of the femoral head. Additionally, local pin tract complication such as infection could occur and would delay surgical treatment. Despite this view, skeletal traction is frequently used for stabilization of acetabulum fractures before surgery.

Preoperative Evaluation for Deep Venous Thrombosis
Multiple trauma patients with orthopaedic injuries, particularly fractures of the pelvis and acetabulum, should be evaluated after resuscitation and hemodynamic stabilization are achieved to determine the risk for development of deep venous thrombosis (DVT). DVT has been reported in 58% of patients with major trauma and 61% of patients with pelvic fractures.[12] The incidence of pulmonary embolism (PE) in this population has been re-

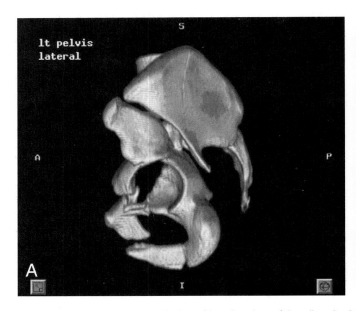

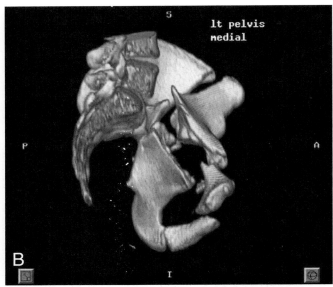

Figure 13 Lateral **(A)** and medial **(B)** views of innominate bone of three-dimensional CT scan of the pelvis.

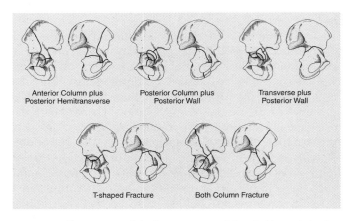

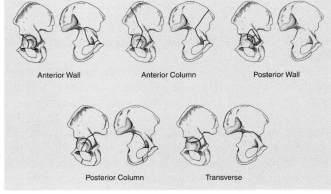

Figure 14 Elementary acetabular fracture patterns. *(Adapted with permission from Letournel E, Judet R (eds): Fractures of the Acetabulum, ed 2. Berlin, Germany, Springer-Verlag, 1993.)*

Figure 15 Associated acetabular fracture patterns. *(Adapted with permission from Letournel E, Judet R (eds): Fractures of the Acetabulum, ed 2. Berlin, Germany, Springer-Verlag, 1993.)*

ported in up to 10% of patients and remains the most common cause of mortality after a traumatic event.[12,13] Duplex ultrasound is the most widely used screening tool for the detection of DVT in the lower extremities. This diagnostic tool has limited use in the proximal venous system. The rates of DVT are likely underdiagnosed. PE has occurred in patients with negative results from screening examinations of the lower extremities; therefore, the etiology of the thrombi is likely the proximal venous system. The detection of DVT in patients with pelvic and acetabular fractures remains a clinical challenge. Physical examination is unreliable and does not address proximal thrombi. Venography is considered the gold standard for use in detecting lower extremity DVT, but is of limited value for the evaluation of venous thrombi that are proximal to the inguinal ligament. Venography is a time-consuming, costly, invasive proce-

dure with associated morbidity. It requires specialized personnel and does not allow for adequate visualization of the proximal venous systems. Magnetic resonance venography (MRV) is potentially an attractive tool for the evaluation of the pelvic veins. MRV has been reported to have sensitivity and specificity rates of 100%.[14] This method is noninvasive, does not involve ionizing contrast, and has three-dimensional capabilities. MRV, however, is costly and time consuming and involves placing patients who are being intensively monitored in the intensive care unit in the scanner device. Computed tomography venography (CTV) appears to have sensitivity and specificity rates comparable to MRV. Most trauma patients routinely undergo evaluation with CT and would only require the addition of contrast medium to obtain a CTV. The incidence of DVT in patients with pelvic and acetabular fractures detected by CTV and

MRV was compared in a prospective study.[14] Positive screening studies were confirmed by selective pelvic venographies. The false positive rate for MRV was 100% and for CTV was 50%. The authors concluded that positive results obtained with these screening studies should be validated by selective pelvic venography.

Other investigators performed a prospective, blinded study to assess the values of preoperative contrast venography and MRV for the detection of DVT in the thigh and pelvis of patients with acetabulum fractures. In 33% of patients, MRV detected asymptomatic thrombi. Forty-two percent of these findings were confirmed with contrast venography; however, contrast venography failed to identify the remaining 58% of thrombi noted with MRV. The authors concluded that MRV was superior to contrast venography for the preoperative evaluation of proximal DVT in patients with an acetabular fracture.[15]

Indications for Surgical Treatment

Patients with displaced acetabular fractures are usually treated with surgical reduction and fixation to allow early ambulation and to decrease the risk of posttraumatic arthritis. Nonsurgical treatment, however, can still be successful for a minority of displaced acetabulum fractures. Indications for nonsurgical treatment are based on the analysis of the fracture configuration. The decision to elect surgical treatment is based on a review of the initial series of plain radiographs and CT scans. Attempts at closed reduction by manipulation under anesthesia or skeletal traction are not useful for the treatment of articular fractures of the acetabulum. Nonsurgical treatment is reserved for those patients with nondisplaced fractures, for patients with tolerable incongruity or displacement, and for patients who have contraindications to surgery (such as local or systemic infection and severe osteoporosis). Many elderly patients, however, even with some degree of osteoporosis, can benefit from surgery. Bone of satisfactory quality can be found for fixation, particularly along the pelvic brim and greater sciatic notch. Relative contraindications include advanced age, associated medical conditions, and associated soft-tissue or systemic injuries.

Displaced fractures that should be considered for nonsurgical treatment include fractures in which (1) a large portion of the acetabulum remains intact and the femoral head remains congruent with this portion of the acetabulum, and (2) there is a secondary congruence present following only moderate displacement of a both-column fracture.

The single column fracture can be treated nonsurgically. The primary requirement is that the femoral head remains stable within the acetabulum. It has been suggested that a stress examination using fluoroscopy be performed on the anesthetized patient as a final confir-mation when nonsurgical treatment is being considered.[16] In patients with posterior wall fractures, indications for surgical stabilization include instability of the hip, associated marginal impaction of the articular surface, and retained osteochondral fragments. If the CT scan (on the CT cut that shows maximal involvement) shows that less than 50% of the width of the posterior articular cartilage is displaced, nonsurgical treatment could be considered if the posterior wall injury is part of a more complex pattern requiring an ilioinguinal approach. Any posterior wall fracture associated with instability of the hip should be considered for open reduction and internal fixation.

To assess the size of the intact portion of acetabulum, it is useful to perform roof arc measurements.[17] Similar determinations can be made from the CT scan. A CT scan of the superior acetabular articular surface from the vertex to 10 mm inferior to the vertex is equivalent to an area described by all three roof arc measurements of 45°. At 10 mm below the acetabular vertex, the subchondral bone appears as a ring or arc. If nonsurgical treatment is to be considered, the femoral head should be congruous with the roof of the acetabulum on three views of the pelvis taken when the patient is not in traction, and all roof arc measurements should be more than 45°, or a CT scan should show no fracture lines involving the superior acetabular articular surface in the superior 10 mm of the acetabulum.[18]

The CT arc measurement technique in assessing fractures for potential open reduction and internal fixation is most applicable for use in the anterior column, and less so in the posterior column. A particularly helpful application is to evaluate the anterior column component of a T-shaped fracture. If the anterior column component is at a low level (below 10 mm of the acetabular vertex) only the posterior portion of the fracture will be treated surgically.

A both-column fracture with secondary congruence presents a unique situation. Because both-column fractures detach all articular segments from the intact ilium, the fracture fragments can remain congruously grouped around the femoral head despite medial and proximal displacement of the femoral head and some rotational displacement of the fragments. CT can be used to assess coverage of the superior portion of the femoral head in its displaced position.

Surgical treatment should be performed within 10 days of the injury so that the fracture fragments remain mobile. Three weeks after injury, bony callus is usually present making reduction of the fracture more difficult.

Biomechanics of Fixation

There has been a relative paucity of data regarding the implants and techniques used for internal fixation of acetabular fractures. Several methods exists for surgical internal fixation of acetabular fractures. The choice of which construct to use depends on fracture pattern, the approach chosen, and surgeon preference. Most studies focus on the relative stiffness of the various constructs. One recent study examined the comparative strength of three methods of fixation of transverse acetabular fractures in a formalin-treated cadaveric pelvic model.[19] The fractures were fixed with anterior and posterior column lag screws, anterior lag screws and a posterior screw and wire construct, or a posterior 3.5-mm pelvic reconstruction plate. The method that used two lag screws had higher stiffness when compared with the other methods; however, the stiffness was not statistically significant. The maximum load to failure was significantly higher in the fixation method using a plate construct. The use of formalin-treated specimens was a limitation of the study.

In a another study, a biomechanical evaluation of various methods of fixation for transverse acetabular fractures in a synthetic pelvic model was presented.[20] In part one of this study, transverse acetabular fractures were fixed with a 10-hole pelvic reconstruction plate and one of four screw configurations. The stiffest construct resulted from two screws on each side of the fracture with one screw placed near the fracture and the other screw placed at the end of the plate. In part two of the study, transverse acetabular fracture fixation methods were compared using combinations of pelvic reconstruction plates and column screws. The stiffest construct combined a posterior column plate with an anterior column screw.[20]

The T-shaped acetabulum fracture fixation methods have been evaluated biomechanically using a cadaveric model. The stability of three fixation techniques, which required anterior, posterior, or combined surgical approaches for T-type acetabular fractures were investigated. The evaluated fixation methods included anterior column plate with anterior-to-posterior lag screw; posterior column plate with posterior-to-anterior lag screw; and dual plating. The investigators found that a plate with a lag screw placed during a single approach provided stability comparable to that achieved with dual plating in a combined approach.[21]

Annotated References

1. Letournel E, Judet R (eds): *Fractures of the Acetabulum*, ed 2. Berlin, Germany, Springer-Verlag, 1993.

2. Routt ML Jr, Simonian PT, Ballmer F: A rational approach to pelvic trauma: Resuscitation in early definitive stabilization. *Clin Orthop* 1995;318:61-74.

3. Matta J: Fractures of the acetabulum: Accuracy of reduction in clinical results managed in patients managed operatively within 3 weeks after injury. *J Bone Joint Surg Am* 1996;78:1632-1645.

4. Hak D, Olson S, Matta J: Diagnosis and management of post and trauma degloving injuries associated with pelvic and acetabular fractures. *J Trauma* 1997;42:1046-1051.

5. Epstein HC, Wiss DA: Posterior fractures dislocation of the hip with fractures of the femoral head. *Clin Orthop* 1985;201:9-17.

6. Siebenrock K, Gautier E, Woo AK, Ganz R: Surgical dislocation of the femoral head for joint debridement and accurate reduction of fractures of the acetabulum. *J Orthop Trauma* 2002;16:543-552.
   In this study, acetabular fracture reduction, femoral head viability, and outcome of selected acetabular fractures that were treated surgically with the Kocher-Langenbeck approach using a trochanteric flip osteotomy and surgical dislocation of the femoral head were evaluated. At a mean follow-up of 35 months, 12 patients showed good to excellent clinical results according to the D'Aubigne score. None of the hip joints developed signs of osteonecrosis of the femoral head despite 7 of the 12 hips sustaining a traumatic hip dislocation.

7. Kregor PJ, Templeman D: Associated injuries complicating the management of acetabular fractures: Review and case studies. *Orthop Clin North Am* 2002;33:73-95.
   In this study, the authors developed treatment strategies for acetabular fractures with associated injuries. This article presents a literature review of associated injuries and presents methods of surgical treatment using multiple case examples.

8. Borrelli J Jr, Goldfarb C, Catalano L, Evanoff BA: Assessment of articular fragment displacement in acetabular fractures: A comparison of computerized tomography and plain radiographs. *J Orthop Trauma* 2002;16:449-456.
   This article presents a retrospective evaluation of CT scans and plain radiographs of patients with displaced acetabular fractures as well as the canine acetabular fracture model. The purpose of the study was to compare the use of plain radiographs and CT scans for assessing articular fracture displacement, particularly step and gap. The radiographs showed poor sensitivity at assessing step deformity compared with CT scans. Some radiographs were also poor at showing step deformities involving single column fractures of the acetabulum. CT scans were more accurate in measuring step and gap displacement than plain radiographs in the canine model.

9. Letournel E: Fractures of the cotyloid cavity: Study of 75 cases. *J Chronic Dis* 1961;82:47-87.

10. Beaule P, Dorey F, Matta J: Letournel classification for acetabular fractures. *J Bone Joint Surg Am* 2003; 85-A:1704-1709.

The study assessed the interobserver and intraobserver reliability of Letournel's acetabular fracture classification system and the effect of CT on its reliability. Surgeons who studied under Letournel, acetabular fracture surgeons, and trauma surgeons initially evaluated AP and Judet radiographs and CT scans, which were randomly selected from an acetabular fracture database. Reviewers classified the fracture pattern first based on the plain radiograph and subsequently in conjunction with the CT scans. Letournel's classification system for acetabular fractures was determined to have substantial reliability. CT did not appear to be essential for the classification of acetabular fractures.

11. *American College of Surgeons Committee on Trauma: Advanced Trauma Life Support for Doctors, Student Course Manual*, ed. 6. Chicago, IL, American College of Surgeons, 1993.

12. Geerts WH, Code KI, Jay RM, Chen E, Szalai JP: Prospective study of venous thromboembolism after major trauma. *N Engl J Med* 1994;331:1601-1606.

13. Webb LX, Rush PT, Fuller SB, Meredith JW: Greenfield filter prophylaxis of pulmonary embolism in patients undergoing surgery for acetabular fracture. *J Orthop Trauma* 1992;6:139-145.

14. Stover MD, Morgan SJ, Bosse MJ, et al: Prospective comparison of contrast-enhanced computed tomography versus magnetic resonance venography in the detection of occult deep vein thrombosis in patients with pelvic and acetabular fractures. *J Orthop Trauma* 2002;16:613-621.

    A prospective evaluation of computed tomographic venography and magnetic resonance venography was performed to determine the rate of pelvic venous thrombosis following acetabular or pelvic fracture. Thirty patients with pelvic or acetabular fractures were prospectively screened with both modalities. Pelvic deep venous thrombosis was detected by computed tomographic venography in two patients (7%) and by magnetic resonance venography in four patients (13%). Positive screening studies were confirmed by invasive pelvic venography. The false-positive rate for computed tomographic venography was 50%, and the false-positive rate for magnetic resonance venography was 100%. The authors concluded that either computed tomographic venography or magnetic resonance venography to screen for asymptomatic thrombi in patients with pelvic fractures was not reliable because of the high false-positive rates.

15. Montgomery KD, Potter HG, Helfet DL: Magnetic resonance venography to evaluate the deep venous system of the pelvis in patients who have an acetabular fracture. *J Bone Joint Surg Am* 1995;77:1639-1649.

16. Tornetta P III: Non-operative management of acetabular fractures: The use of dynamic stress views. *J Bone Joint Surg Br* 1999;81:67-70.

17. Matta JM, Anderson LM, Epstein HC, Hendricks P: Fractures of the acetabulum: A retrospective analysis. *Clin Orthop* 1986;205:230-240.

18. Olson SA, Matta JM: The computerized tomography subchondral arc: A new method of assessing acetabular articular continuity after fracture (a preliminary report). *J Orthop Trauma* 1993;7:402-413.

19. Chang J, Gill S, Zura R, Krause W, Wang G: Comparative strength of three methods of fixation of transverse acetabular fractures. *Clin Orthop* 2001;392:433-441.

    In this biomechanical analysis, plate and screw fixation, lag screw fixation, and lag screw plus wire fixation were compared in a cadaveric model of transtectal transverse acetabular fractures. The authors found significantly greater strength of fixation and maximum strength in the construct that used plate and screw fixation; however, greater stiffness was achieved with lag screw fixation.

20. Shazar N, Brumback R, Novak V, Belkoff S: Biomechanical evaluation of transverse acetabular fracture fixation. *Clin Orthop* 1998;352:215-222.

21. Simonian PT, Routt ML Jr, Harrington RM, Tencer AF: The acetabular T-type fracture: A biomechanical evaluation of internal fixation. *Clin Orthop* 1995;314:234-240.

Chapter 24

Acetabular Fractures: Definitive Treatment and Expected Outcomes

Adam Starr, MD

Berton R. Moed, MD

Indications for Surgical Management

Any fracture of the acetabulum disturbs normal joint mechanics.[1] In its normal state, the hip is incongruous.[2] At low loads, the femoral head articulates with the anterior and posterior portions of the acetabulum, but not with the superior dome. As load increases, the socket elastically deforms, and the femoral head becomes congruous with the entire acetabulum. The ability of the acetabulum to deform is altered by fracture. After internal fixation, the natural structural characteristics of the intact acetabulum are not immediately restored.[3] These characteristics may return as the fracture heals; however, joint irregularities such as step-off or gap will remain unless surgically corrected. Malreductions significantly increase contact pressures at the articular surface,[4] and joint surface contact stress increases as displacement increases.[5] These alterations in joint contact pressure are likely mechanisms of posttraumatic arthrosis. Limiting these abnormalities is the aim of acetabular fracture management.

The goals of surgical treatment of patients with acetabular fracture are to decrease the risk of arthrosis, maximize hip function, and minimize the risk of complications. The surgeon must be able to determine which fractures require surgery and which surgical technique is the most appropriate to accomplish these goals. In some instances, however, nonsurgical care is the most appropriate treatment.

In general, the main indications for surgical acetabular fracture treatment are hip joint instability and joint incongruity. The indications for nonsurgical management are listed in Table 1.

The assessment of hip joint stability is critical when deciding whether to recommend surgical or nonsurgical fracture treatment. Hip joint stability assessment, however, is often based more on subjective impression than objective data. Furthermore, nonsurgical treatment can be catastrophic in patients with a fracture that subsequently proves to be unstable (such as a "small" posterior wall fracture). Dynamic stress views can be used to assess hip stability in patients with fractures that would otherwise meet the criteria for nonsurgical management.[6] The precise amount of stress to be applied, however, remains unknown. Nonetheless, stress testing with the patient under general anesthesia using fluoroscopy is the best method currently available.[6] The index of suspicion for occult instability should increase when other associated fractures of the pelvic ring are present.

Fractures below the weight-bearing dome can be managed without surgery as long as the fractures are stable. Roof arc criteria to define the weight-bearing dome (exclusive of patients with both-column fractures or fractures involving the posterior wall) have been described based on the three standard (AP and two oblique) acetabular radiographic views. The description, however, has varied. Initially, the boundaries of the weight-bearing dome were reported as $\geq 30°$ on the obturator oblique view, $\geq 40°$ on the AP view, and $\geq 50°$ on the iliac oblique view,[7] which was later simplified to $\geq 45°$ on all three radiographic views.[8] The results of biomechanical cadaver studies indicate that more of the posterior column than the anterior column may be necessary to maintain stability.[9] High anterior column displacement leads to increased contact pressures at the joint surface,[3] but intermediate and low anterior column fractures remain stable when tested biomechanically.[9] Conversely, posterior column fractures show great sensitivity to fracture. Published guidelines for roof arc angles that are acceptable for nonsurgical management recommend that fractures with an anterior roof arc angle of $\leq 25°$ and fractures with a posterior roof arc angle of $\leq 70°$ should be treated surgically. The boundary of the medial roof arc angle, measured on the AP view, is described as being $\leq 45°$, and fractures that enter this region are said to affect the weight-bearing dome. In general, this means that any fracture that exits the anterior column through the iliac wing or that exits the posterior column superior to the ischial spine may meet surgical indications.[9]

Regardless of roof arc measurements, both-column fractures may be managed nonsurgically, provided the fragments achieve secondary congruency. Although data from biomechanical studies of both-column fractures

TABLE 1 | Indications for Nonsurgical Management of Acetabular Fractures

Nondisplaced fractures or fractures with less than 2 mm of displacement

Displaced fractures below the level of the weight-bearing dome of the acetabulum but with a stable femoroacetabular relationship (congruency)

Both-column fractures having secondary congruence

Posterior wall fractures, the size and position of which do not affect hip joint stability

Advanced medical problems that make the risk of surgery outweigh its benefits or osteopenia or fracture fragmentation that make adequate reduction or stable fixation unlikely

that have been stabilized with secondary congruence show increased contact pressures,[10] these pressures are not as high as those reported after internal fixation with a step malreduction.[5] Presumably, as healing of both-column fractures takes place and the elastic properties of the acetabulum return to a more normal state, the joint contact pressures diminish, lessening the risk of arthritis. These biomechanical data correlate well with data from clinical studies, which show that both-column fractures that heal with secondary congruency commonly have satisfactory outcomes.[11]

Surgical Approaches

Selection of an appropriate surgical approach is straightforward for fractures involving one acetabular column or wall. For posterior fractures, the Kocher-Langenbeck approach is most commonly used with excellent success.[8,12-15] This approach offers good visualization of the retroacetabular surface and access to the quadrilateral surface, where the columnar fracture reduction can be assessed by palpation. During the approach, care should be taken to protect the blood supply to the femoral head. The short rotators should be divided at least 1 cm from their trochanteric attachment, and the quadratus femoris should not be detached from the proximal femur.[16,17] If distal access to the ischium is needed, the quadratus femoris may be released medially from the ischial tuberosity. Alternatives such as a direct lateral approach[13] or the addition of a trochanteric flip osteotomy[16] may have benefit in selected circumstances. The direct lateral approach may provide additional anterior and superior access when treating patients with more superiorly located posterior wall fractures, and this approach may be used to avoid operating through traumatized posterior soft tissues. The trochanteric flip osteotomy allows for direct visualization of the joint surface after hip dislocation, without compromising the femoral head blood supply.

For patients with anterior fractures, the ilioinguinal exposure is the surgical approach of choice[15] because it affords excellent visualization of the iliac fossa and the entire pelvic brim from the pubic symphysis to the anterior portion of the sacroiliac joint. Additionally, the quadrilateral surface and the inner aspect of the pubic body can be palpated and manipulated through this exposure. Direct visualization and access to the quadrilateral surface can be obtained using the Stoppa modification.[18] Alternatives include the iliofemoral approach for high anterior column fractures[11] and the Smith-Petersen approach for specific atypical variants of the anterior wall fracture.[19] Modifications of the ilioinguinal approach have been described that provide improved access to the joint and anterior wall.[20,21]

For fractures involving more than one column, the choice of surgical approach entails some decision making. Guidelines are provided in Table 2. Complex fractures are easier to reduce through more extensive exposures, and the main goal of surgery is to achieve an anatomic reduction of the joint. However, extended approaches may carry a greater risk for the patient.[22] These risks are predictable and can be minimized if appropriate steps are taken.[22-26] It is possible, however, to treat many patients with complex fractures using a standard anterior or posterior surgical approach.[27,28]

A more extensive approach such as the extended iliofemoral approach or one of its modifications has specific indications. Delayed treatment of fractures can be complicated by the resorption of fracture lines and callus formation that may limit indirect fracture reduction. Extensive exposure may be necessary to clean and mobilize the fracture and directly visualize the joint. Fractures that are displaced high in the superior articular surface may require an extended exposure because an anatomic reduction in this area is critical for a successful result. Both-column fractures with posterior extension into the sacroiliac joint may also require an extended approach or the use of a modification of the ilioinguinal[21] to allow access to the lateral ilium and facilitate reduction. The simultaneous combination of front and back exposures (a Kocher-Langenbeck approach combined with an iliofemoral or an ilioinguinal approach) may be used as an alternative to an extended approach,[29] but the distinct advantages of each approach may be compromised. Sequential front and back exposures are necessitated when the initial approach is not sufficient (either as expected from the preoperative plan or as an unexpected event during surgery) to allow accurate repositioning of the opposite column.

The objective in limiting the use of the surgical exposures that strip the abductor muscle mass from the outer surface of the ilium fractures is to limit exposure-related complications. However, the approach that provides the best chance of achieving an anatomic reduction in the hands of the surgeon should be used. Surgeon experience plays an important role in the decision-making process; therefore, surgeons with limited experi-

TABLE 2 | Surgical Approach General Guidelines

Fracture Type	Recommended Approach	Indicator(s)
Transverse	Kocher-Langenbeck	Major displacement at posterior column
	Ilioinguinal	Major displacement at anterior column
		Fracture angle from high anterior to low posterior
	Extended approach	Major displacement transtectal
		Fracture healing evident (> 15 days old)
Transverse and posterior wall	Kocher-Langenbeck	Use in most patients
	Extended approach	Major displacement transtectal
		Fracture healing evident (> 15 days old)
		Extended posterior wall component
		Associated pubic symphysis disruption
	Simultaneous front and back	Alternative to extended approaches
		Inability to fully visualize a transtectal fracture line is an important limitation
T-shaped	Kocher-Langenbeck	Use in most patients
	Ilioinguinal	Minimal posterior displacement
	Extended approach	Major displacement transtectal
		Wide separation of columns
		Associated pubic symphysis disruption
		Fracture healing evident (> 15 days old)
	Simultaneous front and back	Alternative to extended approaches (as above)
	Sequential front and back	When selected approach fails to reduce the opposite column
Anterior column/wall and posterior hemitransverse	Ilioinguinal	Use in most patients
	Extended approach	Fracture healing evident (> 15 days old) and Wide displacement of posterior column
	Front and back choices	Alternatives to extended approaches
Both columns	Ilioinguinal	Use in most patients
	Extended approach	Posterior column is comminuted
		Fracture healing evident (> 15 days old)
		A displaced fracture line crosses the sacroiliac joint

ence may require a more extensive surgical exposure when treating patients with complex fractures.

Fracture Fixation

The necessary amount of fixation is that which maintains fracture reduction until union. Fixation is most often provided by using 3.5-mm steel cortical screws and malleable steel plates contoured to match the anatomy of the pelvis. Longer screws and specific plate bending instruments are required. A typical fixation construct after reduction will include interfragmentary screws and a plate to buttress the wall fragments or neutralize columnar displacement forces. Plate fixation stiffness is increased by the placement of screws as close to the fracture as possible paired with screws at the ends of the plate.[30] Thorough knowledge of pelvic and joint anatomy will allow for application of these principles and help avoid screw penetration of the joint. Spring plates offer a method for buttressing small peripheral wall fragments without devascularization or screw penetration into the

joint; they can be used in conjunction with lag screws and a standard buttress plate.

Screws placed from one column of the acetabulum to the other (column screws) may be placed through the planned exposure or through small separate percutaneous incisions as part of an open or closed reduction. Placement through small incisions may improve screw direction and effectiveness as well as decrease the extent of required exposure in some patients. Safe screw placement often requires fluoroscopic or computer-assisted guidance.[31-33]

The literature provides limited guidance regarding the best construct for fixation of particular fracture patterns. For transverse fractures, plate fixation of the posterior column coupled with anterior column screw fixation results in a significantly stiffer construct than that provided by plate fixation of the posterior column alone.[30] Although column screw fixation alone has been reported in some patients, plate fixation of transverse fractures has a comparatively higher yield strength.[34] Clinical evaluation has demonstrated that some fractures may be amenable to screw fixation alone and usually consist of large fracture fragments through good bone material with minimal fragmentation.[11]

Closed reduction and percutaneous fixation of acetabular fractures remains an experimental procedure. Reports on small series of patients have shown that the technique can lead to acceptable clinical outcome.[35,36] The method, however, requires multiple surgeons, specialized equipment, and excellent fluoroscopic or computer-assisted guidance to avoid catastrophic injury. Although promising, the risks and indications of this method are not yet fully known.

Acute Total Hip Arthroplasty

Patients older than 40 years have been shown to have outcomes that are comparably worse than those of their younger counterparts, although surgical reconstruction of acetabular fractures in elderly patients can be successful.[11] Care must be taken to reliably identify those patients or fracture types that will do poorly after attempts at open reduction and internal fixation, whether because of the inability to obtain a fracture reduction or inability to maintain reduction until union. One study identified a specific fracture pattern in osteopenic elderly patients in whom the superior articular surface is impacted, creating a characteristic radiographic finding, the "seagull sign."[37] All patients in whom this fracture pattern was identified had poor outcomes in spite of surgical repair. Other studies report several criteria (osteopenia, fragmentation of the joint, and/or associated injuries to the femoral head and neck) that can be used to identify patients who are best managed with acute total hip arthroplasty.[38,39] Using these indications, 79% of patients had good to excellent results at short-term follow-up, despite early cup migration and settling. Although absolute indications for acute total hip arthroplasty in the setting of acetabular fracture are currently unclear, it will likely continue to have a role in the acute treatment of some patients with these injuries.

Complications

Acetabular fracture management can result in predictable complications for which surgeons can help prevent or minimize the impact. Wound infection, nerve palsy, posttraumatic arthritis, osteonecrosis, heterotopic bone formation, and thromboembolism are the most common major complications associated with acetabular fracture care.

Wound infection rates in single surgeon series were reported to be between 2% and 5% of patients.[11,40] Patients with acetabular fractures can have associated soft-tissue injuries that range from minor contusions to closed degloving injuries or open fractures. Soft-tissue injury may force a surgeon to alter the approach or delay surgery until the soft-tissue environment is optimized. In patients with closed degloving injuries, evidence suggests that many of these injuries are colonized with bacteria.[41] Injuries in the surgical field may require open débridement and specialized soft-tissue care,[41] although percutaneous débridement and treatment with antibiotics has been suggested.[42] Infection is more common after extensile exposures likely because of the increased surgical soft-tissue injury and the increased duration of surgery.[11]

Obesity is associated with high postoperative infection rates,[43] probably because of the poor healing capacity of fat and problems associated with wound care in obese patients. Patients with acetabular fractures often have associated injuries[44] and may be immunocompromised because of poor nutrition or because they have undergone multiple blood transfusions. Experienced surgical teams and the use of perioperative antibiotics can minimize the risk of wound complications, even if an extensile exposure is used.[23-25] A first-generation cephalosporin given before surgery followed by 24 hours of antibiotic treatment is sufficient prophylaxis in most patients.

Postoperative infection is best managed with early surgical intervention. If identified early, infection can be managed with débridement of infected tissues and treatment with appropriate antibiotics. Resorbable beads impregnated with antibiotic can be a useful adjunct. Hardware removal may be necessary after fracture union because plates and screws often become colonized with bacteria during wound sepsis.

Nerve palsy may occur from injury or surgery. Careful neurologic examination prior to surgery is mandatory. Nerve deficits may not be noticed during a cursory examination in the emergency department. The peroneal portion of the sciatic nerve is most frequently injured in patients with acetabular fractures. Reported rates of postoperative sciatic nerve injury in large series of patients range from 2% to 6%.[11,40] Maintaining hip extension and knee flexion has been shown to limit intraneural pressure.[45] Various methods of nerve monitoring have been described,[46] although the need for these techniques in pelvic and acetabular fracture surgery is subject to debate.[47,48]

The prognosis for sciatic nerve recovery depends primarily on the severity of initial injury. Recovery of the tibial portion of the nerve is usually more rapid and more complete than recovery of the peroneal portion.[49] The prognosis for recovery of patients with iatrogenic palsy is better than the prognosis for patients with palsy caused by the traumatic injury. Although most patients achieve a functional recovery, residual deficits can often be noted with precise nerve testing. Nerve recovery can be uncomfortable and worrisome for patients. Medications such as gabapentin can help alleviate symptoms of burning pain and dysesthesias. Patient education is also important. During postoperative rehabilitation, patients with foot drop should use an ankle-foot orthotic device to prevent equinus contracture and steppage gait.

The lateral femoral cutaneous nerve is at risk during ilioinguinal exposures. A 12% rate of neuralgia following anterior exposures of the acetabulum has been reported.[11] If the nerve must be sacrificed during surgery, it is recommended that the cut ends be buried in muscle to prevent the formation of a painful neuroma. Although injury to other major nerves, including the femoral and obturator nerves, has been reported, it is rare.[50]

Posttraumatic arthritis results from damage to joint surfaces at the time of injury and from malunion after fracture care. Cartilage injury may be severe enough to lead to arthritis despite anatomic reduction. Even if anatomically reduced, free joint fragments that were initially reduced may settle or be resorbed over time and lead to joint irregularity. The factors under the surgeon's control are quality of reduction and patient selection. The findings of clinical and laboratory studies have indicated that improved quality of reduction is linked to improved joint outcome and that displacements as small as 1 mm may be sufficient to alter the mechanical environment of the joint.[1,5] Studies assessing large series of patients with acetabular fractures treated by various surgeons have shown that arthritis is rare in patients whose fractures are anatomically reduced.[40,51,52]

Intra-articular debris and hardware that penetrates the joint can also lead to arthritis. CT is the best diagnostic imaging modality for evaluating patients for the presence of debris in the joint. Surgeons must be certain that fragments noted on CT scans are identified intraoperatively. Postoperative CT may help define residual fragments and evaluate reduction.[53] The best method for evaluating patients for intra-articular screw penetration is generally thought to be fluoroscopy during surgery.[54,55] With a concave surface such as the acetabulum, the entire screw needs to be visualized outside of the radiographic joint on only one view. This quick and reliable procedure should be carried out intraoperatively at the completion of surgery.

Osteonecrosis occurs in 2% to 4% of patients[11] and is usually associated with femoral head dislocation at injury. If the vascular supply remains intact, prompt reduction should decrease vascular compromise.[13,56] Osteonecrosis of the femoral head is normally visible within 2 years of injury. Osteonecrosis of fractured segments of the acetabulum can also occur, usually because of soft-tissue stripping at the time of surgery. Osteonecrosis of the acetabulum may lead to chondrolysis and joint destruction, but in most patients the segments of bone appear to revascularize.

Extensive heterotopic ossification has a significant adverse effect on early functional outcomes.[57] Heterotopic ossification is more common after extensile exposures, but it also commonly occurs after simple posterior exposure of the acetabulum.[11,40,58,59] The use of prophy-laxis in this patient population is controversial.[60] Necrotic or injured muscle identified during surgery should be removed.[61] Some studies have shown the effects of indomethacin to be equivalent to those of radiation in the prevention of heterotopic bone,[62,63] whereas other studies have shown indomethacin to have no effect.[59,64] Indomethacin increases the risk of long bone nonunion when used as prophylaxis for heterotopic bone,[65] and it must be used with caution in patients with multiple orthopaedic injuries. Patient compliance may also be an issue with its use.[64] Radiation effectively prevents heterotopic ossification, even when an extensile exposure is used.[11,24] Most modern series report a single dose of 600 cGy within 48 hours of surgery,[24] but the precise timing is controversial.[66,67] The risk of sarcoma formation is of concern, but no known articles have been published reporting this complication among patients with acetabular fractures. Because the risk of cancerous degeneration of irradiated tissue increases with time, some radiation oncologists will not use radiation treatment on young patients.

Expected Outcomes

Patient outcomes after treatment of displaced fractures of the acetabulum have been evaluated in several ways. The method most commonly used to assess overall results is a modification of the hip scale developed by Merle D'Aubigne and Postel and adapted by Letournel and Judet. In this clinical grading system, pain, gait, and hip range of motion each have a possible score ranging from 1 to 6 points. The sum of these three scores produces the final clinical score. Clinical results are classified using this method as excellent (score = 18), very good (score = 17), good (score = 15 or 16), fair (score = 13 or 14), or poor (score < 13).[11,13,40,68]

Radiographic assessment is another important measure of acetabular fracture treatment outcome. According to the radiographic outcome criteria most often used, patients with normal-appearing hip joints are classified as having excellent outcomes; those with mild changes and minimal sclerosis and joint narrowing (≤ 1 mm) are classified as having good outcomes; those with intermediate changes and moderate sclerosis and joint narrowing (< 50%) are classified as having fair outcomes; and those with advanced changes are classified as having poor outcomes.[13,40,69] In multiple studies, a strong association has been demonstrated between clinical outcome as measured by the modified Merle D'Aubigne and Postel hip scale and this radiographic grading system.

Three standard plain radiographic views (one AP and two oblique) are routinely used to evaluate acetabular fracture reduction.[11,40] One study showed that the quality of this reduction is strongly associated with the clinical result.[40] Furthermore, using a modified Merle D'Aubigne and Postel hip scale, it was determined that an anatomic reduction (< 2 mm of maximum displacement shown on any of the three views) as opposed to an imperfect (2 to 3 mm of displacement) or poor reduction (> 3 mm of displacement) was a highly significant predictor of a good to excellent clinical result. Therefore, the findings on postoperative radiographic assessment of fracture reduction should correlate with outcome. However, problems with the interpretation of the plain radiographs in measuring displacement can occur, especially regarding the postoperative evaluation of patients with posterior wall fractures.[11,52,70] In these patients, two-dimensional CT provides additional prognostic information regarding fracture displacement parameters.[53] These additional data help confirm the importance of fracture reduction in predicting clinical outcome for all fracture types. The best results are predicated on an anatomic fracture reduction and attaining postoperative congruity between the acetabular roof and femoral head.

It is generally believed that positive outcomes of the surgical treatment of acetabular fractures are achieved by surgeons who dedicate their efforts over an extended period to the treatment of these complex injuries. Surgeon-specific reports of clinical results show overall good to excellent results in 75% of patients with acetabular fractures treated within 3 weeks of injury.[11,40,71] Expected good to excellent clinical outcomes drop to below 50% for patients treated by less experienced surgeons.[72,73] Even in the most experienced hands, delay in surgical treatment beyond 3 weeks can have an adverse effect on clinical outcome.

Although clinical outcomes are often used to assess success in patients who have undergone surgery to treat acetabular fractures, functional outcome assessment should also be used.[74,75] A validated, well-designed, self-reported patient assessment tool, such as the Musculoskeletal Function Assessment questionnaire, is useful for determining general health status. Studies have shown that the Merle D'Aubigne and Postel hip scale, both in its original and modified forms, demonstrate a ceiling effect in the evaluation of patients with acetabulum fractures.[68,76] In other words, there is crowding of the scores at the upper end of the scale, limiting its ability to discern differences among patients with "better" clinical outcomes. Using the Musculoskeletal Function Assessment questionnaire to assess patients, one study reported that the scores were relatively poorer in patients with acetabular fractures compared with those of the normal population, indicating that complete return to a preinjury level of function is uncommon in patients with acetabular fractures, despite a good to excellent Merle D'Aubigne and Postel hip scale score.[68]

Annotated References

1. Olson SA: Biomechanics of acetabular fractures, in Tile M (ed): *Fractures of the Pelvis and Acetabulum*, ed 3. Philadelphia, PA, Lippincott Williams & Wilkins, 2003, pp 46-49.

The author provides an elegant, concise discussion of the state of current understanding of acetabular biomechanics and describes the biomechanical consequences of acetabular fractures, intra-articular contact pressure characteristics, instability of the hip, and the mechanics of acetabular fixation.

2. Afoke NY, Byers PD, Hutton WC: The incongruous hip joint. *J Bone Joint Surg Br* 1980;62:511-514.

3. Konrath GA, Hamel AJ, Sharkey NA, Bay BK, Olson S: Biomechanical consequences of anterior column fracture of the acetabulum. *J Orthop Trauma* 1998;12:547-552.

4. Hak DJ, Hamel AJ, Bay BK, Sharkey NA, Olson SA: Consequences of transverse acetabular fracture malreduction on load transmission across the hip joint. *J Orthop Trauma* 1998;12:90-100.

5. Malkani AL, Voor MJ, Rennirt G, Helfet D, Pedersen D, Brown T: Increased peak contact stress after incongruent reduction of transverse acetabular fractures: A cadaveric model. *J Trauma* 2001;51:704-709.

Articular cartilage step-off of greater than 1 mm led to significantly increased contact stress at the loaded acetabular articular surface. Mean peak pressure measured at 1,335 N of loading in all intact specimens before the osteotomy was approximately 10 MPa. Peak pressure after a transverse acetabular fracture did not change when the fracture was perfectly reduced. At 1 mm of step-off, the peak pressure increased by approximately 20% but was not statistically significant. With step-off of 2 mm or greater, the peak pressure increase was approximately 50% and was statistically significant.

6. Tornetta P III: Non-operative management of acetabular fractures: The use of dynamic stress views. *J Bone Joint Surg Br* 1999;81:67-70.

7. Matta JM, Mehne DK, Roffi R: Fractures of the acetabulum: Early results of a prospective study. *Clin Orthop* 1986;205:241-250.

8. Templeman DC, Olson S, Moed BR, Duwelius P, Matta JM: Surgical treatment of acetabular fractures. *Instr Course Lect* 1999;48:481-496.

9. Vrahas MS, Widding KK, Thomas KA: The effects of simulated transverse, anterior column, and posterior column fractures of the acetabulum on the stability of the hip joint. *J Bone Joint Surg Am* 1999;81:966-974.

10. Levine RG, Renard R, Behrens FF, Tornetta P III: Biomechanical consequences of secondary congruence after both-column acetabular fracture. *J Orthop Trauma* 2002;16:87-91.

11. Letournel E, Judet R: *Fractures of the Acetabulum,* ed 2. New York, NY, Springer-Verlag, 1993.

12. Baumgaertner MR: Fractures of the posterior wall of the acetabulum. *J Am Acad Orthop Surg* 1999;7:54-65.

13. Moed BR, Carr SEW, Watson JT: Results of operative treatment of fractures of the posterior wall of the acetabulum. *J Bone Joint Surg Am* 2002;84:752-758.

    In 100 patients who underwent open reduction and internal fixation to treat an unstable, unilateral posterior wall fracture of the acetabulum, final clinical results were excellent in 55, very good in 25, good in 9, fair in 1, and poor in 10. Risk factors for an unsatisfactory clinical result included delay greater than 12 hours to reduction of an associated hip dislocation, age 55 years or older at the time of injury, intra-articular comminution, and the presence of osteonecrosis.

14. Moed BR, Carr SE, Watson JT: Open reduction and internal fixation of posterior wall fractures of the acetabulum. *Clin Orthop* 2000;377:57-67.

15. Tornetta P III: Displaced acetabular fractures: Indications for operative and nonoperative management. *J Am Acad Orthop Surg* 2001;9:18-28.

16. Siebenrock KA, Gautier E, Ziran BH, Ganz R: Trochanteric flip osteotomy for cranial extension and muscle protection in acetabular fracture fixation using a Kocher-Langenbeck approach. *J Orthop Trauma* 1998;12:387-391.

17. Siebenrock KA, Gautier E, Woo AK, Ganz R: Surgical dislocation of the femoral head for joint debridement and accurate reduction of fractures of the acetabulum. *J Orthop Trauma* 2002;16:543-552.

    This is a well-illustrated, concise description of the use and results of a modification of the Kocher-Langenbeck approach. The approach as described allows hip dislocation for direct inspection of the acetabulum and provides improved access to the posterior column, posterior wall, and supra-acetabular region.

18. Cole JD, Bolhofner BR: Acetabular fracture fixation via a modified Stoppa limited intrapelvic approach: Description of operative technique and preliminary treatment results. *Clin Orthop* 1994;305:20-30.

19. Piriou P, Siguier T, De Loynes B, Charnley G, Judet T: Anterior wall acetabular fractures: Report of two cases and new strategies in operative management. *J Trauma* 2002;53:553-557.

20. Kloen P, Siebenrock KA, Ganz R: Modification of the ilioinguinal approach. *J Orthop Trauma* 2002;16:586-593.

    The authors provide a well-illustrated, concise description of the use and results of a modification of the ilioinguinal approach. The approach as described allows hip dislocation for direct inspection of the acetabulum and provides improved access to the anterior column, anterior wall, and quadrilateral plate.

21. Weber TG, Mast JW: The extended ilioinguinal approach for specific both column fractures. *Clin Orthop* 1994;305:106-111.

22. Stannard JP, Alonso JE: Controversies in acetabular fractures. *Clin Orthop* 1998;353:74-80.

23. Stockle U, Hoffmann R, Sudkamp NP, Reindl R, Haas NP: Treatment of complex acetabular fractures through a modified extended iliofemoral approach. *J Orthop Trauma* 2002;16:220-230.

    In this study, 49 patients with 50 complex acetabular fractures were treated using a modified extended iliofemoral approach. Patients included those with associated acetabular fractures or transverse fractures with a comminuted roof area not sufficiently reconstructible through a single approach. In 80% of patients, the reduction was anatomic with a remaining displacement of $\leq$ 1 mm; eight fractures had a persistent displacement of 2 mm; and two fractures had a poor result with 3-mm displacement. Complications included loss of reduction (8%), heterotopic ossification grade 3 (13%), and femoral head osteonecrosis (4%). At 2-year follow-up, 74% of patients had good or excellent radiographic and clinical results. Two patients had undergone total hip replacement, and two patients with femoral head osteonecrosis were scheduled for arthroplasty.

24. Starr AJ, Watson JT, Reinert CM, et al: Complications following the "T extensile" approach: A modified extensile approach for acetabular fracture surgery-report of forty-three patients. *J Orthop Trauma* 2002;16:535-542.

25. Griffin DB, Beaule PE, Matta JM: Results of 107 complex acetabular fractures operated on through the extended iliofemoral approach, in *Final Program of the 17th Annual Meeting of the Orthopaedic Trauma Association, San Diego, CA, October 18-20, 2001.* Available at: http://www.hwbf.org/ota/am/ota01/otapa/OTA01059.htm. Accessed April 27, 2005.

26. Reilly MC, Olson SA, Tornetta P III, Matta JM: Superior gluteal artery in the extended iliofemoral approach. *J Orthop Trauma* 2000;14:259-263.

27. Helfet DL, Schmeling GJ: Management of complex acetabular fractures through single nonextensile exposures. *Clin Orthop* 1994;305:58-68.

28. Schmidt CC, Gruen GS: Non-extensile surgical approaches for two-column acetabular fractures. *J Bone Joint Surg Br* 1993;75:556-561.

29. Routt ML Jr, Swiontkowski MF: Operative treatment of complex acetabular fractures: Combined anterior and posterior exposures during the same procedure. *J Bone Joint Surg Am* 1990;72:897-904.

30. Shazar N, Brumback RJ, Novak VP, Belkoff SM: Biomechanical evaluation of transverse acetabular fracture fixation. *Clin Orthop* 1998;352:215-222.

31. Crowl AC, Kahler DM: Closed reduction and percutaneous fixation of anterior column acetabular fractures. *Comput Aided Surg* 2002;7:169-178.

32. Brown GA, Willis MC, Firoozbakhsh K, Barmada A, Tessman CL, Montgomery A: Computed tomography image-guided surgery in complex acetabular fractures. *Clin Orthop* 2000;370:219-226.

33. Starr AJ, Reinert CM, Jones AL: Percutaneous fixation of the columns of the acetabulum: A new technique. *J Orthop Trauma* 1998;12:51-58.

34. Chang JK, Gill SS, Zura RD, Krause WR, Wang GJ: Comparative strength of three methods of fixation of transverse acetabular fractures. *Clin Orthop* 2001; 392:433-441.

35. Starr AJ, Jones AL, Reinert CM, Borer DS: Preliminary results and complications following limited open reduction and percutaneous screw fixation of displaced fractures of the acetabulum. *Injury* 2001; 32(suppl 1):SA45-SA50.

36. Zura RD, Kahler DM: A transverse acetabular nonunion treated with computer-assisted percutaneous internal fixation: A case report. *J Bone Joint Surg Am* 2000;82:219-224.

37. Anglen JO, Burd TA, Hendricks K, Harrison P: Operative results and functional outcomes of acetabular fractures in geriatric patients, in *Final Program of the 17th Annual Meeting of the Orthopaedic Trauma Association, San Diego, CA, October 18-20, 2001*. Available at: http://www.hwbf.org/ota/am/ ota01/otapa/OTA01060.htm. Accessed April 27, 2005.

38. Mears DC: Surgical treatment of acetabular fractures in elderly patients with osteoporotic bone. *J Am Acad Orthop Surg* 1999;7:128-141.

39. Mears DC, Velyvis JH: Acute total hip arthroplasty for selected displaced acetabular fractures: Two to twelve-year results. *J Bone Joint Surg Am* 2002;84: 1-9.

40. Matta JM: Fractures of the acetabulum: Accuracy of reduction and clinical results in patients managed operatively within three weeks after the injury. *J Bone Joint Surg Am* 1996;78:1632-1645.

41. Hak DJ, Olson SA, Matta JM: Diagnosis and management of closed internal degloving injuries associated with pelvic and acetabular fractures: The Morel-Lavallee lesion. *J Trauma* 1997;42:1046-1051.

42. Tornetta P III, Normand AN: Percutaneous management of Morel-Lavallee lesions, in *Final Program of the 18th Annual Meeting of the Orthopaedic Trauma Association, Toronto, Ontario, October 11-13, 2002*. Available at: http://www.hwbf.org/ota/am/ota02/ otapa/OTA02425.htm. Accessed April 27, 2005.

43. Russell GV Jr, Nork SE, Routt MLC Jr: Perioperative complications associated with operative treatment of acetabular fractures. *J Trauma* 2001;51:1098-1103.

44. Kregor PJ, Templeman D: Associated injuries complicating the management of acetabular fractures: Review and case studies. *Orthop Clin North Am* 2002;33:73-95.

45. Borrelli J, Ungacta F, Kantor J: Intraneural sciatic nerve pressures relative to the position of the hip and knee, in *Final Program of the 14th Annual Meeting of the Orthopaedic Trauma Association, Vancouver, BC, Canada, October 8-10, 1998*. Available at: http:// www.hwbf.org/ota/am/ota98/otapa/OTA98106.htm. Accessed April 27, 2005.

46. Arrington ED, Hochschild DP, Steinagle TJ, Mongan PD, Martin SL: Monitoring of somatosensory and motor evoked potentials during open reduction and internal fixation of pelvis and acetabular fractures. *Orthopedics* 2000;23:1081-1083.

47. Nork SE, Segina DM, Mills WJ, Routt ML: Iliosacral screws inserted without electrodiagnostic monitoring, in *Final Program of the 15th Annual Meeting of the Orthopaedic Trauma Association, Charlotte, NC,*

October 22-24, 1999. Available at: http://www.hwbf. org/ota/am/ota99/otapo/OTP99080.htm. Accessed April 27, 2005.

48. Haidukewych GJ, Scaduto J, Herscovici D Jr, Sanders RW, DiPasquale T: Iatrogenic nerve injury in acetabular fracture surgery: A comparison of monitored and unmonitored procedures. *J Orthop Trauma* 2002;16:297-301.

49. Fassler PR, Swiontkowski MF, Kilroy AW, Routt ML Jr: Injury of the sciatic nerve associated with acetabular fracture. *J Bone Joint Surg Am* 1993;75: 1157-1166.

50. Gruson KI, Moed BR: Injury of the femoral nerve associated with acetabular fracture. *J Bone Joint Surg Am* 2003;85-A:428-431.

    Of 726 acetabular fractures treated, 4 were identified as having a femoral nerve injury, 2 were iatrogenic, and 2 were traumatic. Patients were followed for a mean of 3.4 years. Motor function returned at an average of 18 weeks, and all patients had returned to grade 4 or 5 motor strength by an average of 10 months. Sensory recovery was incomplete. It was concluded that recovery of femoral nerve function without surgical exploration can be expected in this patient population.

51. Chen CM, Chiu FY, Chuang TY, Lo WH: Treatment of acetabular fractures: 10-year experience. *Chung Hua I Hsueh Tsa Chih* 2000;63:384-390.

52. Chiu FY, Chen CM, Lo WH: Surgical treatment of displaced acetabular fractures: 72 cases followed for 10 (6-14) years. *Injury* 2000;31:181-185.

53. Moed BR, Carr SE, Gruson KI, Watson JT, Craig JG: Computed tomographic assessment of fractures of the posterior wall of the acetabulum after operative treatment. *J Bone Joint Surg Am* 2003;85:512-522.

    In 67 patients who underwent open reduction and internal fixation to treat an unstable posterior wall fracture of the acetabulum, postoperative CT was found to detect the degree of residual fracture displacement more accurately than plain radiography. Furthermore, the accuracy of surgical reduction as assessed on postoperative CT was highly predictive of clinical outcome.

54. Norris BL, Hahn DH, Bosse MJ, Kellam JF, Sims SH: Intraoperative fluoroscopy to evaluate fracture reduction and hardware placement during acetabular surgery. *J Orthop Trauma* 1999;13:414-417.

55. Carmack DB, Moed BR, McCarroll K, Freccero D: Accuracy of detecting screw penetration of the acetabulum with intraoperative fluoroscopy and computed tomography. *J Bone Joint Surg Am* 2001;83: 1370-1375.

56. Yue JJ, Sontich JK, Miron SD, Peljovich AE, Yue JH, Patterson BM: Blood flow changes to the femoral head after acetabular fracture or dislocation in the acute injury and perioperative periods. *J Orthop Trauma* 2001;15:170-176.

57. Murphy D, Kaliszer M, Rice J, McElwain JP: Outcome after acetabular fracture: Prognostic factors and their inter-relationships. *Injury* 2003;34:512-517.

58. Johnson EE, Kay RM, Dorey FJ: Heterotopic ossification prophylaxis following operative treatment of acetabular fracture. *Clin Orthop* 1994;305:88-95.

59. Matta JM, Siebenrock KA: Does indomethacin reduce heterotopic bone formation after operations for acetabular fractures? A prospective randomised study. *J Bone Joint Surg Br* 1997;79:959-963.

60. Morgan SJ, Jeray KJ, Phieffer LS, Grigsby JH, Bosse MJ, Kellam JF: Attitudes of orthopaedic trauma surgeons regarding current controversies in the management of pelvic and acetabular fractures. *J Orthop Trauma* 2001;15:526-532.

61. Russell GV, Rath EMS, Washington WJ, Routt MLC: Gluteus minimus muscle debridement to prevent heterotopic ossification after acetabular fracture, in *Final Program of the 15th Annual Meeting of the Orthopaedic Trauma Association, Charlotte, NC, October 22-24, 1999.* Available at: http://www.hwbf. org/ota/am/ota99/otapo/OTP99085.htm. Accessed April 27, 2005.

62. Burd TA, Lowry KJ, Anglen JO: Indomethacin compared with localized irradiation for the prevention of heterotopic ossification following surgical treatment of acetabular fractures. *J Bone Joint Surg Am* 2001; 83:1783-1788.

    Both local radiation therapy and indomethacin were found to provide effective prophylaxis against heterotopic ossification following surgical treatment of acetabular fractures through a posterior or extensile approach. No significant difference in efficacy between the two prophylactic regimens was detected.

63. Moore KD, Goss K, Anglen JO: Indomethacin versus radiation therapy for prophylaxis against heterotopic ossification in acetabular fractures: A randomised, prospective study. *J Bone Joint Surg Br* 1998;80:259-263.

64. Karunakar MA, Bosse MJ, Hall JM, et al: A prospective randomized double-blind placebo-

controlled trial of the efficacy of indomethacin as prophylaxis for heterotopic ossification after operative treatment of acetabular fractures, in *Final Program of the 19th Annual Meeting of the Orthopaedic Trauma Association, Salt Lake City, UT, October 9-11, 2003.* Available at: http://www.hwbf.org/ota/am/ota03/otapa/OTA03065.htm. Accessed April 27, 2005.

65. Burd TA, Hughes MS, Anglen JO: Heterotopic ossification prophylaxis with indomethacin increases the risk of long-bone nonunion. *J Bone Joint Surg Br* 2003;85:700-705.

66. Childs HA III, Cole T, Falkenberg E, et al: A prospective evaluation of the timing of postoperative radiotherapy for preventing heterotopic ossification following traumatic acetabular fractures. *Int J Radiat Oncol Biol Phys* 2000;47:1347-1352.

67. Haas ML, Kennedy AS, Copeland CC, Ames JW, Scarboro M, Slawson RG: Utility of radiation in the prevention of heterotopic ossification following repair of traumatic acetabular fracture. *Int J Radiat Oncol Biol Phys* 1999;45:461-466.

68. Moed BR, Yu PH, Gruson KI: Functional outcomes of acetabular fractures. *J Bone Joint Surg Am* 2003; 85:1879-1883.

In this study, 150 patients with acetabular fractures had a complete physical examination with modified Merle D'Aubigne score and completion of the Musculoskeletal Function Assessment questionnaire. Despite a significant correlation between scores, the Merle d'Aubigne score data were asymmetric, demonstrating a ceiling effect. The Musculoskeletal Function Assessment scores were relatively high compared with those from the normal population, indicating that complete return to a preinjury functional level is uncommon despite a good to excellent clinical score.

69. Matta JM: Operative treatment of acetabular fractures through the ilioinguinal approach: A 10-year perspective. *Clin Orthop Relat Res* 1994;305:10-19.

70. Borrelli J Jr, Goldfarb C, Catalano L, Evanoff BA: Assessment of articular fragment displacement in acetabular fractures: A comparison of computerized tomography and plain radiographs. *J Orthop Trauma* 2002;16:449-456.

71. Mayo KA: Open reduction and internal fixation of fractures of the acetabulum: Results in 163 fractures. *Clin Orthop* 1994;305:31-37.

72. Wright R, Barrett K, Christie MJ, Johnson KD: Acetabular fractures: Long-term follow-up of open reduction and internal fixation. *J Orthop Trauma* 1994; 8:397-403.

73. Kaempffe FA, Bone LB, Border JR: Open reduction and internal fixation of acetabular fractures: Heterotopic ossification and other complications of treatment. *J Orthop Trauma* 1991;5:439-445.

74. Borrelli J Jr, Goldfarb C, Ricci W, Wagner JM, Engsberg JR: Functional outcome after isolated acetabular fractures. *J Orthop Trauma* 2002;16:73-81.

Standardized muscle strength determination, gait, and motion analysis and completion of a Musculoskeletal Function Assessment questionnaire provided a thorough and revealing evaluation of patients who have undergone open reduction and internal fixation of a displaced acetabular fracture. Functional outcome, as determined by Musculoskeletal Function Assessment questionnaire scores, was considerably poorer in those patients with significantly weaker hip flexion and extension strength compared with those of patients with more desirable Musculoskeletal Function Assessment questionnaire scores. The use of these and similar evaluation instruments may allow determination of factors that negatively affect outcome (hip flexion and extension strength) that otherwise may remain unknown.

75. Matta JM, Olson SA: Factors related to hip muscle weakness following fixation of acetabular fractures. *Orthopedics* 2000;23:231-235.

76. Rice J, Kaliszer M, Dolan M, Cox M, Khan H, McElwain JP: Comparison between clinical and radiologic outcome measures after reconstruction of acetabular fractures. *J Orthop Trauma* 2002;16:82-86.

Overall correlation between the clinical and radiologic outcome grades was good, but agreement between the two grades (the prediction of a specific clinical outcome by a corresponding radiologic outcome) was poor. The authors found that the clinical scoring system was difficult to apply specifically to acetabular trauma in 29% of fractures because of associated injuries. They concluded that the Merle d'Aubigne score has shortcomings as an outcome measure for patients with acetabular fractures.

Chapter 25

Spinal Cord Injury: Pathophysiology and Current Treatment Strategies

Brian K. Kwon, MD, PhD, FRCSC

Alexander R. Vaccaro, MD

Introduction

Paralysis following spinal cord injury remains one of the most functionally devastating impairments known to man. Historically believed to be an ailment without cure, many recent advances in the neurobiologic understanding of spinal cord injury have generated optimism regarding the development of effective therapies. At the same time, as the complexities of the pathophysiology are unravelled, it is becoming increasingly evident that the initial forays into neurobiologic treatment will not be made with the expectation of a cure, but rather with the hope of providing incremental improvements in function. Nevertheless, given the rather dismal prognosis for neurologic recovery in patients with acute and chronic spinal cord injuries, the potential for such improvements represents the source of much hope.

For those individuals with acute injury, the primary focus of research has been on neuroprotective strategies that aim to minimize further neural injury. Such strategies require an advanced understanding of the pathophysiologic processes that are initiated immediately after injury. For those whose injuries are subacute or chronic and the neural damage is more established, therapies to promote axonal regeneration are needed. Such strategies are based on the understanding of the pathology of spinal cord injuries and the obstacles that limit regeneration and functional recovery. The problems that patients with spinal cord injuries encounter are multifaceted, and clearly a great deal more must be learned before realizing the dream of returning such individuals to full physical function.

Pathophysiology of Acute Spinal Cord Injury

The various mechanisms by which the spinal column fails under external loads (such as flexion-extension bending, distraction, and shear) infers that the spinal cord can be subjected to a wide spectrum of forces. Whether these different injury mechanisms result in distinct patterns of neurologic deficit in humans is difficult to establish, al-though this may be largely attributable to both the inherent difficulty in estimating all of the forces involved in a given traumatic incident and the limited precision with which contemporary methods of assessment are able to characterize neurologic function. The findings of animal model studies of spinal cord injury corroborate the experience of clinicians who have recognized that the severity of neurologic impairment is related to the energy delivered to the spinal cord, which in turn is influenced by such factors as velocity, displacement, and time of compression.[1] Patients who survive an initial blunt trauma event and have a functionally complete spinal cord injury usually do not have an anatomically severed spinal cord.[2] Even in many patients with gunshot wounds to the spine, the paraplegia is often caused by the concussive effects of the bullet passing adjacent to rather than through the spinal cord. This anatomically incomplete primary injury caused by the initial mechanical forces on the spinal cord is rapidly followed by a complex array of vascular, biochemical, and molecular responses that are considered, for the most part, to further injure the spinal cord. The concept of neuroprotection is based on the premise that counteracting these secondary injury responses will reduce the overall damage to the spinal cord and ultimately maximize the potential for neurologic recovery. Although such a concept has been well borne out in the findings of animal model studies of spinal cord injury, effective neuroprotection has been somewhat difficult to convincingly demonstrate in humans. Animal studies have shown that significant motor function can be maintained with the sparing of as few as 1.4% to 12% of the total number of axons across the injury site.[3] Although comparable data are not available for humans, the implication from such animal model study data is that even small gains in neuroprotection may provide substantial benefit for patients with spinal cord injury.

Following the acute pathophysiologic sequelae of the injury, the hemorrhage and necrotic debris at the lesion site are removed, and a fluid-filled cavity is usually established over time. This cavity, which sometimes extends over multiple rostral-caudal segments, is surrounded by a gliotic scar, fibrous tissue, and a periphery of spared neural tissue, the amount of which probably depends on the mechanism and severity of the initial injury.[2] Although axons may travel within this spared rim of tissue, many are thought to have lost their myelin sheaths, making them inefficient at conducting action potentials across the injury site. Such axons represent a potential substrate for improved neurologic function if they can be remyelinated or induced to conduct action potentials more effectively via pharmacotherapies. The gliotic scar, the cystic cavitation, and the remaining elements of central nervous system myelin within the spinal cord all present formidable obstacles to axonal regeneration.

Emergent Management

As with all trauma patients, patients with spinal cord injuries need to be initially managed in accordance to Advanced Trauma Life Support principles, with initial emphasis on the airway, breathing, and circulation. It is important to recognize that these patients frequently have multiple injuries that should not be overlooked in the setting of acute paraplegia. Respiratory failure secondary to lost diaphragmatic innervation at C3-C5 or neurogenic shock secondary to the loss of sympathetic cardiovascular tone are life-threatening sequelae of spinal cord injuries that must be identified and managed in the primary survey. The spinal column must be immobilized to prevent further trauma to the cord. The need for such immobilization begins in the field at the site of injury and should be judiciously adhered to in the emergency room during the initial patient evaluation. This includes the use of in-line traction of the cervical spine during intubation and careful log rolling of the patient during the examination of the dorsal axial skeleton.

For patients who are otherwise stable from a trauma perspective, the injury to the spinal cord requires other special considerations in the emergent management. As hypoxia and ischemia are thought to contribute to the pathophysiology of acute spinal cord injury, supplemental oxygen to maximize the systemic oxygenation status is recommended, as is volume support to keep the systolic blood pressure between 80 and 100 mm Hg.[4] The outcomes of such measures at a microvascular and cellular level are somewhat uncertain, given the loss of vascular autoregulation within the spinal cord, but efforts to achieve optimal perfusion and oxygenation have a sound rationale in trauma care.

Patients with a spinal cord injury require a carefully performed and documented neurologic assessment that includes the evaluation of motor strength, light touch and pinprick sensation, perianal motor and sensory function, deep tendon reflexes, and the bulbocavernosus reflex. These form the basis of the American Spinal Injury Association (ASIA) scale of spinal cord injury, which classifies severity of neurologic impairment into five grades (A through E). Although this system helps to classify the severity of injury and prognosticate functional recovery, it is important to realize that it is not a linear scale and that perhaps the most important distinction is whether a patient has a functionally complete (ASIA grade A) versus an incomplete (ASIA grade B, C, or D) injury. Approximately 10% to 15% of patients with an ASIA grade A complete injury will improve sufficiently to be designated as incomplete, whereas only 2% to 3% will achieve functional strength distal to the initial level of injury.[5] Conversely, approximately 75% of patients with incomplete injuries become community ambulators.[6]

Finally, appropriate imaging must be performed to characterize the injury of the spinal column and cord. Screening AP, lateral, and open-mouth odontoid radiographic views of the cervical spine with adequate visualization of the cervicothoracic junction are necessary. Patients with any suspected spinal cord injury should have thoracic and lumbar spine radiographs obtained to identify other injuries to the spinal axis because of the frequent occurrence of noncontiguous spinal injuries, which have been reported to be as high as 10.5% of patients.[7] Although some controversy exists regarding what constitutes adequate screening cervical spine films in the awake and cooperative patient, the presence of a spinal cord injury clearly warrants additional imaging studies with CT and/or MRI.

The Role of Pharmacotherapies in Acute Spinal Cord Injury

Methylprednisolone

Historically, it was generally accepted that the only contemporary treatment strategy for acute spinal cord injuries was high-dose methylprednisolone. Large, prospective, randomized National Acute Spinal Cord Injury Studies (NASCIS) of approximately 1,000 patients established intravenous administration of methylprednisolone to patients within 8 hours of spinal cord injury as the standard of care across North America.[8,9]

The use of high-dose methylprednisolone for patients with acute spinal cord injuries has become the most controversial contemporary issue in neurotrauma today. The widespread use of this agent has come under severe criticism in recent years as the execution, results, and interpretation of the NASCIS 2 and 3 studies have undergone intense scrutiny and critical appraisal. The NASCIS 2 study randomized patients within 24 hours of injury, and the analysis of the motor and sensory recovery between the treatment arms demonstrated no significant benefit to methylprednisolone; that is, the primary outcome was in fact negative. The establishment of the 8-hour cutoff was based on a post hoc analysis of only 66 of 162 patients randomized to receive methylprednisolone and 69 of 171 patients randomized to receive placebo who fit within this 8-hour window. In this group, a small but statistically significant benefit in terms of motor recovery and sensory recovery in the methylprednisolone treated patients was detected. Similarly, the primary outcome of the NASCIS 3 study in which patients were randomized to receive methylprednisolone or placebo within 8 hours of injury was also negative. The recommendation to extend the methylprednisolone infusion to 48 hours for patients between 3 and 8 hours of injury was also based on a post hoc analysis of the data that demonstrated a statistically insignificant ($P = 0.08$) improvement in a functional independence measure for this subset of patients. This study also demonstrated a much higher incidence of wound infection, pulmonary embolism, severe pneumonia, sepsis, and even death secondary to respiratory complications with the steroid use, particularly with patients in the 48-hour protocol.

The controversy surrounding the use of methylprednisolone and its central role in the acute management of spinal cord injuries has prompted a number of extensive reviews on the topic. A review commissioned by the American Association of Neurological Surgeons and the Congress of Neurological Surgeons concluded that the 24- or 48-hour methylprednisolone protocol be recommended only as an option rather than the standard of care because the evidence suggesting adverse effects is more consistent than any suggestion of clinical benefit.[10] A similar review by the Canadian Neurosurgical Society and the Canadian Spine Society concluded that "there is insufficient evidence to support the use of high-dose methylprednisolone within 8 hours following an acute closed spinal cord injury as a treatment standard or as a guideline for treatment".[11]

Despite this, the use of methylprednisolone to treat patients with acute spinal cord injuries remains commonplace in most North American medical centers. It would appear that some clinicians believe that its use is still justified based on the otherwise desperate situation that these patients are in and that even a remote chance of benefit is better than no treatment at all. Given the current medicolegal climate, particularly in the United States, there is undoubtedly enormous pressure on physicians to administer methylprednisolone for the reasonably justifiable fear of being held liable for the patient's almost certain long-term neurologic deficit. Some centers in Canada, however, have officially discontinued the use of methylprednisolone for patients with acute spinal cord injuries. An interesting consideration for the ongoing progress of neuroprotection in patients with spinal cord injuries is that if methylprednisolone continues to be perceived as the standard of care, will future studies of other neuroprotective agents be required to administer methylprednisolone as well, thereby introducing a potentially significant confounder to the study design and interpretation?

Monosialotetrahexosylganglioside

The only other neuroprotective agent to have undergone large, prospective, randomized evaluation is monosialotetrahexosylganglioside (GM1). The systemic administration of gangliosides, sialic acid-containing glycosphingolipids that are highly expressed on the outer surface of cell membranes within the central nervous system, has been found to be neuroprotective in various models of central nervous system injury.[12,13] One study randomized 797 patients to receive placebo, low-dose GM1 (300 mg loading dose and then 100 mg/day for 56 days), or high-dose GM1 (600 mg loading dose and then 200 mg/day for 56 days).[14] All patients received methylprednisolone in accordance to NASCIS 2 findings before receiving GM1. GM1 treatment was not associated with a significantly higher proportion of patients with marked motor recovery at 26 weeks compared with those receiving placebo, but additional analysis of this data did reveal some benefit for motor, sensory, and autonomic function in patients with incomplete injuries. The use of GM1 for patients with acute spinal cord injuries has not been approved by the US Food and Drug Administration.

Other Pharmacotherapies for Acute Spinal Cord Injury

The number of other agents that have undergone randomized controlled human evaluation as neuroprotectants in patients with acute spinal cord injury is small, particularly when compared with the vast number of compounds that are studied in animal models. Naloxone and tirilazad mesylate were evaluated as treatment arms in the NASCIS 2 and 3 studies, respectively, but neither was deemed to promote significant neurologic or functional improvement. Thyrotropin-releasing hormone, an endogenous opioid antagonist, was evaluated in a small trial of 20 patients, but the authors found that it did not confer any benefit over placebo.[15] Nimodipine, a calcium channel blocker, was evaluated in a study that randomized 106 patients to receive nimodipine, nimodipine plus methylprednisolone, methylprednisolone alone, or placebo.[16] In the 100 patients available for follow-up, no significant difference between the four groups was observed.

The Role of Decompression in Acute Spinal Cord Injury

One of the most peculiar aspects of treating patients with acute spinal cord injuries is the inability of surgeons to demonstrate that patients with an earlier decompression of their spinal cord fare better neurologically—this despite the fact that most animal studies suggest that earlier decompression results in improved neurologic outcome. The current understanding of the pathophysiology of acute spinal cord injury seems to indicate that the sooner mechanical pressure is relieved from the spinal cord, the better. Human studies have been conducted and have not demonstrated a significant benefit to early decompression, either via closed reduction maneuvers or surgery.[17] In anticipation of conducting a prospective randomized controlled study, the Surgical Treatment for Acute Spinal Cord Injury Study (STASCIS) group performed a retrospective, multicenter analysis of spinal surgery for patients with acute spinal cord injury and found little agreement among centers regarding both the use and timing of surgical intervention for these patients.[18] Many theories attempt to explain why a benefit to early decompression has not been established. First, it could be that the neurologic injury that many patients sustain is of such a severe nature that no current treatment strategy—surgical or pharmaceutical—will have a significant impact on function. Second, it is difficult to identify exactly what early decompression constitutes. For example, in one study that randomized patients to undergo early versus later surgery and found no benefit to early decompression, decompression was performed more than 24 hours after injury in the patients who underwent early surgery.[17,19] Recognizing that robust evidence is lacking regarding this important issue, a prospective, randomized trial comparing early versus later decompression of cervical spinal cord injuries has recently been initiated. This multicenter study is randomizing patients with cervical spinal cord injuries to undergo either early (< 12 hours after injury) or later (> 24 hours after injury) decompression; when completed, it is expected to provide the most epidemiologically sound argument for or against early surgery.

Spinal Cord Injury Syndromes

Complete Versus Incomplete

In an effort to classify and prognosticate patients with patterns of neurologic injury, several spinal cord injury syndromes have been described. As stated previously, probably the most important distinction to be made is whether the patient has a neurologically complete injury (no sparing of motor and sensory function in the lowest sacral segment) or an incomplete injury (some sacral sensation exists). The ASIA classification system is the most common method for characterizing neurologic injury; the most recent standards were published in 2002 (Figure 1). Surgeons who meet the families of patients with spinal cord injury are commonly asked about a prognosis for neurologic recovery. Clearly, the expected neurorecovery of patients with complete tetraplegia or paraplegia is extremely poor, particularly when complete motor and sensory deficits continue for 1 month after the initial injury.[20] Although the chance of recovering functional motor strength in the lower extremities is negligible, 70% to 85% of patients with complete tetraplegia will regain function in at least one motor level distal to the original level of injury. For example, patients with C6 quadriplegia will possibly regain C7 function, and the associated triceps strength has enormous functional implications because it may allow them to transfer independently.

Patients with incomplete spinal cord injuries fare significantly better in terms of upper and lower extremity motor and sensory function. Most patients with incomplete spinal cord injuries will gain 12 to 14 motor points (as measured by the Medical Research Council muscle grading system) in the lower extremities within the first year after injury. Most of the improvements can be expected to occur in the first 9 months, with very little progress occurring beyond 1 year. In general, muscles that have grade 1 or 2 strength at 1 month after injury will recover to at least a grade 3 strength by 1 year, making them "motor-useful." Approximately half of patients with incomplete tetraplegia and three quarters of those with incomplete paraplegia will achieve sufficient lower extremity function so as to become community ambulators, a feat that requires grade 3 to 5 strength of hip flexors or greater on one side and grade 3 to 5 strength of quadriceps or greater on the other side.

Because patients with incomplete spinal cord injuries represent a somewhat heterogeneous group, it is interesting to consider some of the factors that may influence their neurologic outcome. In a review of more than 400 patients with incomplete cervical spinal cord injuries, it was found that neurologic outcome was favorable in younger patients and those with either a central spinal cord or Brown-Séquard syndrome.[21] Interestingly, the type of fracture, mechanism of injury, early definitive surgery, or early anterior decompression (occurring within 24 hours), decompression of stenosis in the absence of fractures, and the administration of high-dose methylprednisolone did not influence neurologic recovery.

Anterior Cord Syndrome

This syndrome describes patients with an anterior lesion to the spinal cord that predominantly affects the anteriorly positioned spinothalamic and corticospinal tracts, but leaves the dorsal columns intact. Such a lesion can be caused by the central retropulsion of bony fragments or herniated disk material. The prognosis for motor recovery in such patients is limited.[21]

Brown-Séquard Syndrome

This syndrome describes a lesion affecting the lateral half of the spinal cord that causes ipsilateral motor and proprioceptive deficits but contralateral pain and temperature impairment. Such a lesion can also be caused by retropulsed bony fragments and disk material or occur in

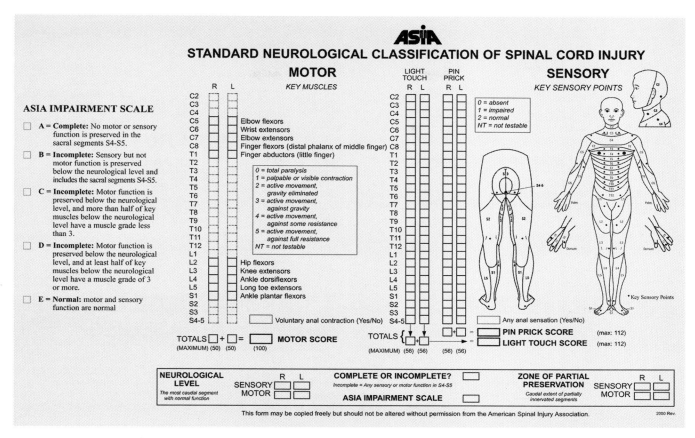

Figure 1 The ASIA Impairment Scale and Assessment Form. Patients with an acute spinal cord injury require a careful neurologic examination that involves motor and sensory testing, and most importantly, an evaluation of function in the lowest sacral segments (S4-S5). The motor score is derived from 10 key myotomes in the upper and lower extremities. Patients are graded based on whether they demonstrate function at S4-S5 (complete versus incomplete) and how much residual motor and sensory function they have maintained (to determine the extent of incompleteness).

patients with penetrating injuries. In general, the prognosis for ambulation in patients with this type of injury is quite favorable, possibly facilitated by spinal cord plasticity in which intact fibers compensate for axons that have been cut on the contralateral side.[22]

Posterior Cord Syndrome

This syndrome describes a lesion affecting the dorsal columns of the spinal cord and causing primarily a proprioceptive loss. Posterior cord syndrome is extremely rare, and little is documented regarding the ultimate prognosis for patients with this type of injury.

Central Cord Syndrome

This is perhaps the most common and most extensively studied pattern of spinal cord injury. It describes a pattern of disproportionately greater upper versus lower extremity motor weakness with variable loss of sensation. The greater upper extremity impairment was originally hypothesized to be related to a somatotopic organization of the corticospinal tracts, with the axons to the lower extremities running more peripheral than those directed to the upper extremities. This hypothesis has

been refuted, and more recent evidence suggests that the disproportionate motor deficit in patients with central cord syndrome simply reflects an injury to the corticospinal tracts that are more responsible for fine motor function in the upper extremity than lower extremity.[23,24]

The optimal management of patients with acute central cord syndrome is somewhat controversial. Many patients, particularly elderly patients with preexisting spondylosis, typically have a central spinal cord injury after low-energy trauma but no significant mechanical instability that warrants acute stabilization. The overall prognosis for neurologic recovery is generally good for patients with this type of injury. Many patients continue to have significant motor impairment and pain, particularly in the hands. For this patient population, it should be determined whether decompression is warranted in the early stages or whether decompression should be postponed until neurologic recovery has reached a plateau. A retrospective evaluation of the surgical management of 50 patients with acute central cord syndrome found that patients with an acute disk herniation or instability achieved greater motor recovery if they underwent decompression within 24 hours.[25] No benefit to early sur-

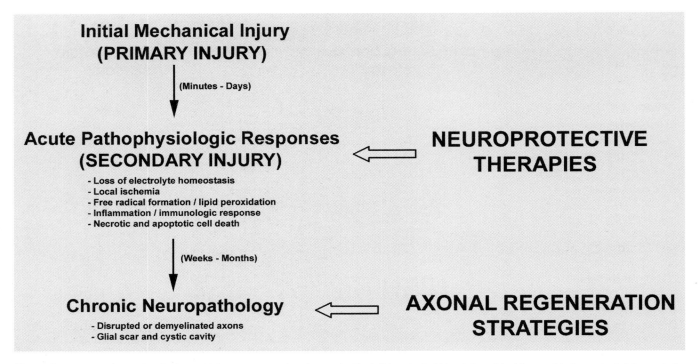

Figure 2 Schematic representation of spinal cord injury responses and repair strategies. The initial mechanical injury (primary injury) is caused by the mechanical damage to the spinal cord. This typically does not transect the spinal cord. Acute pathophysiologic processes are then rapidly activated and are thought to contribute to worsening damage to the spinal cord (secondary injury). Neuroprotective therapies such as methylprednisolone are thought to attenuate these processes and maximize tissue sparing. Over months, these processes lead to a glial cyst and scar at the injury site, and axonal regeneration strategies aim to regrow axons across this region or promote sprouting of intact axons to accommodate for the functional loss.

gery was observed in patients with spinal stenosis or spondylosis, those older than 60 years, and those with bladder dysfunction on initial presentation. These findings suggest that although patients with central cord syndrome have historically done well neurologically, correct optimal management should take into consideration such factors as the mechanism and energy of injury, etiology, and patient age.

Future Directions in Spinal Cord Injury Research

Neuroprotection Strategies

As mentioned previously, the two main neurobiologic streams of research directed toward improving neurologic function after spinal cord injury focus on neuroprotective strategies to minimize secondary damage and maximize the sparing of neural tissue, and axonal regeneration strategies to promote the regrowth of injured axons or the sprouting of spared axons to accommodate for lost fibers (Figure 2). Significant work is also being done in the fields of pain management, functional retraining, and autonomic dysfunction.

Given the current theory of spinal cord repair, it is commonly believed that the greatest impact on neurologic recovery will be achieved through neuroprotective interventions. For orthopaedic surgeons who encounter patients in the acute injury state, these therapies have significant relevance. A greater understanding of the pathophysiology of acute spinal cord injury is facilitating the development of such interventions. For example, the improved understanding of the complex pathways that either promote or inhibit programmed cell death (apoptosis) of neurons and glial cells in the days to weeks following spinal cord injury has led to novel means of arresting the process in animal models. For example, the transgenic overexpression of the antiapoptotic protein Bcl-2 or the in vivo transfection of its gene on a DNA plasmid has been shown to be neuroprotective and to promote functional improvement.[26,27] There is some evidence to suggest that standard pharmacotherapies such as dexamethasone also attenuate the process of apoptosis after spinal cord injuries.[28] It is hoped that additional work in this area will provide clinically effective means of limiting apoptosis in this patient population.

Currently, one of the most intensely studied topics in neuroprotection is the role of inflammatory and immune responses in the pathophysiology of spinal cord injury. Research has demonstrated that some aspects of central nervous system inflammation, in addition to a T cell-mediated immune response to antigens at the spinal cord injury site, may in fact promote functional recovery by clearing cellular debris and secreting neurotrophic factors.[29] A phase 1 human clinical trial in which autologous activated macrophages are injected into the spinal cords of patients with complete thoracic injuries is underway. Other researchers have found that attenuating inflammation facilitates behavioral recovery and that promoting a T cell-mediated immune response can actually worsen neurologic injury and impair functional recovery.[30] These discrepancies highlight the complexities of the inflammatory and immune responses in the pathophysiology of spinal cord injury.

From a clinical standpoint, it is clear that the pathway from drug development at a molecular level in laboratory animals to its actual application in clinical trials of human patients is an extremely long and potentially unsuccessful journey. One of the exciting recent trends in spinal cord injury research is the discovery and characterization of the neuroprotective effects of drugs that are already in human clinical use for other applications and therefore may be safe for use in the treatment of spinal cord injury. Although such pharmacotherapies still require extensive efficacy testing, current applications in humans overcome many important safety issues. Minocycline, for example, is a tetracycline antibiotic that is commonly used in the treatment of acne. Minocycline has been shown to be neuroprotective in various animal models of ischemia, neurodegeneration, and trauma.[31] In a clip compression model of spinal cord injuries, systemic minocycline has been shown to promote animal survival, reduce the area of local spinal cord damage, and improve function on locomotor testing.[31] Erythropoietin is another drug that was found to have significant neuroprotective properties, initially in models of cerebral ischemia, then in models of spinal cord ischemia, and finally in models of traumatic spinal cord injury.[32] A single systemic dose of erythropoietin immediately after blunt spinal cord injury resulted in marked sparing of neural tissue at the injury site and significantly better locomotor function in a rat model.[33] Such promising results will likely justify the initiation of human trials in the foreseeable future.

Axonal Regeneration Strategies

Clinical experience reflects vastly different expectations of axonal regeneration within the central nervous system and the peripheral nervous system. Conceptually, the poor regeneration witnessed in the central nervous system is related to two issues: a limited intrinsic ability of central nervous system neurons to reextend their axons after injury and hostile elements within the central nervous system environment that inhibit axonal growth[34] (Figure 3).

The limited intrinsic capacity of central nervous system neurons to regenerate axons after injury may be closely related to the inability to sufficiently activate the genetic mechanisms necessary for axonal regrowth. The delivery of growth factors may help to stimulate these

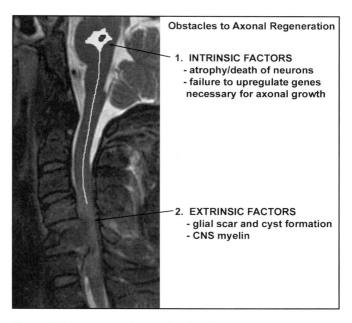

Figure 3 Obstacles to axonal regeneration. This MRI scan helps to illustrate the two principal reasons why axonal regeneration fails in neurons of the central nervous system. First, the central nervous system neurons themselves intrinsically have poor regenerative ability once their axons are disrupted. This may be because of the retrograde atrophy or death of neurons after axotomy and/or the failure to upregulate the genes that are necessary for axonal growth. Second, extrinsic factors at the spinal cord injury site itself are inhibitory to axonal regeneration. Such factors include the hostile glial scar and cyst that develop at the injury site and proteins within central nervous system myelin that are inhibitory to axonal growth.

mechanisms and promote axonal regeneration in patients with either acute or chronic spinal cord injuries.[35,36] Altering levels of intracellular secondary messengers such as cyclic adenosine monophosphate has also been shown to influence the regenerative abilities of neurons.[37]

A great deal has been learned recently about the molecules that inhibit central axonal regeneration. Central nervous system myelin, formed by oligodendrocytes (in contrast to peripheral nervous system myelin, formed by Schwann cells), contains molecules that inhibit axonal growth. The molecules identified and characterized thus far include Nogo, myelin associated glycoprotein, and oligodendrocyte-myelin glycoprotein. Surprisingly, these all appear to bind to the same Nogo receptor, and the subsequent signalling pathways downstream may represent a point of convergence that can be targeted by therapeutic interventions.[38]

The signalling pathways within the axonal tip (the growth cone) are also being extensively studied. Much attention has been placed on the Rho family of small guanosine triphosphatases and their role in mediating the growth cone's response to environmental cues. There is recent evidence to suggest that by manipulating these guanosine triphosphate pathways, axons can be induced to grow or sprout through the otherwise inhibitory central environment.[39]

The other major impediment to central axonal regeneration is the glial scar and cyst that become established at the injury site. Astrocytes comprise a large part of the glial scar, and in addition to forming a physical barrier to axonal growth, they may contribute to the expression of a number of inhibitory molecules. Chondroitin sulfate proteoglycans have been identified within the glial scar as important impediments to axonal growth. The enzymatic degradation of such proteoglycans with chondroitinase ABC was shown to promote axonal sprouting and functional recovery after experimental spinal cord injury.[40] As the molecular components of the glial scar become more clearly characterized, methods to circumvent the barrier and inhibitory effects will have a potential therapeutic role.

The formidable gap created by the cystic lesion at the site of spinal cord injury has invoked much interest in cellular transplantation techniques to serve as "bridges" or matrix for axons to grow through. A number of cellular substrates have been evaluated in this context and appear promising. Fetal tissue transplants were investigated extensively in the 1990s, leading to a small phase I trial of fetal spinal cord tissue transplantation in patients with chronic syringomyelia. The results of this study demonstrated that the technique was feasible and safe, but it did not lead to significant functional recovery.[41] The demonstration that embryonic stem cell transplantation might promote axonal regeneration, remyelination, and functional recovery in animal models of spinal cord injury triggered enormous scientific and public interest over the therapeutic use of embryonic stem cells.[42] Many legal and ethical issues surrounding the use of embryonic stem cells remain unresolved, and this will most certainly influence the progress of this potential therapy in future years. Schwann cell and peripheral nerve transplantation into the spinal cord provides a permissive peripheral nervous system environment that has been shown to encourage the regeneration of injured central nervous system axons. In fact, the demonstration that injured central nervous system axons could grow into the peripheral nervous system environment of peripheral nerve transplants refuted the longstanding view that central nervous system axons lacked any regenerative potential at all. What has limited this otherwise fairly simple therapeutic strategy is the observation that central nervous system axons grow fairly readily into the peripheral nervous system environment of the transplant, but they are reluctant to leave and return to the central nervous system in part because of the inhibitory central nervous system elements discussed previously. This difficulty in crossing the peripheral nervous system to central nervous system barrier has sparked a great deal of interest in olfactory ensheathing glial cells.

These cells ensheathe and accompany regenerating axons from olfactory sensory neurons from the nasal epithelium (peripheral nervous system) into the olfactory bulb (central nervous system). The ability of olfactory ensheathing cells to escort axons across this "peripheral nervous system to central nervous system barrier" has been exploited in numerous transplantation experiments involving acute and chronic spinal cord injuries.[43] Clinical trials in which olfactory ensheathing cells are being transplanted into the spinal cord are underway in various centers around the world.

Summary

Despite enormous scientific and clinical efforts, the prognosis for neurologic recovery in patients with severe spinal cord injuries remains poor. Nevertheless, with an increased understanding of the pathophysiology of acute spinal cord injury and the factors that limit axonal regeneration within the central nervous system, an increasing number of therapeutic strategies are being developed. Although the potential for establishing therapies with some efficacy for this devastating condition has raised a great deal of optimism, goals must remain realistic, and a high level of clinical and epidemiologic rigor must be applied in the human evaluation of these new therapies. The coming years will most certainly be a time of great excitement as the results of numerous human spinal cord injury trials become known and directions for future research are clarified.

Annotated References

1. Kwon BK, Oxland TR, Tetzlaff W: Animal models used in spinal cord regeneration research. *Spine* 2002;27:1504-1510.

   A number of animal models exist in which to develop and evaluate therapeutic strategies for spinal cord injury. This article describes the advantages and disadvantages of injury models in which the spinal cord is sharply or bluntly injured, which can help clinicians interpret studies of a basic science nature. The biomechanical aspects of contusion-type injury models are also discussed.

2. Kakulas BA: A review of the neuropathology of human spinal cord injury with emphasis on special features. *J Spinal Cord Med* 1999;22:119-124.

3. Fehlings MG, Tator CH: The relationships among the severity of spinal cord injury, residual neurological function, axon counts, and counts of retrogradely labeled neurons after experimental spinal cord injury. *Exp Neurol* 1995;132:220-228.

4. Nockels RP: Nonoperative management of acute spinal cord injury. *Spine* 2001;26:S31-S37.

   The author of this article summarizes a number of important nonsurgical considerations in the management of patients with acute spinal cord injuries.

5. Marino RJ, Ditunno JF Jr, Donovan WH, Maynard F Jr: Neurologic recovery after traumatic spinal cord injury: Data from the Model Spinal Cord Injury Systems. *Arch Phys Med Rehabil* 1999;80:1391-1396.

6. Waters RL, Adkins RH, Yakura JS, Sie I: Motor and sensory recovery following incomplete tetraplegia. *Arch Phys Med Rehabil* 1994;75:306-311.

7. Vaccaro AR, An HS, Lin S, Sun S, Balderston RA, Cotler JM: Noncontiguous injuries of the spine. *J Spinal Disord* 1992;5:320-329.

8. Bracken MB, Shepard MJ, Collins WF, et al: A randomized, controlled trial of methylprednisolone or naloxone in the treatment of acute spinal-cord injury: Results of the Second National Acute Spinal Cord Injury Study. *N Engl J Med* 1990;322:1405-1411.

9. Bracken MB, Shepard MJ, Holford TR, et al: Administration of methylprednisolone for 24 or 48 hours or tirilazad mesylate for 48 hours in the treatment of acute spinal cord injury: Results of the Third National Acute Spinal Cord Injury Randomized Controlled Trial. National Acute Spinal Cord Injury Study. *JAMA* 1997;277:1597-1604.

10. Pharmacological therapy after acute cervical spinal cord injury. *Neurosurgery* 2002;50(suppl 3):S63-S72.

    This review commissioned by the American Academy of Neurologic Surgeons and the Congress of Neurological Surgeons summarizes the controversy surrounding the use of methylprednisolone for patients with acute spinal cord injury. The article concludes that there is insufficient evidence to support methylprednisolone usage in this context. The literature on the use of GM1 ganglioside is also reviewed.

11. Hugenholtz H, Cass DE, Dvorak MF, et al: High-dose methylprednisolone for acute closed spinal cord injury: Only a treatment option. *Can J Neurol Sci* 2002;29:227-235.

    This group of Canadian spine surgeons reviewed the existing literature on the use of methylprednisolone to treat patients with acute spinal cord injury and concluded that the evidence (particularly that put forth by the NASCIS 2 and 3 studies) was not sufficient to warrant recommending the use of high-dose steroids as anything more than a treatment option for patients with acute spinal cord injury.

12. Ferrari G, Greene LA: Promotion of neuronal survival by GM1 ganglioside: Phenomenology and mechanism of action. *Ann N Y Acad Sci* 1998;845:263-273.

13. Imanaka T, Hukuda S, Maeda T: The role of GM1-ganglioside in the injured spinal cord of rats: An immunohistochemical study using GM1-antisera. *J Neurotrauma* 1996;13:163-170.

14. Geisler FH, Coleman WP, Grieco G, Poonian D: The Sygen multicenter acute spinal cord injury study. *Spine* 2001;26:S87-S98.

    This prospective, randomized clinical trial of almost 800 patients evaluated the efficacy of GM1 ganglioside for the treatment of acute spinal cord injury. It represents the only large-scale prospective, randomized trial of a neuroprotective agent other than methylprednisolone. For all of the patients who were enrolled, the primary outcome measure was negative, but there appeared to be a treatment benefit in those with incomplete spinal cord injuries.

15. Pitts LH, Ross A, Chase GA, Faden AI: Treatment with thyrotropin-releasing hormone (TRH) in patients with traumatic spinal cord injuries. *J Neurotrauma* 1995;12:235-243.

16. Pointillart V, Petitjean ME, Wiart L, et al: Pharmacological therapy of spinal cord injury during the acute phase. *Spinal Cord* 2000;38:71-76.

    This article presents the results of a prospective, randomized clinical trial that evaluated the calcium channel blocker, nimodipine, with or without methylprednisolone, in the treatment of 100 patients with acute spinal cord injuries. The authors report that their findings failed to demonstrate any significant benefit to the use of nimodipine, but the study may have been underpowered to do so.

17. Fehlings MG, Tator CH: An evidence-based review of decompressive surgery in acute spinal cord injury: Rationale, indications, and timing based on experimental and clinical studies. *J Neurosurg Spine* 1999;91:1-11.

18. Tator CH, Fehlings MG, Thorpe K, Taylor W: Current use and timing of spinal surgery for management of acute spinal surgery for management of acute spinal cord injury in North America: Results of a retrospective multicenter study. *J Neurosurg Spine* 1999;91:12-18.

19. Vaccaro AR, Daugherty RJ, Sheehan TP, et al: Neurologic outcome of early versus late surgery for cervical spinal cord injury. *Spine* 1997;22:2609-2613.

20. Burns AS, Ditunno JF: Establishing prognosis and maximizing functional outcomes after spinal cord injury: A review of current and future directions in rehabilitation management. *Spine* 2001;26:S137-S145.

The authors of this article reviewed a large body of rehabilitation medicine literature to describe the prognosis for neurologic recovery after spinal cord injury of varying degrees of severity.

21. Pollard ME, Apple DF: Factors associated with improved neurologic outcomes in patients with incomplete tetraplegia. *Spine* 2003;28:33-39.

The authors of this article retrospectively reviewed over 400 patients with incomplete traumatic cervical spinal cord injuries to delineate factors that may influence neurologic outcome. They found that patients who were younger and who sustained central cord syndrome or Brown-Séquard type injuries fared the best neurologically. Interestingly, they did not observe any benefit to the use of steroids in these patients.

22. Little JW, Halar E: Temporal course of motor recovery after Brown-Séquard spinal cord injuries. *Paraplegia* 1985;23:39-46.

23. Jimenez O, Marcillo A, Levi AD: A histopathological analysis of the human cervical spinal cord in patients with acute traumatic central cord syndrome. *Spinal Cord* 2000;38:532-537.

This is a study and discussion of the neuropathology and clinical presentation of acute traumatic central cord syndrome. Specifically, the authors histologically examined the cervical spinal cords of patients with acute and chronic central cord syndromes to determine if the loss of alpha motor neurons contributed to the acute hand dysfunction. They found injuries to the lateral corticospinal tract but not a significant reduction in motor neurons, and suggested that the hand dysfunction is more a reflection of the corticospinal tract injury.

24. Levi AD, Tator CH, Bunge RP: Clinical syndromes associated with disproportionate weakness of the upper versus the lower extremities after cervical spinal cord injury. *Neurosurgery* 1996;38:179-183.

25. Guest J, Eleraky MA, Apostolides PJ, Dickman CA, Sonntag VK: Traumatic central cord syndrome: Results of surgical management. *J Neurosurg Spine* 2002;97:25-32.

Studies that evaluate the relationship between surgery and neurologic outcome after spinal cord injury are not common. The authors of this study retrospectively reviewed the outcomes of patients with traumatic central cord syndrome who underwent surgical decompression either within or after 24 hours of injury. Early decompression appeared to be superior to later decompression in those patients whose injuries were related to a traumatic disk herniation or fracture/dislocation, but it did not appear to change the outcome in those patients whose injuries were related to cervical stenosis or spondylosis.

26. Qiu J, Nesic O, Ye Z, et al: Bcl-xL expression after contusion to the rat spinal cord. *J Neurotrauma* 2001; 18:1267-1278.

27. Seki T, Hida K, Tada M, Koyanagi I, Iwasaki Y: Role of the bcl-2 gene after contusive spinal cord injury in mice. *Neurosurgery* 2003;53:192-198.

28. Zurita M, Vaquero J, Oya S, Morales C: Effects of dexamethasone on apoptosis-related cell death after spinal cord injury. *J Neurosurg Spine* 2002;96:83-89.

The authors of this article demonstrated that the administration of dexamethasone in an animal model of acute spinal cord injury was associated with reduced apoptotic death of neurons and glia at the site of spinal cord injury.

29. Hauben E, Schwartz M: Therapeutic vaccination for spinal cord injury: Helping the body to cure itself. *Trends Pharmacol Sci* 2003;24:7-12.

The role of the inflammatory and immunologic responses to spinal cord injury is a matter of considerable debate. The authors of this article discuss how certain aspects of these responses can be manipulated to improve neurologic outcome after spinal cord injury. One such approach, using autologous activated macrophages, has undergone human trials in patients with complete spinal cord injuries.

30. Popovich PG, Jones TB: Manipulating neuroinflammatory reactions in the injured spinal cord: Back to basics. *Trends Pharmacol Sci* 2003;24:13-17.

Although some evidence exists to suggest a beneficial role of the inflammatory and immunologic responses in the treatment of spinal cord injury, the authors of this article reviewed the literature that demonstrates deleterious effects. Their findings are important in that they highlight the incompleteness of the current understanding of the immune system and its role in spinal cord injury. The authors urge caution before initiating clinical trials of therapies that manipulate this response.

31. Wells JE, Hurlbert RJ, Fehlings MG, Yong VW: Neuroprotection by minocycline facilitates significant recovery from spinal cord injury in mice. *Brain* 2003;126:1628-1637.

This article provides the first in vivo demonstration of the neuroprotective effects of minocycline in an animal model of blunt spinal cord injury. The results of this study, which showed decreased secondary injury and improved motor function, raise the exciting possibility that this commonly used drug may be beneficial for the treatment of patients with spinal cord injuries.

32. Goldman SA, Nedergaard M: Erythropoietin strikes a new cord. *Nat Med* 2002;8:785-787.

    The authors of this article review the biologic mechanisms by which erythropoietin may mediate neuroprotection in patients with spinal cord injury and be beneficial in the treatment of other neurologic disorders. The common use of erythropoietin in clinical practice makes it an appealing experimental therapy.

33. Gorio A, Gokmen N, Erbayraktar S, et al: Recombinant human erythropoietin counteracts secondary injury and markedly enhances neurological recovery from experimental spinal cord trauma. *Proc Natl Acad Sci USA* 2002;99:9450-9455.

    This is the first study to demonstrate a significant neuroprotective benefit to the systemic administration of erythropoietin in an animal model of blunt spinal cord injury. The authors demonstrated reduced secondary damage at the site of injury and improved neurologic function on locomotor testing.

34. Kwon BK, Tetzlaff W: Spinal cord regeneration: From gene to transplants. *Spine* 2001;26:S13-S22.

    This article provides a general overview of the neurobiologic strategies that have been developed to promote axonal regeneration after spinal cord injury. Strategies such as neurotrophic factors, myelin inhibition, and cellular transplantation are discussed.

35. Kobayashi NR, Fan DP, Giehl KM, Bedard AM, Wiegand SJ, Tetzlaff W: BDNF and NT-4/5 prevent atrophy of rat rubrospinal neurons after cervical axotomy, stimulate GAP-43 and Talpha1-tubulin mRNA expression, and promote axonal regeneration. *J Neurosci* 1997;17:9583-9595.

36. Kwon BK, Liu J, Messerer C, et al: Survival and regeneration of rubrospinal neurons 1 year after spinal cord injury. *Proc Natl Acad Sci USA* 2002;99: 3246-3251.

    Many therapeutic strategies to promote axonal regeneration in animal models of spinal cord injury lose their efficacy after a short delay in their implementation, raising questions about their applicability in chronic spinal cord injury. The authors of this study applied a growth factor, brain derived neurotrophic factor, to the cell bodies of chronically injured neurons (1 year after spinal cord injury) and demonstrated that axonal regeneration was possible.

37. Qiu J, Cai D, Dai H, et al: Spinal axon regeneration induced by elevation of cyclic AMP. *Neuron* 2002; 34:895-903.

    Failure to regenerate axons after spinal cord injury is related to both the poor intrinsic regenerative ability of central nervous system neurons and to inhibitory elements within the central nervous system environment. The authors demonstrated that the intrinsic ability of a neuron to regenerate can be influenced by levels of intracellular messengers such as cyclic adenosine monophosphate.

38. Kwon BK, Borisoff JF, Tetzlaff W: Molecular targets for intervention in spinal cord injury. *Mol Interv* 2002;2:244-258.

    The authors of this article summarize many of the molecular obstacles that inhibit axonal regeneration and functional recovery after spinal cord injury. The delineation of molecular pathways that mediate such inhibition has led to the discovery of common pathways that are used by numerous agents; such pathways represent potential targets for therapeutic interventions.

39. Fournier AE, Takizawa BT, Strittmatter SM: Rho kinase inhibition enhances axonal regeneration in the injured CNS. *J Neurosci* 2003;23:1416-1423.

    One of the more recent advances in axonal regeneration is the delineation of intracellular signalling pathways at the level of the growth cone, many of which involve the Rho family of guanosine triphosphatases. The authors of this article demonstrate that the inhibitory properties of particular central nervous system myelin proteins (Nogo 66) are mediated through these signalling pathways and that axonal regeneration can be promoted both in vitro and in vivo via pharmacologic manipulation.

40. Bradbury EJ, Moon LD, Popat RJ, et al: Chondroitinase ABC promotes functional recovery after spinal cord injury. *Nature* 2002;416:636-640.

    The glial scar that develops at the site of spinal cord injury is thought to be a major impediment to axonal regeneration and functional recovery. This study demonstrated that the degradation of chondroitin sulfate proteoglycans, a major component of glial scar, could lead to axonal regeneration and/or sprouting and functional recovery in an animal model of spinal cord injury.

41. Wirth ED III, Reier PJ, Fessler RG, et al: Feasibility and safety of neural tissue transplantation in patients with syringomyelia. *J Neurotrauma* 2001;18:911-929.

    This article provides preliminary outcomes of two of eight patients with chronic syringomyelia who underwent fetal tissue transplantations into their spinal cord lesions. The authors report that the two patients did not deteriorate neurologically, and MRI revealed that the fetal tissue was incorporated into the cyst with no adverse effects.

42. McDonald JW, Howard MJ: Repairing the damaged spinal cord: A summary of our early success with embryonic stem cell transplantation and remyelination. *Prog Brain Res* 2002;137:299-309.

Some of the most promising research in the area of stem cell transplantation for the treatment of spinal cord injury was published by McDonald in 1999, and this article discusses the subsequent advances in the use of embryonic stem cells. The authors report that such cells are capable of differentiating into oligodendrocytes and myelinating axons at the spinal cord injury site.

43. Santos-Benito FF, Ramon-Cueto A: Olfactory ensheathing glia transplantation: A therapy to promote repair in the mammalian central nervous system. *Anat Rec B New Anat* 2003;271:77-85.

Olfactory ensheathing glial cells represent a potential cellular substrate for transplantation strategies for spinal cord injuries because of their apparent ability to accompany axons from the permissive peripheral nervous system environment to the inhibitory central nervous system environment. The authors of this article summarize the recent advances in this field of transplantation biology.

Chapter 26

Upper Cervical Spine Injury: Occiput to C2

Thomas J. Puschak, MD

Rick C. Sasso, MD

Introduction

The bony structures of the occiput and upper cervical spine are strong and often not affected by osteoporosis until late in life. Injuries to this area often occur secondary to high-energy trauma from acceleration-deceleration injuries or blunt force trauma to the head and neck. Noncontiguous spinal injuries occur in 10% to 20% of patients with injuries at the craniocervical junction.[1] The occipitoatlantal and atlantoaxial articulations are characterized by minimally constrained joints stabilized by strong ligamentous attachments, allowing a wide range of motion. Traditionally, craniocervical junction injuries have been associated with high mortality rates. Improvements in trauma care in the field have increased the prevalence of patients surviving these injuries long enough to be evaluated in the emergency department. Improved diagnostic imaging has made early diagnosis of these injuries more likely. Although neurologic injury is rare, when present it is generally catastrophic and often fatal.

Relevant Anatomy

Osteology

The occiput is a flat bone that acts as the bony protection of the cerebellum and posterior fossa. It borders the foramen magnum. The occipital condyles are paired semicircular structures that border the foramen magnum anterolaterally and articulate with the superior articular facets on the lateral masses of the atlas. The hypoglossal canal with the XII cranial nerve lies anterior to the occipital condyles. The jugular foramen, containing the internal jugular vein and cranial nerves IX, X, and XI, lies lateral to the condyles. The basion lies at the anterior aspect of the foramen magnum. The clivus extends cranially and anteriorly from the basion and eventually forms the posterior aspect of the sella turcica. The clivus is easily seen on radiographs and is an important landmark in determining occipitocervical alignment.

The atlas is a large ring composed of two large lateral masses connected by an anterior and posterior arch. The lateral masses are wedge shaped and congruent with the occipital condyles. The posterior aspect of the anterior arch has a central indentation where the dens articulates. The transverse ligament attaches on tubercles on the medial aspect of the lateral masses. The posterior arch contains a groove in which the vertebral artery and C1 nerve root lie.

The axis is unique because the dens projects cranially from the body to articulate with the anterior arch of the atlas and transverse ligament. Large lateral masses project laterally from the body. The atlantoaxial joints have a biconvex contour that aids rotation, but is not inherently stable. The lateral masses connect to the posterior elements through pedicles and a narrow bony isthmus, the pars interarticularis. The C2 spinous process is bifid and serves as an attachment of the nuchal ligaments and cranial rotator muscles. The course of the vertebral arteries through the axis is variable and must be understood to minimize injury during surgery.

Ligamentous Anatomy

The main stabilizing ligaments of the craniocervical junction run between the occiput and axis with little connection to the atlas. This relationship helps facilitate rotation at the occipitocervical junction. The ligamentous structures are classified as external or internal.

External ligaments include the ligamentum nuchae, occipitocervical membrane, and atlantoaxial membrane. The ligamentum nuchae is a thick layer of fibers that attaches to the external occipital protuberance and connects to the posterior tubercle of the atlas as well as the spinous processes of the axis and subaxial vertebrae. The occipitocervical membrane is a collection of fibroelastic fibers that runs from the foramen magnum to the anterior and posterior arch of the atlas. A similar group of fibers runs from the atlas to the axis and comprise the atlantoaxial membrane. These membranes provide little structural stability.

The internal craniocervical ligaments are located anterior to the dura in the spinal canal, are situated in three layers, and provide most of the craniocervical stability. The most posterior layer is the tectorial membrane, which is the rostral extension of the posterior longitudinal ligament. This thin ligament attaches to the anterior aspect of the foramen magnum. The middle layer is the cruciate ligament, the lateral projections of which form the transverse atlantal ligament. The transverse ligament attaches to the C1 lateral masses and articulates with the posterior margin of the dens. Vertical triangular bands extend from the transverse ligament up to the anterior foramen magnum and down to the axis. The most anterior layer is the apical and alar ligaments. The alar ligaments are thick, paired structures that connect the dens to the anteromedial aspect of the occipital condyles. The apical ligament is less strong and connects the tip of the dens to the foramen magnum.

Biomechanics

The structures of the occipitocervical junction are designed to safely house the brain stem and upper cervical cord and vessels while providing a wide range of motion. Flexion-extension at the occipitoatlantal joint ranges from 15° to 35°, whereas lateral bending and unilateral rotation are limited to 5°. Flexion-extension at the atlantoaxial joint ranges from 5° to 20° with 40° of lateral rotation to each side. The tectorial membrane and alar ligaments are the main stabilizing structures of the craniocervical junction. Extension is limited by the tectorial membrane and impingement of the occiput on the posterior aspects of the atlas and axis. Flexion is checked by the impingement of the dens on the basion. The tectorial membrane tightens and limits angulation between the atlas and axis in flexion and extension. The alar ligaments limit occipitoatlantal rotation and lateral bending. The alar ligaments and tectorial membranes prevent distraction.

Patient Evaluation

Physical Assessment

Assessment of patients with craniocervical injuries may be difficult because these patients often have associated brain injuries and impaired consciousness. All trauma patients are treated by Advanced Trauma Life Support guidelines. Airway management can be complicated by facial trauma, retropharyngeal hematoma, and vertebral fracture displacement. When intubation is required, the head and neck should be stabilized by an assistant. Severe facial trauma may necessitate fiberoptic intubation or tracheotomy.

After the patient is stabilized and the primary and secondary assessments are completed, a thorough spinal examination is performed. Awake patients will often report suboccipital neck pain, crepitus, and various neurologic symptoms. Patients are often obtunded, and identification of craniocervical injuries is largely radiographic. Patients are log rolled, and the entire spine is inspected for open wounds and palpated for tenderness,

bony step-offs, and hematomas. The results of a detailed neurologic examination are documented. For patients with high cervical injuries, a detailed cranial nerve examination also should be performed.

Radiologic Evaluation

Controversy currently exists regarding the necessity of obtaining radiographs for all awake, asymptomatic patients.[2] Traditionally, three radiographic views are used to assess the cervical spine: an AP subaxial cervical spine view, a lateral cervical spine view, and open mouth odontoid view. Interpretation of these radiographs is often difficult because of soft-tissue shadows, overlying bony structures, artifacts, or poor imaging technique. Occipitocervical dissociations and occipital condyle fractures may be missed because of the oblique orientation of the joint. The clivus normally points toward the dens, and the basion lies within 5 mm of the dens. This relationship can be used to evaluate the status of the occipitoatlantal joint. Retropharyngeal swelling and occipitoatlantal diastasis also suggest occipitoatlantal dissociation. The open mouth odontoid view is useful in identifying dens fractures and C1 ring fractures. Asymmetry of the C1 lateral masses on C2 or abnormally wide spreading of the lateral masses suggests fracture of the C1 ring and possible transverse ligament injury.

CT is far more sensitive than plain radiography in assessing the craniocervical junction. Thin-cut sections with sagittal and coronal reconstructions can easily identify fractures and mild translational or distraction injuries. If a patient requires a head CT scan to assess a closed head injury, a cervical CT scan should also be obtained.

MRI traditionally is not optimal for the initial assessment of trauma patients because of timing logistics. It can be useful in identifying ligamentous injuries, especially when T2-weighted and short tau inversion recovery sequences are obtained. Additionally, MRI is helpful in identifying spinal cord edema, occult fractures, and epidural hematomas.

Occipital Condyle Fractures

Occipital condyle fractures are usually caused by direct trauma to the head or rapid deceleration of the head. Occipital condyle fractures can occur with blunt forces transmitted to the skull through the mandible or from impaction of the cervical spine upward into the fixed skull. Patients with occipital condyle fractures commonly have associated skull base fractures and/or traumatic brain injuries.

Clinical Presentation

Patients are often severely obtunded or unconscious, and the fractures are identified radiographically. Awake patients often report suboccipital pain and occipital headaches. Direct tenderness may not be present because of the deep location of the occipitoatlantal articulation. The neurologic examination is often normal; however, various neurologic deficits including incomplete quadriplegia, respiratory-dependent quadriplegia, cruciate palsy of Bell, and fatal brain stem injury are also associated with occipital condyle fractures. Injury to cranial nerves VI, VII, IX, X, XI, and XII may occur in association with skull base fractures. Patients with unrecognized occipital condyle fractures may present with chronic suboccipital pain.

Radiographic Diagnosis

Occipital condyle fractures are often missed on plain radiographs. Thin-cut CT scans with coronal and sagittal reconstruction are highly accurate in identifying occipital condyle fractures. Head CT scans obtained for evaluation of trauma should include cuts down to the midcervical spine to identify associated upper cervical injuries because up to 30% of patients with occipital condyle fractures will have associated cervical injuries.[3] Although MRI scans are not particularly useful in the evaluation of occipital condyle fractures, they may demonstrate associated craniocervical ligament injuries.

Classification

Occipital condyle fractures are classified based on location, morphology, and presence of ligamentous injury.[4,5]

Type I injuries are comminuted fractures caused by impaction of the condyles into the atlas. This type of injury is usually caused by a direct blow to the head and is a stable injury as long as the contralateral side is not involved.

Type II injuries are condyle fractures with an associated skull base fracture. The fracture may exit through the condyle and into the foramen magnum, or the entire condyle may be separated from the base of the skull. These types of injuries have a similar mechanism to type I injuries and are generally stable unless the entire condyle is separated from the occiput.

Type III injuries are wedge-shaped avulsion fractures resulting from tensile forces on the alar ligaments. The fragments are often displaced medially into the foramen magnum. This type of injury occurs in 30% to 50% of patients with occipitoatlantal dissociation. Type III occipital condyle injuries may be unilateral or bilateral, with three patterns of bilateral injuries: bilateral condyle fractures, unilateral condyle fractures with contralateral occipitoatlantal diastasis, and unilateral condyle fractures with contralateral atlantoaxial diastasis. Unilateral fractures tend to be stable, whereas bilateral fractures require surgical stabilization.

Treatment

Patients with stable type I and type II injuries should be treated with a hard collar or cervicothoracic brace for 6 to 8 weeks. Patients with type II fractures in which the entire condyle is separated from the occiput should be treated with a halo vest for 8 to 12 weeks. Patients with type II injuries that do not respond to external immobilization with collapse resulting in torticollis and/or persistent suboccipital pain should undergo posterior occiput to C2 fusion. Patients with unilateral and nondisplaced type III injuries can be treated in a hard collar or cervicothoracic brace for 6 to 8 weeks. Dynamic radiographs should be used to assess stability after immobilization. Type III injuries with associated atlanto-occipital instability are unstable, and patients with these injuries should be treated with posterior occiput to C2 fusion. Patients with disabling suboccipital pain after treatment of occipital condyle fractures are candidates for late posterior occipitocervical fusion.

Occipitocervical Dissociation

Occipitocervical dissociation typically results from high-energy deceleration-acceleration injuries. The integrity of the alar ligaments, their bony attachments, and the tectorial membrane is lost. Occipitocervical dissociation is associated with a high incidence of craniofacial trauma.

Clinical Presentation

Patients with occipitocervical dissociation are often obtunded or unconscious, and the diagnosis is largely made radiographically. Patients who are awake will have symptoms comparable to those with occipital condyle fractures. Patients with bilateral dislocations and significant occipitoatlantal diastasis usually have brain stem injuries, respiratory arrest, and high mortality rates.

Radiographic Diagnosis

Plain radiographic findings such as retropharyngeal soft-tissue swelling, widening of the space between the occiput and cervical spine, and widening of the space between the basion and dens tip suggest injury to the craniocervical junction. The Powers ratio compares the basion-posterior atlas arch distance with the opisthion-anterior atlas arch distance. If this ratio is greater than one, disruption of the occipitocervical junction is suspected. These landmarks, however, are often difficult to identify on trauma radiographs.

In 98% of normal patients, the distance between the basion and the tip of the dens is less than 12 mm (Figure 1). The posterior axial line is defined as the rostral extent of the posterior cortex of the axis body. The basion also normally lies within 12 mm of the posterior axial line (Figure 2). These radiographic relationships are known as the rule of 12 and are more sensitive than the Powers ratio.

If occipitoatlantal dissociation is suspected, a thin-cut

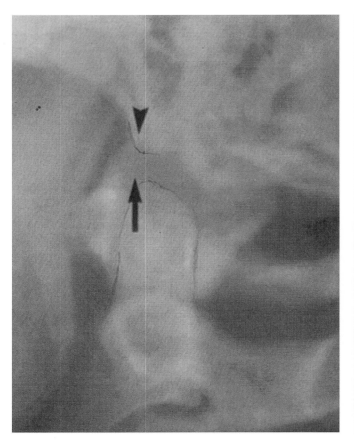

Figure 1 Lateral cervical radiograph demonstrating the normal relationship between the clivus and odontoid tip. The dens tip (*arrow*) lies within 12 mm of the clivus (*arrowhead*).

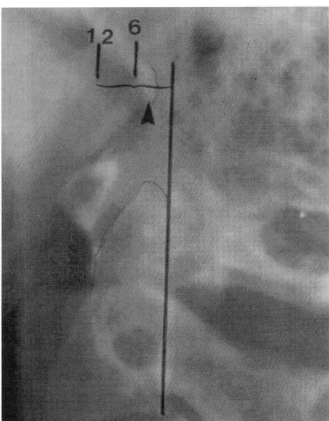

Figure 2 Lateral cervical radiograph on which the posterior axial line has been drawn. This line normally lies within 12 mm of the clivus (*arrowhead*).

CT scan with sagittal reconstruction should be obtained. On sagittal CT scans, the occipitoatlantal joint should be congruous with no more than 2 mm of distraction. Associated atlantoaxial dissociation and widening of the atlantodens interval can also be identified using CT.

Classification

Occipitocervical dislocations are classified by direction of displacement of the occiput. This classification has little prognostic or treatment value. These injuries represent complete ligamentous disruption, and the direction of dislocation often is determined by head position relative to the chest during radiography.

Type I injuries are anterior subluxations of the occiput on the C1 lateral masses. This is the most common type and is frequently seen in children because of the relatively large size of the head compared with the body. Type II injuries are vertical displacement injuries and are subdivided based on involvement at the occipitoatlantal or atlantoaxial joints. Type IIA injuries involve vertical diastasis of the occipitoatlantal joint greater than 2 mm, whereas type IIB injuries involve vertical disruption of the atlantoaxial joint. Type III injuries involve posterior

subluxations of the occiput on the cervical spine and are rarely reported.

Treatment

Once the patient has been resuscitated and stabilized and the dislocation diagnosed, reduction is performed. Because of the severe ligamentous instability, cranial tong traction does not play a significant role in reduction and may be catastrophically harmful. In patients with type I injuries, bolstering the thorax with blankets can allow the head to fall back into reduction. This technique is also useful for patients with type III injuries by placing blankets under the head to translate it forward. Type II injuries are reduced by downward pressure during halo application. Lifting the head of the bed can allow gravity to aid in reduction; however, great care must be taken to make sure that distraction of the head does not occur if the patient slides down in bed. Following reduction and halo vest application, repeat radiographs and CT scan should be obtained to assess reduction.

Halo vest treatment may be attempted in patients with unilateral and bilateral injuries with little displacement on presentation. Close and frequent evaluation of

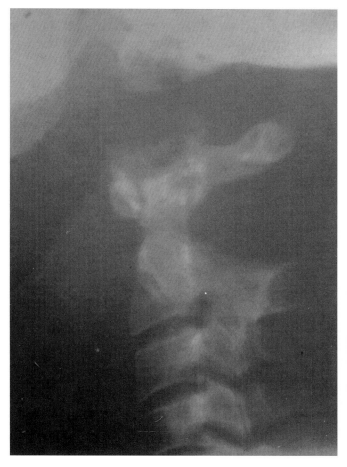

Figure 3 Lateral cervical radiograph showing complete disruption of the occiput-C2 complex. The occipitoatlantal joint is dislocated, and there is significant distraction of the atlantoaxial joint.

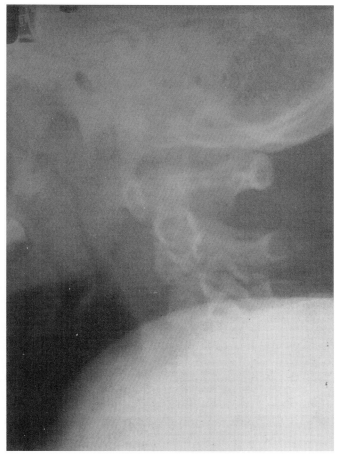

Figure 5 Lateral cervical radiograph of a Jefferson type burst fracture with disruption of the occipitoatlantal joint.

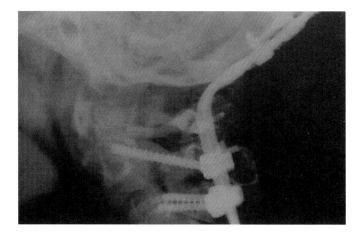

Figure 4 Postoperative lateral cervical radiograph showing reduction and stabilization of occipitoatlantal dislocation.

the reduction must be performed. Patients with bilateral injuries with significant subluxation and all those with dislocation should be primarily stabilized surgically with posterior occiput to C2 fusion to avoid

catastrophic neurologic deterioration from loss of reduction (Figures 3 and 4).

Atlas Fractures

Atlas fractures are common and comprise 10% of all cervical injuries. Atlas fractures are associated with a high incidence of fractures of the axis and atlantoaxial complex (Figure 5). Although neurologic injury is rare in patients with atlas fractures, significant loss of rotational motion often occurs. There are several types of atlas fractures with varying injury mechanisms. Posterior arch fractures occur from extension and axial loading where the posterior arch fails in compression between the occiput and C2 spinous process. Jefferson burst fractures result from a symmetric axial load with the occipitocervical junction in neutral alignment. Isolated lateral mass fractures are caused by nonsymmetrical axial loads. If the head is deviated in the coronal plane, the axial load will be greater on one side, leading to a unilateral lateral mass fracture. Lateral mass and burst fractures may be associated with transverse ligament injuries. Late instability is rare after healing because the transverse ligament fails in tension, with the alar ligaments and facet capsules remaining intact. Instability can be a significant problem in patients with flexion injuries because these secondary restraints are torn in addition to the transverse ligament.

Clinical Presentation

Patients usually have suboccipital pain and local tenderness. Neurologic deficits are rare, but they may be present in patients with concomitant closed head injuries. Patients may have scalp lacerations, facial injuries, and other signs of head trauma. The entire spine should be assessed because other fractures are often present, especially type II odontoid fractures and spondylolisthetic axis fractures.

Radiographic Diagnosis

Retropharyngeal soft-tissue swelling is often seen on lateral cervical radiographs. The lateral masses should lay symmetrically over the C2 lateral masses. In patients with burst fractures, excessive lateral displacement of the atlas lateral masses is commonly observed radiographically. If the lateral displacement of the lateral masses exceeds 6.9 mm on the open mouth view, the transverse ligament is injured. Luxation of the atlantoaxial joint may also be observed on lateral radiographs.

CT can help assess bony and ligamentous anatomy. Posterior C1 arch fractures must be distinguished from congenital posterior arch defects. MRI may be helpful in the evaluation of patients with ligament injuries.

Classification

Atlas fractures are classified according to the location of the fracture and involvement of the alar and transverse ligaments. Anterior arch fractures can be vertical or transverse if created by an avulsion from the longus colli muscles. The Plow fracture is a rare variant of this pattern in which there are bilateral arch fractures with posterior atlantoaxial dislocation. The dens is forced through the anterior arch creating the fracture and dislocation. Patients with these unstable injuries have a high incidence of spinal cord injury. Associated posterior arch injuries are common and must be distinguished from congenital posterior arch defects.

Unilateral lateral mass fractures are stable if the lateral aspect of the C1 ring is intact. Less often, the lateral mass is severely comminuted or dissociated from the ring and may be associated with a contralateral break in the posterior arch. This pattern is comparable to that of the burst fracture. Although fractures of the C1 transverse process are typically stable, they may be associated with vertebral artery injury.

Burst fractures, also known as Jefferson fractures, may be made up of three or four fractures through the anterior and posterior arches. The ring usually splays outward, increasing canal diameter and making neuro-

logic injury rare. As the lateral masses displace, the occipitoatlantal and atlantoaxial joints are disrupted. If the lateral masses are displaced more than 6.9 mm with respect to C2, the transverse ligament is injured and atlantoaxial instability is present. Burst fractures with an intact transverse ligament are typically stable.

Treatment

Patients with stable atlas fractures are treated with external immobilization; however, no prospective data are available to support treatment strategies.[6] Traditionally, patients with isolated anterior and posterior arch and lateral mass fractures have been treated successfully with hard collars, cervicothoracic braces, and halo vests for 8 to 12 weeks with good results. No known study provides conclusive evidence that one of these modes of immobilization is more effective than the others.

Although patients with Plow fractures usually undergo reduction and are immobilized in halo vests, primary posterior C1-2 fusion may be considered for those with significant neurologic deficits or multiple injuries.

The treatment of patients with burst fractures is controversial. If the articular surface of the lateral mass is involved, patients must be made aware of the likelihood of significant loss of rotational motion. Patients with burst fractures with an intact transverse ligament and stable atlantoaxial articulation have been successfully treated with hard collars, cervicothoracic braces, and halo vests for 10 to 12 weeks. Patients with burst fractures associated with transverse ligament injuries and atlantoaxial instability previously treated nonsurgically have the potential for progression of displacement, nonunion, and late atlantoaxial instability. Patients with unstable burst fractures may be successfully treated with halo vest immobilization for 12 weeks; however, frequent evaluation of the lateral masses using open mouth odontoid views must be done. If reduction is not maintained, posterior C1-2 fusion is performed. Once the halo vest is removed, flexion-extension films are obtained. If residual atlantoaxial instability is present, posterior C1-2 fusion is indicated.

Transverse Atlantal Ligament Injuries

Instability from incompetence of the transverse ligament can be caused by various traumatic, infectious, congenital, and inflammatory conditions. This section addresses the evaluation and management of acute traumatic rupture of the transverse ligament and the resulting atlantoaxial instability. The transverse ligament is part of the cruciform ligament of the middle layer of the occipitoatlantoaxial complex. It is the strongest ligament in this complex and is the main structure preventing anterior subluxation of the atlas on the axis. Posterior atlas displacement is prevented by impingement of an intact anterior atlas arch on the dens. Acute rupture of the transverse ligament can occur in association with rapid deceleration-acceleration injuries that produce a significant anterior shear force. Rotational forces may also play a role. An anterior directed force to the back of the head producing anterior translation and forced flexion may also lead to transverse ligament rupture. As noted, the transverse ligament may also be compromised in association with C1 burst fractures and odontoid fractures.

Clinical Presentation

Severe craniofacial trauma is usually associated with these injuries. Patients complain of severe upper cervical pain and limited range of motion because of neck spasm. Symptoms are often elicited or worsened by flexion of the neck. Neurologic examination ranges from normal to transient quadriparesis. Neurologic symptoms may occur late. Complete spinal cord injuries are rare because they are usually fatal at this level. Cardiac and respiratory arrest may occur from injury to the upper cervical cord. Patients may also present with vertigo, syncope, and blurred vision with vertebral artery injury.

Radiographic Diagnosis

The standard method of radiographic evaluation is the lateral cervical radiograph with the beam centered at C2. The anterior atlantodens interval, the distance between the posterior aspect of the anterior C1 arch and the anterior aspect of the dens, is measured. The maximum normal value is 3 mm in adults and 5 mm in children. Trauma cervical spine films are usually taken with patients in the supine position and may be misleading because the head can fall back into extension, reducing the atlantoaxial joint. If the patient is stable and transverse ligament injury is suspected, upright films should be obtained. Protective muscular spasm may prevent radiographic identification on lateral films. If the patient is alert, awake, and cooperative, flexion-extension radiographs may identify the instability. If symptoms persist, dynamic radiographs may need to be repeated in 7 to 10 days once the spasms resolve.

Thin-cut CT scans are useful in visualizing ruptures of the transverse ligament. In addition to evaluating fractures and articular incongruity, they can be used to diagnose transverse ligament injuries in obtunded patients who cannot safely undergo dynamic imaging. Cervical CT scans are also useful in identifying other associated cervical injuries. MRI may be difficult to perform early after injury, but it may be helpful in identification of late presenting injuries. Injuries to the transverse ligament are best viewed on T2-weighted and short tau inversion recovery images.

Treatment

Because midsubstance transverse ligament ruptures have poor healing potential, primary posterior atlantoaxial arthrodesis is indicated for patients with these injuries. Transverse ligament injuries associated with avulsion fractures of the atlas lateral masses may heal with nonsurgical treatment.

Posterior wiring techniques, such as those described by Gallie and Brooks, were the gold standard of posterior fixation for decades. Posterior wiring poorly resists axial rotation, shear, and translation, making halo vest immobilization mandatory for 8 to 12 weeks after surgery. The Magerl transarticular screw technique provides greater stiffness and resistance to translation and rotation, limiting the requirements for external immobilization to a hard collar for 8 to 12 weeks.[7,8] Vertebral artery anatomy must be evaluated with MRI or CT prior to surgery because up to 20% of patients may have anomalies preventing safe screw placement.[9-11] Stabilization of C1-2 by screw fixation of the C1 lateral mass and C2 pedicle is biomechanically similar to the Magerl technique.[12]

Regardless of the technique used, anatomic reduction of the atlantoaxial joint is essential for safe internal fixation. If the C1 arch is not reduced, passage of wires may cause catastrophic neurologic injury because of the relative canal stenosis from vertebral offset. If the atlantoaxial articulation is not reduced prior to screw placement, the resultant screw trajectory will place the vertebral artery at risk.[13]

Odontoid Fractures

Fractures of the dens occur in a bimodal fashion. In young patients, these fractures are a result of rapid deceleration-acceleration injuries and blunt trauma to the head. In the elderly population, they can be caused by simple falls.[14] Neurologic deficits, although rare in most patients with occiput to C2 injuries, occur in up to 20% of patients and are associated with high mortality rates in the elderly. The dens typically fails because of anterior or posterior translational forces. In an anterior directed shear, the transverse ligament tightens along the posterior aspect of the dens. Both structures often fail, resulting in atlantoaxial instability in addition to the dens fracture. In posterior directed shear injuries, the anterior atlas arch directly impinges on the dens and leads to fracture. In the elderly population, increasing thoracic kyphosis leads to a more forward posture of the head and neck, making it more prone to posterior-directed injury during falls. For this reason, dens fractures in elderly patients often occur with posterior displacement and may result in significant canal compromise and spinal cord injury.

Clinical Presentation

Patients may describe a sense of instability of the head and neck and will often support their head with their hands when in an upright position. Patients with minimally displaced fractures may be relatively asymptomatic, whereas others with significant displacement will present with profound spinal cord injuries. Dysphagia is common when a large retropharyngeal hematoma is present.

Radiographic Diagnosis

Odontoid fractures can easily be missed on plain radiographs. The open mouth odontoid and lateral views should be carefully inspected for fracture lines and displacement. If the dens is poorly visualized on plain radiographs, a thin-cut CT scan with coronal and sagittal reconstruction is helpful in diagnosis. Even if the fracture is readily diagnosed on plain radiographs, a cervical CT scan is helpful in identifying additional injuries at other levels.

Classification

The classification of dens fractures is based on the location of the fracture and predicts prognosis and directs treatment. Type I fractures are avulsions of the lateral dens tip resulting from the pull of the alar ligaments. Depending on the amount of ligament injury involved, these fractures may be associated with instability of the occipitocervical junction, which requires careful radiographic evaluation of the occipitocervical junction. Type II fractures occur through the narrow cortical base of the dens. Significant displacement and disruption of the arterial blood supply of the dens can occur in patients with these injuries, impairing healing potential. Type III injuries include extension of the fracture into the body of the axis. The large bony surface area gives this fracture pattern good healing potential. The anterior body fragment may be displaced anteriorly.

Treatment

Treatment of dens fractures varies depending on fracture location, stability, and patient age. Patients with isolated stable type I fractures are treated with a hard collar for 6 weeks. If occipitocervical instability is associated with a type I injury, primary occipitocervical posterior fusion may be indicated.

Treatment of type II injuries has been controversial. Current treatment recommendations are based on nonunion risk factors, patient age, and associated injuries. Nonsurgical management is associated with high nonunion rates, whereas surgical management often results in significant loss of motion. Even when patients are immobilized in halo vests, nonunion rates of 36% to 65% have been reported.[15,16] Various factors that affect the healing prognosis of type II fractures have been identified. Patients with initial fracture displacement greater than 5 mm,[17] severe comminution of the dens waist, and an anterior oblique fracture pattern with anterior dis-

placement are associated with high nonunion rates and should be considered surgical candidates.

The quality of reduction is vital to the success of the nonsurgical treatment of patients with type II injuries. A 20% malreduction results in a 40% decrease in fracture surface area contact. Additionally, halo vests do not completely control motion at the fracture site, and overdistraction of the fracture increases the likelihood of nonunion. Interposition of the transverse ligament at the fracture site may also increase nonunion rates.

Patients with transverse type II fractures that are displaced less than 5 mm with no comminution should be treated in a halo vest for 10 to 12 weeks. Frequent assessment of the reduction of these patients must be performed. Primary direct fixation of the fracture with an anterior odontoid screw may be considered if halo vest immobilization is not tolerated.

Primary surgical stabilization of type II fractures should be performed in patients who will not tolerate halo vest immobilization, for example, polytrauma patients, elderly patients,[18,19] or those with spinal cord or pulmonary injuries. Primary surgical intervention is also recommended for patients with fracture patterns associated with high nonunion rates.

Anterior odontoid screw fixation may be performed in young healthy patients.[20-22] The potential benefit is maintaining atlantoaxial motion. The dens diameter is too small to safely place two 3.5 mm screws in 10% of the population.[23] Although two screws have the potential to provide better rotational stability of the fracture, studies have shown that there is no significant advantage to using a two-screw over a single-screw technique.[24,25] Potential complications include a 5% to 20% incidence of dysphonia and dysphagia, a 10% nonunion rate, and a 50% reduction of atlantoaxial rotation. Anterior odontoid screw fixation is contraindicated for patients with severely comminuted dens fractures, as well as those with an anterior oblique fracture pattern with anterior displacement because the fracture plane is parallel to the trajectory of the screw. These fracture patterns should be stabilized with posterior atlantoaxial arthodesis.[26]

In patients with type III fractures, healing has been predictable with the use of halo vests and cervicothoracic braces. A 15% malunion rate with nonsurgical treatment has been reported.[27,28] Poor results were attributed to the use of cervical orthotic devices rather than halo vest immobilization. Posterior atlantoaxial arthrodesis is generally reserved for patients who do not respond to nonsurgical management.[26] The type III fracture is a relative contraindication to anterior odontoid screw fixation.

Odontoid fractures in the elderly population are associated with morbidity and mortality rates similar to those for patients with hip fractures. Halo vest immobilization is poorly tolerated in elderly patients and may lead to aspiration and death. Primary posterior atlantoaxial fusion should be performed in elderly patients who

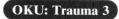

are healthy enough to tolerate surgery. Patients who are too sick or demented to undergo surgery may be treated in a soft collar with an understanding that nonunion will be the outcome.

Traumatic Spondylolisthesis of the Axis (Hangman's Fracture)

Traumatic fractures of pars interarticularis of the axis have been referred to as hangman's fractures because of their resemblance to fractures created during judicial hanging.[29-31] These injuries commonly occur as a result of hyperextension caused by motor vehicle accidents, falls, and diving injuries. Traumatic spondylolisthesis of the axis is a more appropriate descriptive term because the mechanism of injury is different than that of judicial hanging. The mechanism of injury in judicial hanging is distraction-hyperextension. Forensic autopsy findings in judicial hanging cases suggest that death is caused by craniocervical distraction and vertebral artery rupture and not the axis fracture. The more common traumatic spondylolisthesis seen after motor vehicle and diving accidents is caused during hyperextension, compression, and rebound flexion. The pars interarticularis fails because of high bending moments created by extension and axial loading. Once fracture of the pars interarticularis occurs, the C2-3 disk is placed in tension and may fail depending on the stress involved. Although it is unknown whether flexion is a primary force or a rebound phenomenon, flexion forces are thought to result in anterior angulation and translation of the axis body, and in instances of severe injury, dislocation of the C2-3 facet joints.

Clinical Presentation

Patients with this type of injury often have upper cervical pain, decreased range of motion, and associated craniocervical trauma. Neurologic deficits are rare because the canal tends to expand. Patients with an associated C2-3 dislocation often have profound neurologic deficits from spinal cord injury. Associated vertebral artery injuries may occur and are often fatal when bilateral.

Radiographic Diagnosis

Fractures of the pars interarticularis are easily identified on plain radiographs. Cervical CT scans are helpful in identifying whether the fracture extends into the vertebral body. It is important to recognize an atypical hangman's fracture so that displacement of the vertebral body fragment into the spinal canal during reduction is avoided.

Classification

These injuries have been classified into three types based on the mechanism of injury and severity of soft-tissue injury,[32] and this classification system has been modified to describe a fourth type of injury.[33]

Type I injuries are bilateral pars fractures with less than 3 mm of C2-3 subluxation. These injuries are caused by axial loading and hyperextension. They are stable as a result of the maintained integrity of the C2-3 disk.

Type II injuries involve displacement of the pars fracture with anterior translation of the axis body and disruption of the C2-3 disk. Hyperextension and rebound flexion is the mechanism of injury for type II fractures. Type IIA injuries have also been described in which the C2-3 disk space is distracted and the dens and axis body are angulated in flexion. Type IIA injuries are caused by a flexion-distraction mechanism.

Type III injuries involve anterior angulation of the axis body with dislocation of the C2-3 facet joints. The mechanism of injury is primary flexion and rebound extension. These dislocations cannot be reduced by tong traction because the anterior and posterior structures are separated.

Treatment

Reduction of displaced fractures can be performed using tong traction. Traction is started at 10 lb with frequent radiographic assessment performed to avoid overdistraction. Reduction can be adjusted by changing the angle of applied traction. The presence of an atypical hangman's fracture with extension of the fracture into the anterior body must be identified prior to reduction because the anterior body fragment could be angulated into the canal during reduction, with catastrophic results.[34] Type III injuries are irreducible and should be surgically reduced and stabilized.

Type I injuries are stable, and patients can be treated for 6 to 8 weeks in a cervicothoracic orthosis.[35] Upright radiographs in the brace are used to assess the adequacy of reduction.

Type II injuries are unstable, and patients are treated in a halo vest for 8 to 12 weeks. Despite their initial displacement and unstable nature, these injuries heal reliably with good results. The treatment of type IIA injuries is controversial. If they are reducible, they are treated the same as type II injuries. If reduction is not attainable or maintained, prolonged bed rest with traction may be required until the fracture is stable enough to be held in a halo vest.[36] Surgical stabilization is indicated when reduction is not maintainable and in patients who do not tolerate external immobilization. Surgical options include reduction and direct osteosynthesis of the pars fracture with C2 pedicle screws or anterior C2-3 fusion and plate stabilization. The posterior technique potentially preserves motion at C2-3; however, the anterior fusion technique provides more stiffness.

Type III injuries are irreducible, and patients require surgical reduction and stabilization. Removing the top of the C3 facet with a high-speed burr aids in the reduction of the C2-3 joint. Once reduced, the C2-3 segment is stabilized with wires or screw fixation. Screw fixation allows for stabilization of the C2-3 joint along with direct osteosynthesis of the C2 pars fracture. The screws may be connected by plates or rods, and patients are immobilized in a hard collar for 6 weeks. Although wiring techniques are typically used to stabilize the C2-3 joint, halo vest immobilization is often required postoperatively to treat the pars fracture. Once stabilized, type III fractures heal predictably.

Axis Body Fractures

Fractures of the axis body may be variants of odontoid and hangman's fractures or they may resemble fracture patterns comparable to those in the subaxial spine. These fractures occur caudal to the dens and involve the C2 vertebral body. Injury mechanisms are similar to those creating dens and hangman's fractures as well as subaxial fractures.

Clinical Presentation

Awake patients usually report upper cervical pain and tenderness. Neurologic deficits are rare. Dysphagia can occur as a result of retropharyngeal hematoma.

Radiographic Diagnosis

Axis body fractures are easily identified on plain radiographs. Cervical CT scans are useful in evaluation of the spinal canal and atlantoaxial joints, as well as in identifying associated fractures at other levels.

Classification

A classification system for axis body fractures has been described.[37] Type I injuries are teardrop fractures of the anterior-inferior end plate. These injuries are stable unless the vertebral body is displaced more than 4 mm posteriorly. Type II injuries are horizontal cleavage fractures that occur caudal to where a type III odontoid fracture occurs. Type III injuries represent a burst fracture of the axis body, and type IV injuries are vertical shear fractures.

Treatment

Displaced fractures should be reduced using tong traction. Patients with stable fractures may be treated with hard collars or cervicothoracic braces for 6 to 8 weeks. Unstable fractures still have a high healing potential secondary to the large bony surface area, and patients with these injuries may be treated in a halo vest for 6 to 8 weeks. If fracture reduction is not maintained in a halo vest or if there is significant associated atlantoaxial instability, posterior atlantoaxial fusion should be performed. Patients with unstable type I teardrop fractures

should be treated with reduction and posterior C2-3 fusion.

Annotated References

1. Vaccaro AR, An HS, Lin SS, et al: Noncontiguous injuries of the spine. *J Spinal Disord* 1992;5:320-329.

2. Harris MB, Waguespack AM, Kronlage S: 'Clearing' cervical spine injuries in polytrauma patients: Is it really safe to remove the collar? *Orthopedics* 1997; 20:903-907.

3. Hanson JA, Deliganis AV, Baxter AB, et al: Radiologic and clinical spectrum of occipital condyle fractures: Retrospective review of 107 consecutive fractures in 95 patients. *AJR Am J Roentgenol* 2002;178: 1261-1269.
    This is a retrospective radiologic review of correlating diagnostic imaging findings in patients who underwent treatment for occipital condyle fractures. The authors reported that unilateral injuries were treated nonsurgically, whereas bilateral injuries required surgical stabilization. Associated cervical injuries were noted in 31% of patients.

4. Anderson PA, Montesano PX: Morphology and treatment of occipital condyle fractures. *Spine* 1988; 13:731-736.

5. Tuli S, Tator CH, Fehlings MG, Mackay M: Occipital condyle fractures. *Neurosurgery* 1997;41:368.

6. Lee TT, Green BA, Petrin DR: Treatment of stable burst fracture of the Atlas (Jefferson Fracture) with rigid cervical collar. *Spine* 1998;23:1963-1967.

7. Hanson PB, Montesano PX, Sharkey NA, et al: Anatomic and biomechanical assessment of transarticular screw fixation for atlantoaxial instability. *Spine* 1991;16:1141-1145.

8. Naderi S, Crawford NR, Song GS, et al: Biomechanical comparison of C1-C2 posterior fixations. *Spine* 1998;23:1946-1956.

9. Madawi AA, Casey AT, Solanki GA, et al: Radiological and anatomical evaluation of the atlantoaxial transarticular screw fixation technique. *J Neurosurg* 1997;86:961-968.

10. Paramore CG, Dickman CA, Sonntag VKH: The anatomical suitability of the C1-C2 complex for transarticular screw fixation. *J Neurosurg* 1996;85: 221-224.

11. Wright NM, Lauryssen C: Vertebral artery injury in C1/C2 transarticular screw fixation: Results of a sur-

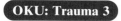
vey of the AANS/CNS section on disorders of the spine and peripheral nerves. *J Neurosurg* 1998;88: 634-640.

12. Hott JS, Lynch JJ, Chamberlain RH, Sonntag VK, Crawford NR: Biomechanical comparison of C1-2 posterior fixation techniques. *J Neurosurg Spine* 2005;2:175-181.

    The authors of this study conducted a biomechanical comparison of transarticular screw fixation with C1 lateral mass–C2 pedicle fixation to stabilize the C1-2 articulation. Both constructs resisted flexion, lateral bending, and axial rotation comparably well. The authors reported that the relative weakness of the C1 lateral mass–C2 pedicle screw technique in extension could be overcome with placement of a structural interspinous graft.

13. Gluf WM, Schmidt MH, Apfelbaum RI: Atlantoaxial transarticular screw fixation: A review of surgical indication, fusion rate, complications, and lessons learned in 191 adult patients. *J Neurosurg Spine* 2005;2:155-163.

    In this retrospective review of 191 consecutive patients who were treated with transarticular screw fixation of C1-2, the authors assessed the rate of fusion, surgery-related complications, and lessons learned. An overall fusion rate of 98% was reported. Although complications were rare, a patient death from bilateral vertebral artery injury was reported.

14. Lakshmanan P, Jones A, Howes J, et al: CT evaluation of the pattern of odontoid fractures in the elderly: Relationship to upper cervical spine osteoarthritis. *Eur Spine J* 2005;14:78-83.

    In this CT scan review of 23 patients older than 70 years with odontoid fractures, the authors assessed fracture patterns and the degree of arthritic change in the atlanto-dens, atlantoaxial, and subaxial joints. They reported that fixation of the dens to the atlas from degeneration of the atlanto-dens joint combined with maintained atlantoaxial joint motion and a stiff spondylitic subaxial spine can result in significant torque forces at the base of the dens from simple, low-energy falls.

15. Anderson LD, D'Alonzo RT: Fractures of the odontoid process of the axis. *J Bone Joint Surg Am* 1974; 56:1663-1674.

16. Schatzker J, Rorabeck CH, Waddell JP: Fractures of the dens (odontoid process): An analysis of thirty-seven cases. *J Bone Joint Surg Br* 1971;53:392-404.

17. Greene KA, Dickman CA, Marciano FF, et al: Acute axis fractures: Analysis of management and outcomes. *Spine* 1997;22:1843-1852.

18. Bednar D, Parikh J, Hummel J: Management of type II odontoid process fractures in geriatric patients. *J Spinal Disord* 1995;8:166-169.

19. Seybold EA, Bayley JC: Functional outcome of surgically and conservatively managed dens fractures. *Spine* 1998;23:1837-1846.

20. Fountas KN, Kapsalaki EX, Karampelas I, et al: Results of long-term follow-up in patients undergoing anterior screw fixation for type II and rostral type III odontoid fractures. *Spine* 2005;30:661-669.

    In this retrospective review of fusion rates in 38 patients treated with anterior odontoid screw fixation for type II odontoid fractures, the rate of stable fracture healing was reported to be high. Only one unstable nonunion and one instrumentation failure occurred.

21. Aebi M, Etter C, Coscia M: Fractures of the odontoid process: Treatment with anterior screw fixation. *Spine* 1989;14:1065-1070.

22. Montesano PX, Anderson PA, Schlehr F, Thalgott JS, Lowrey G: Odontoid fractures treated by anterior odontoid screw fixation. *Spine* 1991;16(suppl 3): S33-S37.

23. Doherty BJ, Heggeness MH: Quantitative anatomy of the second cervical vertebra. *Spine* 1995;20:513-517.

24. Jenkins JD, Coric D, Branch CL: A clinical comparison of one and two-screw odontoid fixation. *J Neurosurg* 1998;89:366-370.

25. Sasso R, Doherty BJ, Crawford MJ, Heggeness MH: Biomechanics of odontoid fracture fixation: Comparison of the one and two screw techniques. *Spine* 1993;18:1950-1953.

26. Jeanneret B, Magerl F: Primary posterior fusion C1/C2 in odontoid fractures: Indications, techniques and results of transarticular screw fixation. *J Spinal Disord* 1992;5:464-475.

27. Clark CR, White AA: Fractures of the dens: A multicenter study. *J Bone Joint Surg Am* 1985;67:1340-1348.

28. Muller EJ, Schwinnen I, Fischer K, et al: Non-rigid immobilization of odontoid fractures. *Eur Spine J* 2003;12:522-525.

    In this study, patients with minimally displaced (> 2 mm fracture gap, > 5 mm translation, > 11° angulation) stable type II and III odontoid fractures were treated with cervical orthotic devices. The authors reported nonunion rates of 25% and 15% for patients with type II and type III fractures, respectively.

29. Brashear R Jr, Venters G, Preston ET: Fractures of the neural arch of the axis. *J Bone Joint Surg Am* 1975;57:879-887.

30. Francis WR, Fielding JW, Hawkins RJ, Pepin J, Hensinger R: Traumatic spondylolisthesis of the axis. *J Bone Joint Surg Br* 1981;63:313-318.

31. Schneider RC, Livingston KE, Cave AJ, et al: Hangman's fractures of the cervical spine. *J Neurosurg* 1965;22:141-154.

32. Effendi B, Roy D, Cornish B, Dussault RG, Laurin CA: Fracture of the ring of the axis: A classification based on the analysis of 131 cases. *J Bone Joint Surg Br* 1981;63:319-327.

33. Levine AM, Edwards CC: The management of traumatic spondylolisthesis of the axis. *J Bone Joint Surg Am* 1985;67:217-226.

34. Starr J, Eismont FJ: Atypical hangman's fractures. *Spine* 1993;:1954-1957.

35. Coric D, Wilson JA, Kelley DL: Treatment of traumatic spondylolisthesis of the axis with nonrigid immobilization: A review of 64 cases. *J Neurosurg* 1996; 85:550-554.

36. Vaccaro AR, Madigan L, Bauerle WB, et al: Early halo immobilization of displaced traumatic spondylolisthesis of the axis. *Spine* 2002;27:2229-2233.
    The authors of this study conducted a retrospective review of early halo placement after reduction of type II and type IIA hangman's fractures and reported that patients with fractures with greater than 12° of angulation on presentation may require extended periods of traction to ensure maintenance of reduction in the halo vest.

37. Benzel EC, Hart BL, Ball PA, Baldwin NG, Orrison WW, Espinosa M: Fractures of the C-2 vertebral body. *J Neurosurg* 1994;81:206-212.

Chapter 27

Lower Cervical Spine Injuries

Jens R. Chapman, MD

Sohail K. Mirza, MD

Introduction

The cervical spine, which is capable of considerable motion and responsible for protecting the neural elements and vascular structures it encompasses, is a structure that is at risk for injury. The dynamics of cervical spine injuries are complex, multifactorial processes. In the trauma setting, the treating physician is charged with effectively analyzing the structural integrity of the cervical spine and treating injuries according to their instability. From an outcomes perspective, the most significant impact is associated with prevention of secondary neurologic deterioration in patients who are initially neurologically intact and optimization of the chances for recovery in patients with an established spinal cord injury.[1] The risk of secondary neurologic injury and long-term patient morbidity has been correlated to undiagnosed spinal injuries.[2] Therefore, an effective spinal clearance algorithm and spinal stabilization measures should be integrated into the overall trauma care pathway to optimize results. Although unprecedented diagnostic and stabilization measures have become available over the past decade, physicians are increasingly challenged with treating elderly patients with considerable comorbidities and complex underlying spinal abnormalities. Thus, familiarity with a variety of treatment strategies and their physiologic impact also represent important covariables to successful outcomes.

Pertinent Anatomy

The lower cervical spine accounts for most of neck flexion-extension motion and left to right bending and about 50% of axial rotation. Conceptually, the lower cervical spine is usually thought of as having two columns: the anterior column, which consists of the entire vertebral body with the intervertebral disks and their ligamentous attachments and includes the anterior and posterior longitudinal ligaments; and the posterior column, which consists of the spinal canal, the posterior arch, and the interspinous ligaments.[3] By subdividing the posterior arch into a left and right facet joint complex, the main structural load-bearing components of the lower cervical spine form a tripod consisting of a vertebral body with intercedent discoligamentous complex and two facet joints. Some degree of structural stability is inferred by the uncovertebral joints and the sagittal inclination of the facet joints. Crucial mechanical stability is, however, provided by the anterior and posterior longitudinal ligaments for the anterior column and interspinous ligaments as well as facet capsules for the posterior column. Integrity of the functional spinal unit is usually preserved if all anterior components and one posterior structural component are intact or if all posterior components and one anterior structural component are intact.[3] Successful management of cervical spine trauma is contingent on identifying disruption of these key osseous and ligamentous structures and weighing their influence on the integrity of the neck as a whole.

Evaluation
Spine Clearance
All patients with suspected spine injury are methodically examined with a history and inspection, palpation, and neurologic evaluation according to the American Spinal Injury Association (ASIA) standards.[4] Based on several large-scale studies, the role of routine cervical screening radiographs has been reevaluated.[2,5,6] It is widely accepted that in the absence of high-energy injury mechanisms patients who are cognitively unimpaired have no neck tenderness and have a normal neurologic examination that requires no routine spine screening radiographs.[6] Plain radiography, especially a lateral cervical spine view covering the skull base to the cervicothoracic junction, continues to be the most widely used diagnostic screening tool for trauma patients. The usefulness of flexion-extension radiographs in an acute posttraumatic setting continues to be controversial. It is generally agreed that in an awake and cooperative neurologically intact patient, flexion-extension views may be of some use in detecting occult ligamentous lesions if such are suspected. In an acute setting, however, factors such as limited neck mobility because of muscle spasms diminish the value of these examinations. Therefore, for patients

with neck pain and normal neurologic and screening radiographs, postprimary clinical and radiographic evaluations are generally recommended after 1 or 2 weeks of protective neck immobilization.[6] Continued challenges regarding neck clearance typically involve cognitively impaired patients. Although dynamic fluoroscopy has been used by some physicians to assess cervical spine stability in sedated and unresponsive patients, this technique has not found widespread acceptance because it is cumbersome to perform and offers limited visualization of the cervicothoracic junction.[7] Most medical centers use a protocol for spine clearance for at-risk patients that includes three separate phases (Figure 1). The first phase uses a helical CT scan of the entire cervical spine with sagittal and coronal reformatted views. The second phase involves a secondary review of all spine imaging studies. Once absence of any radiographic signs of injury is confirmed, the third phase is initiated, which uses upright lateral spine radiographs to assess for the presence of new-onset deformity[7] (Figure 2).

Neuroimaging

Given the inherent limitations of conventional spinal radiographic visualization, especially in the craniocervical and cervicothoracic transition zones, helical cervical spine CT scans are increasingly being validated as the preferred diagnostic modality for at-risk patients. Routine screening CT of the cervical spine has been recommended for patients with head or facial trauma, impaired cognitive status, focal neurologic findings on examination, history of ankylosing spinal disorders, and history of high-energy trauma.[2,5] MRI has been recommended for any patient with cervical spinal cord injury and as a screening tool for patients with ankylosing disorders.[7] In addition to demonstrating acute hemorrhage and spinal cord signal changes, some imaging sequences, such as T2-weighted fat-suppression views, can demonstrate acute ligament injuries of the cervical spine[8,9] (Figure 3).

Vertebral Artery Injuries

For patients with significant cervical spine injuries, such as unstable burst fractures or fracture-dislocations, flow to the vertebral artery may be disrupted in up to 20%.[10] Should imaging tests reveal a displaced fracture involving the foramen transversarium, further assessment with CT angiography or magnetic resonance angiography is recommended. Transcranial Doppler screening may identify clinically relevant flow disruption. Long-term follow-up studies have revealed persistent vertebral artery occlusion beyond 26 months following an initial injury.[10] This finding may be of significance in surgical planning.

Spinal Stability Prediction

Despite important gains in refining neuroimaging tests and making them more widely available, the advent of this technology has not allowed for unequivocal determination of spinal stability or correlation with spinal cord injury. This is because of kinetics of energy dissipation in high-energy injuries, biomechanical factors of vertebral body injury during a traumatic event, and pretraumatic spinal canal diameter relative to spinal cord size. An in vitro study that assessed the axial load failures of the cervical spine demonstrated a transient spinal canal occlusion resulting from a burst fracture of up to 80% during rapid load application, with spontaneous reduction of up to 20% canal occlusion caused by a spontaneous rebound phenomenon of the vertebral body fragments after the initial loading event.[11] Attempts to correlate injury mechanisms with injury patterns have been unsuccessful. In cadaveric impact testing, failure of the vertebral column preceded any deflection of the head by up to 300 ms.[12] The conclusion of these and other studies is that similar injury mechanisms may result in morphologically different injury patterns, thereby significantly limiting attempts at mechanistic injury classification.[13] This also places an additional burden on the treating physician who has to collate clinical and imaging findings into an individual cohesive stability assessment for each injured patient.

Cervical Spine Stability

Correct assessment of the stability of a traumatized cervical spine is critical for spine clearance and injury management. Unfortunately, specific definitions of lower cervical instability remain somewhat vague.[14] The general definition coined by White and Panjabi described spinal instability as the inability of the spine to prevent initial or additional damage to the neural elements, incapacitation deformities, or pain from structural changes.[15] This definition, however, offers little specific guidance to a practitioner charged with the task of managing a cervical spine injury. A scoring system, such as that devised by White and Panjabi, has continued to provide a helpful reference as well as a checklist toward assessing lower cervical stability[15] (Table 1). However, all structural and biomechanical osteoligamentous considerations aside, any patient with neurologic injury in the cervical spine by definition has an unstable neck.

Injury Classification

The ASIA criteria for the classification of spinal cord injuries, which assign a specific functional grade to categories of neurologic function and allow for assignment of a numeric and reproducible motor score to patients with spine injuries, have been widely accepted.[4] In contrast, little or no consensus exists on how to classify the musculoskeletal aspects of lower cervical spine injuries. Concepts used for classification purposes include anatomic, biomechanical, or combined models. Lack of desirable features such as simplicity, interobserver and even in-

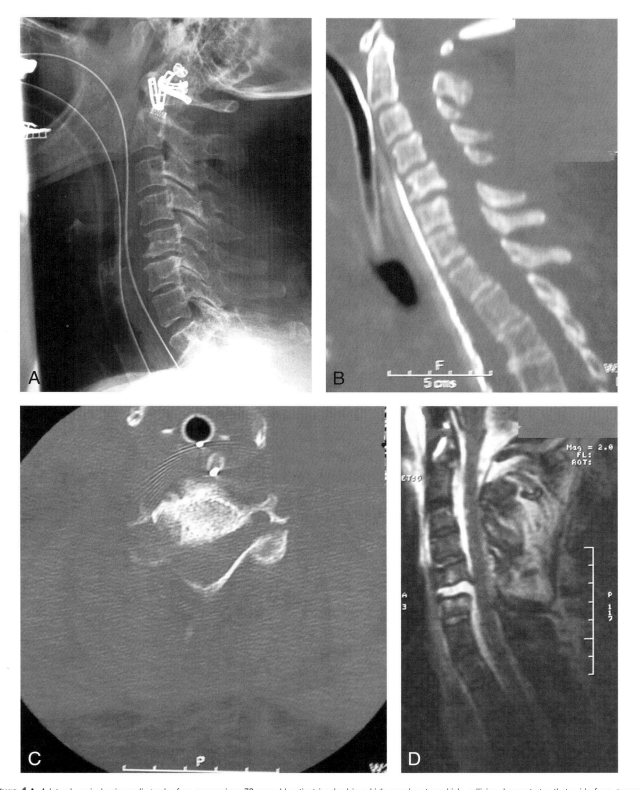

Figure 1 A, A lateral cervical spine radiograph of an unconscious 73-year-old patient involved in a high-speed motor vehicle collision demonstrates that aside from generalized degenerative changes no obvious radiographic abnormalities were detected. **B** and **C,** Based on the patient's risk criteria, routine screening helical CT scans of head and cervical spine were obtained that demonstrate interspinous gapping on the sagittally reformatted midline image at C5-6 and unroofing of the right facet joint on the axial image. **D,** Based on CT scan findings, a sagittally reformatted T2-weighted MRI scan was obtained on which a distractive type fracture dislocation (type C injury) of the C5 on C6 segment can be seen. Seemingly occult ligamentous injuries can be missed on initial recumbent cervical spine screening radiographs. Spine clearance protocols can benefit from institution of a risk-based implementation of routine neurologic imaging studies to minimize the risk of missing injuries.

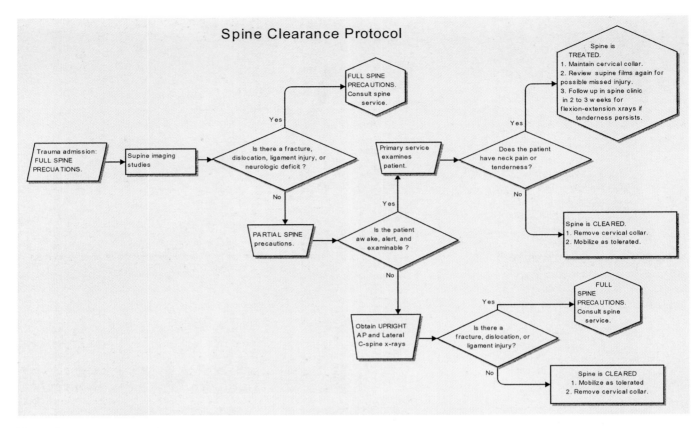

Figure 2 Spine clearance protocol.

traobserver reliability, and relevance toward treatment and outcomes have limited the general acceptance of lower cervical spine classification systems (for example, the often used and comprehensive system described by Allen and associates[13]). Conceptually, the system devised by the AO/ASIF, and accepted by the Orthopaedic Trauma Association, combines widely accepted injury types with some correlation to treatment algorithms.[16] The three basic injury categories consist of type A injuries, which include inherently stable fracture patterns usually caused by axial loading mechanisms; type B injuries, which include bending injuries, such as unilateral or bilateral dislocations with or without fractures; and type C injuries, which are circumferentially destabilized fracture-dislocations. Unfortunately, a multitude of subcategories adds to the complexity of this system, and intricate knowledge of all of these subcategories is not necessarily relevant for specific management decisions.

Emergent Management
Basic Care
Emergent management for patients with lower cervical spine injuries should take into account the potential for spinal cord injury as well as the overall trauma burden and baseline physiologic parameters of the affected patient. Basic common care concepts include immobiliza-

tion on a rigid back board, with full spine precautions and rigid neck collar used during the resuscitation phase, and volume resuscitation, with the goal of maintaining a hematocrit level above 30%, normotension, and normal oxygen saturation. Pharmacologic care for patients with suspected spinal cord injuries includes possible intravenous administration of methylprednisolone as well as administration of intravenous vasopressors in those with neurogenic shock.[1]

Emergent Reduction
Timing the reduction of cervical fracture-dislocations based on performing additional neuroimaging such as MRI has been a controversial topic in the past. Several case reports raised fears that secondary neurologic deterioration may occur as a result of disk or bone fragments being dislodged into the spinal canal during a reduction maneuver.[17] The potential gain of the additional diagnostic insight afforded by MRI has to be balanced with the additional manipulation incurred through multiple patient transfers and the imaging induced time delay in reduction of a compromised spinal cord. Based on the findings of prospective studies, the safety of closed reduction of awake, alert, examinable patients with spinal cord injuries before performing MRI has been established.[18,19] Early reduction of cervical fracture-

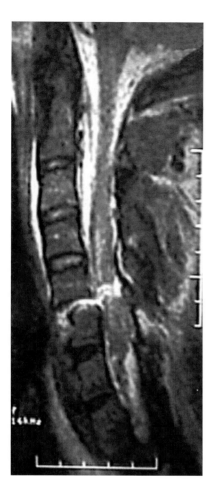

Figure 3 This sagittally formatted T2-weighted MRI scan demonstrates a spinal cord transsection at the C4-5 level in a 17-year-old male who was involved in a motorcycle crash. Outright spinal cord transsections are relatively uncommon; when they do occur, they are typically the result of indirect injury mechanisms.

TABLE 1 | Instability Criteria

Element	Score* (points)
Anterior elements unable to function	2
Posterior elements unable to function	2
Sagittal plane translation > 3.5 mm	2
Sagittal plane rotation > 11°	2
Positive stretch test results?	2
Spinal cord damage	2
Nerve root damage	1
Abnormal disk narrowing	1
Dangerous loading anticipated	1

*A total score of 5 or more indicates instability.
(Adapted with permission from White AA III, Panjabi MM: *Clinical Biomechanics of the Spine.* New York, NY, JB Lippincott, 1990.)

dislocations may improve recovery for patients with spinal cord injury, although the incidence and specific circumstances leading to improvement remain unclear[1,20] (Figure 4).

The true incidence of disk herniation associated with unilateral or bilateral facet dislocations is not known. In a prereduction MRI study, 2 of 11 patients (18%) were found to have a herniated disk, whereas an additional 5 patients demonstrated evidence of disk herniation on postreduction MRI scans.[18] None of these patients experienced secondary neurologic deterioration. In a retrospective study of 82 patients with bilateral and unilateral fracture-dislocations, closed reduction was successful in 97.6% of patients in an average of 2.1 hours.[18] In two patients, emergent surgery was performed for failure to achieve closed reduction. One patient experienced delayed neurologic deterioration by one root level after reduction. Using postreduction MRI, 17 of 76 patients (22%) were found to have a disk herniation and 18 of 76 patients (24%) were found to have disk disruption. Statistically significant improvements of the ASIA motor score were found in patients with complete injuries as well as in those with incomplete injuries. The mean ASIA motor score improved in patients with complete spinal cord injury from an average of 9.8 prereduction to

16.9 within 24 hours after closed reduction. For patients with incomplete spinal cord injury, the mean ASIA motor score improved from 35.8 to 47.7.[18]

Reduction of a dislocated lower cervical spine should be performed in a controlled setting using the principles outlined in Table 2. This includes patient monitoring (cardiovascular, respiratory, and neurologic), incrementally increasing skeletal traction using fluoroscopy or serial radiographs, and providing intravenous analgesia and muscle relaxation. As traction is applied to the cervical spine, radiographs are periodically assessed for overdistraction in any of its segments. Manual reduction attempts are generally discouraged because they can be associated with less controllable forces exerted on the neck. It has been recommended that cervical reduction efforts be abandoned and an emergent MRI scan obtained when a patient's neurologic status deteriorates. Similarly, reduction efforts are usually abandoned when realignment has failed with traction weight amounting to two thirds of the patient's body weight. This weight recommendation, however, is not absolute and depends on individual clamp specifications. For most graphite-based tongs, a fixed limitation of 80 lb has been suggested because of the risk of clamp deformation at higher loads with subsequent clamp pullout.[18,19] In patients with a persistent spinal cord impinging lesion, emergent surgical intervention aimed at effective decompression and stabilization of the affected segment may have to be considered.

Nonsurgical Management

Considerations for treatment involve the presence of neurologic injury, overall injury load of the afflicted patient, and preexistent comorbidities. Factors favoring successful nonsurgical care include absence of neurologic injury, predominantly bony injuries that leave the key

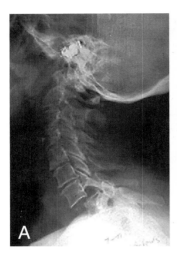
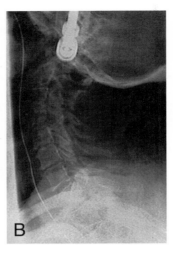
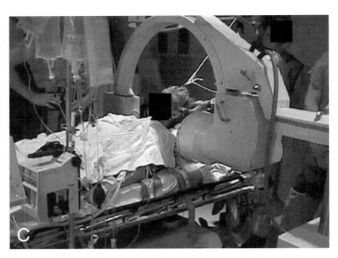

Figure 4 A, Radiograph demonstrating an ASIA A C6 level complete neurologic level in conjunction with a C6-7 bilateral facet dislocation (type B injury) in a 42-year-old man after a barefoot waterskiing injury. The patient presented within 4 hours of the injury. **B,** Radiograph demonstrating that successful emergent reduction of the deformity was achieved at 70 lb using skeletal cervical traction (as described by White and Panjabi) and sequential weight increases and interval checks. During the reduction procedure, the patient experienced gradual return of extremity sensation and motor function and made a full motor and sensory recovery within weeks of the injury. **C,** Photograph showing the typical setup for skeletal cervical traction aimed at reduction of cervical fracture dislocations. Note the C-arm position and elevated pulley setup to facilitate controlled spinal realignment under a monitored setup. Manipulation of cervical dislocations may increase the risk of displacing an intervertebral disk into the spinal canal during reduction efforts.

supportive ligaments intact, and single-system injury scenarios.[21] Choices of nonsurgical care range from activity restrictions for patients with inherently stable injuries to external immobilization with a brace or halo vest or prolonged recumbent skeletal traction for those with severely unstable injuries. Soft collars have no inherent biomechanical stabilizing effects on the lower cervical spine and are usually used for adjuvant management of neck muscle sprains. Rigid neck collars are suitable for external immobilization after surgery and can be considered for patients with minimally deformed compression fractures or apophyseal injuries.[22] Conventional neck collars offer little stabilization to the transition zones, such as the cervicothoracic region.[23] Some additional stability can be provided by thoracic and cranial attachments to rigid neck collars. Nevertheless, injuries treated with such combination devices should be inherently stable because actual wear characteristics of these braces commonly limit their usefulness in real life.

Halo vests provide the most rigid form of external immobilization for patients with cervical spine injuries. Limitations of these devices and complications such as infections, skin breakdown, and respiratory complications in up to 35% of patients have been reported.[24] Loss of fracture reduction with a patient immobilized in a halo vest can occur because of injury type, poor halo ring placement, poor vest fit, and unfavorable patient body habitus. A common phenomenon is the occurrence of snaking, which can be observed as a focal kyphosis in the midcervical spine on a recumbent lateral radiograph, whereas an upright lateral radiograph shows maintained lordosis. For this reason, halo vest assemblies are used primarily to treat patients with upper cervical spine injuries.[21] In general, halo vest treatment is also unsuitable

for extremely obese patients, multiple-trauma patients, patients with chest deformities or chest injuries, and frail elderly patients. Before placement of a halo ring or cranial traction, patients should be assessed for the possible presence of a skull fracture or cranial defect. If applied for a suitable indication and with necessary attention to detail, however, halo vests continue to offer a reasonable nonsurgical management alternative.

Historically, certain types of unstable lower cervical spine injuries have been successfully treated (temporarily or definitively) with prolonged recumbent skeletal cranial traction with the patient positioned in a spinal cord injury bed. This treatment option has largely become obsolete because of the increased morbidity associated with prolonged bed rest as well as cost and quality of life considerations. Should prolonged recumbent skeletal traction be chosen, a detailed care plan should be implemented by an experienced care team. This includes consideration for use of a Rotorest bed (Kinetic Concepts, San Antonio, TX), daily lateral follow-up radiographs, pulmonary care, alimentary support, a deep venous thrombosis prevention program, and a plan and timeline for conversion to a further external immobilization program on conclusion of traction.

Surgical Treatment

The goal of surgical treatment of lower cervical spine injuries is to restore the physiologic parameters of the affected region to the best possible degree. This includes providing effective stabilization and realignment to the injured segments and providing for decompression of compromised neural elements. Ideally, this concept is achieved with the least invasive and atraumatic tech-

TABLE 2 | Reduction Protocol

Exclusion Criteria

Patients with skull fractures

Patients with distractive spinal injury

Most patients with ankylosing cervical spine disorders

Cognitively impaired patients with unknown spinal cord injury status (proceed with caution)

Setup

Supine position on trauma gurney

Pulse oximetry

Blood pressure and electrocardiographic monitoring

Intravenous muscle relaxation and analgesia titrated to provide comfort yet allowing for patient feedback

Static shoulder pull-down (shoulder tape or wrist guards)

C-arm or fluoroscopy in lateral projection

In adults: Gardner Wells tongs (Codman and Shurtleff, Randolph, MA)

Use titanium if anticipated reduction below 100 lb (otherwise stainless steel should be exchanged for titanium following reduction)

For pediatric patients: 4 or 6 pin graphite halo

Pulley system, rope, and weights

Procedure

Baseline lateral C-spine image (save and print for reference)

Baseline weight 10 lb

Increase every 5 min by 5 to 10 lb

Incremental increases of weight followed by repeat images and neurologic evaluation

Stop traction or reduction efforts if patient deteriorates neurologically and obtain emergent MRI scan

Stop if adjacent disk level widens by 1.5 times normal or more

Maximum weight: 80% body weight (stainless steel tongs)

After reduction accomplished reduce weight to 10 to 20 lb and position head in neutral position

Obtain postreduction neuroimaging

---

nique involving the fewest possible motion segments in any arthrodesis construct. Advances in neuroimaging together with refinements of surgical implants for the cervical spine offer unprecedented treatment options. To this end, posterior or anterior surgery alone or combined anterior and posterior treatment paradigms can be considered.

Posterior Surgery

The advantages of this relatively straightforward approach include the ability to perform direct fracture reduction of dislocations, rigid posterior element-based internal fixation, posterior spinal canal and foraminal decompression, multilevel posterior instrumentation (including the transition zones of the craniocervical and cervicothoracic regions), and some degree of kyphotic deformity correction. In general, posterior cervical spine fusions are also reported to have fewer nonunions com-

pared with anterior procedures. The disadvantages of posterior neck surgery include the inherent problems of performing prone position surgery in a medically potentially unstable patient, a trend toward increased blood loss, and myofascial pain.

Although dorsal neural element decompression can be effectively achieved in patients with depressed posterior element fractures or foraminal impingement caused by facet fractures, this technique provides only limited or no anterior cord decompression. In a trauma setting, any neural decompression surgery should generally be accompanied by an arthrodesis of the affected levels with stable internal fixation to maintain physiologic alignment. Current posterior implant options include interspinous cable fixation and posterior plates and screws or rod and screw systems. Interspinous cable fixation has been used for more than five decades to treat patients with interspinous ligament disruption who also have intact posterior bony structures and no herniated intervertebral disks. Interspinous cable fixation offers only limited stability for patients with torsionally unstable spine injuries and is unsuitable for those with deficient posterior elements. Posterior screw purchase in the lower cervical spine has been described for the lateral masses of the C2 through C7 segments.[23,25]

Although different techniques have been described, two techniques have emerged as predominant: one using a screw trajectory starting from the center of the lateral mass and directed in a straight, slightly lateral fashion and the other offering some biomechanical advantages and a decreased risk of nerve root injury by using a more cephalad and laterally directed screw trajectory that results in a slightly longer screw length.[25] Over the past decade, both techniques have been shown to be safe and effective posterior cervical stabilization methods (Figure 5). Because of the absence of suitable lateral masses at the axis and in the cervicothoracic junction, pedicle screw fixation has emerged as the posterior fixation technique of choice for those levels, especially in osteopenic patients. Pedicle screw fixation of the C3 through C6 segments has been described for degenerative stabilization.[23] This technique appears to be largely unnecessary for treatment of lower cervical trauma because of its challenging application technique and the associated increased risk of iatrogenic injury to vertebral artery or neural elements.

Several retrospective studies have reported successful outcomes for more than 95% of patients who were treated with segmental posterior cervical fixation using small reconstruction plates for lower cervical spine trauma and cervicothoracic injuries.[23,25,26] The disadvantages of using posterior cervical plates include increased technical challenges of aligning screw placement over a plate, especially in patients with deformity or those requiring multilevel fixation. The conceptual advantages of posterior rod and screw fixation systems with their fixed

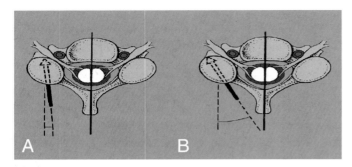

Figure 5 This diagram depicts two widely accepted techniques used for posterior segmental instrumentation of the lower cervical spine. Both techniques use screw anchoring in the lateral masses. The technique described by Roy-Camille **(A)** suggests a straightforward trajectory, whereas the technique presented by Magerl **(B)** favors an upward and outward screw trajectory with improved biomechanical stability and possibly reduced likelihood of nerve root or vertebral artery injury. (Courtesy of Michael Janssen, DO.)

connection systems include their ability to provide multilevel rigid stabilization, especially in patients with deformity or those with osteopenia. To date, however, there have been no known studies conducted to support the use of these more expensive and complex instrumentation systems over posterior cervical plates and screws.

Anterior Surgery

Common trauma indications for anterior subaxial cervical spine surgery typically include unstable burst fractures in metabolically healthy patients as well as patients with previously reduced lower cervical spine fracture-dislocations.

The advantages of anterior surgery for injuries of the lower cervical spine include the ability to perform comprehensive anterior column decompression and reconstruction and stabilization through a relatively atraumatic Smith-Robinson approach with the patient in a supine position. Compared with posterior surgery, anterior cervical decompression and stabilization has been reported to be associated with a trend toward improved neurologic outcomes in patients with spinal cord injury.[21] In a prospective comparison of anterior and posterior cervical surgery, 70% of patients in the anterior cervical surgery group improved at least one Frankel grade compared with patients in the posterior cervical surgery group, in which 57% improved at least one Frankel grade.[26]

The limitations of anterior subaxial trauma surgery include exposure usually restricted to two or three motion segments, poor access to the cervical transition zones, and increased exposure-related morbidity compared with posterior neck procedures. Anterior cervical plating also can result in decreased stiffness in flexion, torsion, and axial loading characteristics compared with segmental posterior stabilization techniques. Compared with posterior procedures, increased rates of nonunion and hardware failure have been reported for patients

who undergo multilevel anterior arthrodesis and for osteopenic individuals.[27]

From a surgical perspective, anterior subaxial neck surgery can be divided into three phases: decompression, anterior column reconstruction, and anterior stabilization. There are several treatment variables available for each of these three phases (Figure 6).

Decompression
Depending on the indication, anterior cervical decompression surgery can be accomplished with either diskectomy or corpectomy. In an acute trauma setting, multilevel anterior corpectomies are rarely if ever indicated. The increased iatrogenic destabilizing effect of a corpectomy relative to a diskectomy should also be considered. Thus, the decompression needs of a patient should be matched with the patient's biomechanical and morphologic circumstances.

Anterior Column Reconstruction
Reconstruction of an anterior column defect can be achieved with a tricortical structural iliac crest graft, structural fibular allograft, or a structural titanium cage with autologous local bone graft core. Anterior column reconstruction options have emerged from concerns over morbidity associated with autologous iliac crest bone graft. However, to date there are no peer-reviewed studies comparing the healing rates of trauma patients who have received autologous iliac crest graft and those who have undergone anterior column corpectomy reconstructions using either fibular allograft or titanium cages.

Anterior Stabilization
If supplemental posterior surgery is not needed, anterior stabilization can be achieved with a low-profile plate and unicortical vertebral body screws, which are rigidly locked into the plate. Rigid anterior plate fixation has minimized the need for supplemental external immobilization with halo vests and improves the ability to maintain physiologic neck alignment until bony healing has been achieved. More recently, dynamic locking plates have been introduced with the stated goal of improved graft healing because of improved load sharing with the graft for patients with degenerative indications; however, these devices have little or no place in the treatment of a traumatically disrupted spinal column.

Results of anterior surgery in patients with subaxial spine trauma have generally been favorable, even in those with flexion-type injuries, despite the inherently more limited biomechanical stiffness of these constructs compared with posterior devices.

Combined Anterior and Posterior Surgery
Since the advent of third-generation anterior and posterior instrumentation systems, combined anterior and posterior surgery for patients with subaxial trauma is rarely needed.[25] In a prospectively randomized study

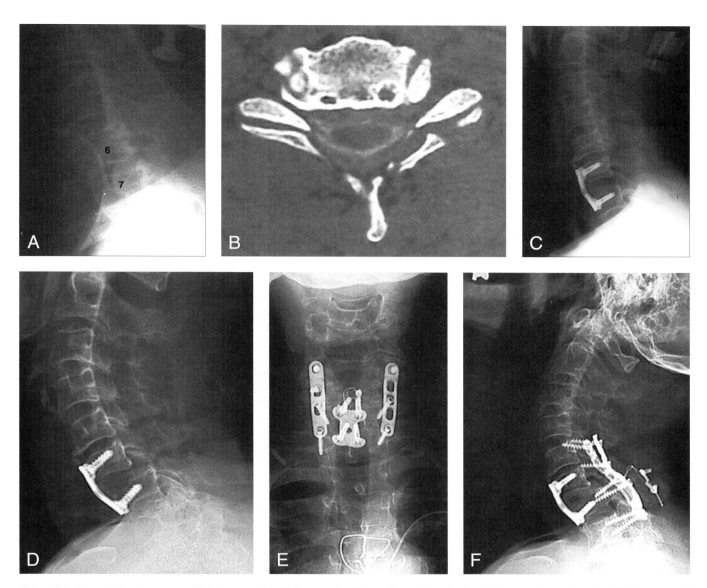

Figure 6 A, Swimmer's view demonstrates mild displacement of the C6-7 segment in a 72-year-old man with neck pain and C7 arm numbness and weakness following a syncopal incident. **B,** CT myelogram was obtained after achieving reduction with skeletal traction (25 lb); MRI was contraindicated because the patient had a pacemaker. This axial image shows a more complex injury pattern, with a left-sided superior facet fracture with comminution into the neural arch. This injury pattern was interpreted as a type B unilateral facet fracture dislocation. Because of persistent C7 radicular deficits and inability of the patient to tolerate nonsurgical care, surgical stabilization of the injury was suggested. **C,** Postoperative lateral radiograph shows that the patient was treated with an anterior cervical diskectomy and arthrodesis and instrumentation using a locking plate C6-7. The patient was then immobilized postoperatively with a Minerva brace. During a routine postoperative visit, the patient reported recurrent arm pain and weakness. **D,** Upright lateral cervical radiograph revealed a loss of reduction, with recurrent anterolisthesis C6 on C7. AP **(E)** and lateral **(F)** radiographs show final healing after the patient underwent a posterior procedure that included wide foraminotomies and posterior segmental instrumentation of C5 through T1. The patient experienced complete symptom relief. Although anterior surgical stabilization is gaining popularity because of its relatively atraumatic technique, it remains biomechanically inferior to posterior segmental surgical stabilization.

of 52 patients, 90% healed successfully with anterior surgery and 100% healed successfully with posterior surgery alone.[26] Exceptions to this generalization are patients with unusually severe fracture-dislocations, fracture malunions, displaced fracture-dislocations in conjunction with ankylosing disorders, and severe multilevel posttraumatic myelopathy combined with cervical stenosis. For some of these patients, staged procedures on separate days can achieve the ultimate treatment goals while lessening the physiologic impact of a same-day combined procedure. The specific approach to choose first largely depends on the individual patient's injury and comorbidities. For instance, most patients with fracture-dislocations or ankylosing spine disease are usually more effectively reduced and stabilized from an initial posterior approach. A supplemental anterior approach can then be performed at a later date. In contrast, patients with kyphotic fracture malunion or a severe burst fracture will usually require an anterior approach first followed by a secondary posterior stabilization and decompression of neural elements as needed.

Timing of Surgical Intervention

The timing of surgical intervention for lower cervical spine trauma remains somewhat controversial, particularly because what constitutes emergent spine care remains poorly defined. Some studies have used a 72-hour threshold as a tidemark for emergent surgery.[19,28] In contrast, some animal studies suggest that a 6-hour timeline to decompression should be used for possible reversal of spinal cord injury.[1] In humans, a trauma-to-treatment window of 8 hours has been established in the second National Acute Spinal Cord Injury Study, which evaluated the use of high-dose methylprednisolone.[20] However, the actual surgical treatment of a patient with a spinal cord injury commonly takes place on a delayed basis. This was shown in a multicenter clinical study that reported 50.7% of surgeons performed spinal cord decompressive surgery after 48 hours following injury.[1] Based on the responses of 36 medical centers in North America, the authors concluded that emergent surgical intervention within 8 hours of injury was not feasible.

If early surgical intervention for cervical spine trauma is chosen, adherence to trauma management principles such as maintenance of spine immobilization, physiologic blood pressure, hematocrit level, and oxygenation as well as atraumatic airway management are recommended. Secondary postresuscitation hypotension has been shown to be particularly damaging in patients with central nervous system injuries and should be avoided as much as possible.[20] To date, several studies comparing early versus delayed surgical intervention for patients with spinal cord injuries have failed to convincingly identify significantly improved neurologic outcomes for either timing group. However, the considerable number of covariables affecting patients with spinal cord injuries compared with the relatively small study populations significantly limits the interpretability of data from these studies. Conversely, the belief that surgical intervention within 72 hours may lead to spinal cord deterioration has largely been refuted in several studies.[28,29] Additional large-scale database evaluations are underway to determine the effect of the timing of surgical intervention on neurologic recovery. Over the past decade, a dramatic shift in the population of cervical spinal cord injury patients (away from younger male individuals and increasingly involving elderly patients) has been observed. This shift has introduced complex new treatment variables and challenges because of commonly encountered comorbidities in the elderly.[30]

With regard to anterior versus posterior surgical approach, a recent prospective comparison study showed no statistically significant differences between anterior and posterior procedures for stabilization of lower cervical spine fracture-dislocations.[26] This study also confirmed that circumferential stabilization for acute cervical trauma in the absence of confounding factors is rarely if ever necessary (Figure 7).

Treatment of Typical Injuries

Type A Injuries

These injuries include inherently stable injuries, primarily apophyseal injuries such as transverse process fractures and isolated spinous process fractures, compression fractures, and burst fractures. Most flexion or extension teardrop fractures retain inherent spinal stability and can be treated with an external orthotic device.[22] After comprehensive injury assessment, external immobilization is recommended and is usually achieved with a rigid neck collar for several months followed by clinical and radiographic reevaluation.

Type B Injuries
Unilateral Facet Dislocations With or Without Fracture

Patients with these injuries usually are treated with closed reduction and postreduction neuroimaging to assess for neural element compression. In a prospective study, 5 of 22 patients (23%) with unilateral facet injuries were found to have a disk herniation. Nerve root injuries are a prevalent form of neurologic injury in this patient population and usually occur on the side of the dislocation.[18] Depending on the degree of disk disruption and possible neural element encroachment, nonsurgical treatment of patients with these injuries can consist of external immobilization with a cervicothoracic brace or halo vest. Surgical treatment can consist of diskectomy and bone grafting with anterior locking plate fixation or posterior foraminotomy and arthrodesis using bone graft as well as segmental stabilization with screw and rod or plate constructs.

Bilateral Facet Dislocations With or Without Facet Fracture

One study reported that these injuries were associated with a disk herniation in 2 of 15 patients (13%).[18,29] Complete spinal cord injuries were found in 30% of patients.[18] Suggested treatment consists of closed reduction followed by neuroimaging for patients with spinal cord injury. Definitive management usually requires surgical stabilization with arthrodesis and rigid stabilization. Surgical stabilization can be accomplished with anterior stabilization for patients with good bone quality or by using posterior segmental stabilization with a screw-based system. For patients with poor bone quality or other causes of insufficient vertebral body screw purchase, an increased risk of secondary loss of reduction has been reported[31] (Figure 8).

Type C injuries

These injuries include complex fractures in patients with associated comorbidities, high-grade burst fractures, and severe fracture-dislocations. Concomitant spinal cord in-

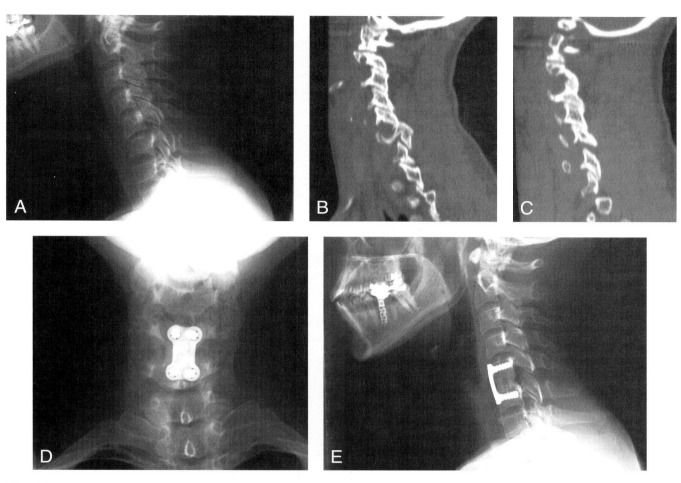

Figure 7 Anterior treatment bilateral facet dislocation. **A,** A lateral radiograph demonstrates a C5-6 facet dislocation (type B injury) in a 36-year-old man after a motorcycle crash. The patient had no discernible spinal cord neurologic injury (ASIA E). **B** and **C,** Because of the injury mechanism, routine screening CT scans of the head and cervical spine were obtained, which allow for rapid and effective visualization of the entire cervical spine. A parasagittal image of the right-sided completely dislodged lateral masses **(B)** and a parasagittal left-sided distracted and disrupted C5-6 facet joint complex **(C)** are shown. The patient was awake and alert and had no evidence of a skull fracture; therefore, closed skeletal reduction was expediently carried out and achieved at 75 lb. On successful reduction, the weight was reduced to 20 lb, with the patient immobilized on a Rotorest bed. Definitive treatment was carried out with anterior cervical diskectomy and fusion using a fibula allograft and anterior cervical locking plate. Although this procedure can be done in a relatively expedient and atraumatic fashion, it is biomechanically inferior to posterior segmental stabilization. Care also must be taken to avoid iatrogenic overdistraction when type C injuries are treated using this technique. Postoperative AP **(D)** and lateral **(E)** radiographs show successful healing of the fusion at 6-month follow-up.

juries are commonly observed in patients with type C injuries.

High-Grade Burst Fractures
High-grade burst fractures are most commonly treated with a corpectomy, anterior strut grafting, and rigid anterior plate fixation. Supplemental posterior fixation may be considered if the patient is osteopenic (Figure 9).

Hyperextension Fractures
Hyperextension fractures are commonly associated with ankylosing spine conditions, such as disseminated idiopathic skeletal hyperostosis or ankylosing spondylitis. In patients with a pretraumatic spinal column kyphosis, fractures in an ankylosing spine often present as hyperextension injuries. The frequently irregular fracture planes typically indicate the presence of a fracture-dislocation with complete structural compromise. Closed reduction attempts should be undertaken with the greatest of care in patients with this type of injury because secondary spinal cord injury can occur with fracture manipulation. If medically feasible, early surgical intervention is frequently desirable because closed reduction is difficult if not impossible to maintain, and epidural hematoma formation can further compromise the spinal cord. Typically, definitive care consists of a multilevel posterior segmental stabilization in association with posterior spinal canal decompression. In patients with an anterior column gap, secondary anterior stabilization can be achieved with a structural bone graft and plate fixation. Given the long lever arms of the spinal column and vertebral osteopenia in patients with ankylosing spinal disorders, isolated anterior fracture stabilization is prone to fixation failure and thus less desirable.[31]

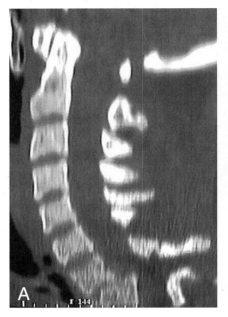

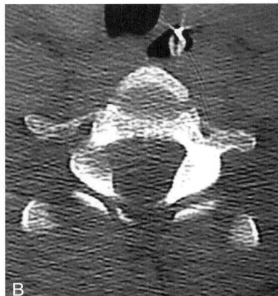

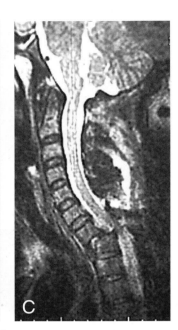

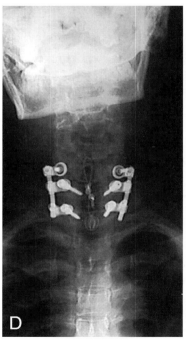

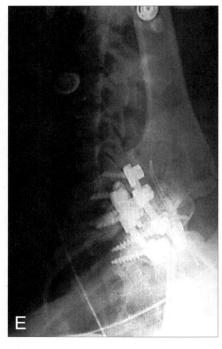

Figure 8 This sagittally reformatted T2-weighted MRI scan **(A)** and axial screening CT **(B)** show a bilateral facet dislocation (type B injury) at C7/T1 (ASIA unknown) in a 32-year-old obese woman with unknown neurologic injury status (ASIA unknown) who presented with loss of consciousness and multiple system injuries after an unrestrained high-speed car crash. Because of the inability to obtain a neurologic status on the patient, an emergent MRI scan **(C)** was ordered to assess for neural element compromise. This study, as represented by a sagittal T2-weighted image, shows no signal changes within the cord but ongoing cord compression. After being unable to achieve closed reduction with 100 lb of traction, the patient underwent emergent posterior open reduction and stabilization. Closed reduction in the cervicothoracic junction can be difficult and is prone to failure. Postoperative AP **(D)** and lateral **(E)** radiographs were obtained after posterior open reduction and decompressive laminectomy of the C7 level. Stabilization was achieved using C6 to T1 rod and screw fixation. The patient was found to have intact spinal cord function (ASIA E) after recovery from head injury. Although anterior stabilization of the cervicothoracic junction is technically possible, posterior segmental fixation is recommended because of ease of access and superior biomechanical characteristics.

Fracture-Dislocation

Unfortunately, these injuries are commonly associated with spinal cord injury. Patients with cervical fracture-dislocations commonly present with significant translational displacement. Closed reduction can be difficult to maintain because of loss of key structural elements such as facet joints. After the best possible closed reduction is achieved and neuroimaging is performed, early surgical care usually involves posterior multilevel segmental instrumentation and arthrodesis. Secondary anterior col-

umn reconstruction may be necessary depending on the reduction result.

Summary

Over the past decade, several important changes have provided a more streamlined approach to the management of patients with lower cervical spine trauma. Increasingly, helical CT scans are used for the rapid and comprehensive evaluation of patients who are at

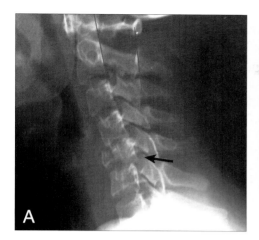
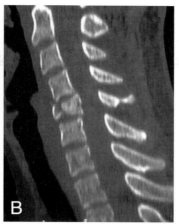
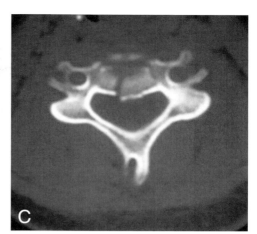

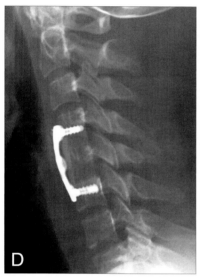
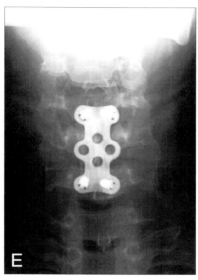

Figure 9 A, A lateral cervical spine radiograph demonstrates a C5 unstable burst fracture (*arrow*) in a 27-year-old man after a diving injury. The patient reported transient loss of motor and sensory function following the incident. By the time of arrival in the emergency room, the patient was found to have normal neurologic function. Sagittal **(B)** and axial **(C)** CT scans were obtained after the patient had been placed on cranial skeletal traction (20 lb). The CT scans show the absence of a major posterior column disruption and the presence of 20% residual canal compromise. After discussion of treatment options, which included consideration of management with a halo vest, the patient elected to proceed with surgery. Postoperative lateral **(D)** and AP **(E)** radiographs show healing of an autologous tricortical graft that had been secured with an anterior cervical locking plate.

risk for spinal injury. Recent literature has generally supported early closed reduction of lower cervical spine fracture-dislocations with skeletal cranial traction as a safe management strategy, provided proper technique and attention to detail are applied. With the option of early indirect closed reduction to achieve effective decompression of a compromised spinal cord, surgical intervention can be delayed until optimum clinical circumstances are present. Despite clear conceptual advantages of spinal cord and neural element decompression toward enhancing chances of neural recovery, actual supportive clinical data remain incomplete.

The availability of anterior cervical locking plates that have achieved good surgical results has shifted the preferred surgical approach for lower cervical spine trauma from a posterior approach to the less traumatic anterior approach, thus allowing for more expedient and atraumatic surgical management of many commonly occurring unstable lower cervical spine injuries. However, the increasing incidence of cervical spine fractures in the growing segment of the elderly popu-lation, which is often afflicted with considerable co-morbidities and complex nontraumatic spine conditions, poses new treatment challenges.[31] The role of more sophisticated surgical stabilization techniques has yet to be sufficiently evaluated.

Annotated References

1. Tator CH, Fehlings MG, Thorpe K, Taylor W: Current use and timing of spinal surgery for management of acute spinal cord injury in North America: Results of a retrospective multicenter study. *J Neurosurg* 1999;91(suppl 1):12-18.

2. Blackmore CC, Emerson SS, Mann FA, Koepsell TD: Cervical spine imaging in patients with trauma: Determination of fracture risk to optimize use. *Radiology* 1999;211:759-765.

3. Nuckley DJ, Konodi MA, Raynak GC, Ching P, Chapman JR, Mirza SK: Neural space integrity of

the lower cervical spine: Effect of anterior lesions. *Spine* 2004;29:642-649.

4. American Spinal Injury Association: *Standards for Neurological and Functional Classification of Spinal Cord Injury, Revised 1992.* Chicago, IL, American Spinal Injury Association, 1992.

5. Blackmore CC, Mann FA, Wilson AJ: Helical CT in the primary trauma evaluation of the cervical spine: An evidence based approach. *Skeletal Radiol* 2000; 29:632-639.

6. Stiell IG, Clement CM, McKnight RD, et al: The Canadian C-spine rule versus the NEXUS low-risk criteria in patients with trauma. *N Engl J Med* 2003; 349:2510-2518.

7. Harris MB, Kronlage SC, Carboni PA, et al: Evaluation of the cervical spine in the polytrauma patient. *Spine* 2000;25:2884-2891.
   This two-part study consisted of a surgeons survey of spine clearance pathways and a prospective study of 153 multiple-traumatized patients, who were evaluated following a standardized protocol using fluoroscopy and CT. 8 of 153 patients could not be adequately evaluated with fluoscopy.

8. Chiu WC, Haan JM, Cushing BM, Kramer ME, Scalea TM: Ligamentous injuries of the cervical spine in unreliable blunt trauma patients: Incidence, evaluation, and outcome. *J Trauma* 2001;50:457-464.

9. Halliday AL, Henderson BR, Hart BL, Benzel EC: The management of unilateral lateral mass/facet fractures of the subaxial cervical spine: The use of magnetic resonance imaging to predict instability. *Spine* 1997;22:2614-2621.

10. Giacobetti FB, Vaccaro AR, Bos-Giacobetti MA, et al: Vertebral artery occlusion associated with cervical spine trauma: A prospective analysis. *Spine* 1997; 22:188-192.

11. Carter J, Mirza SK, Tencer A, et al: Canal geometry changes associated with axial compressive cervical spine fracture. *Spine* 2000;25:46-54.

12. Nightingale RW, McElhaney JH, Richardson WJ, Best TM, Myers BS: Experimental impact injury to the cervical spine: Relating motion of the head and the mechanism of injury. *J Bone Joint Surg Am* 1996;78:412-421.

13. Allen BL, Ferguson RL, Lehman TR, O'Brien RP: A mechanistic classification of closed, indirect frac-tures and dislocations of the cervical spine. *Spine* 1982;7:1-27.

14. Panjabi MM, Lydon C, Vasavada A, et al: On the understanding of clinical instability. *Spine* 1994;19: 2642-2650.

15. White AA III, Panjabi MM: *Clinical Biomechanics of the Spine.* New York, NY, JB Lippincott, 1990.

16. Gertzbein SD: Spine update: Classification of thoracic and lumbar fractures. *Spine* 1994;19:626-628.

17. Farmer J, Vaccaro A, Albert TJ, Malone S, Balderston RA, Cotler JM: Neurologic deterioration after cervical spinal cord injury. *J Spinal Disord* 1998;11: 192-196.

18. Grant GA, Mirza SK, Chapman JR, et al: Risk of early closed reduction in cervical spine subluxation injuries. *J Neurosurg* 1999;90(suppl 1):13-18.
    Successful closed reduction using emergent skeletal traction was achieved in 98 consecutive patients with fracture-dislocation of the lower cervical spine. There was one patient with delayed temporary neurologic deterioration following reduction. Conversely, significant neurologic improvement could be observed following reduction in patients with spinal cord injury.

19. Vaccaro AR, Falatyn SP, Flanders AE, et al: Magnetic resonance evaluation of the intervertebral disc, spinal ligaments, and spinal cord before and after closed traction reduction of cervical spine dislocations. *Spine* 1999;24:1210-1217.

20. Fehlings MG, Tator CH: An evidence-based review of decompressive surgery in acute spinal cord injury: Rationale, indications, and timing based on experimental and clinical studies. *J Neurosurg* 1999; 91(suppl 1):1-11.

21. Fisher CG, Dvorak MFS, Leith J, Wing PC: Comparison of outcomes for unstable lower cervical flexion teardrop fractures managed with Halo thoracic vest versus anterior corpectomy and plating. *Spine* 2002;27:160-166.
    In this retrospective cohort study 45 patients with flexion-teardrop type injuries treated with either halo or anterior corpectomy and fusion were compared in several variables. Of the 24 patients treated with halo vest there were 5 failures, there were no failures in the anterior surgical group. Kyphosis was found to be 11.4° in the halo group compared with 3.5° in the anterior surgery group. There were no differences in the clinical outcomes measures, however.

22. McGuire RA, Degnan G, Amundson GM: Evaluation of current extrication orthoses in immobilization of the unstable cervical spine. *Spine* 1990;15:1064-1067.

23. Chapman J, Anderson PA, Pepin C, Toomey S, Newell DW, Grady MS: Posterior instrumentation of the unstable cervico-thoracic spine. *J Neurosurg* 1996;84:552-558.

24. Garfin SR, Botte MJ, Waters RL, Nickel VL: Complications in the use of the halo fixation device. *J Bone Joint Surg Am* 1986;68:320-325.

25. Adams MS, Crawford NR, Chamberlain RH, Sonntag VKH, Dickman DA: Biomechanical comparison of anterior cervical plating and combined anterior/lateral mass plating. *Spine J* 2001;1:166-170.

  Using a cervical spine burst fracture model posterior plating demonstrated superior biomechanical stiffness. Anterior plating alone failed in a flexion-distraction model. While combined anterior and posterior instrumentation provided superior biomechanical load characteristics, the clinical relevance of this finding for fixation needs was questioned.

26. Brodke DS, Anderson PA, Newell DW, Grady MS, Chapman JR: Comparison of anterior and posterior approaches in cervical spinal cord injuries. *J Spinal Disord Tech* 2003;16:229-235.

  Prospectively randomized study of 52 patients presenting with spinal cord injury treated with anterior or posterior segmental fixation. Both treatment groups were found to be equivalent from a statistical perspective, with trends toward improved neurologic recovery and less pain, but higher nonunion rate in the anterior group.

27. Dvorak MF, Pitzen T, Zhu Q, Gordon JD, Fisher CG, Oxland T: Anterior cervical plate fixation: A biomechanical study to evaluate their effects of plate design, endplate preparation, and bone mineral density. *Spine* 2005;30:294-301.

28. Mirza SK, Krengel WF III, Chapman JR, et al: Early versus delayed surgery for acute cervical spinal cord injury. *Clin Orthop* 1999;359:104-114.

29. Vaccaro AR, Daugherty RJ, Sheehan TP, et al: Neurologic outcome of early versus late surgery for cervical spinal cord injury. *Spine* 1997;22:2609-2613.

30. Irwin ZN, Arthur M, Mullins RJ, Hart RA: Variations in injury patterns, treatment, and outcome for spinal fracture and paralysis in adult versus geriatric patients. *Spine* 2004;29:796-802.

  In this retrospective cohort analysis a comparison of adult (6,029 patients) and geriatric (3.973 patients) was made in regard to mortality rates, treatment and injury characteristics. For the geriatric cohort increased mortality was found to be related to medical comorbidities, cervical spine injuries and paralysis. In the presence of paralysis a mortality rate of nearly 30% was identified.

31. Johnson MG, Fisher CG, Boyd M, Pitzen T, Oxland TR, Dvorak MF: The radiographic failure of single segment anterior cervical plate fixation in traumatic cervical flexion distraction injuries. *Spine* 2004;29: 2815-2820.

Chapter 28

Thoracolumbar Trauma

Christopher M. Bono, MD

Marie D. Rinaldi, BA

Introduction

The thoracolumbar spine is a common site of traumatic injury. It represents a biomechanical transition zone between the rigid thoracic and more mobile lumbar spine. The rib cage provides additional stability to the thoracic spine. Costovertebral articulations along the posterolateral disk space span two vertebrae. Additional ligaments link the medial rib to the anterior aspect of the thoracic transverse processes. The thoracolumbar junction also marks a sagittal alignment transition zone between the kyphotic thoracic spine and the lordotic lumbar region.

Large forces can be concentrated at the thoracolumbar spine during abrupt and dramatic acceleration changes (such as those produced during motor vehicle accidents). Osseous and/or ligamentous components can fail. Injuries can range from isolated, minor vertebral body compression fractures to circumferential osseoligamentous disruption, such as in a fracture-dislocation. The likelihood of neurologic injury is greater with higher-energy lesions.

Approximately 90% of all thoracic and lumbar injuries occur at the thoracolumbar junction. Males between the ages of 15 and 35 years are the most frequently affected. A recent study has demonstrated that the likelihood of severe and multiple level spinal injuries are higher with motorcycle than automobile accidents.[1] Within the military population, the incidence of thoracolumbar fractures in Army pilots has been demonstrated to be about 13%.[2] Helicopter crashes and parachuting accidents were the most common associated traumatic event, accounting for 73% of injuries.[2]

Diagnostic Considerations

Plain Radiographs

Plain radiographs should be obtained if injury is suspected. Often, spinal fractures are inadvertently first detected by CT of the chest or abdomen. However, this does not obviate the need for high-quality plain radiographs. If a thoracolumbar injury is detected, completion radiographs of the entire spine should be obtained because the rate of concomitant, noncontiguous spinal in-

jury can be as high as 12%.[3] AP and lateral thoracic and lumbar views should be obtained. However, dedicated radiographs centered at the T12-L1 junction are invaluable in any patient with a suspected thoracolumbar injury.

Overall alignment can be assessed using lateral radiographs. The thoracolumbar junction is normally neutral (flat or straight) in both the sagittal and coronal planes. Relative kyphosis can be measured using the Cobb method. This measures the angle between the superior end plate of the nearest uninjured cranial vertebra and the inferior end plate of the nearest uninjured caudal vertebra (Figure 1). The percentage of height loss of the injured vertebral body is based on comparing values of the injured segment to those of adjacent cranial and caudal uninjured vertebrae. Anterior and posterior vertebral body height should be measured separately to more accurately detect compression of one or both regions. Although not a steadfast rule, loss of greater than 50% of vertebral height suggests posterior ligamentous complex (PLC) disruption. Posterior vertebral body fragment retropulsion can often be appreciated on lateral radiographs.

Coronal and rotational alignment of the spine can be assessed using AP radiographs. The relative distance between the spinous processes and the pedicles is a reflection of rotation. Coronal angulation or translation suggests high-energy trauma. Interpedicular width should successively increase from caudal to cranial. Abnormal widening suggests lateral displacement of the pedicles, which is often associated with burst fractures.

Computed Tomography

CT revolutionized physicians' ability to detect and assess bony injuries of the spine. Thin-cut slices should be obtained through the level of injury, as well as at normal adjacent levels. Fracture lines extending to the posterior vertebral body distinguish burst from compression fractures. The dimensional effects of retropulsed bone fragments on the spinal canal are easily appreciated. Posterior column injuries, such as facet dislocations, facet

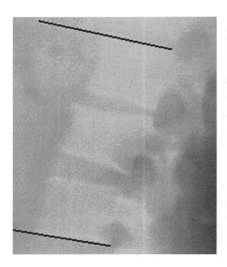

Figure 1 Vertebral body height loss can be appreciated on a lateral radiograph of the thoracolumbar junction. Kyphosis can be assessed using the Cobb method, which measures the angle between the superior end plate of the suprajacent and infrajacent uninjured levels (*black lines*).

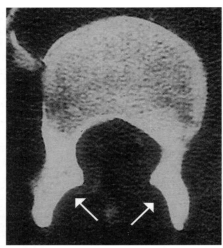

Figure 2 CT scan with empty or naked facet sign (*white arrows*) indicates the presence of facet dislocation.

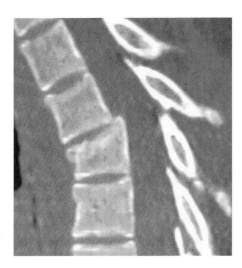

Figure 3 Coronal CT reconstruction demonstrates translation, which is otherwise difficult to appreciate using axial images alone.

fractures, and pedicle fractures, can also be clearly visualized with CT. Lamina fractures that occur concomitantly with a burst fracture are often associated with posterior dural tears and nerve root entrapment. The so-called naked facet is an indication of complete facet dislocation (Figure 2). In the absence of this sign, most other translational deformities can be easily overlooked because they are in the plane of axial CT images. High-quality sagittal and coronal CT reconstructions can facilitate diagnosis of even subtle distraction or translational injuries (Figure 3).

Numerous methods for quantifying canal compromise have been described.[4] However, the superiority or reproducibility of one method versus another has not been clearly demonstrated. Sagittal canal diameter, which is the distance from the posterior aspect of the most posteriorly displaced fragment to the anterior aspect of the lamina, is among the more simple measurements. To arrive at a percentage of canal compromise, this value is compared with the sagittal diameters of uninjured levels above and below the fracture. It has been postulated that this method can underestimate the amount of neural compression and that cross-sectional area measurement is more representative.[4] Unfortunately, this method is cumbersome and difficult to perform using commonly available CT technology. Canal compromise from translational deformity (as in fracture-dislocations) can be underestimated on axial CT images. Sagittal reconstructions are particularly helpful in assessing the spinal canal in these situations. Rotational deformity is best detected by consecutive axial CT images (Figure 4).

Magnetic Resonance Imaging

MRI is superior for evaluating the neural elements, intervertebral disks, and spinal ligaments. MRI can help assess patients with neurologic injury that is incongruous with the skeletal level of injury and for those with soft-tissue injury, if deemed clinically relevant. Compression to the spinal cord or cauda equina can be directly visualized. Nerve root entrapment within a lamina fracture can be seen on axial MRI scans. Intervertebral disk herniation associated with canal compromise is not easily appreciated with CT, and can be better visualized with MRI.

The use of MRI to assess the integrity of the spinal ligaments is becoming more commonplace. In one study, an intact posterior longitudinal ligament (PLL) as visualized using MRI was found to be associated with better canal clearance through posterior distraction instrumentation than if the PLL was disrupted.[5] MRI can also be used to assess the PLC, the integrity of which is an important determinant of burst and compression fracture management. T2-weighted images are more useful than T1-weighted images. Short T1 inversion recovery images may be the most sensitive in detecting edema within the soft tissues, albeit at the expense of decreased image clarity. Findings may vary from mild increased signal between spinous processes on T2-weighted images (indicative of benign ligament sprain) (Figure 5) to bright and expansive signal extending from the tip of the spinous process to the interlaminar interval (indicative of gross PLC disruption). Although these extremes are readily discerned, it is the varying gradations between these extremes that are more difficult to interpret. An MRI grading system has been recently developed to help differentiate these varying degrees of ligamentous injury.[6] The prognostic significance of such a grading system has yet to be demonstrated; however, in one

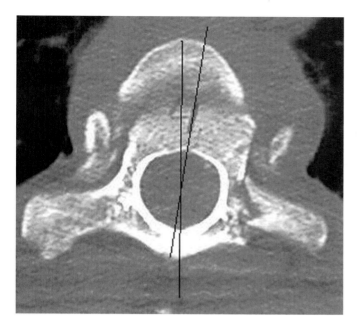

Figure 4 An axial CT scan demonstrates rotational deformity, which is highlighted by the midsagittal lines drawn through the involved vertebra (*black lines*).

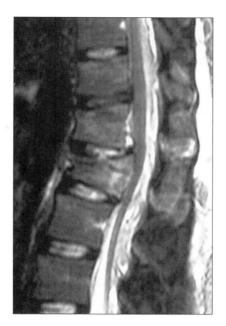

Figure 5 A T2-weighted MRI scan demonstrates mild increased signal within the posterior ligaments in a patient with a T12 burst fracture. This injury is most likely a sprain because the mechanical competence of the PLC is not compromised.

study, PLC disruption was predictive of recurrence of kyphosis in surgically treated patients at final follow-up.[6]

Classification of Thoracolumbar Injuries

Many classification systems for thoracolumbar injuries have been proposed, each with unique advantages and disadvantages.[7] The ideal system should be clinically useful, prognostic, and aid in treatment decision making. Currently, however, there is no universally accepted classification system. Complex systems that attempt to be all-inclusive have led to poor interobserver and intraobserver reproducibility, whereas simpler systems with better reproducibility are useful for only one or two injury patterns. Two of the more widely used systems are the McAfee classification system and the AO/Magerl classification system.[8,9]

McAfee Classification System

The McAfee classification system is an adaptation of the classification system proposed by Denis, which is based on dividing the spine into three distinct columns (Figure 6). Its development was based on analyzing multiplanar CT scans and plain radiographic images of 100 consecutive thoracolumbar injuries.[9] The focus was to postulate the mechanism of failure of the important middle column. It was found that the middle column could fail by axial compression, axial distraction, or translation in the transverse plane. Sagittal CT reconstructions were used to determine if the posterior column had failed, namely by distraction injury to the facet joint.

The importance of the McAfee classification system must be considered in the temporal and technological context in which it was introduced. At that time, spinal instrumentation was limited to sublaminar wiring and the use of hook devices. Sublaminar wiring is effective in maintaining sagittal alignment, but it cannot be used to provide compression or distraction; nonsegmental hook constructs could be placed in either compression or distraction. Because it was recognized that some injuries could be worsened, displaced, or exaggerated with compression or distraction, this system was devised to differentiate between injuries caused primarily by distractive or compressive forces. Thus, the McAfee system classifies injuries based on treatment requirements. The development of modern multiple (claw) hook systems and pedicle screw constructs enables segmental fixation that does not rely on distractive or compressive forces for fixation. Although the McAfee classification system has played an important role in the understanding and treatment of thoracolumbar fractures, it is not all-inclusive. Furthermore, its prognostic value has not been assessed since its development, and interobserver and intraobserver reproducibility values have not been reported.

AO/Magerl Classification System

This comprehensive classification system for thoracolumbar spine fractures was developed with the support of the AO group and later modified.[10] The intent of the system was to be all-inclusive or at least more inclusive than previous systems. Injuries are divided into three general types: type A (compression injuries), type B (distraction injuries), and type C (torsion injuries). These types are divided into subgroups based on fracture morphology by

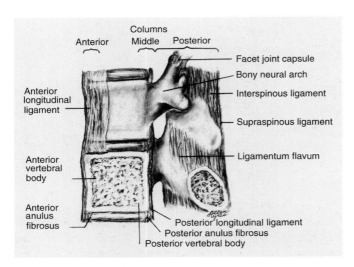

Figure 6 The anatomic structures comprising the three longitudinal columns of stability in the thoracolumbar spine: the anterior column (anterior two thirds of the vertebral body, anterior part of the anulus fibrosus, and anterior longitudinal ligament), middle column (posterior one third of the vertebral body, posterior part of the anulus fibrosus, and posterior longitudinal ligament), and posterior column (facet joint capsules, ligamentum flavum, osseous neural arch, supraspinous ligament, interspinous ligament, and articular processes). *(Adapted with permission from: McAfee P, Yuan H, Fredrickson BE, Lubicky JP: The value of computed tomography in thoracolumbar fractures: An analysis of one hundred consecutive cases and a new classification. J Bone Joint Surg Am 1983;65:461-473.)*

Suggested Injury Nomenclature

Acceptable terminology when referring to the most common injuries includes (1) compression fractures; (2) burst fractures; (3) bending injuries, such as flexion-distraction and Chance injuries; and (4) fracture-dislocations. By convention, compression fractures include those injuries with some degree of vertebral body height loss without involvement of the posterior vertebral body. Burst fractures contain fracture lines that extend through the posterior body without translation or dislocation. Pure dislocations at the thoracolumbar junction are rare and usually occur as a result of a flexion-distraction mecha-

distinguishing between primarily bone or ligamentous failure and identifying the direction of displacement (Figure 7). The AO/Magerl classification system was based on analysis of CT scans and plain radiographs of more than 1,400 consecutive injuries at five trauma centers. Although the AO/Magerl classification system is more inclusive than the McAfee classification system, it is much more complex. Its interobserver reliability has been found to be inversely proportional to its complexity. In a recent study, the mean interobserver agreement was 67% when participants were asked only to classify injuries as type A, B, or C.[11] For some injuries, the kappa statistic was as low as 0.33 (perfect is 1.0). As subgroups were added to the decision process, the interobserver reliability precipitously dropped. Interestingly, the authors found injury classification to be improved if MRI findings were used.

nism. The most classic example is a lap-belt injury in which the facet joints can be subluxated, perched, or jumped. Fracture-dislocations refer to those injuries with a translational component in addition to varying fracture patterns. Importantly, fracture-dislocations can exhibit posterior vertebral body fractures that, on CT scans alone, may appear to have a burst pattern. However, translation on plain radiographs or CT reconstructions helps distinguish the injury types.

Burst and Compression Fractures
Nonsurgical Management

Most thoracolumbar fractures can be treated nonsurgically.[12] The clinical challenge is to predict which fractures can be successfully and safely treated nonsurgically based on injury characteristics. Clear-cut treatment recommendations do not exist, partly because of inconsistent injury description that makes extrapolation of published data difficult.

Various forms of nonsurgical management can be used. Progressive mobilization and observation without an external support device may be used for some minor injuries. External orthotic devices can be used for more substantial fractures. Hyperextension braces (such as a Jewett device) are useful in counteracting sagittal flexion moments, but they offer minimal resistance to rotation or lateral flexion. Custom fit, clam-shell devices, such as a thoracolumbar sacral orthotic device, provide multiplanar support.

In rare circumstances, patients with mechanically unstable fractures are treated nonsurgically by extended bed rest and continued spinal precautions.[13] Some complications of prolonged recumbency, such as decubitus ulcers and pulmonary compromise, can be mitigated with the use of a specially designed bed that continuously oscillates from side to side (RotoRest, Kinetic Concepts, San Antonio, TX). Trapdoor devices allow the posterior skin and integument to be inspected without moving the patient. Chemical thromboprophylaxis should be considered in these patients, but should be delayed 4 to 5 days from injury to avoid epidural hematoma formation at the fracture site.

Compression fractures can be treated nonsurgically if the PLC is intact. Substantial anterior vertebral height loss (> 50%), interspinous process gapping, or more than 30° to 35° of kyphosis suggest a PLC disruption. In such patients, surgical treatment may be considered. MRI is often useful to evaluate posterior ligament injury. For patients with mild compression fractures with minimal height loss (< 10%), movement can be allowed as tolerated without an orthotic device. For patients with more substantial fractures, a Jewett hyperextension brace can be used for 6 to 8 weeks to maintain alignment until healing. Standing radiographs in the brace should be obtained to confirm adequate control (no progression

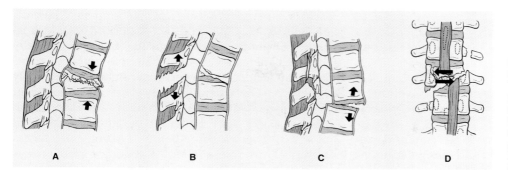

Figure 7 A, Type A fractures are compression injuries of the anterior column (vertebral body). Type B injuries have transverse anterior (**B**) or posterior (**C**) disruption. **D,** Type C fractures are rotational injuries. *(Adapted with permission from Magerl F, Aebi M: A comprehensive classification of thoracic and lumbar injuries, in Aebi M, Thalgott JS, Webb JK (eds): AO ASIF Principles in Spine Surgery. Berlin, Germany, Springer, 1998, p 22.)*

of kyphosis) of the fracture after initial fitting. Follow-up radiographs should be made at monthly intervals (at 1, 2, and 3 months, then 6 months and 1 year) until bony healing occurs.

Burst fractures are higher-energy injuries. Axial load applied to a flexed spine is thought to be the primary mechanism of injury; however, recent in vitro biomechanical evidence suggests that extension moments might also be important.[14] As with compression fractures, an intact PLC should be considered a prerequisite for nonsurgical care. Some studies report that canal compromise greater than 50% is an indication for surgical decompression and/or stabilization. However, scant data are available to support this indication in neurologically intact patients with an intact PLC. Kyphosis greater than 25° to 30° and/or anterior vertebral body height loss of greater than 50% are highly suggestive of posterior ligament injury. Although there are reports in the literature that recommend nonsurgical care for some patients with neurologic deficits, it is recommended that this be reserved for patients who are medically unfit to undergo surgery.

Nonsurgical treatment of burst fractures usually includes a custom-made, form-fitting thoracolumbosacral orthotic device or hyperextension cast. The patient should remain on log-roll precautions until the brace is applied. Before ambulation begins, weight-bearing radiographs with the patient in the brace should be obtained. The kyphotic angle and vertebral body height loss should be measured and compared with initial values. If kyphosis or vertebral body height loss increases, the integrity of the posterior ligaments should be more closely evaluated. In patients with stable injuries, the brace is worn at all times for 3 months. The purpose of the brace is to allow the fracture to heal with minimal additional vertebral body height loss. Follow-up radiographs should be obtained at regular intervals. Patients should be advised of the clinical signs of conus medullaris compression and cauda equina syndrome.

Outcomes

Compression Fractures
A recent review of the records of 85 patients who were treated nonsurgically (physiotherapy and/or braces) for

thoracolumbar wedge (compression) fractures with greater than 3-year follow-up reported a 69% incidence of nonspecific chronic low back pain of varying severity.[15] The degree of kyphosis correlated with pain intensity, but a critical value of kyphosis was not reported. Vertebral body height loss did not correlate with outcome. The use of either bracing or physiotherapy did not influence outcomes. Back pain was the main outcome measure.

Burst Fractures
One study documented results of nonsurgical treatment of stable thoracolumbar burst fractures in 42 patients without neurologic deficit who were followed for 11 to 55 years. Although average kyphosis was 26° in flexion and 17° in extension, kyphosis did not correlate with the degree of pain or function at final follow-up. No instance of neurologic deterioration was reported. Low pain scores (average of 3.5 on visual analog scale) were documented, and no patient used narcotics for pain control. Eighty-eight percent of patients returned to work and were able to resume their preinjury occupations.

Outcomes of another nonsurgically treated group of 38 patients with thoracolumbar burst fractures without neurologic deficit were retrospectively reviewed.[16] Patients with injuries with posterior arch fractures or dislocation or kyphosis greater than 35° were excluded from the study. All patients were permitted early ambulation. Only nine patients were treated in a brace. Average kyphosis increased from 20° to 24° over an average follow-up of 4 years. Thirty-two patients had no pain or mild pain, whereas four patients had moderate pain. Two patients had severe pain, both of whom underwent surgery more than 1 year after injury. There was no correlation between kyphosis or canal compromise and clinical outcome. Seventy-six percent of patients returned to preinjury occupations. Complications included transient hematuria and urinary retention in three and six patients, respectively.

Sixty consecutive neurologically intact patients with thoracolumbar burst fractures treated with an orthotic device were followed for an average of 42 months.[17] Initial and final kyphosis averaged 6° and 8°, respectively. Ninety-one percent had satisfactory functional outcomes and 83% reported slight or no pain and returned to preinjury activity levels. Three patients who developed urinary tract infections were successfully treated with antibiotics.

Another study reported the results of the nonsurgical treatment of 24 neurologically intact patients with burst fractures.[18] Treatment consisted of a thoracolumbosacral orthotic device, Jewett hyperextension brace, or a hyperextension cast and early ambulation. No patient developed a neurologic deficit. A statistically insignificant increase in kyphosis was observed.

Nonsurgical Management of Patients With Neurologic Deficit

Nonsurgical care is sometimes used to manage patients with neurologic compromise. This would be most commonly indicated in patients with a complete neurologic injury who are medically unfit to undergo surgery. One study reported that no patients with a thoracolumbar burst fracture associated with a complete injury (Frankel grade A) demonstrated neurologic recovery, regardless of whether surgical or nonsurgical treatment was used.[19] Other studies have reported comparable recovery rates in patients with neurologic deficits. In an early review of the results in 89 patients, neurologic recovery was documented in 35% and 38% of nonsurgically and surgically treated patients, respectively. The extraspinal benefits of surgical stabilization in patients with complete neurologic injury, such as improved patient mobilization, pulmonary toilet, and pain relief, although intuitive, should be considered on an individual patient basis.

Nonsurgical Versus Surgical Treatment

The results of surgical and nonsurgical treatment have been compared in select groups of patients with clearly defined thoracolumbar injuries. One classic study compared the results of surgical versus nonsurgical management of unstable thoracolumbar fractures in a group of neurologically intact patients.[20] Significantly longer hospital stays were noted in the nonsurgical group (mean, 80 days) versus the surgical group (mean, 30 days); mean duration of immobilization was also longer (67 days for the surgical group versus 18 days for the surgical group). The final degree of kyphosis was greater in the nonsurgical group, but the degree of deformity did not affect functional outcomes. No patient had neurologic deterioration, and there was no difference in pain scores or rates of return to work. From these data, the main benefit of surgical treatment appears to be earlier mobilization in patients with unstable fractures, but the potential risk for secondary neurologic compromise, despite the low incidence reported, remains a concern for most practitioners.

A more recent study prospectively compared outcomes of patients with thoracolumbar burst fractures without neurologic deficit who were treated with either posterior surgery or nonsurgical management.[21] Patients with injuries that involved the posterior arch, such as facet dislocations, were excluded. The nonsurgically managed patients (N = 47) received a course of treatment that included a hyperextension brace and early ambulation. The surgical group (N = 33) underwent short-segment pedicle screw fixation. Although mean outcome scores were better in the surgical group at 3 months, the mean 6-month and 2-year outcome scores were not statistically different. Kyphosis correction was also initially better in the surgical group, but this benefit was not demonstrable at final follow-up. Pain scores followed a similar pattern.

The results of a more recent prospective randomized controlled study comparing surgical and nonsurgical treatment of stable thoracolumbar burst fractures in patients without neurologic deficit have also been reported.[22] Patients with injuries with suspected or confirmed posterior ligamentous disruption were excluded. Nonsurgical care included a brace or cast followed by early mobilization. Surgical treatment was either anterior or posterior surgery. There were no statistical differences in degree of kyphosis, functional outcome, or pain scores between the two groups; however, surgically treated patients tended to have higher pain scores and more complications.

These results strongly suggest that nonsurgical management consisting of bracing and early mobilization is an effective treatment method for patients with thoracolumbar burst fractures without posterior ligamentous injury; however, these studies lack clear recommendations regarding how to determine the integrity of the PLC.

Surgical Treatment

Surgical treatment includes stabilization with or without decompression. Surgical goals are to restore and maintain spinal alignment and provide stability until solid bony fusion is achieved. In patients with neurologic deficit and canal compromise, decompression is targeted at maximizing the space available for the neural elements. Anterior and posterior procedures can be used for both stabilization and decompression.

Compression Fractures

In the rare instance that a compression fracture is associated with posterior ligament injury, posterior stabilization is the preferred method of treatment. The surgical goal is to correct kyphosis until solid fusion is achieved. Posterior pedicle screw or hook constructs can be used. Before surgical stabilization, the surgeon should be confident of the diagnosis. An anterior procedure is rarely indicated to stabilize a compression fracture.

Burst Fractures

Significant controversy exists regarding the indications and optimal method of surgical treatment of patients with thoracolumbar burst fractures. This is particularly true for patients without neurologic deficit. Posterior surgery alone has been advocated by some, whereas others advocate anterior or combined anterior and posterior surgery.[23] In patients with neurologic deficit (in particular those with incomplete deficits), it is generally agreed that a decompressive maneuver is warranted. Indirect reduction of displaced vertebral body fragments can be achieved through distraction and realignment with posterior instrumentation; however, this appears to be more effective if the PLL is intact and if surgery is performed early (within 2 to 4 days after injury). Direct fragment removal through an anterior approach offers better anatomic decompression, but the neurologic benefits of this technique have not been conclusively established. Techniques have also been developed to remove vertebral body fragments and perform interbody fusion through a posterior approach, but these procedures are not widely performed. Various anterior and posterior instrumentation options are available.

Suggested Surgical Indications

A progressive neurologic deficit is an indication for urgent decompression. Progressive kyphotic deformity is a result of mechanical instability, which warrants surgical stabilization. Injury characteristics that are highly suggestive of PLC disruption and therefore provide relative surgical indications are progressive kyphotic deformity, kyphosis greater than 25° to 30°, and (3) vertebral body height loss greater than 50%. Patients with neurologic deficit associated with at least 25% canal compromise can benefit from surgical decompression.

Posterior Surgery

Stabilization

Posterior surgery is used primarily to stabilize burst fractures in neurologically intact patients. Stabilization can be achieved using a variety of constructs. Compressive forces placed along posterior constructs can be corrective; however, it is not a recommended form of treatment in patients with posterior vertebral body comminution (burst fractures) because of the risk of causing intrusion of bony fragments into the canal. Pedicle screws are among the more popular methods of fixation. If reduction is desired, distraction can be applied. They enable short-segment fusion with a theoretic advantage of three-column stability over hook constructs. At a minimum, the level above and below the fracture should be included in the fusion (short-segment instrumentation); some studies have advocated using two levels above and below[24] (Figure 8). Short-segment instrumentation can result in rates of pedicle screw breakage or failure as high as 50%, which is thought to be the result of continued cyclic loading amplified by anterior column deficiency.[25] Transpedicular intracorporeal bone grafting was intro-

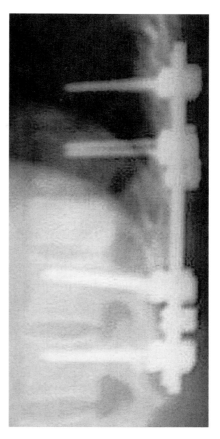

Figure 8 Radiograph showing long-segment posterior instrumentation. This type of instrumentation may be more effective in maintaining kyphotic correction when used to stabilize thoracolumbar burst fractures. Hardware failure is more likely with short-segment instrumentation.

duced in an attempt to reconstitute the vertebral body height, but this has not diminished the rate of hardware failure with short-segment pedicle screw stabilization.[25,26] Although a useful option, posterior stabilization using hooks and rods is used less frequently because it requires the inclusion of at least two to three segments above and below the injury. Sublaminar wire constructs are typically not used in the stabilization of unstable burst fractures.

Indirect Decompression

A number of posterior methods of decompressing the spinal canal have been advocated. Simple decompressive laminectomy has fallen out of favor because it causes further posterior destabilization and can lead to progressive kyphotic deformity. Indirect reduction, which relies on longitudinal distraction along the fractured segment, works through ligamentotaxis of the displaced posterior vertebral fragments. With distraction, an intact PLL and/or posterior anulus are thought to pull the fragments back into place. One study that used this technique in 22 patients with junctional (T11 to L2) burst fractures reported an average 28% improvement in canal compromise.[27] Although patients with an incomplete neurologic injury improved an average of 1.8 Frankel grades, the rate of neurologic recovery or injury could not be predicted based on the amount of canal clearance. A cadaveric study found that the posterior vertebral height, posterior vertebral body angle, and cross-diagonal angle showed significantly higher correlations with canal encroachment.[28] Interestingly, extension of the motion segment (a commonly performed maneuver used to reduce burst fractures) did not affect canal clearance.

Indirect reduction has not been uniformly endorsed, however, because disruption of the PLL appears to compromise its effectiveness. One study documented an average improvement in canal compromise of only 19% (from 57% preoperatively to 38% postoperatively) after posterior distractive instrumentation was performed in 30 patients.[29] Independent of canal clearance, incomplete (Frankel grades B through D) injuries improved one or more grades. Although the authors thought that disruption of the PLL was a contributing factor to the modest effects on canal clearance, the integrity of the PLL was not assessed with MRI. From these findings, it was inferred that more than 50% canal compromise might be indicative of PLL disruption and that decompression should be performed through an anterior approach in these patients.

A greater delay from injury to operation is thought to compromise the efficacy of indirect canal clearance. One study found that surgery performed within 1 week of injury resulted in an average 33% improvement in canal compromise. Surgery done 1 or 2 weeks after injury resulted in average 24% and 0% improvements, respectively.[30] As in other studies, all incomplete injuries improved by one or more Frankel grades regardless of canal clearance. Improved canal clearance has been reported in patients stabilized within 4 days (from 56% to 38%) compared with those stabilized more than 4 days after injury (from 52% to 44%).

Direct Canal Decompression Through a Posterior Approach

Methods of anterior canal decompression through an all-posterior approach have been developed. A posterolateral approach has been described that was used to reduce the displaced vertebral body segments to clear the spinal canal in 31 patients.[31] The technique included removal of the facet joint and/or pedicle to gain access to the posterior vertebral body. Statistically significant decreases in canal compromise were achieved, as measured by CT, with neurologic improvement reported in 96% of patients. Stabilization with a pedicle screw construct and fusion was used.

Concomitant Lamina Fracture

The combination of a lamina fracture and burst fracture can be associated with a dural tear (37% of patients) or entrapped nerve roots (13% of patients). Posterior lam-inectomy has been recommended for exploration and dural repair or freeing of nerve roots before any planned anterior procedure.[32,33]

Anterior Surgery

Anterior decompression is the most direct and effective method of clearing the spinal canal in patients with a burst fracture. Most of the injured vertebral body along with the suprajacent and infrajacent disks can be removed. Retropulsed fragments are carefully removed to relieve pressure on the spinal cord or cauda equina. The highest rates of neurologic recovery have been reported after anterior decompressive surgery for burst fractures in patients with incomplete neurologic injuries.[34] One report documented a median change of two Frankel grades in patients undergoing anterior decompression within 48 hours.[34]

As this maneuver destabilizes the spine, the vertebral body defect must be replaced with a supportive strut that will also allow bony fusion. Structural autograft (such as rib, fibula, iliac crest, or allograft struts) can be used. More recently, titanium mesh cages filled with harvested morcellized cancellous autograft iliac crest or salvaged bone from the corpectomy have become popular. Anterior column reconstruction (strut grafting) should be stabilized by anterior instrumentation, posterior instrumentation, or both. Numerous constructs can be used for anterior stabilization. In vitro biomechanical studies have compared various anterior devices.[35] Among the more rigid devices are plates with fixed-angle vertebral body screws and cross-linked rod-screw-staple designs, such as the Kaneda system. In general, anterior instrumentation and fusion leads to better maintenance of alignment than stand-alone posterior procedures.

In an early report, anterior surgery was performed in 35 patients with thoracolumbar burst fractures and neurologic injury.[36] Iliac crest autograft struts were used to reconstruct the anterior column. A modified anterior Harrington rod-screw system spanning from the vertebral bodies above and below the fractured segment was used. High rates of neurologic recovery were documented in patients with incomplete injuries, whereas patients with complete neurologic damage showed no improvement. Of 21 patients with incomplete loss of bowel or bladder function initially, 19 showed some improvement. Twelve of 13 patients who were treated early (within 10 days of injury) recovered useful bladder function. Five of 8 patients who were treated late (more than 10 days after injury) gained useful bladder function without incontinence. In another study, anterior plating techniques were used in conjunction with anterior decompression and strut grafting to treat a variety of thoracolumbar fractures and excellent maintenance of alignment and rates of neurologic recovery were reported.[37]

Another study reported the use of stand-alone instrumentation with a plate in 12 patients with thoracolumbar burst fractures.[38] In 10 patients, postoperative kyphosis correction was maintained at 1-year follow-up; the other two patients had 10° to 20° of correction loss. Both of these patients had preoperative kyphosis angles greater than 50°, suggesting that anterior fixation alone may not be sufficient to stabilize injuries with significant posterior ligamentous injury. However, this occurrence may have been related to the implant, which has demonstrated a high rate of fatigue failure as a stand-alone implant.

In the largest series to date, 150 consecutive patients with thoracolumbar burst fractures were treated with a single-stage anterior decompression, strut grafting, and instrumentation using the Kaneda rod-sleeve-staple device.[39] Canal clearance was nearly 100%. A 93% fusion rate was reported. Instances of pseudarthroses were successfully treated using posterior instrumentation and fusion. Ninety-five percent of patients (142) improved at least one Frankel grade.

Influence of Timing on Neurologic Outcomes

The timing of surgery may influence the rate of neurologic recovery. In a study of 22 patients with thoracolumbar burst fractures, anterior decompressive surgery performed within 48 hours of injury resulted in a mean improvement of two Frankel grades and complete resolution of bowel and bladder function in 44% of patients.[40] Surgery 48 hours after injury improved Frankel scoring by only one grade, with no patient recovering complete bowel or bladder function. Although this study was not randomized, these data offer some evidence that early anterior decompressive surgery may benefit neurologic outcome.

Delayed Decompression

For a variety of reasons, not all patients undergo early decompressive surgery. Residual canal stenosis can be present for long periods (weeks to years) in some patients. In consideration of this specific scenario, one study examined the effects of late decompression in patients with burst fractures. In 49 patients with conus medullaris or cauda equina level injuries, neurologic improvement (Frankel grade and bladder control) was statistically better when patients underwent decompression within 2 years after injury.[41] The overall rate of bladder improvement was 50% for patients with fractures at or below T12. These data suggest that substantial improvements in Frankel grade and bladder/bowel function can be expected even with long periods of neurologic compression after burst fracture.

Combined Anterior and Posterior Surgery

In some patients, combined anterior and posterior surgery can be performed. The specific indications and benefits of this maneuver remain unclear. Advantages include nearly complete canal clearance, immediate stability, and high fusion rates. However, the added morbidity of the combined procedures is a potential disadvantage. In a recent retrospective review, the results of combined anterior and posterior surgery were compared with those of posterior surgery alone for the treatment of patients with thoracolumbar burst fractures.[23] Although the method of treatment did not affect neurologic recovery, combined anterior and posterior surgery resulted in better maintenance of kyphosis correction. Interestingly, loss of correction was not associated with a higher rate of back pain. Combined anterior and posterior techniques have also been advocated to maximize canal decompression and overall construct stability, but PLC disruption is an important determining factor for combined surgery.

Anterior Versus Posterior Surgery

Few studies have compared anterior and posterior surgical methods. An early comparison of these methods with decompression was reported for patients with incomplete neurologic injury. Although not all of the 59 patients in the study had burst fractures, neurologic recovery was related to the adequacy of canal clearance. Motor, sensory, and bladder improvement was statistically better in the anterior than posterior surgery group. Posterior surgery included posterolateral decompression through a transpedicular approach and stabilization, whereas anterior surgery entailed a full corpectomy at that level of injury. Regarding bladder function specifically for patients with conus level lesions, 70% of patients in the anterior group improved, whereas only 12% in the posterior group showed improvement. The posterior group was treated an average of 6.4 days from injury, whereas no patient in the anterior group underwent surgical treatment within 30 days of injury. In contrast, motor recovery was not statistically affected by the choice of approach. More recently, the results in mechanically unstable thoracolumbar burst fractures without neurologic deficit have been analyzed.[42] Although anterior and posterior procedures resulted in equivalent clinical results, less blood loss and shorter surgery times were documented for posterior procedures.

Less Invasive Methods

Less invasive methods of surgically treating patients with thoracolumbar burst fractures have been developed; however, few reports evaluating these methods appear in the literature. One study used a thoracoscopic approach to perform corpectomy, anterior column reconstructions, and anterior instrumentation in this patient population.[43] Although low, incidences of vascular injury and neurologic deterioration were noted that were higher than those for open surgery. The efficacy and advantages of the thoracoscopic approach to treating spinal fractures remains to be demonstrated, not only because of the steep learning curve for performing such procedures, but also because of the increasing number of reports of equivalent results achieved using nonsurgical treatment.

Neurologic Outcomes and Canal Compromise

The relationship between canal compromise (as measured using CT) and neurologic injury has been extensively investigated. Deficit severity does not appear to be predictable based on the amount of residual canal stenosis but is probably more influenced by the instantaneous canal compromise that occurs at the time of neurologic impact, which is substantially more than what is detectable on initial imaging. Furthermore, there is no consensus of optimal method of measurement of canal compromise.

One group studied canal remodeling in 115 patients treated with posterior distraction instrumentation (two levels above and below injured vertebra) by measuring the midsagittal diameter and the cross-sectional area of the spinal canal.[44] They found a mean canal clearance ranging from 49% to 72% of normal immediately postoperatively. At final follow-up, the mean canal measurements were 87% of normal. Importantly, canals with greater amounts of initial compromise demonstrated greater amounts of clearance. These findings strongly suggest that direct decompression (anterior or posterior) may not be necessary in neurologically intact patients with varying degrees of canal compromise. Canal clearance was not statistically different between patients who underwent surgery early (within 3 days of injury) or late (more than 3 days after injury). Another study retrospectively reviewed the CT scans and plain radiographs of 83 patients with thoracolumbar burst fractures that were treated surgically or nonsurgically with at least a 12-month follow-up.[45] They found that the spinal canal underwent substantial remodeling, regardless of the type of treatment. None of the patients worsened neurologically during the follow-up period. The authors concluded that, in neurologically intact patients, the spinal canal can undergo natural resorption and clearance.

In one review, the amount of canal compromise was greater in patients with neurologic deficit (mean, 52%) than in those who were neurologically intact (35%).[46] However, the average amount of canal clearance was not significantly different for those who demonstrated neurologic recovery (20%) and those who did not (23%). A more important predictor of neurologic deficit was the presence of posterior ligamentous disruption (61% versus 25% for patients with and without neurologic deficit, respectively). Unfortunately, the study did not specify the method used to determine the integrity of the PLC. In an analysis of various radiologic canal measurements in patients with burst fractures and neurologic deficit, the only measurement that correlated statistically with neurologic status was the sagittal-to-transverse ratio.[47] The absolute cross-sectional area, sagittal canal diameter, and

transverse diameter by themselves were not correlative. Another group found that 25%, 50%, and 75% canal compromise corresponded to a 0.29, 0.51, and 0.71 predictive value, respectively, for the presence (but not severity) of a neurologic deficit.[48] In a similar study, 45% canal compromise and posterior column injury was predictive of the presence of neurologic injury at the L1 level.[49] Again, the severity of deficit could not be correlated. By measuring the cross-sectional area of the canal, one study found that 1.0 cm^2 was the critical level below which all patients had some degree of neurologic deficit, whereas patients with a canal area of 1.0 cm^2 to 1.25 cm^2 had no or incomplete neurologic injuries.[50]

Bending Injuries: Flexion-Distraction and Chance Injuries

In contrast to dislocations of the cervical spine, pure dislocations at the thoracolumbar region are rare. The most common mechanism of injury is thought to be flexion-distraction forces, which is often associated with patients wearing lap seat belts. Improperly worn, high-riding lap seat belts can concentrate high-energy forces along an apex that is anterior to the thoracolumbar junction during head-on collisions. This potentiates distractive forces along the entire vertebral segment. This is distinguished mechanistically from flexion-compression injuries in which the axis of flexion is about the spinal canal, resulting in anterior compressive and posterior tensile forces.

Flexion-distraction injuries can have varying fracture patterns of the vertebral body and posterior elements. By convention, they are distinguished from fracture-dislocations by the absence of translation, although these injuries are often confused. Flexion-distraction injuries can be purely ligamentous, osseoligamentous, or purely osseous. Fractures are typically transverse. In some patients, a fracture line can be noted from the tip of the spinous process, through the laminae, and exiting the midanterior aspect of the vertebral body. In pure ligamentous injuries, the facet joints can be subluxated or in some patients frankly dislocated (perched or locked).

Almost two thirds of patients with thoracolumbar flexion-distraction injuries have a neurologic deficit, presumably from distraction of the neural elements. A perforated viscus is a commonly associated nonspinal injury that is thought to be secondary to sudden increases of pressure within the intestines from abdominal compression. In some patients, the abdominal injury is discovered first, and the spine injury can be missed. An ecchymotic region along the abdomen is suggestive of this injury pattern.

Nonsurgical treatment is infrequently used to treat thoracolumbar flexion-distraction dislocations. In patients with purely bony flexion-distraction injuries, hyperextension casting or bracing may be an option. This

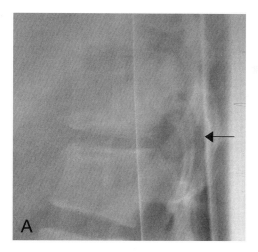
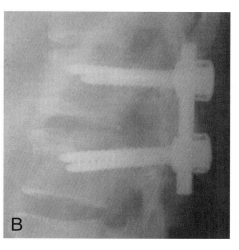
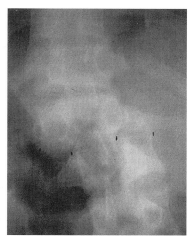

Figure 9 Preoperative **(A)** and postoperative **(B)** radiographs showing a flexion-distraction injury of the thoracolumbar junction. Although mild compression of the vertebral body was noted, the more significant finding is the perched facets (*black arrow*).

Figure 10 Radiograph showing a thoracolumbar fracture-dislocation. This type of injury can have various bony fracture patterns and are distinguished from other injuries by the presence of translational deformity, a sign of high-energy trauma. The black points mark the lateral borders of the dislocated end plates.

should be continued until bony union is radiographically and clinically confirmed, usually at approximately 3 to 4 months. Most other flexion-distraction injuries should be treated surgically. Because the spine flexes about an anterior axis of rotation, the anterior longitudinal ligament is usually intact and there is little, if any, vertebral body comminution. In most patients, anterior surgery (which necessitates resection of the anterior longitudinal ligament) will further destabilize the spine. Therefore, posterior compressive instrumentation and fusion is the most common treatment. Because the intervertebral disk can be ruptured in patients with severe injuries, care must be taken not to overcompress the construct, which can cause loose disk fragments to be expelled into the spinal canal. Short-segment pedicle screw or hook constructs are effective means of stabilizing these injuries (Figure 9).

In 15% of patients, a burst fracture configuration occurs in conjunction with a flexion-distraction mechanism.[51] Intervertebral disk herniations can occur in approximately 5% of patients and may also warrant anterior diskectomy for decompression.

Studies of flexion-distraction injuries in the thoracolumbar spine are relatively sparse, but most suggest that patients typically have good outcomes with regard to pain resolution. One study evaluated 17 patients with flexion-distraction injuries of the thoracolumbar spine, 82% of whom were treated nonsurgically.[52] Approximately 80% of these patients had mild or no pain at follow-up, but only 65% were able to return to preinjury activities. The patients with significant alterations of their activity choices had multiple concomitant injuries in addition to spinal trauma.

Another study advocated the use of nonsurgical treatment if specific radiographic criteria were met.[53] In this series, 85% of patients with less than 15° of initial kyphosis and no neurologic deficit healed well after ex-

tension casting. Patients with greater than 15° of kyphosis, neurologic deficits, or purely ligamentous injuries underwent surgical treatment. Twelve of 13 patients had good results at 1 year.

Another study reviewed a series of thoracolumbar flexion-distraction injuries that were treated surgically with short-segment (single-level) fusions. Fourteen of 16 patients (87%) had little or no pain at follow-up.[54] A more recent study reviewed the surgical treatment of 23 patients with flexion-distraction injuries of the thoracolumbar spine. Short-segment posterior pedicle screw instrumentation was used, and the patients used a thoracolumbosacral orthosis for 3 months postoperatively. Final average kyphosis improved from 9.5° to 5.4°, and pain was absent or mild for all but two patients.

Fracture-Dislocations

Thoracolumbar fracture-dislocations are typically high-energy injuries with an associated high rate of complete neurologic deficit.[55,56] In patients with complete neurologic deficits, surgery is indicated to stabilize the spine, which can facilitate patient transfers, mobilization, and pulmonary care. Injuries can occur from a variety of mechanisms, including flexion, shear, and extension forces[56] (Figure 10). Fractures can be realigned through postural reduction in the prone position in the operating room. In some patients, misalignment must be reduced using an open procedure and direct manipulation. In patients who are neurologically intact or incompletely injured, this must be performed carefully so as not to cause additional neurologic injury.

In most patients, posterior instrumentation and fusion are sufficient for fracture-dislocations.[55,56] In patients with extensive vertebral body comminution, compression, or fragments displaced into the spinal canal, a combined anterior and posterior approach might be used; however, anterior stand-alone procedures should be avoided. A recent report demonstrated excellent maintenance of alignment in 15 patients who were stabilized using short-segment pedicle screw instrumentation.[55]

Complications

Surgical timing is an important consideration, especially when dealing with patients with multiple trauma or those with incomplete neurologic deficits. In a retrospective chart review of patients with spinal fractures (including cervical, thoracic, and lumbar injuries), those with injuries that underwent fixation within 3 days of injury had a lower rate of pneumonia and shorter hospital stays than those that underwent fixation more than 3 days after injury.[57] Although these two groups were not randomized and the late fixation group could have included patients that were more severely injured, the Injury Severity Scale scores were not statistically significantly different. Moreover, the average age, Glasgow Coma Scale score on admission, and chest injury score were significantly higher in the late fixation group.

In a prospective study of 75 consecutive polytrauma patients with spine fractures, anterior surgery performed within 24 hours (urgent group) of injury was associated with significantly greater blood loss than when performed between 24 and 72 hours (early group).[58] In contrast, patients who underwent posterior surgery exhibited comparable blood loss regardless of the timing of the surgery. There were no reports of thromboembolism, neurologic deterioration, pressure sores, deep wound infections, or systemic sepsis in either the early or urgent group.

Another study reported a 10% incidence of wound infections after surgery for patients with thoracolumbar fractures.[59] Although this retrospective study did not include a control group, the authors believed that this rate was higher than that reported in the literature for patients who undergo elective thoracolumbar procedures. A complete neurologic deficit was a statistically significance risk factor for infection. Other possible risk factors, such as concomitant distant site infections or potential bacteremic sources such as open fractures, were not included in the analysis.

Summary

Although the optimal treatment of thoracolumbar fractures remains unclear, several treatment principles can be recommended after an in-depth review of the literature. Fracture stability remains difficult to definitively determine; however, the value of MRI in evaluating the integrity of the PLC appears to be increasing. In patients who are neurologically intact and have an intact PLC,

nonsurgical treatment will likely be successful. Ligamentous instability, with or without neurologic deficit, is likely better treated with surgical stabilization. The most effective means of canal decompression for patients with burst fractures is via an anterior approach; however, the superiority of this approach in maximizing neurologic recovery remains to be proved.

Annotated References

1. Robertson A, Branfoot T, Barlow IF, et al: Spinal injury patterns resulting from car and motorcycle accidents. *Spine* 2002;27:2825-2830.

   This retrospective study of 22,858 patients (including 1,121 motorcyclists and 2,718 car occupants) was conducted to determine spinal injury patterns and clinical outcomes in patients involved in automotive accidents. The authors found that spinal injury occurred in 126 motorcyclists (11.2%) and 383 car occupants (14.1%). Mean Injury Severity Scores were 18.8 and 15.1, respectively. Isolated spinal injuries occurred in 30 motorcyclists (23.8%) and 130 car occupants (33.9%). The thoracic spine was most commonly injured in motorcyclists (54.8%), and the cervical spine was most commonly injured in car occupants (50.7%). Overall, motorcyclists were more severely injured, had more extremity trauma, a higher mortality rate, and a spinal injury pattern consistent with forced hyperflexion of the thoracic spine, which led the authors to conclude that the predominance of cervical injuries and higher incidence of neck and facial injuries in car occupants may reflect abdominothoracic seat belt restraint and that the high frequency of multilevel injuries reaffirms the need for vigilance in patient assessment.

2. Belmont PJ, Taylor KF, Mason KT, et al: Incidence, epidemiology, and occupational outcomes of thoracolumbar fractures among U.S. Army Aviators. *J Trauma* 2001;50:855-861.

3. Vaccaro AR, An HS, Lin S, et al: Noncontiguous injuries of the spine. *J Spinal Disord* 1992;5:320-329.

4. Frank E, Bonsell S: The accuracy of anterior-posterior measurements in the assessment of spinal canal compromise in burst fractures. *Neurol Res* 1994;16:410-412.

5. Brightman R, Miller C, Rea G, et al: Magnetic resonance imaging of trauma to the thoracic and lumbar spine. The importance of the posterior longitudinal ligament. *Spine* 1992;17:541-550.

6. Oner FC, van Gils APG, Faber JAJ, et al: Some complications of common treatment schemes of thoracolumbar spine fractures can be predicted with magnetic resonance imaging. *Spine* 2002;27:629-636.

   This prospective cohort study was conducted to assess the predictive value of MRI findings for patients with thoracolumbar spine fractures. Fifty-three patients with 71 fractures were assessed with MRI in a prospective fashion. Twenty-four patients with 39 fractures were treated nonsurgically and 29 patients with 32 fractures were treated surgically according to an established treatment protocol. MRI scans were obtained within 1 week of injury and at 2-year follow-up. Pain scores were obtained at the 2-year follow-up. The authors found that an overall unfavorable outcome in the nonsurgically treated group was related to the progression of kyphosis, which in most patients was predictable with the use of MRI. In the surgically treated group, recurrence of the kyphotic deformity was predictable by the lesion of the PLL complex and evidence of end-plate comminution and vertebral body involvement on MRI scans. They recommend using MRI to develop reliable prognostic criteria for patients with these injuries.

7. Mirza SK, Mirza AJ, Chapman JR, et al: Classifications of thoracic and lumbar fractures: Rationale and supporting data. *J Am Acad Orthop Surg* 2002;10: 364-377.

   This article provides a basic overview of the most commonly used classification systems for thoracolumbar spine fractures. The rationale, key components, and advantages and disadvantages of each classification system are discussed.

8. Magerl F, Aebi M, Gertzbein S, Harms J, Nazarian S: A comprehensive classification of thoracic and lumbar injuries. *Eur Spine J* 1994;3:184-201.

9. McAfee P, Yuan H, Fredrickson BE, et al: The value of computed tomography in thoracolumbar fractures: An analysis of one hundred consecutive cases and a new classification. *J Bone Joint Surg Am* 1983; 65:461-473.

10. Gertzbein S, Crowe P, Fazl M, et al: Canal clearance in burst fractures using the AO internal fixator. *Spine* 1992;17:558-560.

11. Oner FC, Ramos LM, Simmermacher RK, et al: Classification of thoracic and lumbar spine fractures: Problems of reproducibility. A study of 53 patients using CT and MRI. *Eur Spine J* 2002;11:235-245.

12. Weinstein JN, Collalto P, Lehmann TR: Thoracolumbar "burst" fractures treated conservatively: a long-term follow-up. *Spine* 1988;13:33-38.

13. Burke DC, Murray DD: The management of thoracic and thoracolumbar injuries of the spine with neurological involvement. *J Bone Joint Surg Br* 1976; 58:72-78.

14. Langrana NA, Harten RD, Lin DC, et al: Acute thoracolumbar burst fractures: A new view of loading mechanisms. *Spine* 2002;27:498-508.

15. Folman Y, Gepstein R: Late outcome of nonoperative management of thoracolumbar vertebral wedge fractures. *J Orthop Trauma* 2003;17:190-192.

16. Shen WJ, Shen YS: Nonsurgical treatment of three-column thoracolumbar junction burst fractures without neurologic deficit. *Spine* 1999;24:412-415.

17. Aligizakis A, Katonis P, Stergiopoulos K, et al: Functional outcome of burst fractures of the thoracolumbar spine managed non-operatively with early ambulation, evaluated using the load sharing classification. *Acta Orthop Belg* 2002;68:279-287.

18. Chow GH, Nelson BJ, Beghard JS, et al: Functional outcome of thoracolumbar burst fractures managed with hyperextension casting or bracing and early mobilization. *Spine* 1996;21:2170-2175.

19. Dendrinos GK, Halikias JG, Krallis PN, Asimakopoulos A: Factors influencing neurological recovery in burst thoracolumbar fractures. *Acta Orthop Belg* 1995;61:226-234.

20. Willen J, Lindahl S, Nordwall A: Unstable thoracolumbar fractures: A comparative clinical study of conservative treatment and Harrington instrumentation. *Spine* 1985;10:111-122.

21. Shen WJ, Liu TJ, Shen YS: Nonoperative treatment versus posterior fixation for thoracolumbar junction burst fractures without neurologic deficit. *Spine* 2001;26:1038-1045.

   In this prospective nonrandomized study, the authors reported that outcome scores were better in the surgical group at 3 months, but the 6-month and 2-year scores were not statistically different. Kyphosis correction was initially better in the surgical group, but not at final follow-up. Pain scores followed a similar pattern.

22. Wood K, Butterman G, Mehbod A, et al: Operative compared with nonoperative treatment of a thoracolumbar burst fracture without neurological deficit. *J Bone Joint Surg Am* 2003;85-A:773-781.

   In this randomized prospective study of neurologically intact patients with stable burst fractures, the authors reported no statistical differences in kyphosis, functional outcome, or pain scores between those patients who underwent surgical or nonsurgical treatment. Patients who were treated surgically tended to have higher pain scores and more complications.

23. Been HD, Bouma GJ: Comparison of two types of surgery for thoraco-lumbar burst fractures: Combined anterior and posterior stabilisation vs posterior instrumentation only. *Acta Neurochir (Wien)* 1999;141:349-357.

24. Akbarnia BA, Crandall DG, Burkus K, et al: Use of long rods and a short arthrodesis for burst fractures of the thoracolumbar spine: A long-term follow-up study. *J Bone Joint Surg Am* 1994;76:1629-1635.

25. Alanay A, Acaroglu E, Yazici M, et al: Short-segment pedicle instrumentation of thoracolumbar burst fractures: Does transpedicular intracorporeal grafting prevent early failure. *Spine* 2001;26:213-217.
    In this prospective randomized study of 20 patients, kyphosis progression and the incidence of screw failure was reported to be similar for fractures treated with and without transpedicular bone grafting (50% and 40%, respectively).

26. Knop C, Fabian HF, Bastian L, et al: Late results of thoracolumbar fractures after posterior instrumentation and transpedicular bone grafting. *Spine* 2001;26: 88-99.

27. Starr J, Hanley E: Junctional burst fractures. *Spine* 1992;17:551-557.

28. Isomi T, Panjabi MM, Kato Y, et al: Radiographic parameters for evaluating the neurological spaces in experimental thoracolumbar burst fractures. *J Spinal Disord* 2000;13:404-411.

29. Katonis P, Kontakis G, Loupasis G, et al: Treatment of unstable thoracolumbar and lumbar spine injuries using Cotrel-Dubousset instrumentation. *Spine* 1999; 24:2352-2357.

30. Scheffer MM, Currier BL: Thoracolumbar burst fractures, in Levine AM, Eismont FJ, Garfin SR, et al (eds): *Spine Trauma*. Philadelphia, PA, WB Saunders, 1998, pp 428-451.

31. Silvestro C, Francaviglia N, Bragazzi R, et al: Near-anatomical reduction and stabilization of burst fractures of the lower thoracic or lumbar spine. *Acta Neurochir (Wien)* 1992;116:53-59.

32. Cammisa FP Jr, Eismont FJ, Green BA: Dural laceration occurring with burst fractures and associated laminar fractures. *J Bone Joint Surg Am* 1989;71: 1044-1052.

33. Denis F, Burkus J: Diagnosis and treatment of cauda equina entrapment in the vertical lamina fractures of lumbar burst fractures. *Spine* 1991;16:S433-S439.

34. Kostuik J: Anterior fixation for fractures of the thoracic and lumbar spine with or without neurologic involvement. *Clin Orthop* 1984;189:103-115.

35. Brodke DS, Gollogly S, Bachus KN, et al: Anterior thoracolumbar instrumentation: Stiffness and load sharing characteristics of plate and rod systems. *Spine* 2003;28:1794-1801.

36. Esses SI, Botsford DJ, Kostuik JP: Evaluation of surgical treatment for burst fractures. *Spine* 1990;15: 667-673.

37. Haas N, Blauth M, Tscherne H: Anterior plating in thoracolumbar spine injuries: Indication, technique, and results. *Spine* 1991;16:S100-S111.

38. Ghanayem AJ, Zdeblick TA: Anterior instrumentation in the management of thoracolumbar burst fractures. *Clin Orthop* 1997;335:89-100.

39. Kaneda K, Taneichi H, Abumi K, et al: Anterior decompression and stabilization with the Kaneda device for thoracolumbar burst fractures associated with neurological deficits. *J Bone Joint Surg Am* 1997;79:69-73.

40. Clohisy J, Akbarnia B, Bucholz R, et al: Neurologic recovery associated with anterior decompression of spine fractures at the thoracolumbar junction (T12-L1). *Spine* 1992;17:S325-S330.

41. Transfeldt E, White D, Bradford D, et al: Delayed anterior decompression inpatients with spinal cord and cauda equina injuries of the thoracolumbar spine. *Spine* 1990;15:953-957.

42. Stancic MF, Gregorovic E, Nozica E, et al: Anterior decompression and fixation versus posterior reposition and semirigid fixation in the treatment of unstable burst thoracolumbar fracture: Prospective clinical trial. *Croat Med J* 2001;42:49-53.

43. Khoo LT, Beisse R, Potulski M: Thoracoscopic-assisted treatment of thoracic and lumbar fractures: A series of 371 consecutive cases. *Neurosurgery* 2002;51(suppl 5):S104-S117.

44. Wessberg P, Wang Y, Irstam L, et al: The effect of surgery and remodelling on spinal canal measurements after thoracolumbar burst fractures. *Eur Spine J* 2001;10:55-63.

45. Dai LY: Remodeling of the spinal canal after thoracolumbar burst fractures. *Clin Orthop* 2001;382:119-123.

46. Kim NH, Lee HM, Chun IM: Neurologic injury and recovery in patients with burst fracture of the thoracolumbar spine. *Spine* 1999;24:290-294.

47. Vaccaro AR: Combined anterior and posterior surgery for fractures of the thoracolumbar spine. *Instr Course Lect* 1999;48:443-449.

48. Fontijne WP, de Klerk LW, Braakman R, et al: CT scan prediction of neurological deficit in thoracolumbar burst fractures. *J Bone Joint Surg Br* 1992;74:683-685.

49. Hashimoto T, Kaneda K, Abumi K: Relationship between traumatic spinal canal stenosis and neurological deficits in thoracolumbar burst fractures. *Spine* 1988;13:1268-1272.

50. Rasmussen P, Rabin M, Mann D, et al: Reduced transverse spinal area secondary to burst fractures: Is there a relationship to neurologic injury? *J Neurotrauma* 1994;11:711-720.

51. Eismont FJ: Flexion-distraction injuries of the thoracic and lumbar spine, in Levine AM, Eismont FJ, Garfin SR, et al (eds): *Spine Trauma*. Philadelphia, PA, WB Saunders, 1998, pp 402-413.

52. LeGay D, Petrie D, Alexander D: Flexion-distraction injuries of the lumbar spine and associated abdominal trauma. *J Trauma* 1990;30:436-444.

53. Anderson PA, Henley MB, Rivara FP, et al: Flexion-distraction and chance injuries to the thoracolumbar spine. *J Orthop Trauma* 1991;5:153-160.

54. Triantafyllou S, Gertzbein S: Flexion-distraction injuries of the thoracolumbar spine: A review. *Orthopedics* 1992;15:357-364.

55. Razak M, Mahmud MM, Hyzan MY, et al: Short segment posterior instrumentation, reduction and fusion of unstable thoracolumbar burst fractures: A review of 26 cases. *Med J Malaysia* 2000;55:9-13.

56. Denis F, Burkus J: Shear fracture-dislocation of the thoracic and lumbar spine associated with forceful hyperextension (lumberjack paraplegia). *Spine* 1992; 17:156-161.

57. Croce MA, Bee TK, Pritchard E, et al: Does optimal timing for spine fracture fixation exist. *Ann Surg* 2001;233:851-858.

58. McLain RF, Benson DR: Urgent surgical stabilization of spinal fractures in polytrauma patients. *Spine* 1999;24:1646-1654.

59. Rechtine GR, Cahill D, Chrin AM: Treatment of thoracolumbar trauma: Comparison of complications of operative versus nonoperative treatment. *J Spinal Disord* 1999;12:406-409.

Chapter 29

Lumbosacral Trauma

Carlo Bellabarba, MD

Timothy P. McHenry, MD

Introduction

The structural integrity of the sacrum is crucial for maintaining pelvic and spinal column alignment as well as protecting lumbosacral neurologic function. Injuries to the sacrum may result in pain, deformity, and significant loss of lower extremity, bowel, bladder, and sexual function. Consequently, treatment of these injuries needs to optimize both structural and neurologic outcome and requires a thorough understanding of both nerve decompression and skeletal reconstruction. Comprehensive knowledge of the relationship of the sacrum to pelvic neurovascular and visceral structures is also necessary. The severity of sacral fractures varies widely from insufficiency fractures in osteopenic patients to complex fracture patterns caused by high-energy injury mechanisms such as motor vehicle collisions or falls from heights. The management of a specific sacral fracture must be tailored to the particular injury pattern.

Patient Evaluation

The evaluation of patients with sacral fractures must evolve through various phases, all of which have their particular emphasis.

Initial Evaluation

The forces required to cause a fracture of the sacrum are usually of such magnitude that emergent resuscitation becomes the top priority. The initial evaluation of patients with sacral fractures, which is essentially the same as those with pelvic fractures, requires a team approach (see chapter 21). Initial resuscitation follows Advanced Trauma Life Support guidelines to address immediate life-threatening conditions and maintain cardiopulmonary and hemodynamic stability. Patients with associated anterior-posterior compression pelvic ring injuries may benefit from the application of a circumferential pelvic antishock sheet or anterior external fixator in the resuscitative phase to reduce pelvic volume and provide provisional pelvic stability.

Early determination of neurologic status is of paramount importance in patients with sacral fractures. This includes a careful evaluation of sacral root function because most patients with transverse sacral fracture components will have cauda equina deficits. In fact, the presence of sacral root deficits is frequently central to the clinical diagnosis of transverse sacral fractures, which are more commonly missed in neurologically intact patients. The fact that sacral root injuries are less clinically obvious than more rostral neurologic injuries mandates a thorough examination of the perirectal region. Perianal sensation, anal sphincter tone, voluntary perianal contraction (when possible), and the integrity of the bulbocavernosus reflex arc should be evaluated. In the unresponsive patient, perineal somatosensory-evoked potentials and anal sphincter electromyography may provide important evidence suggesting the presence of sacral plexus injury. Rectal and vaginal examination also allow for detection of unrecognized open sacral fractures. The identification of either cauda equina deficits or an open fracture is important in determining injury prognosis and the potential urgency of surgical intervention.

Radiographic Evaluation

Because of the sagittal inclination of the sacrum and the juxtaposition of the iliac wings, sacral fractures can be difficult to visualize on plain radiographs. This is particularly true of injuries without obvious pelvic asymmetry in which sacral fractures and transverse components in particular are often overlooked. However, these injuries are detectable on careful scrutiny of AP pelvic radiographs.[1,2] Abnormalities in the contour of the sacral foramina and sacral arcuate line and the presence of a "paradoxical inlet" view of the sacrum on the AP pelvic view (Figure 1) strongly indicate the presence of a sacral fracture with kyphotic deformity. The increasing use of sophisticated imaging techniques such as CT for the routine initial assessment of patients with abdominal and pelvic trauma has facilitated the detection of previously unrecognized sacral fractures. The detection of a sacral fracture merits a full radiographic evaluation of the pelvis. Additional pelvic views include inlet and outlet views, and a dedicated CT scan should be obtained. A

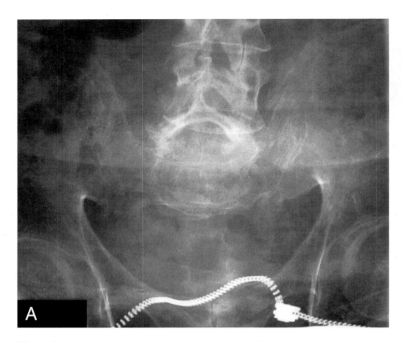
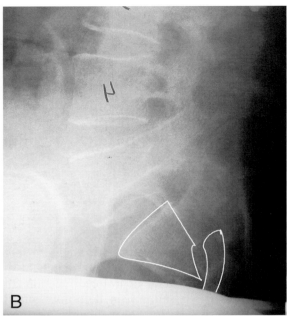

Figure 1 Paradoxical inlet view of the sacrum. AP radiograph **(A)** of the pelvis demonstrates a paradoxical inlet appearance of the sacrum caused by flexion deformity of the upper sacrum, which is evident on the lateral sacral radiograph **(B)** in a patient with a Roy-Camille type 2 Denis zone III sacral U fracture.

dedicated fine-cut CT scan of the sacrum with two-dimensional sagittal and coronal reformations is recommended to provide detailed information on the fracture configuration, resulting instability pattern, and extent of sacral canal and neuroforaminal compromise[3] (Figure 2).

Fracture Classification

Depending on its location and configuration, a sacral fracture can impair stability of the pelvic ring, lumbosacral junction, or the sacrum alone. Sacral fractures have been classified according to their potential for associated sacral root injury[4,5] (Figure 3). The most common fractures involve the sacral ala exclusively and are classified as zone I injuries, with a 5.9% rate of neurologic injury, mainly to the L5 root. Zone II injuries, which involve the neuroforamina but do not extend medially into the sacral canal, have a 28% incidence of neurologic injury. Any fracture extending into the sacral canal is defined as a zone III injury. Although much less common, zone III injuries have the highest rate of neurologic injury (57%), which consists mainly of cauda equina syndrome (76%). Although the implications of zone I injuries pertain mainly to posterior pelvic ring stability, some zone II fractures and many zone III injuries may affect both posterior pelvic ring and lumbosacral stability.

Zone II sacral fractures can be subclassified according to their effect on lumbosacral stability. As per the classification system proposed by Isler in 1990 (Figure 4), the lumbosacral junction is stable in Isler type 1 injuries because the longitudinal sacral fracture extends lateral to the L5-S1 facet joint and the lumbosacral articulation

therefore remains within the stable component of the sacrum.[6] Once the longitudinal fracture extends into (Isler type 2) or medial to (Isler type 3) the L5-S1 facet joint, the joint either becomes associated with the unstable sacral fragment or (with comminution) is completely dissociated from the sacrum, and the possibility of lumbosacral instability ensues. This unstable pattern was noted in almost 40% of unstable vertical sacral fractures.[6,7]

Because zone III injuries constitute a wide array of potential injury types with various possible fracture configurations and displacement patterns,[8] a subjective or descriptive classification system can aid in conceptualizing and verbally describing multiplanar sacral injuries (Figure 5). Most injuries in which a transverse fracture of the sacrum is identified have associated longitudinal or vertical injury components, usually in the form of bilateral transforaminal fractures that extend rostrally to the lumbosacral junction to produce the so-called sacral U fracture.[3,9] Variations from the classic longitudinal fracture pattern result in H-, Y-, and lambda-type fracture variants, among others, in which the central upper sacral segment (to which the remainder of the spine is attached) is dissociated from the pelvis and peripheral sacrum and results in spinopelvic dissociation (Figure 6).

To account for the broad range in severity and direction of displacement in zone III sacral fractures, those with transverse components have been further subclassified according to presumed injury mechanism. Four fracture types that are characterized by the extent of angulation, displacement, and comminution have been

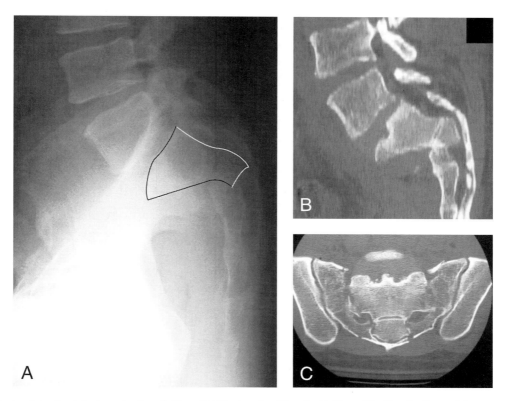

Figure 2 Sacral U fracture-dislocation. Lateral sacral radiograph **(A)**, sagittal CT reformation **(B)**, and axial CT scan **(C)** of Roy-Camille type 2 Denis zone III sacral U fracture.

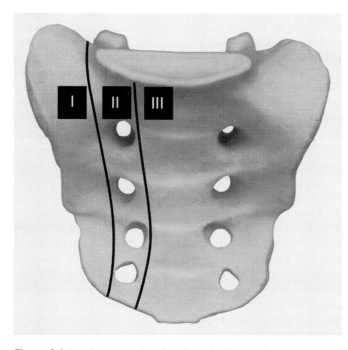

Figure 3 Schematic representation of the Denis classification of sacral fractures.

injuries had no associated sagittal plane translation, type 2 injuries resulted in posterior translation of the upper fracture fragment relative to the lower fragment. Type 3 injuries are likely associated with an extension moment and have complete anterocaudal translation of the upper sacrum relative to the lower fracture fragment. Type 4 injuries are segmentally comminuted fractures of the sacrum without significant translation or angulation and are thought to be caused by direct axial loading of the neutrally positioned spine.

Injury Biomechanics

The normal continuity of load transmission from the lumbosacral spine to the lower extremities is therefore disrupted after injury, a situation that is not relieved by the sitting position. Therefore, physiologic loads on the sacrum cannot be alleviated by restricted weight bearing without recumbency. The tendency is for the spine and upper sacral segment to displace anterocaudally, with associated sagittal plane rotation resulting in shortening and sacral kyphosis.

Neurologic Injury

Injury to sacral nerves may be caused by a variety of mechanisms and manifest as monoradiculopathies, multiple but unilateral radiculopathies, and, with bilateral sacral root involvement, incomplete and complete cauda

described[10,11] (Figure 7). Although all were thought to result from an axial load, type 1 and type 2 injuries were caused by a flexion moment that resulted in kyphotic angulation at the transverse fracture site. Whereas type 1

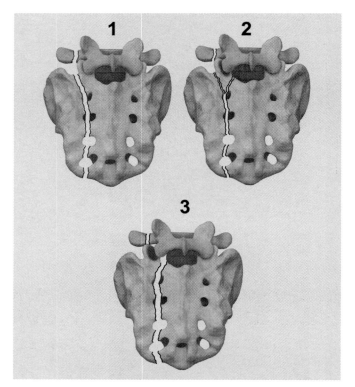

Figure 4 Schematic representation of the Isler classification of three types of zone II sacral fractures with lumbosacral injury.

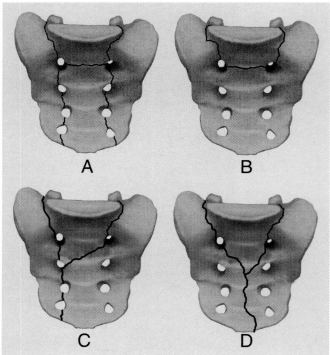

Figure 5 Schematic representation of the four types of complex Denis zone III sacral fractures. **A,** Sacral H fracture. **B,** Sacral U fracture. **C,** Sacral Y fracture. **D,** Sacral lambda fracture.

equina syndrome.[4,5,12] Nerve root dysfunction may present as potentially reversible neural injuries caused by contusion, by compression and traction that result from fracture angulation and translation, or by direct compression by bony fragments within the sacral spinal canal or the ventral foramina. Nerve root transection or avulsion can also occur, causing an irreversible neurologic deficit.[3,13] These deficits may also occur on a delayed basis in a time frame of hours to months after the initial trauma, secondary to root compression from an evolving epidural hematoma, fracture instability, or callus formation. Documentation of accurate serial neurologic evaluations is therefore of utmost clinical importance and should clearly establish the pattern and severity of any neurologic deficit. For lower extremity deficits, this requires a strength grading from 0 to 5 of all key muscle groups. The formal neurologic injury severity grading scheme presented in Table 1 is somewhat analogous to the American Spinal Injury Association classification system for spinal cord injuries and is a useful tool for assessing the neurologic status of patients with sacral root deficits.[4]

Treatment Options

The treatment options discussed in this chapter focus primarily on Denis zone III sacral injuries with lumbosacral instability patterns. Treatment options for Denis zone I, zone II, and the few zone III injuries that constitute mainly the posterior component of pelvic ring disruptions are discussed in detail in chapter 22.

If left untreated, a sacral injury can result in painful deformity or loss of neurologic function. Late corrective surgery is usually far more complex and associated with generally worse outcomes compared with appropriately timed early intervention. Efficient use of clinical, radiographic, and neurophysiologic diagnostic measures and careful follow-up is therefore important to assure timely detection of these injuries and maintenance of acceptable fracture alignment.

Given these circumstances, nonsurgical treatment may be considered for patients with predominantly isolated, closed, osseous injuries with retained lumbosacral stability. Conversely, surgical realignment and fixation of the unstable lumbopelvic junction, with adjunctive decompression of compromised lumbosacral roots, may be considered if it is in the patient's best interest to provide the best potential environment for early and safe mobilization, to provide the best possible environment for recovery of sacral root deficits, or to protect against the complications of late fracture displacement.

Because of the relative infrequency of Denis zone III injuries, commonly associated multisystem injuries, and the relatively recent evolution of rigid lumbopelvic fixation techniques, there are few objective data in the literature to support any specific treatment protocol. There-

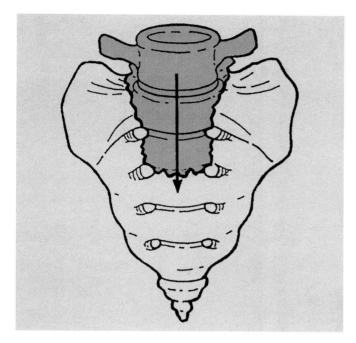

Figure 6 Schematic representation of the two major fracture fragments in Denis zone III sacral fractures with longitudinal and transverse components (sacral U fracture). The central upper sacral fragment and remainder of the spine *(shaded area)* are dissociated from the peripheral sacral fragment and both hemipelves. *(Adapted with permission from Hunt N, Jennings A, Smith M: Current management of U-shaped sacral fractures or spino-pelvic dissociation.* Injury 2002;33:123-126.)

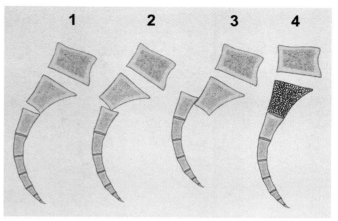

Figure 7 Roy-Camille and associates[11] and Strange-Vognsen and Lebech[10] subclassification of Denis zone III sacral fractures.

TABLE 1	Gibbons Classification of Cauda Equina Impairment	
Type	**Neurologic Deficit**
1	None
2	Paresthesias only
3	Lower extremity motor deficit
4	Bowel/bladder dysfunction

fore, the potential benefits of surgery should be carefully weighed against the potential risks of surgical management.

Nonsurgical Treatment

The treatment of sacral fractures has traditionally involved recumbency followed by progressive weight bearing over a period of approximately 3 months.[14] Bifemoral traction has also been used in an attempt to achieve the best possible fracture stability and alignment available via closed methods. Although surgical complications can be avoided by using closed treatment methods that have been shown to provide reliable fracture healing, potential disadvantages include life-threatening pulmonary and thromboembolic complications associated with prolonged recumbency, the development of decubitus ulcers, the inability to reliably relieve sacral canal and neuroforaminal compression, and the potential for late instability, deformity, and (progressive) neurologic deficits.

Surgical Treatment

Although the surgical treatment of sacral fractures is only supported by class III evidence, multiply injured patients with severe displacement or neurologic deficits are often best treated surgically.[3-5,9,13,15-21]

Timing

The timing of surgical intervention is dictated by many factors. Although the presence of an open fracture or neurologic deficit may dictate the need for expeditious surgical intervention, the multiply injured patient's physiologic status is the main determinant of the timing of surgical intervention. Therefore, although desirable from a neurophysiologic standpoint, emergent decompression of compromised neural elements is rarely feasible or safe in the acutely traumatized patient. Based on retrospective data, effective neurologic decompression within 2 weeks of injury appears to minimize the likelihood of permanent compression-induced neurologic deterioration.[5] This may allow for meaningful neurologic recovery in a time frame that is more in line with a patient's physiologic tolerance.

Decompression

In patients with sacral root deficits, decompression alone has been advocated as a method for theoretically enhancing the possibility of neurologic recovery while minimizing the potential for complications associated with the more extensive dissection and greater surgical time required for surgical stabilization.[21,22] The validity of this approach, however, is compromised by the fact that sacral root compression is largely a function of fracture displacement and angulation, both at the neuroforaminal

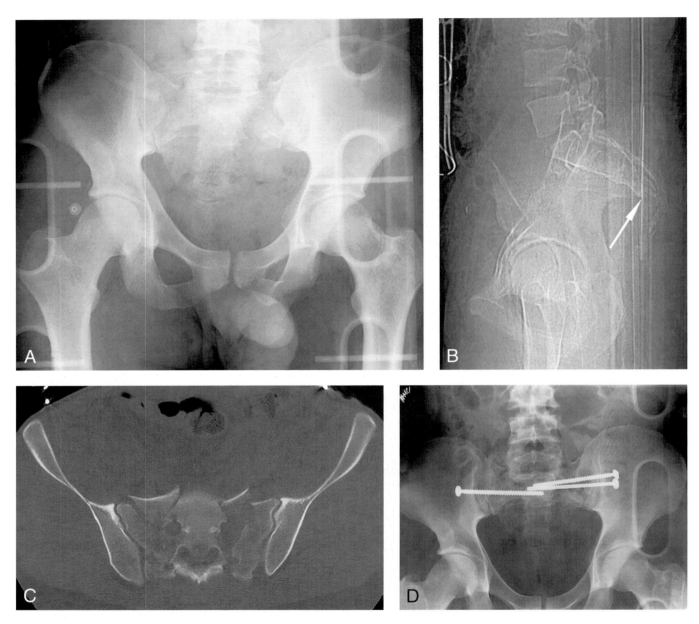

Figure 8 Failure of iliosacral screw fixation for treatment of Roy-Camille type 1 Denis zone III sacral U fracture. AP pelvic radiograph **(A)**, lateral sacral radiograph **(B)**, and axial CT scan **(C)** at S1 of a 19-year-old man with a Denis zone III sacral U fracture with a low S3-4 transverse fracture component (*white arrow*) and mild sacral angulation without translation (Roy-Camille type 1). Because of the relatively mild fracture displacement, the patient's labile intracranial pressure, multiple injuries, and a severe degloving lesion over his posterior pelvis, the patient was stabilized percutaneously with bilateral iliosacral screw fixation, as demonstrated on postoperative AP pelvic radiograph **(D)**. Despite the patient not bearing weight postoperatively, anterocaudal displacement of the fracture occurred, with bending of the iliosacral screws, as noted on AP pelvic radiograph **(E)**, lateral sacral radiograph **(F)**, and axial CT scan **(G)**, which demonstrate the anterocaudally displaced position of the L5 transverse process and L5-S1 facet joints anterior to the sacral ala. Reduction and stabilization with lumbopelvic fixation restored lumbopelvic alignment and realignment of iliosacral screw tracts as shown on AP pelvic radiograph **(H)**, lateral sacral radiograph **(I)**, and axial CT scan **(J)**.

and sacral canal levels. The compression cannot be addressed by laminectomy and foraminotomy alone. It is unlikely that the sacral roots can be comprehensively decompressed without fracture realignment and stabilization.[3]

When used in conjunction with reduction and stabilization of both transforaminal and transverse sacral fracture components, laminectomy can be performed through a posterior approach, which allows for neuroforaminal and sacral canal decompression. The posterior approach also allows access to the often kyphotic and translated upper sacral body. Reduction can be achieved by various techniques. Disimpaction of the upper and lower sacral fracture fragments often requires prying them apart with an elevator inserted into the transverse fracture. Once mobilized, the upper sacrum can be reduced by securing it with a Schanz screw, usually inserted between the S1 and S2 roots, which can then be used as a joystick to reduce the

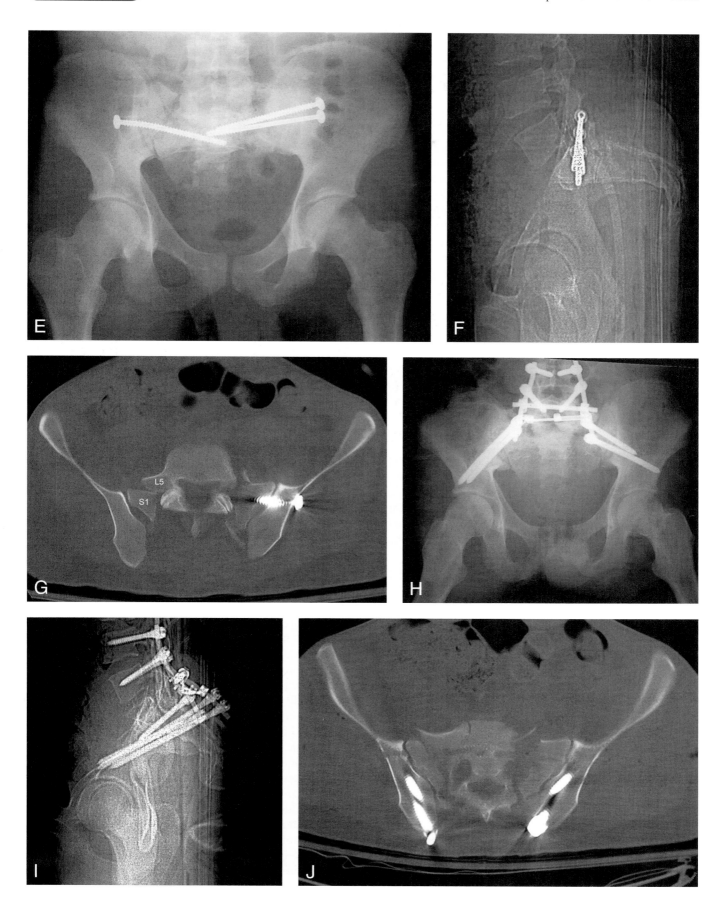

sagittal plane angulation.[3,13] Traumatic dural tears can also be repaired as necessary.

Stabilization

Percutaneous iliosacral screw fixation is the least invasive of surgical stabilization methods, but it carries the disadvantage of not allowing for reduction of sacral angulation. Safely feasible only in minimally displaced fractures, this technique is less biomechanically sound than lumbopelvic stabilization methods (Figure 8). Nevertheless, in a series of 13 patients who had minimal sacral angulation and displacement, one study found in situ iliosacral screw fixation to be safe and effective.[17] Weight bearing was restricted for 12 weeks postoperatively, and patients required 8 to 12 weeks of bracing postoperatively with a thoracolumbosacral orthotic device with a thigh extension.

Posterior fixation with sacral bars and posterior tension band plate are largely ineffective in stabilizing the injury pattern typically seen in Denis zone III sacral fractures with a transverse component. As with iliosacral screws alone, these techniques are limited in their ability to neutralize sagittal plane rotational forces.[1,23]

Sacral alar plates can be used to stabilize the transverse fracture component in a more appropriate plane.[11,19] A disadvantage is that these plates must rely on often suboptimal fixation into the frequently comminuted or osteopenic sacral ala to neutralize the considerable loads across the lumbopelvic junction. This technique can be combined with iliosacral screw fixation to enhance stabilization across the longitudinal fracture components. Weight bearing must be restricted for 2 to 4 months postoperatively using this technique.

Lumbopelvic fixation offers a biomechanically validated method that meets the necessary criteria for providing suitably stable low-profile fixation of complex sacral fractures with lumbosacral instability by connecting solid points of fixation rostral (lumbosacral pedicles) and caudal (iliac wings) to the injury[1,15,20,24] (Figure 9). Variants of this type of fixation have been previously described for the treatment of pelvic injuries with Denis zone II sacral fractures, in which they are particularly valuable if lumbosacral instability is present (Isler types 2 and 3).[25,26] Clinical data regarding the usefulness of this relatively new technique for treating Denis zone III sacral fractures are beginning to emerge. Preliminary findings suggest a negligible rate of fixation failure, but with infectious and wound-related complications that approach 20%.[13] These findings do not, however, appear to adversely affect longer-term results. The advantage of this method of fixation has been a reliable healing rate without displacement or loss of fixation despite aggressive sacral root decompression and immediate, unrestricted weight bearing.

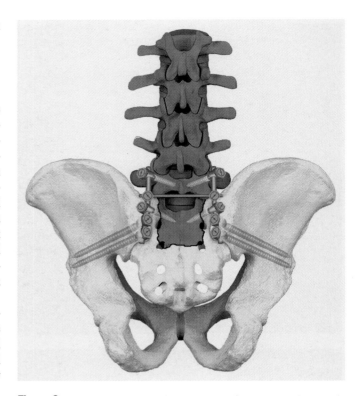

Figure 9 Schematic representation of how lumbopelvic fixation secures the two main fracture fragments in Denis zone III sacral U fractures and their variants.

Insufficiency Fractures

Sacral U insufficiency fractures may occur for several reasons, with the common pathway being severe osteopenia.[27,28] These fractures are frequently missed on plain radiographic evaluation of the pelvis, and symptoms may be present for many months prior to diagnosis. Additional investigation using technetium bone scanning and CT may be necessary to establish the diagnosis.[27] These fractures can be extremely unstable and disabling, particularly because pain is rarely relieved with sitting. Pseudarthrosis may develop, leading to potentially lifelong pain and activity restriction. Along with treatment of the underlying cause of osteopenia, restricted weight bearing alone may be appropriate for 6 to 12 weeks in patients with timely diagnosis. Patients with progressive fracture displacement, neurologic deficits,[29] delayed diagnosis, and impending or established pseudarthrosis, or those who cannot tolerate recumbency because of their physiologic condition or inadequate pain relief are candidates for surgical stabilization.[30] Lumbopelvic fixation, with the possible addition of iliosacral screws, and bone grafting of pseudarthroses appears to offer the most biomechanically sound fixation option.[1] This treatment method and variations thereof have been shown to provide reliable early pain relief with immediate unrestricted weight bearing.[30] Unlike the high-energy injury patient population in whom formal arthrodesis of the ilium to the lumbosacral spine is not routinely performed, the benefits of obtaining fusion of the pelvis to the lumbosacral spine most likely outweigh the disadvantages in elderly patients with a pathologic fracture.

Summary

Based on both musculoskeletal and neurologic concerns, complex Denis zone III sacral fractures with associated lumbosacral instability have functional consequences that can be severe in magnitude and broad in their implications. These injuries are challenging to diagnose and treat. Advanced imaging modalities have facilitated early diagnosis and improved understanding of these multiplanar fractures and their patterns of instability. Sophisticated instrumentation techniques have enhanced the ability of physicians to stabilize these injuries and have permitted a more aggressive approach to decompression. Despite these advances, the relative low incidence of these injuries and the many confounding factors that influence functional outcomes have hampered the ability of physicians to objectively determine the best treatment method, which, consequently, remains unclear.

Annotated References

1. Schildhauer TA, Ledoux WR, Chapman JR, Henley MB, Tencer AF, Routt ML Jr: Triangular osteosynthesis and iliosacral screw fixation for unstable sacral fractures: A cadaveric and biomechanical evaluation under cyclic loads. *J Orthop Trauma* 2003;17:22-31.

   The authors compared triangular osteosynthesis and standard iliosacral screw osteosynthesis for unstable transforaminal sacral fractures. They found that triangular osteosynthesis provided significantly greater stability than iliosacral screw fixation under in vitro cyclic loading conditions that simulate the early stages of postoperative patient mobilization.

2. Ebraheim NA, Sabry FF, Tosic A: Radiographic evaluation of transverse sacral fractures. *Orthopedics* 2001;24:1071-1074.

   In this cadaveric study, plain radiographic analysis was used on sacral U fractures that had been created and marked with radio-opaque material and resulted in findings that may facilitate early identification of these fractures.

3. Chapman JR, Schildhauer TA, Bellabarba C, Nork SE, Mirza SK: Treatment of sacral fractures with neurologic injuries. *Top Spinal Cord Inj Rehabil* 2002;8:59-78.

   This review article provides an overview of the current methods of evaluation and treatment of complex sacral fractures.

4. Gibbons KJ, Soloniuk DS, Razack N: Neurological injury and patterns of sacral fractures. *J Neurosurg* 1990;72:889-893.

5. Denis F, Davis S, Comfort T: Sacral fractures: An important problem. Retrospective analysis of 236 cases. *Clin Orthop* 1988;227:67-81.

6. Isler B: Lumbosacral lesions associated with pelvic ring injuries. *J Orthop Trauma* 1990;4:1-6.

7. Oransky M, Gasparini G: Associated lumbosacral junction injuries (LSJIs) in pelvic fractures. *J Orthop Trauma* 1997;11:509-512.

8. Bellabarba C, Stewart JD, Ricci WM, DiPasquale TG, Bolhofner BR: Midline sagittal sacral fractures in anterior-posterior compression pelvic ring injuries. *J Orthop Trauma* 2003;17:32-37.

   The authors of this prospective series evaluated 10 patients with type A pelvic fractures and Denis zone III sacral fractures consisting of a midline fracture through the sacrum. This unusual injury pattern was noted to comprise 0.6% of pelvic fractures and 1.4% of sacral fractures treated during a 10-year period. Nine patients were treated with reduction, anterior pelvic stabilization, and early weight bearing. One patient with a minimally displaced injury was treated nonsurgically. All fractures healed without displacement, and there were no objective neurologic deficits attributable to sacral root injury. The authors concluded that patients with sagittally oriented midline fractures of the sacrum that extend into the spinal canal (Denis zone III) as part of displaced, vertically stable anterior-posterior compression pelvic injuries have a low incidence of neurologic deficit attributable to sacral root or plexus injury.

9. Hunt N, Jennings A, Smith M: Current management of U-shaped sacral fractures or spino-pelvic dissociation. *Injury* 2002;33:123-126.

   The authors assessed four patients with sacral U fractures who were treated using a variety of fixation systems, and they present a clinical overview of current concepts regarding the evaluation and treatment of patients with complex sacral fractures.

10. Strange-Vognsen HH, Lebech A: An unusual type of fracture in the upper sacrum. *J Orthop Trauma* 1991; 5:200-203.

11. Roy-Camille R, Saillant G, Gagna G, Mazel C: Transverse fracture of the upper sacrum: Suicidal jumper's fracture. *Spine* 1985;10:838-845.

12. Kutsy RL, Robinson LR, Routt ML: Lumbosacral plexopathy in pelvic trauma. *Muscle Nerve* 2000;23: 1757-1760.

After review of the electrophysiologic data from 22 consecutive patients with pelvic trauma who were referred for electromyography, the authors of this study report that lumbosacral plexopathy was significantly more common in patients with sacral fractures (incidence of 2.03%) than among the entire population of patients with pelvic and acetabular fractures (overall incidence 0.7%).

13. Bellabarba C, Schildhauer TA, Mirza SK, et al: Decompression and lumbar fixation for sacral fracture-dislocations with neurologic deficits, in *Final Program of the Annual Meeting of the Orthopaedic Trauma Association, October 9-11, 2003, Salt Lake City, UT*. Available at: http://www.hwbf.org/ota/am/ota03/otapa/OTA03959.htm. Accessed May, 2005.

This retrospective case series describes 18 patients with cauda equina syndrome and complex sacral fractures causing dissociation of the vertebral column from the pelvis who were treated with posterior sacral decompression and lumbopelvic fixation. The authors found that although lumbopelvic fixation provided healing without loss of alignment in all patients despite early weight bearing, this technique resulted in significant soft-tissue complications. Neurologic recovery occurred in 83% of patients.

14. Phelan ST, Jones DA, Bishay M: Conservative management of transverse fractures of the sacrum with neurological features: A report of four cases. *J Bone Joint Surg Br* 1991;73:969-971.

15. Hessmann MH, Rommens PM: Transverse fracture-dislocation of the sacrum: A diagnostic pitfall and a surgical challenge. *Acta Chir Belg* 2002;102:46-51.

The authors discuss the evaluation and treatment of two patients with transverse sacral fracture-dislocations and neurologic deficits and provide an overview on the current evaluation and treatment of patients with this type of injury. One of the patients was treated with lumbopelvic fixation and healed successfully. The other patient experienced failure of iliosacral screw fixation.

16. Suzuki K, Mochida J: Operative treatment of a transverse fracture-dislocation at the S1-S2 level. *J Orthop Trauma* 2001;15:363-367.

The authors report on a patient with an S1-S2 sacral fracture-dislocation that was treated with posterior decompression, in situ lumbopelvic fixation without reduction, and supplementary S1-S2 cannulated screw fixation. The patient healed successfully and had marked improvement in neurologic function.

17. Nork SE, Jones CB, Harding SP, Mirza SK, Routt ML Jr: Percutaneous stabilization of U-shaped sacral fractures using iliosacral screws: Technique and early results. *J Orthop Trauma* 2001;15:238-246.

The authors of this retrospective review evaluated the early results of fluoroscopically guided supine iliosacral screw fixation in 13 patients with minimally displaced sacral U fractures and absence of bowel or bladder dysfunction. This technique was limited to patients who had primarily sacral kyphotic deformities without significant translation. Neurologic decompression was not performed, and patients did not bear weight in a thoracolumbosacral orthotic device with a thigh extension for 12 weeks after fixation. All fractures healed clinically and radiographically, with no significant change in kyphosis. Screw disengagement without a change in position of the sacral fracture was noted in the only patient treated with a single unilateral screw. Some resolution of neurologic deficits occurred in all patients who did not have an associated spinal cord injury associated with a more rostral spine fracture. The authors concluded that early percutaneous iliosacral screw fixation is an effective treatment for sacral U fractures with primarily angulatory deformities.

18. Hessmann M, Degreif J, Mayer A, Atahi S, Rommens PM: Transverse sacral fracture with intrapelvic intrusion of the lumbosacral spine: Case report and review of the literature. *J Trauma* 2000;49:754-757.

This case report describes a patient with an S1-S2 fracture-dislocation and L4-5 flexion distraction injury that was successfully treated using posterior decompression and L4-S2 posterior pedicle screw and rod instrumentation. The authors recommend treatment of sacral fractures according to guidelines similar to those accepted for other patients with unstable spine fractures and neurologic deficits.

19. Taguchi T, Kawai S, Kaneko K, et al: Operative management of displaced fractures of the sacrum. *J Orthop Sci* 1999;4:347-352.

20. Strange-Vognsen HH, Kiaer T, Tondevold E: The Cotrel-Dubousset instrumentation for unstable sacral fractures: Report of 3 patients. *Acta Orthop Scand* 1994;65:219-220.

21. Fisher RG: Sacral fracture with compression of cauda equina: Surgical treatment. *J Trauma* 1988;28:1678-1680.

22. Fountain S, Hamilton RD, Jameson RM: Transverse fractures of the sacrum: A report of six cases. *J Bone Joint Surg Am* 1977;59:486-489.

23. Griffin DR, Starr AJ, Reinert CM, Jones AL, Whitlock S: Vertically unstable pelvic fractures fixed with percutaneous iliosacral screws: Does posterior injury pattern predict fixation failure? *J Orthop Trauma* 2003;17:399-405.

The authors of this retrospective study of 62 consecutive patients who were treated with iliosacral screws for type C pelvic fractures over 5 years investigated the failure rate of percutaneous iliosacral screw fixation of vertically unstable pelvic fractures. The authors found a significantly higher failure of fixation in patients whose posterior injury consisted of a sacral fracture (4 of 30 patients) than in patients whose posterior injury consisted of dislocation or fracture-dislocation of the sacroiliac joint (0 of 32 patients). The authors concluded that although percutaneous iliosacral screw fixation is a useful technique in the management of vertically unstable pelvic fractures, a vertical sacral fracture should make the surgeon more wary of fixation failure and loss of reduction.

24. Schildhauer TA, McCulloch P, Chapman JR, et al: Anatomic and radiographic considerations for placement of transiliac screws in lumbopelvic fixations. *J Spinal Disord Tech* 2002;15:199-205.

    The authors of this radiographic study used CT to determine the available paths that allow for iliac screw placement with maximum diameter and length and found that the posterior-superior iliac spine to anterior-inferior iliac spine path had the largest bony canal lengths.

25. Schildhauer TA, Josten C, Muhr G: Triangular osteosynthesis of vertically unstable sacrum fractures: A new concept allowing early weight-bearing. *J Orthop Trauma* 1998;12:307-314.

26. Josten C, Schildhauer TA, Muhr G: Therapy of unstable sacrum fractures in pelvic ring: Results of osteosynthesis with early mobilization [in German]. *Chirurg* 1994;65:970-975.

27. Soubrier M, Dubost JJ, Boisgard S, et al: Insufficiency fracture: A survey of 60 cases and review of the literature. *Joint Bone Spine* 2003;70:209-218.

    This retrospective review of 55 women and 5 men with 91 insufficiency fractures over an 8-year period was conducted to determine the location, risk factors, and most useful imaging technique for identifying these fractures. The authors found that fractures occurred most commonly in the pelvic girdle (30.7%, 28 of 91 patients) and in the sacrum (29.6%, 27 of 91 patients). Osteoporosis without additional risk factors was present in half of the patients. Other risk factors included fluoride treatment, rheumatoid arthritis, osteomalacia, corticosteroid treatment, and hyperparathyroidism. Plain radiography identified the fracture in 65% of patients, whereas scintigraphy was positive in 87.5%. The authors concluded that scintigraphy is a more reliable screening tool for insufficiency fractures than plain radiography.

28. Weber M, Hasler P, Gerber H: Insufficiency fractures of the sacrum: Twenty cases and review of the literature. *Spine* 1993;18:2507-2512.

29. Finiels PJ, Finiels H, Strubel D, Jacquot JM: Spontaneous osteoporotic fractures of the sacrum causing neurological damage: Report of three cases. *J Neurosurg* 2002;97(suppl 3):380-385.

    The authors report three instances of nerve root compromise in elderly women with sacral insufficiency fractures. Based on a literature review, they estimated the incidence to be approximately 2%, but suspect that these injuries are underreported. Sphincter dysfunction and lower-limb paresthesias are the most common symptoms and are often overlooked. The neurologic manifestations were delayed in some patients. A full recovery is normally thought to ensue with healing of the fracture.

30. McGee AM, Bache CE, Spilsbury J, Marks DS, Stirling AJ, Thompson AG: A simplified Galveston technique for the stabilisation of pathological fractures of the sacrum. *Eur Spine J* 2000;9:451-454.

    This is a retrospective case series of six patients who were treated with lumbar pedicle screws and a threaded iliac bolt for fixation of sacral insufficiency fractures caused by malignant neoplasms. Neurologic decompression was performed as required, and patients were allowed to bear weight as tolerated postoperatively. The authors report that they had no surgical complications using this technique.

Chapter 30

Spinal Injury: Special Considerations

Daniel T. Altman, MD

Robert A. Gallo, MD

John M. Flynn, MD

Jonathan S. Erulkar, MD

James J. Yue, MD

Pediatric Spinal Trauma

Pediatric spinal trauma represents an entity distinct from adult trauma. Because of anatomic differences in children and adults, pediatric spinal injuries are less frequent than adult spinal injuries but are associated with a higher mortality rate given their propensity to occur in the upper cervical spine.[1] In addition to a broad range of anatomic variation, poor patient communication and unique radiographic variants frequently make diagnosis difficult.

Anatomy

A clear understanding of normal pediatric spine anatomy is a prerequisite for any discussion of spinal trauma. The fundamental difference in pediatric cervical spines is the relative increased elasticity of ligamentous structures, including interspinous ligaments, posterior joint capsules, and cartilaginous end plates. Increased ligamentous laxity allows the spinal column to absorb and distribute traumatic forces and thus protect the osseous structures from injury.[2] However, when combined with the normal anterior wedging of the vertebral bodies and horizontally oriented facets, this elasticity subjects the cervical spine to greater mobility with flexion and extension.[2-5] A relative lack of developed neck musculature and a larger head size contribute to increased torque and make children more susceptible to injuries of the upper cervical spine.[2,6,7] Beginning at age 8 years and extending to adolescence, the pediatric spine adopts a more adult-like configuration, replete with ossified bony structures, rectangular vertebral bodies, and vertically oriented facets.[5,8]

The pediatric vertebral column also features numerous synchondroses and cartilaginous growth areas between adjacent ossification centers. The synchondroses are radiolucent but can be differentiated from fractures by the presence of subchondral sclerosis and smooth, regular patterns of lucency.[9,10] Although most vertebral bodies share similar patterns of development, the atlas and axis display slightly different patterns of growth.[8-13] All segments possess a central ossification center (centrum) that forms the vertebral body and two posterolateral neural arches that develop into the posterior elements. The synchondroses and the age ranges in which they appear and closure occurs are outlined in Table 1.

Background

The epidemiology of spinal injuries directly correlates with the anatomic configuration of the spine. Up to 80% of pediatric vertebral injuries occur within the cervical spine.[2,14] As the spinal column matures and the fulcrum of force moves caudally from C2-C3 in young children to C5-C6 in adults, the location of injury follows this migration.[1,14-16] Generally, children age 8 years and younger have a higher incidence of injuries to the upper cervical spine (C1-C4) than older children, whose injuries are more evenly distributed throughout the cervical spine.[1,2,14,17] Because of the more cephalad location of injury, younger children are more likely to have associated closed head injuries and increased mortality rates.[8,10] The increased laxity of the pediatric spinal column distributes forces such that multiple injuries occur at noncontiguous levels of the cervical spine in 24% of all children diagnosed with a cervical spine injury.[18]

TABLE 1 | Normal Vertebral Synchondroses

Synchondrosis (Bordering Ossification Centers)	Age of Appearance (years)	Age of Closure (years)
Atlas		
Neural (neural arches posteriorly)	Birth	3
Neurocentral (centrum, neural arch)	Birth	7
Axis		
Neural (neural arches posteriorly)	Birth	3
Basilar odontoid (odontoid, neural arch)	Birth	6
Apical odontoid (odontoid body and tip)	2	11
Subaxial Vertebrae		
Neural (neural arches posteriorly)	Birth	4
Neurocentral (centrum, neural arch)	Birth	6
Secondary (spinous, transverse, and mammillary processes)	Variable	20

Just as a difference in location of injury occurs between younger and older children, a dichotomy exists in regard to the mechanism of injury: all children more commonly have injuries secondary to motor vehicle collisions (as a passenger, pedestrian, or bicyclist), whereas older children more often experience sports-related injuries.[2,19] Overall, motor vehicle accidents account for half of all injuries, sports activities cause nearly one third, and falls and nonaccidental injuries cause the remainder.[2,11,19] Among the motor vehicle-related injuries, pedestrian and bicycle accidents have more associated injuries and patients have an overall poorer prognosis.[19] With the exception of those that occur while diving, sports-related injuries experienced by older children and caused by lower energy forces generally have a better prognosis than those involving motor vehicle collisions.[2]

The data on mechanism and associated cervical spine injuries have led to several preventive measures to reduce the risk and severity of injury. Several studies correlating craniocervical injuries and death associated with airbag deployment led to the recommendation that children age 12 years and younger sit in the back seat of a motor vehicle.[20-24] Similarly, a series of odontoid fractures was attributed to children sitting in a car seat facing forward.[25] The authors concluded that rapid deceleration caused extreme hyperflexion of the neck and resultant odontoid fractures. This study contributed to the practice of placing children younger than 8 years and weighing less than 80 lb in a car seat facing posteriorly.[25] Finally, a study reporting the assessment of several children with flexion-distraction fractures and abdominal injuries caused by lap belts substantiated the need for shoulder harnesses and proper lap belt placement over the proximal thigh instead of the abdomen.[17,26,27] Despite case reports involving seat belts and other protective devices, approximately 80% of cervical spine injuries involve improperly restrained young children (75%) and unrestrained older children and adolescent passengers (87%).[19,28]

Initial Management and Evaluation

Guidelines involving immobilization have recently evolved based on improved understanding of the pediatric spine. Because of a relatively greater head circumference than chest circumference, children immobilized on regular flat long boards are subjected to a flexion posture (a prominent occiput forces the head forward and into anterior translation).[12,16,17,29] Therefore, thoracic elevation via mattress pads or an occipital recess built into the board is necessary to obtain neutral alignment.[12,16]

The initial evaluation of children with trauma shares similarities with adult protocols. Although history and symptomatology may be more elusive in the pediatric population, physical examination findings are typically equivalent to those of adults. In children with suspected injuries, repeated physical examination is crucial because of difficulties in obtaining a thorough history and physical examination.[12] Nearly 85% of pediatric cervical spine injuries are associated with midline cervical tenderness (most sensitive), paraspinous muscular tenderness, torticollis, and/or cervical muscle spasm.[30] Isolated sensory deficits (40% of neurologic injuries) are the most common neurologic findings.[30]

The need for radiographic imaging is determined by history and physical examination findings. Mechanism alone (for example, head injury caused by a fall down a flight of stairs) is enough to prompt the use of diagnostic imaging. If a child is somnolent, nonconversant, and/or has midline cervical tenderness, torticollis, neurologic deficit, or painful distracting injuries, then a cervical spine series consisting of AP, lateral, and odontoid views should be obtained.[30] Additionally, if the child demonstrates unexplained hypotension and is younger than 8 years, diagnostic imaging is warranted.[31,32]

Lateral cervical spine radiographs alone are insufficient and miss 21% of injuries,[10,30] whereas the combination of the three views has a sensitivity of 91%.[30,33-37] Voluntary flexion-extension views in the cooperative adolescent and CT (sensitivity of 94%) should be reserved for further elucidation of equivocal radiologic findings or for those children with suspected injury but without evidence of abnormalities on plain radiographs.[32]

Because there is a potential for significant soft-tissue injury without osseous injury in this patient population, MRI is a valuable adjunctive tool for detecting pediatric spine injuries. Vertebral growth centers, ligaments, muscles, intervertebral disks, and/or the spinal cord can be imaged using MRI, which helps diagnose those "occult" injuries that are not detectable using plain radiography and account for 40% to 70% of pediatric spine injuries.[15,38] One children's institution proposed that MRI is indicated for an obtunded or nonverbal child with a mechanism of injury that is suspicious for cervical spine injury, when plain radiographs and/or CT scans are equivocal, in patients with neurologic symptoms without radiographic findings, or when physicians are unable to clear the cervical spine based on imaging and physical examination within 3 days after the injury.[1-4,39]

Normal Anatomic Radiographic Variants

Any evaluation of a pediatric lateral cervical spine film should begin with assessment of the four lines corresponding to the anterior and posterior vertebral bodies, spinolaminar junction, and tip of the spinous processes.[8,12] These lines should assume a smooth contour. Any variant should alert the physician to the possibility of traumatic injury.

The ligamentous laxity of the pediatric spinal column was historically a source of consternation when evaluating radiographs because normal pediatric variants often fall outside of accepted adult ranges. Confusion in evaluating radiographs gave rise to the entities of "pseudo-Jefferson fracture" and the "pseudosubluxation of C2-C3." The "pseudo-Jefferson fracture," visualized on odontoid views, represents physiologic lateral displacement of the lateral masses up to 6 mm, which is considered normal until age 7 years.[10] The most common pseudoinjury is pseudosubluxation at C2-C3 and can occur in almost 50% of children younger than 8 years.[40,41] Pseudosubluxation can be as marked as 4 mm of anterior displacement, but as opposed to traumatic C2-C3 subluxation, corrects with extension.[12] Swischuk's line, which is drawn along the spinolaminar line from C1-C3, normally passes within 1.5 mm of the posterior arch of C2.[8,41] Any increase in this distance is considered abnormal.

In adults, the transverse and alar ligaments are assumed to be intact if the atlanto-dens interval measures

3 mm or less; in children, this value can be as wide as 5 mm before ligamentous insufficiency is suspected.[8,40] When uncertainty arises, the space available for the spinal cord, which normally divides the area within the C1 ring equally among the odontoid, spinal cord, and subarachnoid space, aids in determining whether significant pathology exists.[8] Other subtle radiographic differences in children are the absence of lordosis without injury and physeal plates that have smooth, regular lucencies with subchondral sclerotic borders.[9,42-44]

Spinal Cord Injury Without Radiographic Abnormality

Spinal cord injury without radiographic abnormality (SCIWORA) is believed to be caused by longitudinal distraction with hyperflexion or hyperextension of the immature, elastic spinal column.[4,6] These forces result in a spinal cord that is stretched from distraction or contused from a transient vertebral displacement with subsequent realignment.[6] The elasticity of the young spinal column allows 5 cm of stretch before rupturing, whereas the adult spinal cord, tethered by the brachial plexus and the cauda equina, tolerates only 5 to 6 mm of distraction before injury.[2,3,45,46]

Because of the pathogenesis of the injury, children younger than 8 years are more prone to SCIWORA.[6] This injury manifests in several ways, ranging from short-lived paresthesias and/or motor weakness to complete spinal cord injury; progression can occur as late as 48 hours after injury.[6] Neurologic status at presentation is the best predictor of outcome, with more severe neurologic deficits associated with poorer outcomes.[2,3] Regardless of injury severity, all patients with this type of injury have an increased susceptibility to recurrent SCIWORA because of destabilization of the spinal column resulting from the inciting event.[6]

Although SCIWORA is still defined by absence of bony or ligamentous injuries using plain radiographs and CT scans, MRI can often pinpoint the exact injuries of the spinal cord and related structures.[6,47] Typical findings include mild hemorrhage or edema of the spinal cord, and identifiable lesions were found in 50% of patients with SCIWORA who underwent MRI.[48,49] Transection, epidural hematoma, and traumatic disk herniation account for the remainder of instances.[50,51] MRI offers some prognostic value in that a normal MRI scan is associated with better recovery of function regardless of the severity of neurologic dysfunction at presentation.[48,49]

Acute treatment generally involves maintenance of blood pressure during spinal shock and institution of standard adult steroid protocol (methylprednisolone at 30 mg/kg given within the first 8 hours after the injury followed by 5.4 mg/kg/h for 24 to 48 hours, depending on the initial time of presentation).[8,17,52,53] Long-term treatment involves 12 weeks of hard collar immobilization, with an additional 12 weeks of avoiding activities that require significant neck flexion and extension.[4,54]

Occipitoatlantoaxial Injury

The use of MRI has also helped to refine understanding of the pathologies of craniocervical junction injuries, which represent the most lethal (50% mortality) of cervical spine injuries.[55] These injuries, currently viewed as a continuum ranging from mild to severe, include isolated muscular abnormalities, prevertebral soft-tissue swelling, apical ligament abnormality, unilateral or bilateral facet joint abnormality, and tectorial membrane abnormalities.[55] The status of the tectorial membrane determines the stability of the injury.[55]

Young children, who possess small occipital condyles and horizontally oriented occipitoatlantal joints, are more apt to suffer craniovertebral dislocations with sudden decelerations.[55-58] Up to 60% of these unstable injuries are often initially undiagnosed.[59]

Traditionally, a Powers ratio greater than 1 suggests occipitoatlantal injury.[60] The Powers ratio is limited to identifying anterior occipitoatlantal trauma, and fails to quantify vertical and posterior dislodgement. More recently, a C1-2:C2-3 ratio measured as the shortest distance between these spinous processes has been proposed and is thought to represent a tectorial membrane abnormality if greater than 2.5.[55]

Initial management consists of halo vest application for patients with unstable injuries.[55] Most of these injuries will require fusion from the occiput to C2 because the osseous structures fail to provide stability lost by ligamentous disruption.[55] Fusion is carried to C2 because of a clear association between craniocervical injury and atlantoaxial instability regardless of neurologic status. Adjunctive halo vest stabilization is necessary following fusion.

Odontoid Fractures

Odontoid fractures, especially in young children, can often elude diagnosis. Nearly one third of patients in a recent study had a delayed diagnosis that was discovered after the child reported persistent neck stiffness as late as 4 months after injury.[25] In children younger than 6 years, fractures almost uniformly occur at the synchondrosis between the odontoid process and body of C2.[8,25] The typical mechanism is hyperflexion, with the odontoid process displaced anteriorly. Although rare, neurologic injury can occur following major anterior displacement of the upper cervical spine with the apical fragment.[25] Initial reduction of these fractures is obtained by extending the neck in the halo vest. Contrary to the nonunion problems prominent in adult patients with odontoid fractures, synchondrosis disruptions heal without complications because the synchondrosis is located inferior to the level of vascular supply to the lower dens.[10]

Definitive treatment with a halo vest alone is associated with dramatically fewer complications than surgical intervention. The most common complication is infection of a pin.[8,12] Because of the relatively thin skull size in children younger than 10 years, the use of at least five pins is advocated. Multiple pins decrease the necessary torque generated per pin and allow for the simple removal of a single infected pin without having to insert another. A preapplication CT scan is recommended to determine the thickest areas (usually anterolaterally and posterolaterally) for pin site placement.[8,12]

Atlantoaxial Rotatory Subluxation

Atlantoaxial rotatory subluxation is a rotational abnormality of the atlantoaxial joint caused by the anterior facet of C1 locking on the facet of C2.[9,10] This disorder is far more common in children than their adult counterparts because of the combination of horizontally oriented facets and increased laxity of the ligaments and joint capsules of the C1-2 facets.[17] In addition to trauma, respiratory infections can also cause this abnormality.

Clinically, the child's head adopts a "cock-robin" appearance and is rotated to one side and tilted to the other.[9,32] Subtle radiographic findings, including loss of a defined craniocervical junction and a lateral mass of C1 rotated anterior to the odontoid with or without a normal atlanto-dens interval,[9,10] make CT, especially a dynamic study, a more useful modality for detecting and determining the severity of this injury.[10,61-67] Atlantoaxial injuries have been classified into four categories: type I (simple rotatory displacement without anterior shift of C1), type II (rotatory displacement with an anterior shift of 5 mm or less), type III (rotatory displacement with an anterior shift of greater than 5 mm), type IV (rotatory displacement with a posterior shift).[68]

Type I injuries, the most common, typically reduce spontaneously; therefore, only supportive treatment is indicated. Anteriorly displaced subluxations require correction with halter traction and immobilization in a reduced position for 6 weeks.[9,32] Rarely, a C1-C2 fusion is necessary for patients with neurologic deficiencies, irreducible or recurrent displacement, and subluxation that is present for longer than 3 weeks.[8,9,17,32]

Lower Cervical Spine Injuries

Lower cervical spine injuries typically occur in older children because of a decrease in the relative size of the head and a consequent shift in the fulcrum of force to the lower cervical levels. Fractures of the lower cervical spine are rare in children younger than 8 years.[2] Most fractures and dislocations in the lower cervical spine can be treated with halo immobilization. The use of laminectomy for these injuries, however, remains controversial.[32]

Thoracolumbar Spine Fractures

As with fractures of the lower cervical spine, reports of thoracolumbar injuries are scarce in the literature. Orthopaedists assume that the Denis three-column classification system is relevant in children, particularly older children, although the validity of this scheme has not been specifically studied in the pediatric population.[69]

Lap seat belt injuries have garnered attention secondary to published case reports.[70] These injuries are flexion-distraction injuries caused by a rapid deceleration. An improperly worn lap seat belt creates a fulcrum anterior to the normal axis and thus renders the spine more prone to flexion and distraction.[71] In this setting, all elements posterior to the fulcrum are tensioned beyond their limits and eventually fracture and/or rupture. Ecchymosis signifying the location of the lap belt can be identified in most patients. One study estimated that 50% of lap seat belt injuries are associated with intra-abdominal injuries such as colonic tears.[26] Reduction can usually be obtained by hyperextension of the lumbar spine and immobilization with a brace or cast. Surgical stabilization should be undertaken for patients with concomitant bowel injuries, neurologic deficits, and mechanical instability, especially those with purely soft-tissue injuries.[72]

Child Abuse

With hyperflexion as occurs in the shaken baby syndrome and the anatomic milieu of the pediatric spine, upper cervical and thoracolumbar spine injuries may be more common in this syndrome than previously realized.[73,74] A report of the autopsy findings of five battered children with shaken baby syndrome despite no evidence of direct cranial trauma revealed an epidural and/or subdural hemorrhage at the craniocervical junction in one child and contusions of the upper cervical spine in the other four children.[75] These findings prompted the conclusion that high cervical trauma, not intracranial injury, may contribute to death in the shaken baby syndrome.[75]

As with the appendicular skeleton, atypical patterns of force, such as the axial loading, flexion, and rotation required to cause a circumferential fracture of the thoracolumbar spine, are highly suspicious for abuse, especially in young children.[17,76] In these fractures, which are associated with metaphyseal fractures at other locations, the centrum of the vertebral body separates from the disk and growth centers and rotates into the spinal canal.[17,76] The ensuing spinal cord compression causes rapid-onset high-level tetraplegia from disruption of the craniocervical region and in the subaxial spine.

Birth Injuries

Flaccid quadriplegia occurs in approximately 1 in 60,000 child births.[77] Although all spinal cord injuries in this population manifest as "spinal shock" (flaccid with no spontaneous motion nor tendon reflexes), two distinct entities based on location of injury are defined.[78] Upper cervical spinal cord injuries, the most common type of spinal cord injury in neonates, are linked to cephalic presentation and the use of forceps for rotational maneuvers,[78,79] whereas cervicothoracic injuries typically occur in the setting of breech presentations.[80] Most neonates with upper cervical injuries require mechanical ventilation, which is typically long-term if the first respiratory effort occurs after the first day of life.[78]

Bedside ultrasound is surprisingly accurate when compared with MRI studies and therefore represents the diagnostic modality of choice in the evaluation of suspected birth-related spinal cord injury.[17,81] An external immobilization device consisting of a thermoplastic molded device contoured to the occiput, neck, and thorax and secured with Velcro straps across the forehead and torso has been developed to immobilize the neonatal spinal column.[82]

Ballistic Trauma to the Spine

Ballistic injuries to the spine have challenged surgeons treating patients in the military and civilian arenas for generations. Much of the early information regarding firearm-related spinal cord injury was generated from military experience with high-velocity missile wounds. However, military and civilian gunshot injuries often differ in several ways. For example, military wounds are primarily high-velocity injuries, whereas civilian injuries result from low-velocity injuries caused by handguns. Military wounds are therefore associated with a higher degree of tissue damage and contamination. For these reasons, evaluation and treatment of military and civilian gunshot injuries may be quite different. Nevertheless, clinicians treating patients with ballistic spinal injuries are faced with similar challenges, including optimal evaluation of injury, indications and benefits of surgical intervention, and the risks of short-term and long-term complications.

Epidemiology

Gunshot wounds to the spine have become an increasingly significant cause of spinal cord injury in the US civilian population. In 1998, gunshot injuries accounted for 21.8% of all spinal cord injuries.[83] Gunshot wounds are the second leading cause of traumatic quadriplegia and paraplegia behind only motor vehicle accidents.[84]

Penetrating wounds account for a larger proportion of spinal cord injuries in urban settings than in rural settings. Victims of gunshot wounds to the spine are predominantly young men. Two prospective series found ethnic distribution of urban gunshot spinal cord injury patients to be approximately 47% black, 45% Hispanic, 4% white, and 4% of miscellaneous ethnicities.[83,85,86] The likelihood of a spinal cord injury from a gunshot wound was higher in those with previous gunshot wounds (30%) or those with prior involvement with the criminal justice system (52%).[87]

These studies also identified several other characteristics of civilian gunshot injuries to the spine. First, civilian gunshot injuries are typically caused by handguns. More than twice as many patients are shot in the back as the front. The thoracic spine is the most frequently involved region of injury, followed by the lumbar and cervical spine.[88,89]

Firearm-related injuries to the spine often result in disability and significant cost to society. Gunshot trauma is the third most costly etiology of injury and fourth most expensive form of hospitalization. It has been reported that gunshot injuries account for 24% of orthopaedic admissions, 32% of orthopaedic inpatient days, 26% of all orthopaedic trauma cases, 15% of all fractures requiring surgical intervention, and 14% of all orthopaedic surgery cases done at a Level 1 trauma center.[85,90]

It has been estimated that medical care costs range from $28,000 to $33,000 per gunshot wound for patients requiring hospitalization.[91] Given the potential for non-orthopaedic injury, long-term hospitalization, and rehabilitation needs associated with such injuries, the cost of gunshot injuries to the spine can be divided into direct costs and indirect costs. Direct costs refer to the actual expenditure of funds and costs associated with care. These direct costs including acute care, rehabilitation care, and lifetime care costs. One study reported that the average cost of acute care and rehabilitation for gunshot-related spinal cord injuries was $137,118 per patient.[92] The authors of this study found that the total cost of treating gunshot-related spinal cord injuries over an 11-year period was $78 million. They went on to estimate that the total lifetime costs of patients treated at their center was between $312 and $390 million (in 1991 dollars).[93] Another study examined the direct costs of acute and rehabilitation care in an adolescent population with gunshot-related spinal cord injuries.[94] The authors estimated an average direct cost for acute care to be $142,710 for quadriplegic patients and $87,750 for paraplegic patients.

Indirect costs refer to the value of lost productivity or expenditures that have not occurred. By their nature, indirect costs are more difficult to evaluate than direct costs. There is little information on the indirect costs of gunshot-related spinal cord injuries; however, any such estimation can be undertaken by obtaining patient employment and income data before and after such injuries.

Ballistics

A bullet causes tissue damage through direct or permanent crush of tissue (permanent cavity), elastic deformation caused by passage of the bullet (temporary cavity), and transmitted shock waves.[85,87,95] Permanent cavity is the primary destructive factor for low-velocity bullets

($< 1,000$ ft/s). Temporary cavitation becomes a more significant injury mechanism with high-velocity bullets ($> 1,000$ ft/s). In addition to direct damage, high-velocity bullets may injure the spinal cord by transmitting shock waves without direct penetration of the spinal cord.

The wounding potential of a bullet is based on several characteristics. These ballistic characteristics include size, velocity, design, and composition.[96] The wounding capacity of a gunshot depends on the energy of the projectile on impact. The energy of a projectile is determined by the following equation of kinetic energy:

$$\text{Energy} = \tfrac{1}{2} \, \text{Mass} \, (\text{Velocity})^2$$

In accordance with this equation, a doubling of velocity leads to a quadrupling of the kinetic energy. By convention, bullet wounds are classified as low-velocity injuries (such as those caused by a handgun) or high-velocity injuries (such as those caused by a rifle). Ultimately, tissue injury reflects the amount of energy transferred from projectile to tissue. This transfer energy depends on the properties of the bullet as well as those of the target.

In addition to mass and velocity, several other factors affect the wounding potential of a gunshot. Tissue injury is also affected by the amount of fragmentation of a bullet as well as the yaw (or end-over-end rotation) as the bullet moves through tissue. As such, tissue damage also depends on the material properties (density, specific gravity, elasticity, and thickness) of the injured tissues.[97]

Patient Evaluation

The evaluation of patients with a gunshot wound to the spine includes a thorough history, physical examination, and radiographic evaluation. Several aspects of the history that are particularly helpful in determining the possible severity of injury (but are often unavailable) include the type of weapon and bullet as well as the possible trajectory of the bullet. If conscious and communicative, the patient should be questioned about current neurologic symptoms as well as those that may occur after the injury.

A detailed physical examination is of particular importance. First, the patient should be examined for entry and exit wounds, and the soft tissue should be palpated for turgor and crepitus. This examination may provide clues to the extent of tissue damage as well as potential injuries to adjacent organ systems. Neurologic evaluation should follow the guidelines of the American Spinal Injury Association to carefully define the patient's neurologic level, complete versus incomplete injury status, and zone of injury.

Radiographic evaluations provide information regarding the corresponding vertebral level of injury. Radiographic evaluation is important to define the fracture pattern and degree of comminution. In addition, radiographs may aid in the identification of retained bullet

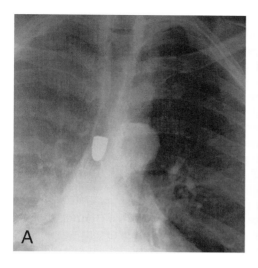
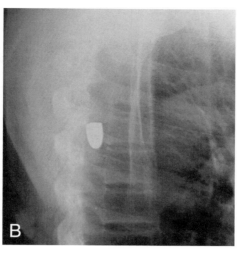

Figure 1 AP **(A)** and lateral **(B)** radiographs of a patient with a retained bullet within the thoracic spinal canal.

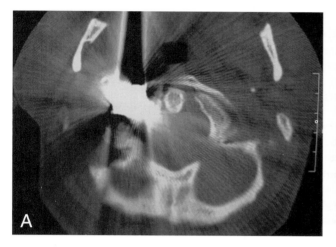
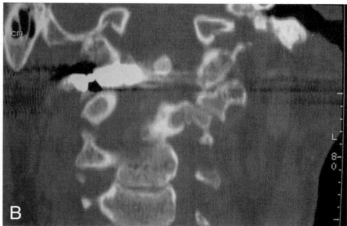
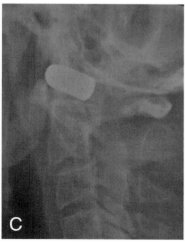

Figure 2 Axial CT scan **(A)**, coronal CT reconstruction image **(B)**, and lateral radiograph **(C)** of a patient with a retained bullet within the upper cervical region. CT can often help locate ballistic fragments and identify at-risk structures.

fragments, in the assessment of spine stability, and in the evaluation of the bullet pathway (Figure 1). CT scans will often help to further evaluate the extent of spinal cord injury and the encroachment of bone or bullet fragments into the spinal cord (Figure 2).

MRI is not routinely indicated for the initial evaluation of gunshot-related wounds to the spine. Although MRI has been performed safely in patients with gunshot injuries to the spinal cord, it has had minimal effect on their acute management.[95,98]

Spine Stability

Most civilian gunshot-related injuries of the spine are stable. Nevertheless, it is possible that a gunshot wound may produce instability in the spine. In a review of 12 cervical gunshot-related spine injuries, 4 were unstable and treated with a halo vest followed by a rigid brace.[99] In addition, 24 patients with thoracic and lumbar gunshot-related injuries were evaluated and only 1 was found to have an unstable injury that required brace treatment. Given the low likelihood of spinal instability from gunshot-related injuries, recent studies have concluded that prehospital stabilization with thoracolumbar braces unnecessarily delays transportation of patients with gunshot wounds to the thorax.[100]

Although surgical stabilization for gunshot wounds is rarely indicated, severe bone comminution and previous laminectomy may predispose patients to posttraumatic instability.

Surgical Indications and Complications

Much of the early data regarding the treatment of ballistic injuries to the spine were obtained from military experience with high-velocity and grossly contaminated wounds. The surgical tenets of wartime treatment include débridement of the missile track and devitalized tissue, spinal cord decompression, visualization of the spinal cord to determine prognosis, removal of retained fragments, and tight dural closure.[85,87,93,95,98] Such surgical intervention addresses concerns for a variety of possible complications, including neurologic compromise, infection, toxicity, and pain. The civilian experience has been much more variable.[101] The differences in surgical management outcomes for civilian and military gunshot-related injury to the spine have been attributed to differences in ballistic energy and associated injury contamination.

There is little evidence demonstrating significant neurologic recovery with surgical intervention in civilian patients with gunshot-related injuries to the spine. Several authors have examined the effects of decompressive laminectomy in these patients and determined that it is not effective in improving neurologic recovery.[102]

It is generally agreed that the surgical removal of bullets from within the canal is indicated for patients who are demonstrating neurologic deterioration.[89,102-104] Some authors also advocate surgical intervention in patients with persistent incomplete injuries with evidence of neural compression.[101] One study found significant motor improvement in patients who underwent bullet removal from the spinal canal below the T12 level; however, they reported no improvement in those who underwent bullet removal from the cervical or thoracic regions.[98,105] This difference was attributed to the likelihood of nerve root damage in the lumbar canal as opposed to spinal cord injury in the thoracic and cervical regions. Other studies have found no

improvement of neurologic recovery and increased complication rates (such as infection and fistula formation) with surgical intervention.[106]

From military experience, infection prevention was cited as an indication for surgical intervention, particularly in patients with colon perforation. Several studies have reviewed the treatment of civilian patients with transcolonic gunshot wounds to the spine and concluded that early removal of the bullet was not necessary to prevent infection.[88,107] In addition, retained bullets in civilian patients with gunshot-related injuries do not present a significant risk factor for infectious complications. Current recommendations include routine use of broad-spectrum antibiotic therapy for 72 hours after injury and for 7 to 14 days after concurrent injury to a contaminated alimentary tract.[107]

Although rare, neurologic deterioration has been reported to result from migration of bullet fragments within the spinal canal.[108] In addition, late neurologic symptoms have been reported in patients with canal narrowing secondary to fibrous tissue reaction to retained bullet fragments.[109] In both instances, surgical removal of the retained fragment and associated fibrous tissue is indicated.

Lead toxicity caused by retained bullet fragments in the spinal canal and intervertebral disk space has also been reported.[110] Although rare in patients with gunshot-related injuries to the spine, symptoms of lead intoxication (and high blood serum lead levels) are indications for medical treatment and surgical excision of retained fragments. Recent animal studies have suggested that copper jacketed bullets within the spinal canal should be removed because of the highly toxic effects of copper on neurologic tissues.[111]

Chronic pain is a common problem for patients with gunshot-related injury to the spine. Although often cited as a surgical indication for treatment or prevention of chronic pain, studies have shown that removal of the retained fragment does not typically relieve pain symptoms.[112]

Annotated References

1. Nitecki S, Moir CR: Predictive factors of the outcome of traumatic cervical spine fracture in children. *J Pediatr Surg* 1994;29:1409-1411.

2. Kokoska ER, Keller MS, Rallo MC, Weber TR: Characteristics of pediatric cervical spine injuries. *J Pediatr Surg* 2001;36:100-105.

   The authors assessed the mechanisms and patterns of 408 cervical spine injuries relative to outcome. They demonstrated that children in motor vehicle-related accidents, especially those who were not properly restrained, tended to have worse outcomes than older children with sports-related injuries.

3. Pang D, Wilberger JE: Spinal cord injury without radiographic abnormalities in children. *J Neurosurg* 1982;57:114-129.

4. Pang D, Pollack IF: Spinal cord injury without radiographic abnormality in children: The SCIWORA syndrome. *J Trauma* 1989;29:654-664.

5. Swischuk LE, Swischuk PN, John SD: Wedging of C3 in infants and children: Usually a normal finding and not a fracture. *Radiology* 1993;188:523-526.

6. Kriss VM, Kriss TC: SCIWORA (spinal cord injury without radiographic abnormality) in infants and children. *Clin Ped* 1996;119-124.

7. Patel JC, Tepas JJ III, Mollitt DL, Pieper P: Pediatric cervical spine injuries: Defining the disease. *J Pediatr Surg* 2001;36:373-376.

   In this study, the authors reviewed a 10-year series of 1,098 children with cervical spine injuries. They found that upper cervical spine injuries were equally prevalent among younger and older children and carry a higher mortality rate than lower cervical spine injuries.

8. Copley LA, Dormans JP: Cervical spine disorders in infants and children. *J Am Acad Orthop Surg* 1998;6:204-214.

9. Fielding JW, Hensinger RN: Fractures of the spine, in Rockwood CA, Wikins KE, King RE (eds): *Fractures in Children, Volume 3*. Philadelphia, PA, JB Lippincott Company, 1984, pp 683-732.

10. Lustrin ES, Karakas SP, Ortiz AO, et al: Pediatric cervical spine: Normal anatomy, variants, and trauma. *Radiographics* 2003;23:539-560.

    This article details the normal anatomic configuration and radiographic appearance of the normal pediatric spine and contrasts this constellation with findings in patients with traumatic cervical spine injuries.

11. Ogden JA: Ogden JA: *Injury in the Child*. Philadelphia, PA, Lea & Febiger, 1982, pp 385-422.

12. Dormans JP: Evaluation of children with cervical spine injury. *Instr Course Lect* 2002;51:401-410.

13. Sullivan JA: Fractures of the spine in children, in Green NE, Swiontkowski MF (eds): *Skeletal Trauma in Children,* ed 3. Philadelphia, PA, WB Saunders, 2003, pp 344-370.

14. Eleraky MA, Theodore N, Adams M, Rekate HL, Sonntag VK: Pediatric cervical spine injuries: Report of 102 cases and review of literature. *J Neurosurg* 2000;92(suppl 1):12-17.

    The authors of this retrospective clinical study compared cervical spine injuries of children birth to age 9 with those between the ages of 10 to 16 years. The authors noted higher levels of cervical spine injuries among younger children and an increasing trend towards surgical fixation of these injuries.

15. Hill SA, Miller CA, Kosnik EJ, Hunt WE: Pediatric neck injuries. A clinical study. *J Neurosurg* 1984;60:700-706.

16. Herzenberg JE, Hensigner RN, Dedrick DK, Phillips WA: Emergency transport and positioning of young children who have an injury of the cervical spine: The standard backboard may be hazardous. *J Bone Joint Surg Am* 1989;71:15-22.

17. Loder RT: Pediatric spinal trauma, in Fardon DF, Garfin SR, Abitbol JJ, Boden SD, Herkowitz HN, Mayer TG (eds): *Orthopaedic Knowledge Update: Spine 2*. Rosemont, IL, American Academy of Orthopaedic Surgeons, 2002, pp 291-297.

18. Williams C, Bernstein T, Jelenko C: Essentiality of the lateral cervical spine radiograph. *Ann Emerg Med* 1981;10:198-204.

19. Brown RL, Brunn MA, Garcia VF: Cervical spine injuries in children: Review of 103 patients treated consecutively at a level I pediatric trauma center. *J Pediatr Surg* 2001;36:1107-1114.

    The authors of this retrospective review of 103 consecutive cervical spine injuries found that predictors of mortality include younger age, motor vehicle-related mechanisms, C1 dislocations, Injury Severity Scores greater than 25, and associated closed head injuries.

20. Willis BK, Smith JL, Falkner LD, Vernon DD, Walker ML: Fatal air bag mediated craniocervical trauma in a child. *Pediatr Neurosurg* 1996;24:323-327.

21. Cooper JT, Balding LE, Jordan FB: Airbag mediated death of a two-year-old child wearing a shoulder/lap belt. *J Forensic Sci* 1998;43:1077-1081.

22. Marshall KW, Koch BL, Egelhoff JC: Air bag-related deaths and serious injuries in children: Injury patterns and imaging findings. *AJNR Am J Neuroradiol* 1998;19:1599-1607.

23. McCaffrey M, German A, Lalonde F, Letts M: Air bags and children: A potentially lethal combination. *J Pediatr Orthop* 1999;19:60-64.

24. Mehlman CT, Scott KA, Koch BL, Garcia VF: Orthopaedic injuries in children secondary to air-

bag deployment. *J Bone Joint Surg Am* 2000;82:895-898.

25. Odent T, Langlais J, Glorion C, Kassis B, Bataille J, Pouliquen JC: Fractures of the odontoid process: Report of 15 cases in children younger than six years. *J Pediatr Orthop* 1999;19:51-54.

26. Gallagher DJ, Heinrich SD: Pediatric Chance fracture. *J Orthop Trauma* 1990;4:183-187.

27. Black BE: Spine trauma, in Sponseller PD (ed): *Orthopaedic Knowledge Update: Pediatrics 2*. Rosemont, IL, American Academy of Orthopaedic Surgeons, 2002, pp 133-139.

28. Givens TG, Polley KA, Smith GF, Hardin WD: Pediatric cervical spine injury: Three-year experience. *J Trauma* 1996;41:310-314.

29. Nypaver M, Treloar D: Neutral cervical spine positioning in children. *Ann Emerg Med* 1994;23:208-211.

30. Baker C, Kadish H, Schunk JE: Evaluation of pediatric cervical spine injuries. *Am J Emerg Med* 1999;17:230-234.

31. Bohn D, Armstrong D, Becker L, Humphreys R: Cervical spine injuries in children. *J Trauma* 1990;30:463-466.

32. Management of pediatric cervical spine and spinal cord injuries. *Neurosurgery* 2002;50(suppl 3):S85-S99.
    This review article presents the results of an analysis of all available reports of diagnosis and treatment to determine guidelines for the management and treatment of pediatric cervical spine injuries.

33. Shaffer MA, Doris PE: Limitation of the cross table lateral view in detection of cervical spine injuries: A prospective analysis. *Ann Emerg Med* 1981;10:508-513.

34. Doris PE, Wilson RA: The next logical step in the emergency radiographic evaluation of cervical spine trauma: The five-view trauma series. *J Emerg Med* 1985;3:371-385.

35. Cadoux CG, White JD: High-yield radiographic considerations for cervical spine injuries. *Ann Emerg Med* 1986;15:236-239.

36. Ross SE, Schwab CW, David ET, Delong WG, Born CT: Clearing the cervical spine: Initial radiographic evaluation. *J Trauma* 1987;27:1055-1060.

37. Freemyer B, Knopp R, Piche J, Wales L, Williams J: Comparison of five-view and three-view cervical spine series in evaluation of patients with cervical trauma. *Ann Emerg Med* 1989;18:818-821.

38. Orenstein JB, Klein BL, Gotschall CS, Ochsenschlager DW, Klatzko MD, Eichelberger MR: Age and outcome in pediatric cervical spine injury. *Pediatr Emerg Care* 1994;10:132-137.

39. Flynn JM, Closkey RF, Mahboubi S, Dormans JP: Role of magnetic resonance imaging in the assessment of pediatric cervical spine injuries. *J Pediatr Orthop* 2002;22:573-577.
    The authors of this article report that MRI scans obtained in obtunded or nonverbal children with suspected cervical spine injuries, equivocal plain films, neurologic symptoms without radiographic abnormalities, and inability to clear the cervical spine within 3 days confirmed the plain radiographic diagnosis in two thirds of patients and altered the diagnosis in one third of patients.

40. Cattell HS, Filtzer DL: Pseudosubluxation and other normal variations in the cervical spine in children. *J Bone Joint Surg Am* 1965;47:1295-1309.

41. Swischuk LE: Anterior displacement of C2 in children: Physiologic or pathologic. *Radiology* 1977;122:759-763.

42. Juhl JH, Miller SM, Roberts GW: Roentgenographic variations in the normal cervical spine. *Radiology* 1962;78:591-597.

43. Fineman S, Borrelli FJ, Rubinstein BM, Epstein H, Jacobson HG: The cervical spine: Transformation of the normal lordotic pattern into a linear pattern in neutral posture. *J Bone Joint Surg Am* 1963;45:1179-1183.

44. Weir DC: Roentgenographic signs of cervical injury. *Clin Orthop Relat Res* 1975;109:9-17.

45. Leventhal HR: Birth injuries of the spinal cord. *J Pediatr* 1960;56:447-453.

46. Scher AT: Trauma of the spinal cord in children. *S Afr Med J* 1976;50:2023-2024.

47. Khanna AJ, Wasserman BA, Sponseller PD: Magnetic resonance imaging of the pediatric spine. *J Am Acad Orthop Surg* 2003;11:248-259.
    The authors of this article reviewed the role of MRI in assessing pediatric spine disease, including trauma, infections, and neoplasms.

48. Davis PC, Reisner A, Hudgins PA, Davis WE, O'Brien MS: Spinal injuries in children: Role of MRI. *AJNR Am J Neuroradiol* 1993;14:607-617.

49. Grabb PA, Pang D: Magnetic resonance imaging in the evaluation of spinal cord injury with radiographic abnormality in children. *Neurosurgery* 1994;35:406-414.

50. Ahmann PA, Smith SA, Schwartz JF, Clark DB: Spinal cord infarction due to minor trauma in children. *Neurology* 1975;25:301-307.

51. Walsh JW, Stevens DB, Young AB: Traumatic paraplegia in children without contiguous spinal fracture or dislocation. *Neurosurgery* 1983;12:439-445.

52. Bracken MB, Collins WF, Freeman DF, et al: Efficacy of methylprednisolone in acute spinal cord injury. *JAMA* 1984;251:45-52.

53. Bracken MB, Shepherd MJ, Collins WF, et al: A randomized, controlled trial of methylprednisolone or naloxone in treatment of acute spinal cord injury: Results of the Second National Acute Spinal Cord Injury Study. *N Engl J Med* 1990;322:1405-1411.

54. Spinal cord injury without radiographic abnormality. *Neurosurgery* 2002;50(suppl 3):S100-S104.
    Fifteen articles on spinal cord injuries without radiographic abnormality were reviewed to create standard diagnostic, therapeutic, and prognostic standards.

55. Sun PP, Poffenbarger GJ, Durham S, Zimmerman RA: Spectrum of occipitoatlantoaxial injury in young children. *J Neurosurg* 2000;93(suppl 1):28-39.
    In this study, 71 consecutive injuries of the occipitoatlantoaxial region were evaluated. Based on MRI findings, the authors proposed that these injuries occur in a stepwise fashion, with instability occurring with disruption of the tentorial membrane.

56. Bucholz RW, Burkhead WZ: The pathological anatomy of fetal atlanto-occipital dislocations. *J Bone Joint Surg Am* 1979;61:248-250.

57. Kaufman RA, Carroll CD, Buncher CR: Atlantooccipital junction: standards for measurement in normal children. *AJNR Am J Neuroradiol* 1987;8:995-999.

58. Papadopoulos SM, Dickman CA, Sonntag VK, Rekate HL, Spetzler RF: Traumatic atlantooccipital dislocation with survival. *Neurosurgery* 1991;28:574-579.

59. Kenter K, Worley G, Griffin T, Fitch RD: Pediatric traumatic atlanto-occipital dislocation: Five cases and a review. *J Pediatr Orthop* 2001;21:585-589.
    Five patients with atlanto-occipital dislocations that occurred over a 10-year period were retrospectively reviewed by the authors. A synopsis of the parameters used to diagnose this injury is also provided.

60. Powers B, Miller MD, Kramer RS, Martinez S, Gehweiler JA Jr: Traumatic anterior atlanto-occipital dislocation. *Neurosurgery* 1979;4:12-17.

61. Kowalski HM, Cohen WA, Cooper P, Wishoff JH: Pitfalls in the CT diagnosis of atlantoaxial rotatory subluxation. *AJR Am J Roentgenol* 1987;149:595-600.

62. Phillips WA, Hensinger RN: The management rotatory atlanto-axial subluxation in children. *J Bone Joint Surg Am* 1989;71:664-668.

63. Murray JB, Ziervogel M: The value of computed tomography in the diagnosis of atlanto-axial rotatory fixation. *Br J Radiol* 1990;63:894-897.

64. Scapinelli R: The three-dimensional computed tomography in infantile atlantoaxial rotatory fixation. *J Bone Joint Surg Br* 1994;76:367-370.

65. Cowan IA, Inglis GS: Atlanto-axial rotatory fixation: Improved demonstration using spiral CT. *Australas Radiol* 1996;40:119-124.

66. Roche CJ, O'Malley M, Dorgan JC, Carty HM: A pictorial review of atlanto-axial rotatory fixation: Key points for the radiologist. *Clin Radiol* 2001;56:947-958.

67. Roche C, Carty H: Spinal trauma in children. *Pediatr Radiol* 2001;31:677-700.

68. Fielding JW, Hawkins RJ: Atlantoaxial rotatory fixation (fixed subluxation of the atlanto-axial joint). *J Bone Joint Surg Am* 1977;59:37-44.

69. Denis F: Three column spine and its significance in classification of acute thoracolumbar spinal injuries. *Spine* 1983;8:817-831.

70. Chance GQ: Note on type of flexion fracture of spine. *Br J Radiol* 1948;21:452-453.

71. Anderson PA, Henley MB, Rivara FP, Maier RV: Flexion-distraction and Chance injuries to thoracolumbar spine. *J Orthop Trauma* 1991;5:153-160.

72. Gertzbein SD, Court-Brown CM: Rationale for management of flexion-distraction injuries of lumbar spine. *J Spinal Disord* 1989;2:176-183.

73. Rooks VJ, Sisler C, Burton B: Cervical spine injury in child abuse: Report of two cases. *Pediatr Radiol* 1998;28:193-195.

74. Ghatan S, Ellenbogen RG: Pediatric spine and spinal cord injury after inflicted trauma. *Neurosurg Clin N Am* 2002;13:227-233.
    The authors of this article reviewed their own experiences with pediatric spine injuries and correlated their results with the findings in the literature. They suggested that spinal cord injuries may be more prominent than previously realized.

75. Hadley MN, Sonntag VK, Rekate HL, Murphy A: The infant whiplash-shake injury syndrome: A clinical and pathologic study. *Neurosurgery* 1989;24:536-540.

76. Carrion WV, Dormans JP, Drummond DS, Christofersen MR: Circumferential growth plate fracture of the thoracolumbar spine from child abuse. *J Pediatr Orthop* 1996;16:210-214.

77. Vogel LC: Unique management needs of pediatric spinal cord injury patients: Etiology and pathophysiology. *J Spinal Cord Med* 1997;20:10-13.

78. MacKinnon JA, Perleman M, Kirpalani H, Rehan V, Sauve R, Kovacs L: Spinal cord injury at birth: Diagnostic and prognostic data in twenty-two patients. *J Pediatr* 1993;122:431-437.

79. Menticoglou SM, Perleman M, Manning FA: High cervical spinal cord injury in neonates delivered with forceps: Report of 15 cases. *Obstet Gynecol* 1995;86:589-594.

80. Bresnan MJ, Abrams LF: Neonatal spinal cord transaction secondary to intrauterine hyperextension of neck in breech position. *J Pediatr* 1974;84:734-737.

81. Fotter R, Sorantin E, Schneider U, Ranner G, Fast C, Schober P: Ultrasound diagnosis of birth-related spinal cord trauma: Neonatal diagnosis and follow-up and correlation with MRI. *Pediatr Radiol* 1994;24:241-244.

82. Pang D, Hanley ED: Special problems of spinal stabilization in children, in Cooper PR (ed): *Management of Posttraumatic Spinal Instability: Neuro-surgical Topics No. 3.* Park Ridge, IL, American Association of Neurological Surgeons, 1990, pp 181-206.

83. Nobunaga AI, Go BK, Karunas RB: Recent demographic and injury trends in people served by the Model Spinal Cord Injury Care Systems. *Arch Phys Med Rehabil* 1999;80:1372-1382.

84. Kane T, Capen DA, Waters R, Zigler JE, Adkins R: Spinal cord injury from civilian gunshot wounds: The Rancho experience 1980-1988. *J Spinal Disord* 1991;4:306-311.

85. Waters RL, Sie IH: Spinal cord injuries from gunshot wounds to the spine. *Clin Orthop* 2003;408:120-125.
    This article is a review of the epidemiology, ballistics science, patterns of neurologic injury and recovery, and complications of spinal cord injuries caused by gunshot wounds.

86. Waters RL, Adkins RH, Yakura J, Sie I: Profiles of spinal cord injury and recovery after gunshot injury. *Clin Orthop* 1991;267:14-21.

87. Ragucci MV, Gittler MM, Balfanz-Vertiz K, Hunter A: Societal risk factors associated with spinal cord injury secondary to gunshot wound. *Arch Phys Med Rehabil* 2001;82:1720-1723.
    The authors conducted a survey study of 56 patients admitted to a spinal cord injury rehabilitation hospital for spinal injury caused by gunshots. Most respondents were found to have previous involvement in the criminal justice system and only one had a previous social service intervention.

88. Heary RF, Vaccaro AR, Mesa JJ, Balderston RA: Thoracolumbar infections in penetrating injuries to the spine. *Orthop Clin North Am* 1996;27:69-81.

89. Waters RL, Hu SS: Penetrating injuries of the spinal cord: Stab and gunshot injuries, in Frymoyer JW (ed): *The Adult Spine: Principles and Practice.* New York, NY, Raven Press, 1991, pp 815-826.

90. Brown TD, Michas P, Williams RE, et al: The impact of gunshot wounds on an orthopedic surgical service in an urban trauma center. *J Orthop Trauma* 1997;11:149-153.

91. Violence in America: A public health crisis. The role of firearms: The Violence Prevention Task Force of the Eastern Association for the Surgery of Trauma. *J Trauma* 1995;38:163-168.

92. Garland D, Wharton G: Spinal cord injury care: Funding for the future. *Orthopedics* 1994;17:675-678.

93. McKinley WO, Jackson AB, Cardenas DD, DeVivo MJ: Long-term medical complications after traumatic spinal cord injury: A regional model systems analysis. *Arch Phys Med Rehabil* 1999;80:1402-1410.

94. Carrillo E, Gonzalez J, Camillo L, et al: Spinal cords in adolescents after gunshot wounds: An increasing phenomenon in urban North America. *Injury* 1998;29:503-507.

95. Smugar SS, Schweitzer ME, Hume E: MRI in patients with intraspinal bullets. *J Magn Reson Imaging* 1999;9:151-153.

96. DeMuth WE: Bullet velocity and design as determinants of wounding capacity: An experimental study. *J Trauma* 1966;6:222-232.

97. Eismont FJ, Lattuga S: Gunshot wounds of the spine, in Browner BD, Jupiter JB, Levine AM, Trafton PG (eds): *Skeletal Trauma: Basic Science, Management, and Reconstruction*, ed 3. Philadelphia, PA, WB Saunders, 2003, pp 983-1003.

98. Finitsis SN, Falcone S, Green BA: MR of the spine in the presence of metallic bullet fragments: Is the benefit worth the risk? *AJNR Am J Neuroradiol* 1999;20:354-356.

99. Isiklar ZU, Lindsey RW: Low velocity civilian gunshot wounds of the spine. *Orthopedics* 1997;20:967-972.

100. Cornwell EE III, Chang DC, Bonar JP, et al: Thoracolumbar immobilization for trauma patients with torso gunshot wounds: Is it necessary? *Arch Surg* 2001;136:324-327.

    This is a retrospective analysis of data from a state trauma registry. The authors assessed the data of 1,000 patients with torso gunshot injuries and concluded that prehospital thoracolumbar immobilization is rarely beneficial for patients with this type of injury.

101. Benzel EC, Hadden TA, Coleman JE: Civilian gunshot wounds to the spinal cord and cauda equina. *Neurosurgery* 1987;20:281-285.

102. Stauffer ES, Wood RW, Kelly EG: Gunshot wounds of the spine: The effects of laminectomy. *J Bone Joint Surg Am* 1979;61:389-392.

103. Bartlett CS: Clinical update: Gunshot wound ballistics. *Clin Orthop* 2003;408:28-57.

    The author of this article provides a comprehensive review of ballistics injury. The various factors affecting energy transfer of projectile to target as well as the evaluation of tissue damage are discussed.

104. Heiden JS, Weiss MH, Rosenberg AW, Kurze T, Apuzzo MLJ: Penetrating gunshot wounds of the cervical spine in civilians. *J Neurosurg* 1975;42:575-579.

105. Waters RL, Adkins RH: The effects of removal of bullet fragments retained in the spinal canal: A collaborative study by the National Spinal Cord Injury Model Systems. *Spine* 1991;16:934-939.

106. Aarabi B, Alibaii E, Taghipur M, Kamgarpur A: Comparative study of functional recovery for surgically explored and conservatively managed spinal cord missile injuries. *Neurosurgery* 1996;39:1133-1140.

107. Roffi RP, Waters RL, Adkins RH: Gunshot wounds to the spine associated with perforated viscus. *Spine* 1989;14:808-811.

108. Wu WQ: Delayed effects of relational foreign bodies in the spinal cord. *Surg Neurol* 1986;25:214-218.

109. Karim NO, Nabors MW, Golocovsky M, Cooney FD: Spontaneous migration of a bullet in the spinal subarachnoid space causing delayed radicular symptoms. *Neurosurgery* 1986;18:97-100.

110. Grogan DP, Bucholz RW: Acute head intoxication from a bullet in an intervertebral disc space: A case report. *J Bone Joint Surg Am* 1981;63:1180-1182.

111. Tindel NL, Marcillo AE, Tay BK, Bunge RP, Eismont FJ: The effect of surgically implanted bullet fragments on the spinal cord in a rabbit model. *J Bone Joint Surg Am* 2001;83-A:884-890.

    In this study, copper, aluminum, and lead fragments were implanted in intradural and extradural locations of 17 New Zealand white rabbits. Histologic analysis revealed that intradural copper produced major destruction of adjacent axons and myelin. The authors recommended removal of copper fragments from the spinal cord even in the absence of neurologic deficits.

112. Richards JS, Stover SL, Jaworski T: Effects of bullet removal on subsequent pain in persons with spinal cord injury secondary to gunshot wound. *J Neurosurg* 1990;73:401-404.

Section 5

Lower Extremity

Section Editors:
Mark C. Reilly, MD
David C. Teague, MD

Chapter 31

Hip Dislocations and Femoral Head and Neck Fractures

Sean E. Nork, MD

Lisa K. Cannada, MD

Hip Dislocations

Hip dislocations and fracture-dislocations occur across all age groups and most frequently are the result of motor vehicle accidents. These injuries represent an orthopaedic emergency requiring prompt reduction of the hip to protect the femoral head blood supply from further disruption. Associated injuries occur frequently, especially fractures of the acetabulum and femoral head. Posterior dislocations occur much more commonly than anterior dislocations.

The commonly assumed mechanism of a dashboard impact as the primary cause of injury was challenged in a recent study reviewing 48 patients with hip dislocations after head-on motor vehicle crashes.[1] Interestingly, the right hip was involved in 45 patients (93.8%). Furthermore, in patients with associated ipsilateral foot or ankle injuries, more than 90% of the injuries were located on the right side. If a dashboard impact alone were the primary mechanism of injury, a more equal distribution between right- and left-sided injuries would be expected. The authors hypothesized that the right leg position (flexion, adduction, and internal rotation) while the driver presses on the brake pedal may contribute to the observed increased incidence of right-sided hip dislocations in their patient population.

Because of the usual posteriorly directed force that occurs during a motor vehicle crash, posterior dislocations occur more commonly than anterior dislocations, and associated acetabular fractures occur in most patients. Associated injuries occur frequently and have been reported to occur in 95% of patients with a traumatic hip dislocation secondary to a motor vehicle crash.[2] Sciatic nerve injuries occur in approximately 10% of patients after posterior hip dislocations, most commonly involving the peroneal division. In one study, 70% of patients had an associated acetabular fracture, whereas other extremity fractures were identified in 39%. More importantly, despite improved safety systems including passenger restraints, associated closed-head, thoracic, craniofacial, and abdominal injuries were observed frequently (at 24%, 21%, 21%, and 15%, respec-

tively), suggesting the need for general surgical evaluation in patients sustaining traumatic posterior hip dislocations.

Urgent reduction of a posteriorly dislocated hip, in addition to providing patient comfort and minimizing further stretching of the sciatic nerve, maximizes femoral head perfusion. Closed reduction in the emergency department is recommended after sufficient patient sedation and muscle relaxation. If a closed reduction is unsuccessful, further radiologic evaluation to determine the cause is necessary. An associated femoral head fracture and/or a small posterior wall rim avulsion fracture should alert clinicians to the possibility of an associated labral avulsion, which can become a mechanical block to relocation. Failure to obtain a closed reduction is an indication for urgent open reduction. The value of this procedure was confirmed in a study evaluating the relationship between length of time to relocation and the severity of associated nerve injuries. The incidence of major sciatic nerve injuries was higher in patients transferred with the hip still dislocated, and patients with an associated nerve injury had a significantly longer time to relocation than those without.[3]

Plain radiographs after reduction must be obtained and scrutinized for joint congruency and the presence of associated fractures (especially femoral head, femoral neck, or posterior wall acetabular fractures). CT may be useful in ensuring that the acetabulum is free of injury or debris. Immediate weight bearing may be allowed, but appropriate hip precautions are recommended for 6 weeks following dislocation. Osteonecrosis of the femoral head is a potentially devastating complication that occurs in fewer than 10% of patients who undergo prompt reduction of a posterior hip dislocation.

Femoral Head Fractures

Fractures of the femoral head are associated with dislocations of the hip and occur in between 6% and 16% of posterior hip dislocations.[4,5] Femoral head fractures associated with posterior hip dislocations are thought to be produced by contact of the femoral head on the posterior acetabular rim during the dislocation. The location, comminution, and displacement patterns are related to the hip position at impact as well as the energy and load application of the traumatic event.

Anatomy and Classification

In addition to the joint capsule, the ligamentum teres represents a strong attachment between the acetabulum (cotyloid fossa) and femoral head (fovea centralis). Additionally, the ligamentum teres arterial branch from the obturator artery supplies approximately 10% to 15% of the femoral head blood supply. In pure hip dislocations, this structure is obligatorily torn. However, in patients with an associated femoral head fracture after a posterior hip dislocation, the ligamentum teres may remain contiguous with the femoral head segment if the fracture exits cephalad to the fovea centralis.

Several authors have classified femoral head fractures. The most frequently used system, the Pipkin classification, reflects the fracture location and the commonly observed associated injuries to the hip joint (Figure 1). According to this scheme, type I fractures are infrafoveal and are characterized by disruption of the ligamentum teres from the femoral head fragments. Type II fractures are suprafoveal and are characterized by maintenance of the ligamentum teres attachment to the fracture fragment. The type III and IV patterns are characterized by an associated femoral neck or acetabular fracture, respectively. This classification is limited, however, because the fracture location (the distinction between infrafoveal versus suprafoveal) is not reflected in the type III and IV injury patterns.

Femoral head fractures typically involve the anteromedial aspect of the femoral head. The size and extent of the fractures are extremely variable. Impaction of the intact cancellous surface of the dislocated segment of the femoral head is commonly observed because this portion of the head typically rests on the retroacetabular surface. An associated avulsion of the acetabular labrum from the posterior acetabular rim is frequently observed and may prevent a closed reduction in these injuries.

Diagnostic Evaluation and Reduction

The initial radiographic evaluation of any patient with a suspected hip dislocation should include a screening AP pelvic radiograph. This radiograph should be carefully scrutinized for any associated injuries including fractures of the acetabulum, femoral neck, and femoral head. Because of the anteromedial location of most femoral head fractures, Judet oblique radiographs (particularly the obturator oblique view) will demonstrate the fracture well. After a careful evaluation to ensure there are no further associated injuries, a prompt reduction of the dislocated hip should be performed. Pharmacologic muscle relax-

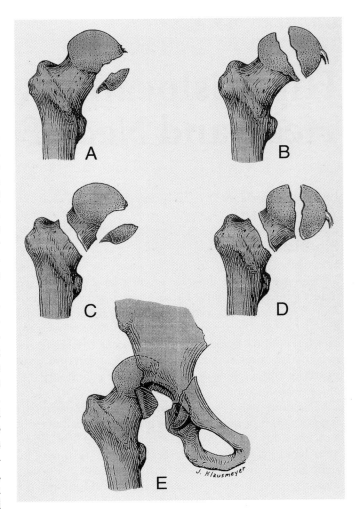

Figure 1 Classification of femoral head fractures. **A,** Infrafoveal fracture (Pipkin I, Brumback IA). **B,** Suprafoveal fracture (Pipkin II, Brumback IIA). **C** and **D,** Infrafoveal fracture or suprafoveal fracture associated with a femoral neck fracture (Pipkin III, Brumback IIIB). **E,** Any femoral head fracture configuration associated with an acetabular fracture (Pipkin IV, Brumback IB or IIB). *(Reproduced with permission from Swiontkowski MF: Intracapsular hip fractures, in Browner BD, Jupiter JB, Levine AM, Trafton PG (eds): Skeletal Trauma: Basic Science, Management, and Reconstruction, ed 2. Philadelphia, PA, WB Saunders, 1998, p 1756.)*

ation is a necessary part of any closed reduction, and use of a general anesthetic should be considered. However, if a general anesthetic is not available or impractical, a reduction attempt with the patient under conscious sedation is a reasonable alternative. Reduction maneuvers in the emergency department should be limited to a single attempt in a relaxed patient. Iatrogenic femoral neck fractures have been reported after forceful attempts. If a closed reduction is unsuccessful, open reduction should be performed immediately.

Radiographic confirmation of a successful closed reduction is established with AP and lateral hip radiographs or AP and Judet oblique pelvic radiographs. CT should then be used routinely to evaluate these injuries. CT scans should be scrutinized for the presence of intraarticular debris, the congruency of reduction, and any associated fractures. A treatment plan can then be formulated based on these images.

Treatment

The treatment of fractures of the femoral head depends on several factors, including patient age, associated injuries, amount of the femoral head involved, and location of the fracture relative to the weight-bearing dome. Closed treatment can be considered for isolated, small, infrafoveal fractures (Pipkin type I). The CT scan should be carefully evaluated to ensure that the hip is concentrically reduced and there is no associated intra-articular debris. Closed management consists of restricted weight bearing with posterior hip precautions followed by progressive weight bearing as tolerated. However, even in infrafoveal fractures, surgical treatment may be necessary. Malunited inferomedial femoral head fractures blocking hip motion have been reported in several patients after nonsurgical treatment.[6,7] In these studies, excision of the inferomedial fragment through an anterior surgical exposure was successful in restoring motion. It has been postulated that primary fragment excision may have prevented this complication.

Most displaced femoral head fractures require surgical treatment to ensure an anatomic reduction. This includes most (if not all) suprafoveal fractures and large infrafoveal fractures that contribute to hip joint instability. Because suprafoveal fractures involve the portion of the femoral head that corresponds to the weight-bearing dome of the acetabulum, even minor incongruities in this location are unlikely to be tolerated by the hip joint.

The surgical approach for fixation of these injuries remains controversial. However, because of the anteromedial fracture location and the posterior blood supply to the hip, anterior approaches may optimize fracture reduction and minimize the risk for further vascular compromise. The surgical approach most commonly advocated for treatment of these fractures is the Smith-Petersen anterior exposure.[8-10] Depending on the location of the cephalad extent of the fracture, an anterior surgical dislocation may be necessary to accurately reduce and stabilize the femoral head injury. An anterior T-shaped capsulotomy is made parallel to the acetabular rim, avoiding damage to the femoral head blood supply. An effort should be made to retain any soft-tissue attachments to the fractured femoral head fragment. An alternative exposure is a digastric trochanteric osteotomy with an anterior surgical dislocation, resulting in a similar level of femoral head visualization. In either approach, a thorough knowledge of the femoral head blood supply is necessary to ensure its preservation and avoid iatrogenic injury. The femoral head fracture can then be stabilized using implants that are countersunk below the articular surface. Given the peripheral loading characteristics observed in the hip joint,[11] multiple small implants are

usually of adequate size to maintain the reduction until union (Figure 2).

Although rare, an associated femoral neck fracture (Pipkin type III) further complicates the management of these injuries. Frequently, the anteromedial fragment is the only portion of the femoral head that remains in the acetabulum, and the remaining femoral head is usually dislocated posteriorly, with minimal associated soft-tissue attachments. Very few reports have been published to guide the management of patients with this injury combination. Prosthetic replacement should be a consideration if soft-tissue attachments to the head fragments are lacking. If open reduction is performed, successful surgical management requires reduction and fixation of both injuries simultaneously. This can be accomplished through either a Watson-Jones (Figure 3) or a Smith-Petersen approach.

In patients with combined femoral head and acetabular fractures, each injury should initially be considered separately to determine the individual needs for surgical fixation. Most of the associated acetabular fractures that occur in combination with fractures of the femoral head are small, posterior rim acetabular fractures and represent an avulsion of the acetabular labrum. The decision to stabilize an associated posterior wall (or rim) acetabular fracture should usually be based on the acetabular fracture characteristics alone. If, however, the femoral head fracture is not fixed or if fragment excision is performed, smaller acetabular fractures may require fixation because of the overall hip joint instability pattern produced by this combination of injuries.

Clinical Results

The long-term treatment outcomes for patients with femoral head fractures remain unknown because most published reports include a small number of patients and combine differing injury patterns and multiple surgical exposures, which make deriving useful conclusions challenging.

An older study retrospectively reviewed the surgical outcomes of 24 patients with Pipkin type I or type II injuries.[9] At a minimum 2-year follow-up, the anterior exposure was associated with decreased surgical time, improved visualization, and no instances of osteonecrosis when compared with using a posterior surgical exposure. However, patients who underwent anterior exposure were found to have a greater incidence of heterotopic ossification. A recent study confirmed these findings and reported that, compared with an anterior approach, the use of the Kocher-Langenbeck approach resulted in a 3.2-fold increase in osteonecrosis.[8] Improved fracture reduction also was noted after the anterior approach. More recently, the surgical outcomes of 30 patients with femoral head fractures were retrospectively evaluated and fragment excision was found to be appropriate in the treatment of small infrafoveal fractures, open reduction

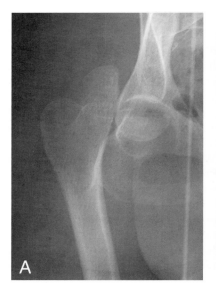
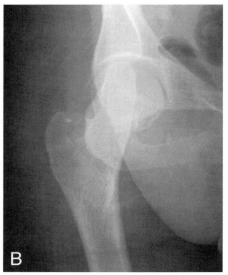
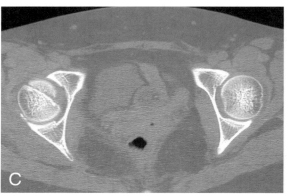
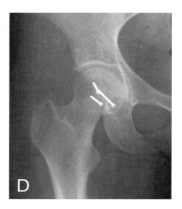

Figure 2 The injury radiograph **(A)** and postreduction radiograph **(B)** demonstrate the presence of a suprafoveal fracture in a 24-year-old female patient with a left hip fracture-dislocation caused by a motor vehicle collision. **C,** CT scan clearly shows the anteromedial fracture locations and the fracture displacement. **D,** Postoperative radiograph of the same patient. An anterior (Smith-Petersen) approach combined with an intraoperative anterior hip dislocation was used to accurately reduce and stabilize the femoral head fracture.

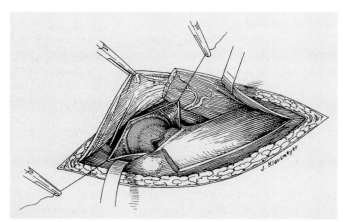

Figure 3 Schematic representation of the Watson-Jones anterolateral exposure to the hip for open reduction of femoral neck fractures. The interval between the tensor fasciae latae and the abductors is bluntly developed, and the vastus lateralis is elevated off the intertrochanteric ridge. The capsule is divided anteriorly along the axis of the neck of the femur and transversely released from its insertion into the proximal part of the femur. With sutures as retracting aids, the fracture can be visualized. A bone hook can be used to disimpact the fracture by applying a laterally directed force, and a blunt instrument can be inserted to improve the reduction (lift the proximal fragment anteriorly). The insertion area for internal fixation devices on the lateral aspect of the proximal end of the femur is easily exposed. *(Reproduced with permission from Swiontkowski MF: Intracapsular hip fractures, in Browner BD, Jupiter JB, Levine AM, Trafton PG (eds): Skeletal Trauma: Basic Science, Management, and Reconstruction, ed 2. Philadelphia, PA, WB Saunders, 1998, p 1790.)*

appropriate for the treatment of larger infrafoveal and suprafoveal fractures, and arthroplasty appropriate for the treatment of comminuted fractures involving large portions of the femoral head.[10]

Complications

The complications observed in patients with femoral head fractures reflect the combined effects of the injury and the surgical treatment. These complications include heterotopic ossification, aseptic necrosis, failure of fixation, and posttraumatic arthritis. Although ectopic bone can occur after an anterior hip exposure for the treatment of a femoral head fracture, functionally significant ectopic bone requiring excision is rarely encountered. It is typically located directly over the anterior hip joint in the region of the rectus tendon and the iliocapsularis muscle. Sharp dissection during the anterior surgical exposure may help minimize this complication. Aseptic necrosis is a potential complication after any traumatic hip injury, and its incidence is likely increased with delayed reduction of a hip joint dislocation. The integrity of the ligamentum teres and its effect on the subsequent development of aseptic necrosis is not clearly understood. The impact of the surgical incision of an intact ligamentum teres is also unknown, but it does not appear to increase the rate of aseptic necrosis of either the intact or fractured segments of the femoral head. Although this complication is uncommon (0 to 23% of patients[8,9,12,13]), it has devastating long-term implications, and preoperative counseling is paramount. Fixation failure occurs rarely in the absence of osteonecrosis or nonunion. The risk of posttraumatic arthritis should be minimized with an accurate and anatomic reduction of the femoral head. However, fracture comminution and peripheral impaction are common and theoretically may contribute to uneven load distribution and acetabular wear. Long-term studies are needed to estimate the frequency of this complication.

Femoral Neck Fractures in Young Patients

Although femoral neck fractures occur more commonly in elderly patients after a fall, they can occur in young patients after a high-energy traumatic event. The mechanisms of injury in younger patients typically include motor vehicle accidents, motorcycle accidents, falls from a height, and injury occurring while participating in high-impact athletic activities. Early diagnosis and treatment are required in young patients because devastating complications occur with some frequency. An understanding of the fracture pattern, associated injuries, biomechanics of fixation, and local anatomy is important in the initial assessment of these patients.

Diagnosis

The clinical presentation of patients with a femoral neck fracture is variable depending on the fracture type and associated mechanism of injury. In patients with stress fractures, nondisplaced fractures, or impacted fractures, groin or buttock pain may be the only initial clinical indicator of injury. However, in patients with an acute and displaced femoral neck fracture, limb shortening and external rotation combined with severe pain are the typical presenting signs and symptoms. In unresponsive or unconscious patients, a high index of suspicion for a femoral neck fracture is necessary; such patients frequently require multiple clinical evaluations, even when the initial radiographs fail to demonstrate evidence of a fracture.

The initial radiographic evaluation includes AP and lateral plain radiographs of the hip. Ideally, the AP view should be taken with the limb held in approximately 10° to 15° of internal rotation to compensate for the anteversion of the femoral neck. This positions the femoral neck on its longest viewable axis to assist with the identification of nondisplaced fractures. In patients with a fracture, however, pain may limit the amount of limb rotation and, hence, the quality of the initial radiographic evaluation. The lateral radiograph helps evaluate frac-

ture displacement if present. A cross-table lateral radiograph is recommended over a frog-lateral radiograph to minimize patient discomfort and the stresses on the femoral neck.

If there is a clinical suggestion of injury to the hip but no evidence of injury on plain radiographs, additional diagnostic studies are required to eliminate the possibility of an occult or nondisplaced femoral neck fracture. MRI has been shown to be both sensitive and specific in the early diagnosis (within 24 hours of injury) of occult fractures of the femoral neck. A technetium bone scan may also be obtained if MRI is unavailable or contraindicated, although 72 hours may be needed before the results of this test are determined.

CT of the abdomen and pelvis is frequently part of the initial evaluation of young patients involved in traumatic accidents. Although a CT scan is not necessary for the routine evaluation of the femoral neck, if obtained for other evaluations, it may reveal an occult injury. In a study of 14 femoral neck fractures that were identified as being associated with an ipsilateral femoral shaft fracture, 8 femoral neck fractures were not visible on initial AP pelvic radiographs.[14] In 6 of these 8 fractures, the fracture was visible on the preoperative CT scan, confirming the usefulness of this study in identifying occult neck fractures.

Vascular Anatomy

The femoral head receives its blood supply from the medial and lateral femoral circumflex vessels, obturator artery, and metaphyseal perforating vessels. The relative contributions of these vessels to the total blood supply of the femoral head have been described previously.[15-17] The lateral epiphyseal artery (the terminal branch of the medial femoral circumflex vessel) is the primary blood supply and runs along the posterosuperior aspect of the femoral neck before terminating into two to four retinacular branches that enter the femoral head.[18] A precise understanding of the vascular anatomy is necessary for safe surgical treatment of hip dislocations and femoral neck fractures.

Classification

Useful fracture classification systems ideally facilitate communication, influence treatment, and predict results. However, many systems are difficult to use and have poor reproducibility. Classification systems most frequently used include the Garden (Figure 4), Orthopaedic Trauma Association/AO (Figure 5), and the Pauwels (Figure 6) schemes.

The Garden classification, based on the recognition of fracture displacements evident on AP pelvic radiographs, includes four stages. Stage I fractures are incomplete with impaction or valgus positioning. Stage II fractures are complete but nondisplaced. Stage III fractures

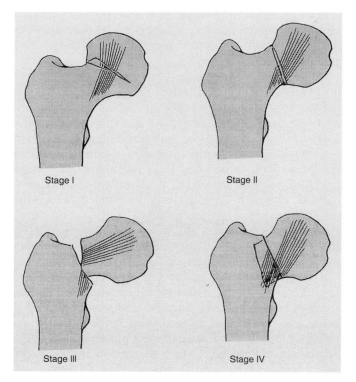

Figure 4 Schematic representation of the Garden classification of femoral neck fractures. Stage I is an incomplete, impacted fracture in valgus malalignment (generally stable). Stage II is a nondisplaced fracture. Stage III is an incompletely displaced fracture in varus malalignment. Stage IV is a completely displaced fracture with no engagement of the two fragments. The compression trabeculae in the femoral head line up with the trabeculae on the acetabular side. Displacement is generally more evident on the lateral view in stage IV. For prognostic purposes, these groupings can be lumped into nondisplaced/impacted (stages I and II) and displaced (stages III and IV), as the risks of nonunion and aseptic necrosis are similar within these grouped stages. *(Reproduced with permission from Swiontkowski MF: Intracapsular hip fractures, in Browner BD, Jupiter JB, Levine AM, Trafton PG (eds): Skeletal Trauma: Basic Science, Management, and Reconstruction, ed 2. Philadelphia, PA, WB Saunders, 1998, p 1775.)*

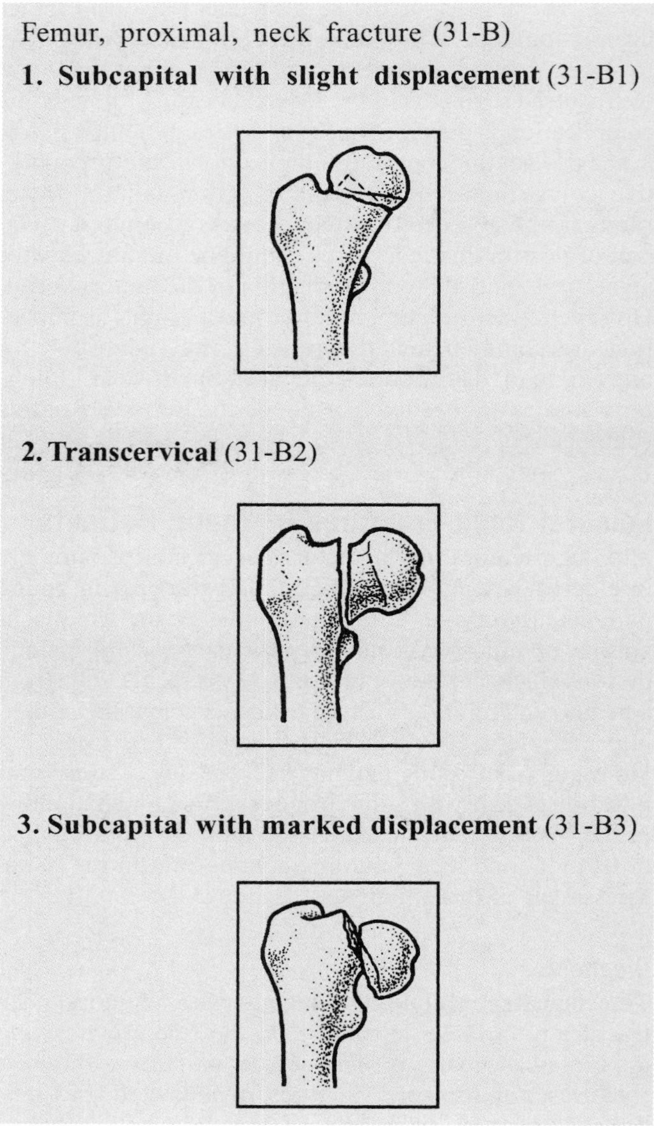

Femur, proximal, neck fracture (31-B)

1. Subcapital with slight displacement (31-B1)

2. Transcervical (31-B2)

3. Subcapital with marked displacement (31-B3)

Figure 5 Schematic representation of the Orthopaedic Trauma Association/AO classification of femoral neck fractures. *(Reproduced with permission from Orthopaedic Trauma Association Committee for Coding and Classification: Fracture and dislocation compendium. J Orthop Trauma 1996;10(suppl 1):32-33.)*

are complete fractures with only partial displacement. Stage IV fractures are characterized by complete displacement. Realignment of the bony trabeculae between the femoral head and the acetabulum occurs in patients with stage IV fractures because the posterior retinacular attachments to the femoral head are lost. A recent report simplified the Garden classification by distinguishing only nondisplaced (stages I and II) and displaced (stages III and IV) femoral neck fractures, which substantially improved both interobserver and intraobserver reliability.[19]

The Orthopaedic Trauma Association/AO classification for femoral neck fractures has nine groups that can be further divided based on fracture displacements and comminution. This system has been criticized for being too complex as well as nonpredictive from a treatment or outcomes perspective.[20] Poor intraobserver and interobserver reliability and limited predictive value was again identified in a recent study reviewing the radiographic classification of these injuries. Restructuring the nine groups into three categories (nondisplaced fractures, basilar fractures, and displaced fractures) resulted in ex-

cellent interobserver and intraobserver reliability and improved prediction of treatment and outcome.

The Pauwels classification is a biomechanical model based on the angle of the femoral neck fracture line relative to the horizontal (type I is up to 30°, type II is between 30° and 50°, and type III is 50° and higher). Because compressive forces dominate in Pauwels type I fractures, the fracture configuration is considered relatively stable. In Pauwels type II fractures, a shearing force is present but may be neutralized with internal fixation. The real theoretic challenge exists in Pauwels type III fractures in which the dominant force is shear that tends to cause varus angulation and inferior translation of the femoral head segment.[21] The Pauwels clas-

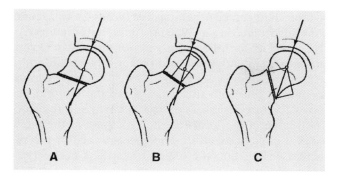

Figure 6 Schematic representation of the Pauwels classification of femoral neck fractures. **A,** In type I patterns, the fracture is relatively horizontal (< 30°) and compressive forces caused by the hip joint reactive force predominate. **B,** In type II patterns, shear forces at the fracture are predicted. **C,** In type III patterns, when the fracture angle is 50° or higher, shear forces predominate. Arrows indicate joint reactive force. *(Adapted with permission from Bartonicek J: Pauwels' classification of femoral neck fractures. J Orthop Trauma 2001;15:359-360.)*

sification has led authors to recommend treatment based on the femoral neck inclination and its potential association with subsequent fracture nonunion.

Treatment

Intracapsular femoral neck fractures in young patients (typically those younger than 50 years) are approached differently than those that occur in elderly patients. The physiologic age of a patient is certainly more important than chronologic age. High-energy femoral neck fractures in patients in the fifth or sixth decade of life require differentiation from the typical low-energy osteoporotic fractures that can occur in elderly patients. The mechanism of injury, fracture pattern, fracture displacement, patient age, and associated injuries will all contribute to the decision-making process regarding treatment.

Intracapsular femoral neck fractures in young patients can be orthopaedic surgical emergencies. Many clinical studies and animal studies demonstrate the effects of a femoral neck fracture on blood flow to the femoral head.[15,22-27] Early surgical reduction and stabilization may improve femoral head blood flow, thereby limiting osteonecrosis to that caused by the injury itself. One recent study reported the results of the early surgical management of femoral neck fractures in elderly patients and the relationship between surgical timing and osteonecrosis.[22] In surviving patients, the rate of osteonecrosis was significantly decreased in those who underwent surgical treatment within 6 hours of injury (10.5%) compared with those who underwent surgical treatment longer than 6 hours after injury (20%). The authors of this study concluded that early surgical intervention is advantageous because it relieves compression trapping of the retinacular vessels, facilitates intraosseous drainage of the femoral head through the reduced cancellous surfaces, and restores the physiologic position of the femoral neck and associated vasculature. Although this study was conducted using elderly patients, the anatomic principles are applicable to younger patients.

Femoral Head Perfusion and Vascular Issues

The blood supply to the femoral head has been previously described.[15,17] These anatomic studies have defined the blood supply to the femoral head and demonstrate the intracapsular location of the vessels that are important for perfusion and femoral head viability. After a fracture of the femoral neck, disruption of some or all of these vessels may occur. In a recent latex injection study, the relationship of the medial femoral circumflex artery to the hip capsule and the posterior muscular attachments has been further elucidated and both the extracapsular and intracapsular segmental branches have been better defined.[18]

Femoral head viability after a fracture of the femoral neck potentially depends on two separate mechanisms that determine femoral head perfusion. Continued and potentially reversible sources of impaired femoral head perfusion include vascular kinking and intracapsular tamponade. Despite femoral neck fracture displacement, capsular integrity and retinacular vessel integrity may exist. The fracture displacement may further compromise femoral head blood flow by kinking the ascending branches of the femoral circumflex vessels. Additionally, capsular distention and pressure can impair femoral head flow, especially when the capsule is completely intact.

Just as it is impossible to determine the integrity of the capsule based on injury radiographs, so too is it impossible to predict intracapsular pressures without additional monitoring. Several studies have demonstrated significant elevations in capsular pressures after a femoral neck fracture. In one such study, the femoral head blood flow of 55 patients with intracapsular femoral neck fractures was prospectively monitored using an intraosseous pressure transducer.[23] In 75% of patients, an increased intracapsular pressure secondary to hemarthrosis was observed. The mean pressures increased from 26 mm Hg in the first 6 hours after injury to 46 mm Hg 7 to 24 hours after injury. Elevated pressures were observed for up to 2 weeks after injury, and no difference was found between displaced and nondisplaced fractures.

Methods for monitoring femoral head blood flow after fracture include dynamic MRI, laser Doppler evaluation, intraosseous pressure monitoring, and direct visualization of blood flow after intraoperative drilling of the femoral head.[23-26,28] One group of authors that used laser Doppler evaluation to demonstrate hemodynamics in the femoral head reported the presence of high sinusoidal flow in intertrochanteric fractures, normal hips, and nondisplaced (Garden stages I and II) femoral neck fractures.[28] However, in 100% of Garden stage IV and 33% of Garden stage III femoral neck fractures, femoral head blood flow measurements were low and nonsinusoidal. In another study, dynamic MRI of the femoral head was performed on 22 patients with a subcapital femoral neck fracture as well as on 10 patients with normal hips and 10 patients with intertrochanteric fractures.[26] The authors reported comparable perfusion with the unaffected side in patients with intertrochanteric fractures and nondisplaced (Garden stages I and II) femoral neck fractures. However, in patients with displaced (Garden stages III and IV) femoral neck fractures, vascular impairment was commonly observed. In a more recent study, dynamic MRI was used to demonstrate normal healing in 19 patients who had some femoral head perfusion.[25] These findings were in contrast to complications identified in 79% of patients with absent perfusion, which included osteonecrosis and nonunion. This information may be of increased importance in elderly or medically compromised patients when the decision to perform arthroplasty versus fixation is unclear. However, the combined findings support the theory that ongoing vascular compromise after displaced femoral neck fractures may contribute to aseptic necrosis.

Hip position has a significant influence on intracapsular pressure. Because the capsular integrity cannot be reliably determined based on the injury radiographs or the initial displacement, hip positioning and its potential effect may be important in all patients with femoral neck fractures. Because flexion, abduction, and external rotation combine to produce the lowest intracapsular hip joint pressures, whereas extension and internal rotation produce the highest intracapsular pressures, maintaining the leg in its normal "antalgic" position with minimal traction until definitive fixation can be accomplished has been recommended.[23,27]

Surgical Treatment

After an appropriate evaluation and attention to life-threatening or limb-threatening injuries, surgical stabilization of the femoral neck fracture should proceed without delay. A closed reduction in the operating room can be done by first flexing the hip in abduction, followed by hip extension and internal rotation while traction is applied. Fluoroscopic evaluation can be used to assess the reduction. In the rare instance where an anatomic reduction is obtained using closed methods, percutaneous stabilization of the femoral neck fracture can be done. Although the decision to perform an additional percutaneous capsulotomy to relieve any ongoing intracapsular vascular disruption should be made at the surgeon's discretion, it should be considered particularly when the hip capsule is likely to be intact. When an adequate closed reduction is not obtained, open reduction should be done. This scenario is commonly observed in younger patients with high-energy fracture patterns as opposed to elderly patients who have experienced a fall from a standing position. Adequate visualization of the femoral neck is necessary for an accurate assessment of the re-

duction. This can be accomplished through a transgluteal (Hardinge) lateral, a Watson-Jones anterolateral approach, or a Smith-Petersen anterior approach. Comminution is frequently observed posteriorly and inferiorly, making the anterior reduction most accurate. A capsular opening in line with the long axis of the femoral neck allows fracture visualization for cleaning and reduction. Knowledge of the local vascular anatomy of the medial femoral circumflex artery and the entrance of the retinacular vessels into the femoral head is a necessity before performing a capsulotomy or placing retractors superiorly and posteriorly.[18] Clamp applications between the femoral head and greater trochanter frequently assist with reduction during fixation. Temporary stabilization with multiple strategically placed Kirschner wires is frequently necessary, especially in patients with comminuted and unstable fracture patterns.

Fixation Methods and Biomechanical Studies

Fixation of a femoral neck fracture should allow for maintenance of reduction during healing, allow some dynamic compression across the fracture site, and ensure rotational stability. Multiple treatment options include multiple cancellous lag screws, a sliding hip screw with or without a derotational screw, a 130° blade plate, or combinations thereof. Three cancellous lag screws are generally adequate for the fixation of most transcervical and subcapital femoral neck fractures. However, the presence of posterior comminution may be associated with a lower resistance to displacement and a lower axial load to failure, necessitating placement of additional fixation. In a biomechanical cadaver study evaluating the use of cancellous lag screws in osteoporotic patients, the enhanced biomechanical strength of a fourth screw was demonstrated in the treatment of fractures with associated posterior comminution.[29] The location of these implants within the femoral neck is potentially more important than the number of implants. One study demonstrated impressive results with two screws used to stabilize displaced femoral neck fractures in elderly patients.[30] When both screws were placed within 3 mm of the femoral neck cortex, nonunion occurred in only 2 of 18 fractures (11.1%). When only one screw was positioned within 3 mm of the femoral neck cortex, nonunion occurred in 9 of 22 patients (40.9%). Nonunion occurred in 5 of 5 (100%) patients when neither screw was properly positioned. Although it is not yet known whether these data can be extrapolated to a younger patient population with increased bone density in the femoral neck, the biomechanical principles of screw placement are nonetheless important.

Certain fracture patterns such as vertical femoral neck fractures and fractures at the basicervical location have been more problematic, necessitating further study. Most biomechanical studies have been conducted using osteoporotic specimens, making extrapolation of data to a younger patient population difficult. However, the basic mechanical principles can be applied. One such study demonstrated a correlation between fixation failure and increasing fracture angle (that is, more vertical fractures).[31] Additionally, the progression of the fracture angle from transcervical to basicervical was reported to be associated with a lower force to failure.

Fixation of vertically oriented femoral neck fractures remains challenging because shear forces across the fracture dominate and predispose fractures to redisplacement. Although implants such as multiple cancellous lag screws encourage controlled collapse along the long axis of the screws, the body weight deforming force vector is directed vertically and relatively parallel to the fracture plane. In a recent biomechanical study, four different constructs were tested to determine the dynamic and static stability in a vertically oriented fracture model (Pauwels type III fractures).[32] Fixation with a sliding hip screw and an additional derotational screw was found to be mechanically superior to fixation with a dynamic hip screw alone, multiple cancellous lag screws, or a 130° blade plate with derotational screw. Another study demonstrated less inferior femoral head displacement and a greater load to failure in cadaver specimens that were stabilized with a sliding hip screw compared with three cannulated cancellous lag screws placed in a vertically oriented femoral neck fracture pattern.[33] Despite these and other biomechanical evaluations of these vertically oriented fracture patterns, the minimum fixation strength necessary for union remains unknown. The impact of increased cancellous bone density (seen in younger patients) on healing and maintenance of reduction also remains unknown. Nonetheless, clinical experience combined with these evaluations should alert surgeons to consider additional fixation methods in the treatment of these particularly difficult fracture patterns.

Outcomes in Young Patients

The early clinical results of the surgical management of femoral neck fractures in young patients have been demonstrated in three studies.[34-36] Combining their results, osteonecrosis occurred in 10.4% of patients, whereas nonunion occurred in 4.5%. Compared with historical studies that evaluated the treatment of displaced femoral neck fractures in young patients, this represents a significant improvement. Although the factors contributing to the improved results are not defined, the improved results are likely a combination of early treatment, anatomic reduction, stable fixation, and respect for the femoral head vascular supply. Depending on surgeon experience and expertise, a variety of implants were used, including a 130° blade plate,[34] multiple cancellous lag screws,[35,36] and a sliding hip screw.[36] No conclusions can be drawn regarding the type of fixation, the need for open reduction, or the timing of fixation, but these results compare favorably and are consistent with the re-

sults of a previous study that emphasized early fixation of femoral neck fracture in young patients.[37]

Complications
Osteonecrosis
Osteonecrosis of the femoral head after a femoral neck fracture is a particularly devastating complication in young patients because there is no reliable and functionally acceptable salvage procedure if collapse occurs. Although elderly patients can remain asymptomatic despite radiographic evidence of osteonecrosis, young patients usually require a secondary reconstructive procedure because of debilitating hip pain. It has been suggested that a higher initial radiographic displacement may be associated with an increased risk for development of osteonecrosis; however, no large study in young patients has been able to quantify or define the relative risk factors. Factors such as timing of surgical stabilization, intracapsular hematoma, displacement, surgical approach, patient age, and type of fixation have all been implicated as potential causes. One study that included 71 patients with osteonecrosis who were treated with internal fixation after a femoral neck fracture found a higher rate of osteonecrosis in patients with displaced fractures.[38] Additionally, more than 30% of the instances of osteonecrosis did not become apparent until more than 3 years after the injury.

Treatment alternatives after collapse are limited and consist of reconstructive osteotomies, hip arthrodesis, joint arthroplasty, and vascularized fibular transplantations. The indications for and results of these secondary surgical reconstructive procedures depend on several patient, social, and anatomic issues.

Nonunion
Historically, the rate of nonunion after surgical fixation of femoral neck fractures in young patients has been as high as 30%. More recent reports of nonunion have been much more favorable, with rates averaging less than 10%.[34-36] The source of these improved results is unclear, but it may be related to an improved understanding of the fracture patterns, the biomechanics of fixation, the surgical timing, and the need for an accurate reduction.

Treatment options for nonunion include revision stabilization with compression, muscle-pedicle grafting, free vascularized osseous transfer, intertrochanteric osteotomy, and prosthetic replacement. Use of intertrochanteric osteotomy for the treatment of a femoral neck nonunion has demonstrated consistent results with predictable union.[39] However, this procedure requires careful preoperative planning and an understanding of the optimal biomechanical environment for healing. In most instances, femoral neck nonunions in young patients represent a biomechanical failure with shear forces overwhelming the compressive forces at the site of the fracture. This may be associated with limb shortening and failure of fixation. A valgus-producing intertrochanteric osteotomy converts a portion (depending on the angle of correction) of these shear forces into compressive forces by reorienting the proximal femoral segment, effectively making the nonunion inclination more horizontal.[39]

Failure of Fixation

Early failure after surgical fixation of a femoral neck fracture is uncommon. Risk factors for this complication include fracture comminution, varus reduction, inferior offset, and the type and location of fracture fixation. Careful attention to the technical details at the time of surgical stabilization can help to minimize the level of risk of fixation failure to that resulting from patient-related issues.

Summary

Hip dislocations, femoral head fractures, and femoral neck fractures in young patients are typically the result of high-energy mechanisms and require prompt identification and management. An improved understanding of the local anatomy, typical injury patterns, and commonly observed associated injuries has improved the subsequent treatment. The normal and pathologic anatomy of femoral head perfusion has influenced the timing, surgical approach, and treatment of femoral head and femoral neck injuries. The complications that can occur after these injuries can be minimized with attention to detail and prompt treatment in some circumstances.

Annotated References

1. Monma H, Sugita T: Is the mechanism of traumatic posterior dislocation of the hip a brake pedal injury rather than a dashboard injury? *Injury* 2001;32:221-222.

    The authors of this study reported that most patients (45 of 48) with posterior hip dislocation after a head-on motor vehicle collision had right-sided injuries. These findings call into question the commonly held belief that these injuries are the result of an impact with the dashboard. The authors present an alternative hypothesis.

2. Hak DJ, Goulet JA: Severity of injuries associated with traumatic hip dislocation as a result of motor vehicle collisions. *J Trauma* 1999;47:60-63.

3. Hillyard RF, Fox J: Sciatic nerve injuries associated with traumatic posterior hip dislocations. *Am J Emerg Med* 2003;21:545-548.

    This 12-year retrospective study of 106 patients was conducted to determine whether reduction of traumatic hip dislocations before transfer reduced sciatic nerve injury. The authors found that a significantly longer relocation time was needed in patients with a major nerve injury, and a higher incidence of complete motor deficits was noted in patients who were transferred with the hip still dislocated.

4. Epstein HC: Posterior fracture-dislocations of the hip: Long-term follow-up. *J Bone Joint Surg Am* 1974;56:1103-1127.

5. Thompson VP, Epstein HC: Traumatic dislocation of the hip: A survey of two hundred and four cases covering a period of twenty-one years. *J Bone Joint Surg Am* 1951;33:746-778.

6. Sontich JK, Cannada LK: Femoral head avulsion fracture with malunion to the acetabulum: A case report. *J Orthop Trauma* 2002;16:49-51.

    The authors report an unrecognized infrafoveal femoral head fracture that resulted in symptomatic malunion requiring débridement.

7. Yoon TR, Chung JY, Jung ST, Seo HY: Malunion of femoral head fractures treated by partial ostectomy: Three case reports. *J Orthop Trauma* 2003;17:447-450.

    Three patients with previous posterior hip fracture-dislocations and malunited inferomedial femoral head fractures were reviewed. The authors report that resection of the fragments using the Smith-Petersen approach allowed return of hip motion without osteonecrosis.

8. Stannard JP, Harris HW, Volgas DA, Alonso JE: Functional outcome of patients with femoral head fractures associated with hip dislocations. *Clin Orthop* 2000;377:44-56.

    In this study, 26 patients surgically treated for a femoral head fracture were reviewed to determine the predictors of outcome and radiographic results. Although retrospective data were used, it was reported that, compared with an anterior approach, the use of a Kocher-Langenbeck posterior approach was associated with a 3.2-fold increase in osteonecrosis. Better visualization and reduction was obtained with a Smith-Petersen anterior exposure.

9. Swiontkowski MF, Thorpe M, Seiler JG, Hansen ST: Operative management of displaced femoral head fractures: Case-matched comparison of anterior versus posterior approaches for Pipkin I and Pipkin II fractures. *J Orthop Trauma* 1992;6:437-442.

10. Yoon TR, Rowe SM, Chung JY, Song EK, Jung ST, Anwar IB: Clinical and radiographic outcome of femoral head fractures: 30 patients followed for 3-10 years. *Acta Orthop Scand* 2001;72:348-353.

    The authors retrospectively evaluated outcomes in 30 patients with femoral head fractures and concluded that fragment excision was appropriate for those patients with small infrafoveal fractures, open reduction was appropriate for those with larger infrafoveal and suprafoveal frac-

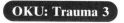

tures, and arthroplasty was appropriate for those with comminuted fractures involving large portions of the femoral head.

11. Konrath GA, Hamel AJ, Guerin J, Olson SA, Bay B, Sharkey NA: Biomechanical evaluation of impaction fractures of the femoral head. *J Orthop Trauma* 1999;13:407-413.

12. Brumback RJ, Kenzora JE, Levitt LE, Burgess AR, Poka A: Fractures of the femoral head. *Hip* 1987;27: 181-206.

13. Marchetti ME, Steinberg GG, Coumas JM: Intermediate-term experience of Pipkin fracture-dislocations of the hip. *J Orthop Trauma* 1996;10: 455-461.

14. Yang KH, Han DY, Park HW, Kang HJ, Park JH: Fracture of the ipsilateral neck of the femur in shaft nailing: The role of CT in diagnosis. *J Bone Joint Surg Br* 1998;80:673-678.

15. Sevitt S: Avascular necrosis and revascularisation of the femoral head after intracapsular fractures: A combined arteriographic and histological necropsy study. *J Bone Joint Surg Br* 1964;46:270-296.

16. Swiontkowski MF: Intracapsular fractures of the hip. *J Bone Joint Surg Am* 1994;76:129-138.

17. Trueta J, Harrison MHM: The normal vascular anatomy of the femoral head in adult man. *J Bone Joint Surg Br* 1953;35:442-461.

18. Gautier E, Ganz K, Krugel N, Gill T, Ganz R: Anatomy of the medial femoral circumflex artery and its surgical implications. *J Bone Joint Surg Br* 2000;82: 679-683.

    The precise anatomy of the medial femoral circumflex artery, its branches, and the associated soft-tissue structures of the posterior femoral neck are described. The extracapsular and intracapsular course of the medial femoral circumflex is described, as well as the relationship with the tendons of the obturator externus and obturator internus. The authors conclude that an improved understanding of the vascular anatomy of the proximal femur should increase the safety of commonly used posterior approaches to the hip.

19. Oakes DA, Jackson KR, Davies MR, et al: The impact of the Garden classification on proposed operative treatment. *Clin Orthop* 2003;409:232-240.

    The authors of this article simplified the Garden classification system into nondisplaced and displaced categories, significantly improving its usefulness.

20. Blundell CM, Parker MJ, Pryor GA, Hopkinson-Woolley J, Bhonsle SS: Assessment of the AO classification of intracapsular fractures of the proximal femur. *J Bone Joint Surg Br* 1998;80:679-683.

21. Bartonicek J: Pauwels' classification of femoral neck fractures: Correct interpretation of the original. *J Orthop Trauma* 2001;15:358-360.

    The authors identify the commonly misquoted angles described by Pauwels and present the correct values.

22. Szita J, Cserhati P, Bosch U, Manninger J, Bodzay T, Fekete K: Intracapsular femoral neck fractures: The importance of early reduction and stable osteosynthesis. *Injury* 2002;33(suppl 3):C41-C46.

    The authors of this article previously reviewed and reported their results on early surgical management of femoral neck fractures in elderly patients and the relationship between surgical timing and osteonecrosis. In their surviving patients, the rate of osteonecrosis was significantly lower in those who underwent surgical treatment within 6 hours of injury (10.5%) compared with those who underwent surgical treatment longer than 6 hours after injury (20%).

23. Bonnaire F, Schaefer DJ, Kuner EH: Hemarthrosis and hip joint pressure in femoral neck fractures. *Clin Orthop* 1998;353:148-155.

24. Gill TJ, Sledge JB, Ekkernkamp A, Ganz R: Intraoperative assessment of femoral head vascularity after femoral neck fracture. *J Orthop Trauma* 1998;12: 474-478.

25. Hirata T, Konishiike T, Kawai A, Sato T, Inoue H: Dynamic magnetic resonance imaging of femoral head perfusion in femoral neck fracture. *Clin Orthop* 2001;393:294-301.

    Dynamic MRI was used to evaluate femoral head perfusion in 36 patients with femoral neck fractures. In 19 patients with either normal (n = 11) or impaired (n = 6) blood flow, healing occurred without complications. In contrast, complications occurred in 15 of 19 patients with absent femoral head perfusion based on dynamic MRI; this included osteonecrosis in 10 patients and nonunion in 5.

26. Konishiike T, Makihata E, Tago H, Sato T, Inoue H: Acute fracture of the neck of the femur: An assessment of perfusion of the head by dynamic MRI. *J Bone Joint Surg Br* 1999;81:596-599.

27. Maruenda JI, Barrios C, Gomar-Sancho F: Intracapsular hip pressure after femoral neck fracture. *Clin Orthop* 1997;340:172-180.

28. Sugamoto K, Ochi T, Takahashi Y, Tamura T, Matsuoka T: Hemodynamic measurement in the femoral

head using laser Doppler. *Clin Orthop* 1998;353:138-147.

29. Kauffman JI, Simon JA, Kummer FJ, Pearlman CJ, Zuckerman JD, Koval KJ: Internal fixation of femoral neck fractures with posterior comminution: A biomechanical study. *J Orthop Trauma* 1999;13:155-159.

30. Lindequist S, Tornkvist H: Quality of reduction and cortical screw support in femoral neck fractures: An analysis of 72 fractures with a new computerized measuring method. *J Orthop Trauma* 1995;9:215-221.

31. Stankewich CJ, Chapman J, Muthusamy R, et al: Relationship of mechanical factors to the strength of proximal femur fractures fixed with cancellous screws. *J Orthop Trauma* 1996;10:248-257.

32. Bonnaire FA, Weber AT: Analysis of fracture gap changes, dynamic and static stability of different osteosynthetic procedures in the femoral neck. *Injury* 2002;33(suppl 3):C24-C32.

33. Baitner AC, Maurer SG, Hickey DG, et al: Vertical shear fractures of the femoral neck: A biomechanical study. *Clin Orthop* 1999;367:300-305.

34. Broos PL, Vercruysse R, Fourneau I, Driesen R, Stappaerts KH: Unstable femoral neck fractures in young adults: Treatment with the AO 130-degree blade plate. *J Orthop Trauma* 1998;12:235-239.

35. Gautam VK, Anand S, Dhaon BK: Management of displaced femoral neck fractures in young adults (a group at risk). *Injury* 1998;29:215-218.

36. Verettas DA, Galanis B, Kazakos K, Hatziyiannakis A, Kotsios E: Fractures of the proximal part of the femur in patients under 50 years of age. *Injury* 2002;33:41-45.

37. Swiontkowski MF, Winquist RA, Hansen ST Jr: Fractures of the femoral neck in patients between the ages of twelve and forty-nine years. *J Bone Joint Surg Am* 1984;66:837-846.

38. Jakob M, Rosso R, Weller K, Babst R, Regazzoni P: Avascular necrosis of the femoral head after open reduction and internal fixation of femoral neck fractures: An inevitable complication? *Swiss Surg* 1999;5:257-264.

39. Marti RK, Schuller HM, Raaymakers EL: Intertrochanteric osteotomy for non-union of the femoral neck. *J Bone Joint Surg Br* 1989;71:782-787.

Chapter 32

Fractures of the Proximal Femur

James Powell, MD

Douglas R. Dirschl, MD

Introduction

Peritrochanteric and subtrochanteric fractures comprise the extracapsular fractures of the proximal femur. Peritrochanteric fractures include intertrochanteric fractures, reverse obliquity fractures, and intertrochanteric fractures with subtrochanteric extension. Subtrochanteric fractures include those in which the main fracture line is entirely distal to the trochanteric region. Annually, approximately 150,000 Americans experience one of these fracture types. Whereas most of these patients are elderly and the fracture is the result of a low-energy fall, there is an increasing number of younger patients who experience high-energy fractures of the proximal femur. The role of the orthopaedic surgeon in the treatment of these injuries involves not only secure surgical stabilization, but also provision for immediate rehabilitation, early return to function, and optimization of patient outcomes.

Peritrochanteric Femur Fractures

Diagnosis and Classification

High-energy injuries nearly always result in significant soft-tissue injury, fracture displacement, and comminution. In both high- and low-energy injuries, the typical appearance of the injured limb is one of shortening and external rotation. Abrasion and/or bruising of the soft tissues may be present over the affected trochanteric region. Neurologic or vascular injury is rare after these fractures, but the neurovascular status of the affected limb should be carefully assessed.

Displaced proximal femur fractures are almost always apparent on routine AP and lateral radiographs of the hip. If subtrochanteric extension of the fracture is present, the entire femur should be radiographically assessed to determine whether a segmental fracture is present. Nondisplaced fractures can be a diagnostic challenge because the fracture line may not be apparent on the initial radiographs. AP radiographs taken with the hip in internal rotation may demonstrate an occult or nondisplaced fracture line. Additional diagnostic testing for an occult fracture can include a technetium Tc 99m bone scan or MRI[1] (see chapter 31).

The classification of peritrochanteric fractures, paralleling that of many other fractures, has undergone some changes in recent years. Classification schemes such as the Evans-Wales system have been shown to be useful for describing fractures, but they have been shown to have less than optimal interobserver reliability. The Orthopaedic Trauma Association (OTA) classification system is sometimes used (Figure 1); however, it also has been shown to have less than optimal interobserver reliability. Most surgeons have greatly simplified the classification of these injuries by referring to fractures as either stable or unstable. Stable injuries are those that have an intact medial buttress when reduced, and the fracture itself can resist compressive loads. An unstable fracture, by contrast, will not have a medial buttress to resist compressive loads, and the implant chosen to stabilize the fracture must resist the entire compressive load in the early phases of healing.

Treatment

Critical to the successful treatment of all fractures of the proximal femur is adequate reduction. Not only does accurate reduction of the fracture restore mechanics of the hip joint and the muscles attaching to the proximal femur, but it will also reduce stress on the surgical implant and lead to more rapid and complete fracture healing. Reduction of the fracture should restore the normal neck-shaft angle in both anteroposterior and lateral planes, restore normal rotational alignment of the femur, and eliminate any translation between the proximal fragment and the femoral shaft. Reduction of all intervening comminuted fragments is not necessary, and excessive stripping at the time of surgery to reduce and stabilize these fragments may delay fracture healing. Excessive shortening and collapse of proximal femoral fractures results in shortening of the limb and a decrease in femoral offset, both of which reduce the lever arm of the hip abductors, effectively weakening them, and resulting in a more prominent antalgic gait. With accurate reduc-

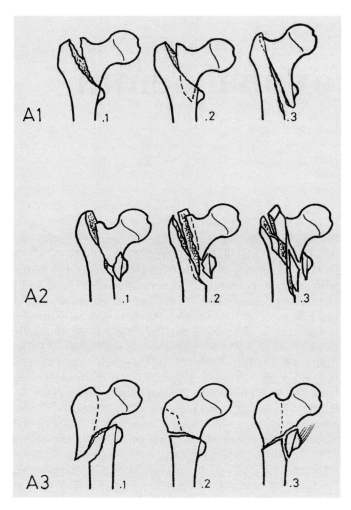

Figure 1 The Müller/AO classification of peritrochanteric femur fractures (incorporated into the *Fracture and Dislocation Compendium* of the Orthopaedic Trauma Association). **Top row,** Extra-articular fracture, trochanteric area, peritrochanteric, simple. **Middle row,** Extra-articular fracture, trochanteric area, peritrochanteric, multifragmentary. **Bottom row,** Extra-articular fracture, trochanteric area, intertrochanteric. *(Reproduced with permission from Müller ME, Nazarian S, Koch P, Schatzker J (eds): The Comprehensive Classification of Fractures of Long Bones. Berlin, Germany, Springer-Verlag, 1990, p 121.)*

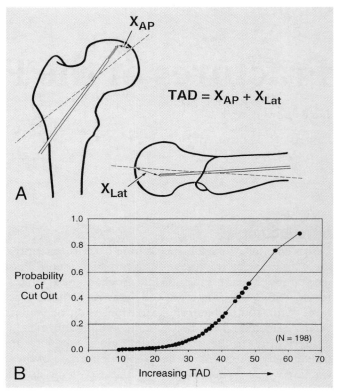

$$TAD = X_{AP} + X_{Lat}$$

Figure 2 The tip-apex distance (TAD) is estimated by combining the distance from the guide-pin tip to the apex of the femoral head on the AP and lateral fluoroscopic views **(A)**. The risk for cutout failure increases dramatically when TAD exceeds a threshold of 25 mm **(B)**. *(Reproduced with permission from Baumgaertner MR, Brennan MJ: Intertrochanteric femur fractures, in* Orthopaedic Knowledge Update: Trauma 2. *Rosemont, IL, American Academy of Orthopaedic Surgeons, 2000, pp 125-131.)*

tion and appropriate choice and application of the surgical implant, excessive collapse can usually be avoided.

The sliding hip screw with a side plate and three or four screws in the femoral shaft continues to be the preferred implant for the treatment of most stable and unstable intertrochanteric femur fractures. These devices are familiar to nearly all orthopaedic surgeons and are in wide use worldwide. Successful treatment with these devices requires accurate fracture reduction, bone contact across the intertrochanteric fracture line, and deep and central positioning of the lag screw in the femoral head. The tip-apex distance has been shown to be a strong predictor of failure of these devices by cutout of the screw from the femoral head.[2] Studies have shown that the risk of failure approaches zero with a tip apex distance less than 25 mm (Figure 2). Sliding hip screws have the highest success rates in the treatment of intertrochan-

teric fractures; failure rates for these devices are high when they are used to treat reverse obliquity fractures or fractures with subtrochanteric extension.

Modifications to the implant and/or the technique of insertion of the sliding hip screw have been made in an effort to further decrease the number of treatment failures. The Medoff sliding plate (Wright Medical, Arlington, TN) adds to the sliding hip screw the capacity for sliding/compression along the axis of the femoral shaft. This device has been shown to have a lower rate of implant failure when used to treat unstable fractures, but the failure rate was equivalent to that of the sliding hip screw when used to treat stable fractures.[3,4] Recently, a compression plate for percutaneous insertion during the surgical repair of proximal femur fractures was introduced.[5] One of the justifications for using this device is that the minimally invasive surgical approach, with no visualization of the fractured bone surfaces, will result in less trauma to the patient and a lower rate of nonunion of the fracture. A prospective, randomized trial comparing this device and a classic compression hip screw reported less surgical blood loss and longer surgical times with the percutaneous device, but no difference was

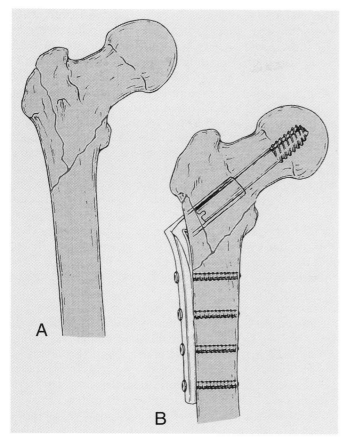

Figure 3 A, Reverse oblique intertrochanteric fracture. Lateral comminution is common. **B,** Telescoping of the sliding hip screw does not promote interfragmentary compression because of the parallel orientation of the fracture plane. Stability requires secure impaction of the fracture, with either osteotomy of the distal piece to provide mechanical engagement or an implant that resists progressive medial displacement of the shaft. *(Adapted with permission from Baumgaertner MR, Chrostowski JH, Levy RN: Intertrochanteric hip fractures, in Browner BD, Jupiter JB, Levine AM, Trafton PG (eds): Skeletal Trauma, ed 2. Philadelphia, PA, WB Saunders, 1998, pp 1833-1881.)*

reported between the two devices in terms of fracture healing, implant failures, or complications.[6]

Plate and screw implants with a 95° angle (the dynamic condylar screw [Synthes, West Chester, PA] and the 95° blade plate) are most commonly used to treat fractures of the distal femur, but they can also be successfully used to treat fractures of the proximal femur. These devices are difficult to insert appropriately in the proximal femur, and they offer no advantage over the sliding hip screw in the treatment of intertrochanteric fractures. For reverse obliquity fractures, in which the fracture line is parallel to a typical sliding hip screw (Figure 3), the 95° screw-plate devices offer improved proximal fixation and stability of the fracture. In fractures with significant medial comminution, however, an intramedullary device may offer greater stability.

Intramedullary devices that incorporate a lag screw directed through the nail into the femoral head offer certain theoretic advantages over screw and plate devices. The intramedullary implant itself can serve as a

buttress against lateral translation of the proximal fracture fragment, and the intramedullary location of the junction between the nail and the lag screw makes the implant stronger at resisting bending forces than a screw-plate implant, in which the junction between the plate and screw are farther from the axis of rotation for bending forces. Fracture of the femoral shaft at the tip of the intramedullary device was the major complication of the first generation of these short, stiff devices,[7] but redesign of the initial devices and introduction of a variety of other new devices have decreased the incidence of this complication. Newer devices are less stiff than the early devices, and long nails are now available to avoid the stress concentration at the tip of the nail associated with shorter devices.[8-10] A biomechanical study has indicated that the forces required to initiate sliding of the hip screw in many of these devices is greater than that of the classic hip compression screw,[11] but it is unknown whether this biomechanical difference has an impact on treatment outcomes. Two recent prospective, randomized trials comparing compression hip screws to intramedullary devices for the treatment of intertrochanteric fractures concluded that there was no difference in outcomes between the two groups.[12,13] The rate of complications, including femoral shaft fracture and screw cutout, however, were higher in the intramedullary nail group. Both studies concluded that the routine use of an intramedullary device to treat intertrochanteric fractures could not be recommended, and that intramedullary devices were most appropriate for the treatment of reverse obliquity fractures and fractures with subtrochanteric extension.

Calcar-substituting hemiarthroplasty or total joint arthroplasty remains a viable treatment option in patients with severely comminuted or pathologic fractures of the proximal femur.[14] The significantly greater surgical and metabolic insult of arthroplasty surgery, the generally good results achieved with newer implants and techniques for fracture stabilization, and the introduction of intramedullary implants have resulted in arthroplasty generally being reserved for the salvage of failures after internal fixation of fractures in elderly patients.[15,16]

Reverse Obliquity Fractures, Highly Comminuted Fractures, and Fractures With Subtrochanteric Extension

The reverse obliquity fracture pattern (Figure 3), the highly comminuted unstable intertrochanteric fracture (OTA type A2), and the fracture with subtrochanteric extension (OTA type A3) make up a group of fractures with a much higher risk of treatment complications and poorer outcomes than traditional intertrochanteric fractures. These fracture patterns represent a disproportionately high percentage of proximal femoral fractures in younger patients. Treatment considerations for these high-energy injuries are necessarily different than in lower-energy intertrochanteric fractures in elderly patients. In particular, the rate of excessive collapse, nonunion, or implant failure with sliding hip screw devices in these fracture patterns has been shown to be as high as 70%.[17] Careful surgical planning, optimization of the patient's medical condition, availability of appropriate implants and equipment, and experience in the treatment of these fractures are necessary to provide optimal care to patients with these fractures. Current recommendations are for the use of 95° screw-plate or intramedullary devices to treat highly comminuted, reverse obliquity, and fractures with subtrochanteric extension. In contrast to the short intramedullary devices that are commercially available for the treatment of intertrochanteric fractures, the devices used to treat these high-energy, unstable fracture patterns should be sized to fill the entire length of the femoral intramedullary canal—short intramedullary implants should not be used to treat patients with these unstable fracture patterns. To achieve good outcomes, care must be given to the details of accurate reduction and to the appropriate positioning and insertion of the implant. One study reported a 46% failure rate in the treatment of fractures with a nonanatomic reduction and an 80% failure rate in fractures with substandard positioning of the implant.[17] A more recent study that compared the use of an intramedullary device and a 95° screw-plate device to treat these high-energy fracture patterns reported shorter surgical times, less blood loss, shorter hospital stays, and fewer reoperations in the intramedullary device group.[18]

Subtrochanteric Femur Fractures

Fractures of the subtrochanteric portion of the femur present difficulties in reduction and stabilization. By definition, the subtrochanteric area extends from the lesser trochanter to the junction of the upper and middle third of the diaphysis. One definition includes the 5 cm of the proximal femur from the lesser trochanter distally. Proximally, extension of the fracture into the intertrochanteric area is common and frequently complicates decision making in terms of implant choice as well as reduction and stabilization from a technical perspective.

There are many large muscular forces that act to cause displacement of the various fracture fragments. The gluteus minimus and medius, which insert at the greater trochanter, pull the proximal fragment into an abducted position. The iliopsoas flexes and externally rotates the proximal fragment if the lesser trochanter is attached. The fracture will typically deform into a varus position because of the insertion of the adductors and hamstrings, which also cause a relative shortening. The short external rotators, including the piriformis, the superior and inferior gemellus, and the obturator internus, cause the proximal fragment in most subtrochanteric femur fractures to assume an externally rotated position.

The pull of these muscles should be considered when attempting to reduce the distal fragment to the proximal. For these reasons, reduction of these fractures through closed means may be difficult. Many surgeons choose to treat these fractures with the patient's limb in traction on a fracture table, but even this often leaves the proximal fragment flexed and abducted. Although open reduction can be easily achieved as part of the surgical procedure for implanting a 95° plate and screw device, an open reduction is unnecessarily invasive when fracture stabilization with an intramedullary device is planned. In this situation, the insertion of a temporary Steinmann pin into the proximal fragment allows the surgeon to manipulate the proximal fragment into an acceptable position by using the pin as a lever to cause adduction and extension of the fragment. After the intramedullary device and the proximal locking screws have been inserted, the Steinmann pin can be removed.

There are high compressive forces on the medial cortex of the femur in the subtrochanteric area and significant tensile forces laterally. Because fractures in this area are frequently comminuted medially, any implants used to stabilize fractures require the ability to resist significant bending moments in varus. In contradistinction to the intertrochanteric area, the subtrochanteric area is predominantly made up of cortical bone and a delay in union can occur. The implant used to stabilize a fracture in this area needs to have a sufficient fatigue life to permit union without implant failure.

Diagnosis and Classification

Subtrochanteric femur fractures have been categorized into two major types, each with two subgroups.[19] Type I fractures do not have extension into the piriformis fossa. In type IA fractures, the lesser trochanteric fragment is intact. Purchase can be obtained with a standard antegrade interlocking nail with an oblique locking screw. Type IB fractures have involvement of the lesser trochanter. Use of a conventional femoral interlocking nail is precluded in the treatment of this type of fracture because purchase cannot be obtained by the proximal locking screw. Fractures in this category will typically be stabilized with a cephalomedullary nail, which relies on retrograde screw insertion along the axis of the neck up into the head; however, satisfactory results with plating techniques involving fixed-angle devices have been reported.[8,17,18] Closed intramedullary nailing affords the biologic advantage of minimal devascularization of the fracture compared with more laterally placed plates. This is a particular advantage in instances in which the posterior medial cortex cannot be restored.

Type II fractures involve extension of the subtrochanteric fracture up into the piriformis fossa. A nondisplaced fracture into this area may be difficult to see and diagnostic imaging should include a satisfactory lateral projection. Type IIA fractures extend from the lesser

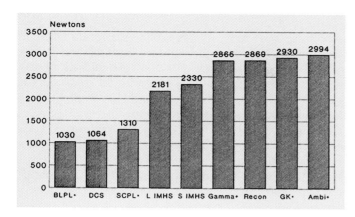

Figure 4 A comparison of the strength of several intramedullary and extramedullary implants in unstable subtrochanteric fractures. BLPL = blade plate, DCS = dynamic condylar screw, SPCL = screw plate, L IMHS = long intramedullary hip screw, S IMHS = short intramedullary hip screw, GK = Gross Kempf intramedullary nail, AMBI = AMBI/Classic compression hip screw. *(Reproduced with permission from Kraemer WJ, Hearn TC, Powell JN, Mahomed N: Fixation of segmental subtrochanteric fractures: A biomechanical study. Clin Orthop 1996;332:71-79.)*

trochanter into the piriformis fossa, but no significant comminution or major fracture of the lesser trochanter is present. Type IIB fractures have significant comminution involving the greater trochanteric area and significant loss of the medial femoral cortex, including the lesser trochanter.

Treatment

Implant Selection Biomechanics

Many types of implants are currently available for the treatment of subtrochanteric fractures; these can be broadly categorized as either extramedullary or intramedullary implants. Several biomechanical studies comparing these types of implants have been conducted. Early investigations involved axial load and bending tests to assess implant stiffness and strength.[20-22] In general, intramedullary implants were found to be almost twice as strong as the extramedullary implants (Figure 4). All three of these studies used an identical testing protocol. The blade plate, dynamic condylar screw, and screw plate all were reported to be significantly less strong than the Gamma nail (Stryker Orthopaedics, Mahwah, NJ), reconstruction nail, and Grosse-Kempf nail, all of which are intramedullary implants. One plate and screw implant that was tested was a standard telescoping screw plate implant (AMBI/Classic, Smith & Nephew, Memphis, TN), which is a compression hip screw specifically designed for the treatment of subtrochanteric fractures. The authors found that the three nails and the AMBI/Classic implant were able to withstand a load of roughly three times body weight.

Other studies have assessed some of the newer implants that are available for the treatment of subtrochanteric fractures. One study compared the intramedullary

hip screw and the Medoff sliding plate system.[23] The Medoff sliding plate is a biaxial plating system that allows collapse along the axis of the lag screw and also permits collapse in the axis of the shaft of the femur. Both two- and three-part subtrochanteric models were tested, with a simulated abductor load applied to a reverse oblique pattern for both the two- and three-part fractures. The intramedullary hip screw and the Medoff sliding plate system provided comparable stability for the treatment of two- and three-part reverse oblique subtrochanteric femur fractures. In the three-part model, displacement of the proximal fragment occurred with the Medoff sliding plate system. A more recent biomechanical analysis of the Medoff sliding plate system compared it with the Gamma nail and the AMBI/Classic implant in both an intertrochanteric and segmental subtrochanteric fracture model.[24] Failure of the Medoff sliding plate system in the subtrochanteric model resulted from permanent deformation of the sliding plate proximal to the interface with the distal base plate. The load to failure was roughly half that of the Gamma nail and the AMBI/Classic implant. The authors, therefore, suggested caution with the use of the Medoff sliding plate system in the treatment of patients with highly unstable subtrochanteric fractures.

Current biomechanical literature suggests that an intramedullary implant is the preferred treatment modality in patients with unstable subtrochanteric fracture because of its greater strength. A plate and screw system specifically designed for the subtrochanteric model (such as the AMBI/Classic) is also a treatment alternative.

Clinical Outcomes

Multiple reports have been published in the literature that assess the use of plating techniques in the treatment of subtrochanteric fractures. One such report included 30 patients whose subtrochanteric fractures were treated using the Medoff sliding plate system, 29 of whom were available for 1-year follow-up.[25] The patient in whom biaxial collapse was permitted healed with greater deformity. Three patients who were originally treated with uniaxial collapse were secondarily converted by dynamization to permit biaxial collapse. A randomized multicenter study of 107 elderly patients who underwent fixation of subtrochanteric fractures compared the efficacy of the Medoff sliding plate with that of three other load-bearing screw-plate devices (the Dynamic Hip Screw [Synthes, Paoli, PA] alone, the dynamic condylar screw, and the Dynamic Hip Screw with trochanteric sliding plate).[26] Of the 55 patients treated with the Medoff sliding plate, 1 had fixation failure versus 8 of 55 patients who were treated with the other plating systems.

Three more recent studies that assess plating techniques have been published. One of these studies reports the results of using the dynamic condylar screw for the treatment of subtrochanteric fractures in a consecutive series of 58 patients, 11 of whom had high-energy mechanisms of injury and 47 of whom had low-energy mechanisms of injury.[27] Ten of the 11 patients with high-energy mechanisms of injury achieved fracture union primarily, whereas implant failure occurred in 11 of 47 patients with low-energy mechanisms of injury; the implant failures generally occurred in older patients. The authors concluded that the dynamic condylar screw device is a satisfactory implant for the stabilization of subtrochanteric fractures caused by high-energy mechanisms, but the implant had a high failure rate in elderly patients in whom weight bearing could not be minimized. Another study reported a 100% union rate using a dynamic condylar screw and biologic reduction techniques for 31 consecutive patients with high-energy subtrochanteric femur fractures.[28] One other recent study reported the technique of using a fixed low-angle plate for submuscular subtrochanteric fracture fixation.[29] In this consecutive series of 20 young patients with high-energy mechanisms of injury, reconstruction was virtually anatomic when compared with the contralateral side, and no mechanical failures were reported.

Another group of authors reported on their use of an unreamed AO femoral intramedullary nail with a spiral blade to treat 80 consecutive patients with nonpathologic fractures of the femur.[30] They found a 21% mechanical complication rate and a 9% revision rate for the patients in their series with subtrochanteric fractures. They concluded that this implant should not be used to treat patients with an intertrochanteric extension or reverse obliquity fractures. They also recommended caution when considering the use of this device in elderly patients with osteoporosis. Another group of authors reported the use of a cephalomedullary nail for the stabilization of 45 Russell-Taylor type IB subtrochanteric femoral fractures; 100% of patients achieved union, but 61% healed in varus.[31] The authors recommended that reduction of the proximal fragment be carefully undertaken before the preparation of the canal and implant insertion. Another study reported the results of stabilization of 52 intertrochanteric-subtrochanteric Russell-Taylor type IIB fractures.[32] Of the 43 patients who were available for follow-up, all were found to be healed at an average of 4.3 months. Four of these 43 patients healed in varus, and greater than 1 cm of shortening occurred in two of those patients. The authors concluded that an excellent radiologic result did not necessarily translate into an excellent functional result. Another study compared the results of treating 25 patients who underwent fixation with a 95° screw-plate device and 17 patients who underwent stabilization with a spiral locked blade.[33] One nonunion was reported in the plated group, and two varus malunions were reported in the spiral locked blade group.

Summary

Accurate reduction of proximal femoral fractures (length, neck-shaft angle, and rotation) is critical to achieve optimal outcome. For adult patients of all ages with stable intertrochanteric fractures, there appears to be no advantage of using intramedullary implants over the traditional compression hip screw devices. In patients with highly unstable intertrochanteric fractures, reverse obliquity fractures, and fractures with subtrochanteric extension, the rate of loss of reduction and failure with sliding hip screw devices is high, and the use of 95° screw-plate devices or long intramedullary devices is recommended.

Currently, most subtrochanteric fractures, particularly type IA and IB fractures, are successfully treated using intramedullary nailing. Care must be taken, however, to avoid a varus malreduction and malunion. Selected fractures with high-energy mechanisms of injury can be satisfactorily reconstructed using biologic plating techniques and 95° screw-plate devices to achieve restoration of normal hip mechanics. In patients with combined intertrochanteric-subtrochanteric fractures, such as type II fractures in elderly patients, the long Gamma nail has been used to achieve satisfactory outcomes.

Annotated References

1. Rizzo PF, Gould ES, Lyden JP, Asnis SE: Diagnosis of occult fracture about the hip: Magnetic resonance imaging compared with bone-scanning. *J Bone Joint Surg Am* 1993;75:395-401.

2. Baumgaertner MR, Curtin SL, Lindskog DM, Keggi JM: The value of the tip-apex distance in predicting failure of fixation of peritrochanteric fractures of the hip. *J Bone Joint Surg Am* 1995;77:1058-1064.

3. Watson JT, Moed BR, Cramer KE, Karges DE: Comparison of the compression hip screw with the Medoff sliding plate for intertrochanteric fractures. *Clin Orthop* 1998;348:79-86.

4. Olsson O, Ceder L, Hauggaard A: Femoral shortening in intertrochanteric fractures: A comparison between the Medoff sliding plate and the compression hip screw. *J Bone Joint Surg Br* 2001;83:572-578.
   This prospective, randomized study compared 54 patients who were treated with the Medoff sliding plate and 60 patients who were treated with the compression hip screw for intertrochanteric fractures. At 4-month follow-up, the Medoff sliding plate group showed significantly more femoral shortening than the compression hip screw group, but less medialization of the femoral shaft. The authors concluded that biaxial dynamization with the Medoff sliding plate was safe and could minimize the rate of postoperative fixation failure.

5. Gotfried Y: Percutaneous compression plating for intertrochanteric hip fractures: Treatment rationale. *Orthopedics* 2002;25:647-651.

6. Kosygan KP, Mohan R, Newman RJ: The Gotfried percutaneous compression plate compared with the conventional classic hip screw for the fixation of intertrochanteric fractures of the hip. *J Bone Joint Surg Br* 2002;84:19-22.

   This prospective, randomized trial of 111 patients compared use of the Gotfried percutaneous compression plate and the classic hip screw in the fixation of intertrochanteric hip fractures. Blood loss was reported to be less in the percutaneous compression plate group, but surgical time was significantly longer. No differences in complication rates and outcomes occurred between the two groups at 6-month follow-up. The authors concluded that the advantages of using a percutaneous compression plate device seem to be more theoretical than practical.

7. Parker MJ, Pryor GA: Gamma versus DHS nailing for extracapsular femoral fractures: Meta-analysis of ten randomized trials. *Int Orthop* 1996;20:163-168.

8. Leung KS, So WS, Shen WY, Hui PW: Gamma nails and dynamic hip screws for peritrochanteric fractures: A randomized prospective study in elderly patients. *J Bone Joint Surg Br* 1992;74:345-351.

9. Hardy DC, Descamps PY, Krallis P, et al: Use of an intramedullary hip-screw compared with a compression hip-screw with a plate for intertrochanteric femoral fractures: A prospective, randomized study of one hundred patients. *J Bone Joint Surg Am* 1998;80:618-630.

10. Rantanen J, Aro HT: Intramedullary fixation of high subtrochanteric femoral fractures: A study comparing two implant designs, the Gamma nail and the intramedullary hip screw. *J Orthop Trauma* 1998;12:249-252.

11. Loch DA, Kyle RF, Bechtold JE, Kane M, Anderson K, Sherman RE: Forces required to initiate sliding in second-generation intramedullary nails. *J Bone Joint Surg Am* 1998;80:1626-1631.

    This biomechanical study was conducted to identify the forces required to initiate sliding in a variety of devices for stabilization of proximal femoral fractures (the Russell-Taylor [RT] Recon Nail [Smith & Nephew, Paoli, PA], ZMS nail [Zimmer, Warsaw, IN], Gamma nail, intramedullary hip screw, and conventional sliding hip screw). In all testing configurations, the sliding hip screw and intramedullary hip screw required lower forces to initiate sliding than the other devices. The Gamma nail required the largest forces to initiate sliding.

12. Adams CI, Robinson CM, Court-Brown CM, McQueen MM: Prospective randomized controlled trial of an intramedullary nail versus dynamic screw and plate for intertrochanteric fractures of the femur. *J Orthop Trauma* 2001;15:394-400.

    The authors of this prospective, randomized, controlled trial comparing the Gamma nail and sliding hip screw in the treatment of 399 patients with intertrochanteric fractures report that at 1 year after fracture, there was no difference between the groups in functional outcome. There was, however, a higher but nonsignificant rate of most postoperative complications in the Gamma nail group. Four femoral shaft fractures were in the Gamma nail group, and no femoral shaft fractures were in the sliding hip screw group.

13. Ahrengart L, Tornkvist H, Fornander P, et al: A randomized study of the compression hip screw and Gamma nail in 426 fractures. *Clin Orthop* 2002;401:209-222.

    This prospective, randomized trial compared the Gamma nail and compression hip screw in the treatment of 426 patients with intertrochanteric fractures. Postoperative walking ability was found to be no different between the two groups at 6 months after surgery. Although cephalic position of the lag screw and screw cutout occurred more frequently in the Gamma nail group, this group had less loss of fracture position.

14. Haentjens P, Casteleyn PP, De Boeck H, Handelberg F, Opdecam P: Treatment of unstable intertrochanteric and subtrochanteric fractures in elderly patients: Primary bipolar arthroplasty compared with internal fixation. *J Bone Joint Surg Am* 1989;71:1214-1225.

15. Haidukewych GJ, Berry DJ: Salvage of failed internal fixation of intertrochanteric hip fractures. *Clin Orthop* 2003;412:184-188.

    In this retrospective review of 20 patients who were treated over a 19-year period for salvage of failed internal fixation of intertrochanteric fractures, a variety of methods were used to secure internal fixation at the time of revision surgery; autograft was used in 17 patients. Nineteen of 20 patients healed by 27-month follow-up; 16 of the patients who healed reported no pain.

16. Haidukewych GJ, Berry DJ: Hip arthroplasty for salvage of failed treatment of intertrochanteric hip fractures. *J Bone Joint Surg Am* 2003;85-A:899-904.

    This is a retrospective case series of 60 patients who were treated over 13 years with arthroplasty for failure of intertrochanteric fracture internal fixation. Thirty-two patients had total hip arthroplasty, and 28 had hemiarthroplasty. Forty-four patients were followed for 2 to 15 years; 39 of these patients reported no pain or mild pain, and 40 were ambulatory. The authors concluded that hip arthroplasty was an effective salvage procedure after failed treatment of an intertrochanteric fracture.

17. Haidukewych GJ, Israel TA, Berry DJ: Reverse obliquity fractures of the intertrochanteric region of the femur. *J Bone Joint Surg Am* 2001;83-A:643-650.

    This is a retrospective case series of 55 reverse obliquity fractures that were treated with open reduction and internal fixation over 11 years. Sixty-eight percent of the fractures healed after the index operation, and 32% either failed to heal or had a failure of fixation. Failure occurred in 6 of 19 fractures that were treated using sliding hip screws, 2 of 15 fractures that were treated with blade plates, 3 of 10 fractures that were treated with dynamic condylar screws (95°), and 0 of 3 fractures that were treated with intramedullary hip screws. Overall, 46% of nonanatomically reduced fractures and 80% of fractures with non-ideally placed implants resulted in failure. The authors concluded that intramedullary and 95° screw-plate devices were superior to sliding hip screws in treating this type of fracture, and suggested that adequate reduction and ideal implant position were critical to a good outcome.

18. Sadowski C, Lubbeke A, Saudan M, Riand N, Stern R, Hoffmeyer P: Treatment of reverse oblique and transverse intertrochanteric fractures with use of an intramedullary nail or a 95-degree screw-plate. *J Bone Joint Surg Am* 2002;84-A:372-381.

    In this prospective, randomized study of 39 patients with OTA type 31-A3 fractures that were treated with either a dynamic condylar screw (95° screw-plate device) or an intramedullary nail, patients treated with an intramedullary nail had shorter surgical times, fewer blood transfusions, and shorter hospital stays. Implant failure or nonunion was noted in 7 of 19 patients who were treated with a dynamic condylar screw, but only in 1 of 20 patients who were treated with an intramedullary nail.

19. Russell T, Taylor J: Subtrochanteric fractures of the femur, in Browner B, Jupiter J, Levine A, Trafton P (eds): *Skeletal Trauma*. Philadelphia, PA, WB Saunders, 1992, pp 1883-1926.

20. Tencer A, Johnson K, Johnston D, et al: A biomechanical comparison of the various methods of stabilization of subtrochanteric fractures of the femur. *J Orthop Res* 1984;2:297-305.

21. Kraemer W, Hearn T, Powell J, et al: Fixation of segmental subtrochanteric fractures. *Clin Orthop* 1996;332:71-79.

22. Mahomed N, Harrington I, Kellam J, Maistrelli G, Hearn T, Vroemen J: Biomechanical analysis of the Gamma nail and sliding hip screw. *Clin Orthop* 1994; 304:280-288.

23. Kummer F, Olsson O, Pearlman C, et al: Intramedullary versus extramedullary fixation of subtrochanteric fractures. *Acta Orthop Scand* 1998;69:580-584.

24. Mahomed M, Harrington I, Hearn T: Biomechanical analysis of the Medoff sliding plate. *J Trauma* 2000; 48:93-103.

    In this biomechanical analysis of the Medoff sliding plate in human cadaveric femurs, results were compared with the AMBI plate and the Gamma nail. Findings demonstrated that the Medoff plate was stiffer than the other two implants for intertrochanteric fractures and segmental subtrochanteric fractures. The ultimate load to failure was lower than for the AMBI plate or the Gamma nail. The authors concluded that because the implant failed at loads of 50% less than other devices, it was at greater risk of failure in patients with an unstable subtrochanteric fracture.

25. Ceder L, Lunsjo K, Olsson O, et al: Different ways to treat subtrochanteric fractures with the Medoff sliding plate. *Clin Orthop* 1998;348:101-106.

26. Lunsjo K, Ceder L, Tidermark J, et al: Extramedullary fixation of 107 subtrochanteric fractures: A randomized multicenter trial of the Medoff sliding plate versus 3 other screw-plate systems. *Acta Orthop Scand* 1999;70:459-466.

27. Kulkarni S, Moran C: Results of dynamic condylar screw for subtrochanteric fractures. *Injury* 2003;34: 117-122.

28. Vaidya S, Dholakia D, Chatterjee A: The use of a dynamic condylar screw and biologic reduction techniques for subtrochanteric femur fractures. *Injury* 2003;34:123-128.

    In this study, 31 consecutive patients (mean age, 32.6 years), most of whom had high-energy subtrochanteric femur fractures, were treated with a dynamic condylar screw using a biologic plating technique. The union rate was 100%; 2 patients had a fracture malunion.

29. Neher C, Ostrum R: Treatment of subtrochanteric femur fractures using a submuscular fixed low angle plate. *Am J Orthop* 2003;32(suppl 9):29-33.

30. Broos P, Reynders P: The use of the unreamed AO femoral intramedullary nail with spiral blade in nonpathologic fracture of the femur: Experience with eighty consecutive cases. *J Orthop Trauma* 2002;16: 150-154.

    In this study, 80 patients were treated with an AO femoral intramedullary nail with spiral blade. Twenty-one percent failed before bony union and revision surgery was necessary in 9% of patients. All complications occurred in elderly women with Seinsheimer fracture type IIC or V.

The authors concluded by recommending that elderly women with reversed oblique fractures or subtrochanteric fractures with intertrochanteric component not be stabilized using this method.

31. French B, Tornetta P: Use of an interlocked cephalomedullary nail for subtrochanteric fracture stabilization. *Clin Orthop* 1998;348:95-100.

32. Barquet A, Francescoli L, Rienzi D, Lopez L: Intertrochanteric-subtrochanteric fractures: Treatment with the long Gamma nail. *J Orthop Trauma* 2000; 14:324-328.

The authors of this multicenter trial assessed 52 patients with intertrochanteric-subtrochanteric femur fractures in nonpathologic bone that were treated by closed reduction and internal fixation with a long Gamma nail. At follow-up, 43 patients were available for review. All fractures healed at an average of 4.3 months. One set of distal locking bolts fractured. Most patients returned to preinjury status on functional assessment.

33. Herscovici D Jr, Pistel WL, Sanders RW: Evaluation and treatment of high subtrochanteric fractures. *Am J Orthop* 2000;29(suppl 9):27-33.

Chapter 33

Fractures of the Femoral Diaphysis

Robert F. Ostrum, MD

Gary S. Gruen, MD

Boris A. Zelle, MD

Evaluation

Fractures of the femoral shaft often are the result of a high-energy injury. Although the fractured extremity may be the most obvious abnormality, the surgeon must be aware of the potential for other injuries. Usually, a traction splint is applied to the lower extremity first. Palpation of pulses is an important part of the initial examination. If the pulse is absent, it may return when the traction splint is applied. Measuring the Doppler arterial pressure index (API) with a blood pressure cuff is a noninvasive method of determining the presence of an arterial injury in the limb without an arteriogram. Ninety-four percent of patients with an API of less than 0.9 have positive angiographic findings, whereas those with an API greater than 0.9 have no injury or only minor injuries.[1]

A secondary survey of all extremities, the pelvis, and the spine is necessary to locate associated fractures. A detailed neurologic examination both proximal and distal to the fracture should be performed and documented in the conscious patient. Compartment syndrome, although uncommon, should be considered in those patients who are at high risk for this condition or in patients in whom an examination is not possible. All patients with femoral shaft fractures who present to the trauma center or emergency department should have an AP and lateral chest radiograph. The patient's pulmonary status and possible compromising factors may alter the timing of surgery and the postoperative course of treatment. An AP radiograph of the pelvis also is included in the initial evaluation. The femoral neck should be closely examined to determine if there is an associated femoral neck fracture. Radiographs of the femur should always include both the knee and the hip. However, because the hip is often resting in external rotation, the use of a radiograph to exclude a femoral neck fracture may be compromised. A CT scan of the abdomen and pelvis, which is often performed in a multiply injured patient, may show a fracture of the femoral neck that is not visible on plain radiographs.

Isolated femoral shaft fractures do not typically cause hypotension and shock. A trauma patient with a diaphyseal femoral fracture who presents in shock must be thoroughly examined to determine the cause of the hypotension. Bilateral femoral shaft fractures may result in blood loss within the thigh compartments that is sufficient to cause a drop in blood pressure; however, these patients usually have a higher degree of multisystem trauma.

Associated injuries to the patient and the injured extremity must be recognized and considered before treatment of the femoral fracture. The presence of an associated ipsilateral femoral neck or acetabular fracture may alter the treatment of the femoral shaft fracture. In patients with an unstable pelvic fracture, the use of a fracture table with a post and traction may be contraindicated. A temporary external fixator may be considered for patients with pulmonary or intracerebral trauma. Although difficult to assess on presentation, the ipsilateral knee should be examined for hemarthrosis and instability, which also may have an effect on the type of fixation performed along with considerations for future treatments.

Treatment

The treatment of femoral shaft fractures depends on several factors including fracture location, fracture pattern, size of the intramedullary canal, presence of other implants, soft-tissue injury, and the general condition of the patient. For most femoral shaft fractures the insertion of an antegrade locked intramedullary nail is the preferred treatment.

Traction

Although an osseous union can occur in a femoral shaft fracture that has been treated with traction, this method has several significant disadvantages such as malalignment, knee stiffness, and prolonged immobilization. However, the application of traction still plays a role in the treatment of femoral shaft fractures in children. In adult patients, traction is recommended only in patients who are unable to undergo surgery.

External Fixation

Temporary external fixation may be useful, particularly in patients with severe soft-tissue damage.[2] To reduce the risk of a medullary infection from the external pin sites, early conversion to an intramedullary nail is preferred.[3] Because external fixation is associated with a limited systemic inflammatory response compared with intramedullary nailing, temporary external fixation is also recommended in patients with unstable general health, such as those with multiple trauma and patients with severe pulmonary compromise.[4]

Plate Fixation

Plate fixation is used in special circumstances including the treatment of ipsilateral femoral neck and shaft fracture, in corrective osteotomy, and for fractures in skeletally immature adolescents. Soft-tissue stripping, which may result in a decreased vascular supply to the bone, is a major concern with plate fixation of the femur. Submuscular plating techniques with minimal deep dissection have been recommended for fractures undergoing femoral plating.[5,6]

Intramedullary Nailing

Reamed intramedullary nails are the gold standard in the treatment of femoral diaphyseal fractures and are associated with a high union rate and a low complication rate. The most recent generation of femoral nails is suited for use in all diaphyseal fractures as well as being applicable for treating subtrochanteric and supracondylar femoral fractures without compromising results. The decision to insert the nail from an antegrade or retrograde portal depends on a variety of factors that must be considered before surgery. Current percutaneous techniques may lead to less blood loss and may improve the patient's overall functional outcome. Open fractures treated with reamed antegrade intramedullary nailing after appropriate wound débridement have achieved excellent results.

Antegrade Versus Retrograde Nailing

Since 1940, antegrade nailing has been the standard for stabilizing femoral diaphyseal fractures. However, retrograde femoral nailing increased in popularity. Relative indications for the use of retrograde nailing in patients include morbid obesity, pregnancy, ipsilateral femoral neck and shaft fracture, bilateral femoral fractures, floating knee, and ipsilateral acetabular fracture.[7]

Several more recent studies have shown the usefulness of the retrograde approach and its ability to achieve good rates of union and excellent knee function.[7-13] In one study, 45 femoral shaft fractures were treated using an unreamed retrograde nail inserted 1 cm anterior to

the anterior cruciate ligament.[8] In the latter part of the study a percutaneous technique was used. A 95.5% union rate was achieved following the primary procedure. In another study, unreamed retrograde nails were used to treat a variety of femoral diaphyseal fractures.[9] Using a tendon splitting incision, a femoral distractor, and an unreamed nail, a union rate of 86% was obtained. The three nonunions did not heal after dynamizing and required exchange to a larger reamed antegrade nail to obtain a union. In a second study using unreamed canal filling retrograde nails, a protocol for dynamization was used at 6 to 12 weeks if little callus was seen. Thirty-three of 35 fractures healed.

In a prospective analysis, 61 fractures were treated with a 10-mm retrograde nail. Fifty-two percent of the fractures had Winquist 3 or 4 comminution, and 26% were open. Following the index procedure, 85% of the fractures healed. However, one bone graft and five dynamizations were required to achieve a 95% union rate. No differences in knee motion were found when a continuous passive motion machine was used. Although none of the 16 open fractures became infected, one patient with thigh fasciotomies developed a deep infection, which led to a septic knee. The use of a uniform size, 10-mm nail (even with reaming) led to lower union rates than those seen with canal-sized implants.

Three studies have compared antegrade and retrograde nailing.[11-13] The medical records of 283 patients with 293 femoral shaft fractures were reviewed.[12] Follow-up data were obtained on 104 fractures treated with retrograde nailing and 94 fractures treated with antegrade nailing. Union was achieved in 88% of the fractures treated with retrograde nailing and 89% of the fractures treated with antegrade nailing. These patients were treated using both a reamed and an unreamed technique without a standard protocol for the insertion method. The incidence of delayed unions, malunions, and nonunions were the same in both groups. The group treated with retrograde nailing had a higher incidence of knee pain, whereas the group treated with antegrade nailing had significantly more hip pain. The authors did not discuss the etiology of the knee pain.

In a prospective randomized clinical trial, the outcomes of 38 antegrade and 31 retrograde nailings were compared.[13] No differences in surgical time, blood loss, or transfusion requirements were found between the two groups. All fractures in both groups healed. A greater incidence of shortening and malrotation in the group that had retrograde nailing was reported; however, this finding was attributed to the use of a fracture table for patients treated with the antegrade nails and to the use of no traction for patients treated with the retrograde technique. A prospective study of 100 fractures treated with 10-mm nails that were inserted retrograde (54) and 10-mm nails inserted antegrade (46) showed that a greater number of the retrograde nails required dynamization compared with the antegrade inserted nails.[11] Eighty percent of the 10-mm retrograde nails and 56% of the 10-mm antegrade nails were undersized. The use of a retrograde nail that was undersized in diameter in relationship to the canal was shown to be related to delayed union in a linear regression analysis. Symptoms caused by distal screws were statistically higher in the retrograde group. There were no differences in surgical times, blood loss, knee motion, or time required to establish the starting point. When secondary procedures were included, 98% of the retrograde group healed and 100% of those treated with antegrade nailing also had fracture union.

In all of the three previous studies higher incidence of knee pain was noted in the retrograde group, whereas there was a greater incidence of thigh pain in the antegrade group.[11-13] Most of the knee pain was secondary to the use of the distal screws; however, most authors did not distinguish secondary traumatic knee pain from pain caused by hardware. Knee motion in patients treated with retrograde and antegrade nailing was equal in all of these studies. Most knees obtained greater than 120° of knee motion when there were no other associated ipsilateral limb injuries. Heterotopic ossification, myositis ossificans, arterial repair, large displaced shaft fragments, dislocated knees, and traumatic hemarthrosis were all given as causes for the decreased knee motion.[7-13]

Results of these studies show that reamed antegrade and retrograde nailing have very high union rates that are not statistically different.[8,11,12] The biology and morphology of the femoral shaft fracture are a greater determinant of fracture union than the point of insertion of the femoral intramedullary nail. Reamed, canal-filling implants had fewer complications and secondary surgeries than their unreamed counterparts. Unreamed nails with retrograde insertion had a higher incidence of delayed union and nonunion. Knee pain is more common in patients treated with retrograde nailing and may often be hardware related. Thigh pain has been reported more often in patients treated with antegrade nailing.

The method of antegrade femoral intramedullary nailing continues to be modified. Percutaneous approaches have increased in popularity. This technique uses a small skin incision made just distal to the iliac crest (more proximal than with the open technique) to allow proper alignment of the guide pin and rod in line with the femoral shaft. The starting site at the piriformis fossa is still considered optimal for antegrade nails; errors made by moving this entry portal too anterior can lead to increased hoop stresses in the proximal femur. Moreover, the treatment of high subtrochanteric fractures through a piriformis approach can be difficult and may result in varus malunion. In high subtrochanteric fractures, the proximal fragment may be abducted and externally rotated. In such instances, the use of the piriformis starting point may increase the risk of varus malunion. Several intramedullary nails have recently

been designed with a frontal plane 4°-angulation in the proximal fourth of the nail to allow for an off-axis trochanteric starting point. These nails seem to be effective in the treatment of femoral shaft fractures; however, the effect of a large entry hole on the abductor muscle insertion site is currently unknown and remains a concern.

Malunion

Intraoperative shortening of the limb with femoral nailing is attributable to the technique and not to the implant used. Postoperative shortening should be avoided by statically locking all femoral nails. With the use of a fracture table, proper limb length can be maintained during nailing. Intramedullary nailing without a fracture table is equally effective and results in a decrease in both setup time for the surgery and time under anesthesia for the patient. However, without a fracture table, limb length must be determined and restored by other means, especially in patients with comminuted and axially unstable fractures. Length determination can be accomplished in the operating room by placing a radiopaque ruler on the intact limb and using the fluoroscope to measure the distance from the intercondylar notch to the top of the lesser trochanter for retrograde nailing and from the epiphyseal scar distally to the tip of the greater trochanter for antegrade nailing. When antegrade nailing is done without a fracture table, it may be necessary to interlock the nail distally before proximally interlocking the nail. Following distal screw insertion through a free hand technique, the nail and screw construct is pounded distally to restore length. The technique of retrograde nail insertion may lead to limb shortening in unstable fracture patterns. When this occurs, insertion of the distal screws through the insertion jig with a "back slapping" of the nail will restore femoral length. Although possible, it is rare to overdistract the femoral fracture because the iliotibial band resists stretching beyond its normal length. Once obtained, the femoral length must be maintained while free-hand proximal locking of the nail is performed. A femoral distractor or temporary external fixator can be very effective in establishing or maintaining length. Rotation must also be determined before locking. By using an image intensifier and matching the orientation of the distal femur to the lesser trochanter (when compared with the uninjured femur), rotational malreduction can be minimized. The clinical significance of femoral malrotation is unknown but small rotations can probably be accommodated because of the normal rotational arc of the hip joint.

Nonunion

Primary union after reamed intramedullary nailing with canal-filling implants should be approximately 95% to 100% successful. In studies of retrograde nailing using smaller diameter, noncanal-filling implants, the incidence of delayed union and nonunion was higher.[7,9-11] Femoral fractures treated with unreamed smaller diameter antegrade nails took longer to heal than those treated with reamed nails. The time to union was 80 days for patients in the reamed group and 109 days for the unreamed group ($P = 0.002$) with the fractures of the distal one third of the shaft showing the greatest difference. A higher rate of technical complications was found in the unreamed group.[14] Delayed union may respond to dynamization but there must be an axially stable fracture pattern and an implant that nearly fills the medullary canal. Care must be taken, however, not to allow a dynamized nail to penetrate the knee joint if shortening occurs. If the morphology of the fracture site suggests length or rotational instability, then exchange nailing may be more appropriate. Exchange nailing may be performed after retrograde nailing although several authors have recommended antegrade nailing after removal of the retrograde nail. In one study of exchange nailing of the femur for nonunion, union was reported in only 53% of patients.[15] Another study found a significant association between patients who smoke and failure to achieve union after exchange nailing.[16]

Postoperative Weight Bearing

The size, type, and number of distal interlocking screws as well as the fracture morphology and its axial stability will determine the ability of the fracture-nail construct to withstand weight bearing. Two distal screws usually are used for distal one third femoral shaft fractures and comminuted fractures with little or no axial stability. A 1999 study[17] showed that two distal interlocking screws were significantly stronger than one. Patients with statically locked comminuted femoral shaft fractures who immediately bore weight showed no hardware failure; only one dynamization was required to achieve union.

Outcome

Union rates are close to 100% when reamed, canal-filling antegrade or retrograde femoral nails are used in the treatment of femoral shaft fractures. Patients treated with retrograde nailing tend to have a higher incidence of postoperative knee pain and effusion, which resolves after several weeks. Pain caused by the placement of distal screws is seen in some patients because of the lack of soft-tissue coverage on the femoral condyles.[7,11,12] Screw removal may be necessary following union. Knee motion does not appear to be compromised after retrograde nailing. It is unknown if there are long-term consequences from using an intra-articular starting point. Antegrade nailing also has inherent complications with up to 40% of patients experiencing proximal hip and thigh pain after antegrade nailing. There was a strong correlation to the development of heterotopic bone at

the trochanter and not all patients obtained relief after nail removal.[18] Trendelenburg gait is another possible complication and can be severe enough to interfere with activities of daily living and the ability to work.

For patients treated with antegrade or retrograde nailing who do not have associated injuries around the extremity, knee motion should return to near normal by 12 weeks after surgery. Some multiply injured patients and others with head injuries may have decreased motion caused by the development of heterotopic bone around the hip, knee, or within the quadriceps. The inability to cooperate with early active range-of-motion rehabilitation may lead to a stiff knee. Fractures of the distal third of the femur can result in limited knee range of motion if fibrosis develops in the patella and the suprapatellar pouch.

Evaluation of the Femoral Neck

In 1953, the combination of fractures of the ipsilateral proximal femur and the femoral shaft was initially described.[19] Ipsilateral fractures of the proximal femur and the femoral shaft are often the result of high-energy injuries, especially vehicle crashes and falls from a height.[20] It has been speculated that the injury mechanism includes longitudinal compressive forces on the femur, as is seen in dashboard injuries. The femoral neck may be subjected to shear forces when the residual energy that is not dissipated by the femoral shaft is absorbed by the proximal femur.[21] The high incidence of associated ipsilateral knee injuries (approximately 20% to 40%) further substantiates the likelihood of this mechanism. Approximately 2.5% to 9% of all femoral shaft fractures are associated with an ipsilateral proximal femur fracture.[20,21] In particular, comminuted and open femoral shaft fractures seem to be associated with an ipsilateral proximal femoral fracture.[22,23] In approximately 20% to 30% of patients, the associated femoral neck fracture is overlooked during the initial assessment.[22] The clinical assessment may be complicated in patients with concomitant injuries who may be sedated and intubated when examined in the emergency department. The presence of an associated ipsilateral femoral shaft fracture predisposes the proximal femur to external rotation. The superimposition of the greater trochanter and the femoral neck on the AP radiograph may mask the femoral neck fracture. The initial radiographic assessment of patients with femoral shaft fractures should always include high-quality AP and lateral views of the ipsilateral hip joint. Many associated proximal femoral fractures are vertically oriented, transcervical neck fractures that are often nondisplaced or minimally displaced.[20-22] Abdominal or pelvic CT scans may be obtained as part of the advanced trauma life support protocol; the femoral neck should be carefully scrutinized. All patients who undergo intramedullary nailing of their femoral shaft fracture also should have postoperative conventional radiographs of their hip joint.

The high incidence of ipsilateral knee injuries associated with combined neck-shaft fractures requires a detailed examination of the ipsilateral knee joint. In addition to preoperative and postoperative radiographs of the knee joint, the ipsilateral knee joint must be carefully evaluated for ligamentous instabilities. This evaluation is often best performed on the anesthetized patient while in the operating room following the fixation of the femoral fractures.

Considerations in Patients With Multiple Trauma

Survival rates in patients with multiple trauma are determined by various factors such as injury severity, the individual biologic response to the injury, and the clinical treatment. It has been shown that the surgical treatment strategy within the first 24 hours after injury has a major impact on outcome for these patients.[4,24] In severely injured patients, the risk of developing multiple organ failure can be as high as 75%.[25] Recent studies have shown that surgical treatment following severe trauma may cause an unfavorable immunologic response, resulting in adverse clinical outcomes.[24] This impact of surgical injury management has been described as the second hit phenomenon, with the initial trauma representing the first hit and the surgical burden being the second hit.[24] Therefore, the timing and the type of initial surgery have gained importance. To reduce the adverse effects of the second hit, the principles of damage control orthopedics (DCO) were introduced.[26] Originally, the term damage control was used to describe the treatment of patients with severe abdominal injuries.[27] The principles of damage control include the immediate surgical treatment of major injuries with significant blood loss, followed by secondary definitive repair of injuries when the patient's general condition has been stabilized.[27] These treatment principles were adapted for multiple-trauma patients with multiple long bone fractures who are at risk for multiple organ failure. In these patients, temporary external fixation of long bone fractures and pelvic injuries is performed as an emergency procedure. After adequate resuscitation, the patient is taken back to the operating room for definitive fracture stabilization. The principles of DCO are used to minimize the second hit in multiple-trauma patients who are at risk for multiple organ failure. Recent clinical studies suggested that following the principles of DCO may significantly reduce the morbidity and mortality of multiply injured patients.[4] The identification of patients who should be treated according to DCO principles is difficult, and the inclusion criteria are still considered controversial. Patients who appear to be at higher risk to deteriorate if treated with extensive early surgical care include hemodynamically unstable patients with complicated resuscitation and those with significant head trauma, severe chest trauma with bi-lateral lung contusion, coagulopathy, and hypothermia ($< 32°C$).[4] Future immunologic and genetic investigations may provide parameters that identify patients who are clinically at high risk for posttraumatic complications.

Head Injury

One study showed there was increased fluid administration and a higher incidence of intraoperative hypotension and hypoxia in patients with head injury who underwent early fracture fixation.[28] The authors also found that these patients had a lower Glasgow Coma Scale score at the time of discharge and warned that hypoxemia and intraoperative hypotension associated with early fracture fixation may contribute to a poor neurologic outcome.

Other studies have refuted these conclusions. In one study of early and delayed pelvic and lower extremity fixation in patients with head injuries, there was no evidence to suggest that early fixation had detrimental effects on the central nervous system.[29] In another study, two groups of patients with head injuries were examined to determine whether a delay in femoral fracture fixation increased pulmonary complications and whether immediate nailing increased the incidence of complications to the central nervous system.[30] A logistic regression analysis showed that a delay in femoral fracture fixation increased the incidence of pulmonary complications in patients with head injuries. More importantly, the results supported the fact that early fixation of the femur did not increase the incidence of complications involving the central nervous system.

Medullary Reaming

The use of intramedullary reaming and early femoral nail insertion in patients with associated injuries is a controversial subject. Reaming is performed before femoral intramedullary nailing to allow for easy placement of a larger, more rigid implant. It has been shown that reaming decreases the major endosteal blood flow to the cortex for about 12 weeks in dogs, perhaps longer in humans. However, higher union rates and a lower incidence of secondary revision surgery has been found in patients who underwent reamed nailing when compared with those who had unreamed nailing.[14]

In one study, lung function was stable and the pulmonary arterial pressure did not increase in the group with unreamed femoral nailing, whereas potentially harmful disturbances in lung function and increases in pulmonary arterial pressure did occur in the group of patients treated with reamed nailing.[31] In another study, results showed that in patients with pulmonary injury the placement of a reamed nail within the first 24 hours after injury led to a higher incidence of adult respiratory distress syndrome (ARDS) (33% versus 7.7%) and a higher mortality rate (21% versus 4%) than in those patients in whom a nail was placed more than 24 hours after injury.[32]

The results of animal studies raised additional questions when it was shown that the mere opening of the piriformis fossa resulted in the release of a large number of emboli and that the insertion of an unreamed nail led to higher pressures and more emboli than the passage of a reamed nail.[33] Several animal studies suggested that although intramedullary reaming is associated with fatty emboli, the lung's physiologic parameters were not significantly different between reamed and unreamed nailing. Results from one study found no differences in intrapulmonary shunting, venous oxygen saturation, the pulmonary vascular resistance index, pulmonary wedge pressure, mean arterial pressure, the cardiac index, or the alveolar arterial oxygen gradient in a sheep model.[34] It was that in either a normal lung or one in an ARDS–like state, the fat embolization of reamed intramedullary nailing had no clinically significant effect in a resuscitated sheep model. Therefore, these animal studies suggest that the fat embolization caused by reaming may result in no significant lung permeability complications or compliance disturbances.[33,34]

Other studies have suggested that in the multiply injured patient the pulmonary injury itself and its level of severity were the major determinants of morbidity and mortality rather than the femoral shaft fracture, its treatment, or timing of the surgery.[35-37] In a study of severely injured patients (injury severity score > 40), the incidence of ARDS was 17% when nailing was done within 24 hours after injury versus 75% when femoral nailing was delayed.[37] Other studies (using a definition of ARDS as a $Pao_2 < 70$ on $FiO_2 = 40\%$ with concomitant pulmonary radiographic changes) have not shown adverse outcomes following nailing of the femoral fracture within the first 24 hours after injury. In fact, early intramedullary nailing of the femur has been associated with lower morbidities and mortalities. A comparison of pulmonary complications in patients with multiple trauma including chest injury and femoral shaft fractures was performed to determine if plating had a beneficial effect over reamed intramedullary nailing of the femoral fracture.[35] Results showed no adverse effects with reference to ARDS, pulmonary embolism, multiple organ failure, pneumonia, or death when comparing acute reamed nailing to plating of the femoral shaft fracture.

Special Circumstances

Ipsilateral Femoral Neck and Shaft Fractures

Multiple treatment options exist for ipsilateral femoral neck and shaft fractures including single implants that simultaneously address both injuries (for example, cephalomedullary nails) or combined procedures that address each injury separately. Depending on the characteristics and location of each fracture, the combination of a medullary implant (with antegrade or retrograde nailing) or a plate with a sliding hip screw or multiple cancellous screws can be used successfully. Although a single implant may initially appear to be an attractive option, a high incidence of femoral neck nonunion was identified in one study.[23] Because the nail entry site is frequently in close proximity to the cephalad extension of the femoral neck fracture, cephalomedullary implants have the added risk of worsening fracture displacement or inducing femoral neck varus deformity. Furthermore, the sliding characteristics of the femoral neck fixation is questionable, carrying a theoretical risk for neck nonunion. This concern has led to the recommendation that the treatment of intracapsular femoral neck fractures be prioritized, particularly as multiple successful options have been demonstrated for femoral shaft fracture stabilization.[23] Depending on the characteristics of the femoral neck fracture, it can first be stabilized with multiple cancellous lag screws or a sliding hip screw. The femoral shaft component can then be stabilized with either a plate or a retrograde nail if appropriate (Figure 1). In the event that an ipsilateral nondisplaced femoral neck fracture is identified after antegrade femoral nailing, strategic screw placement anterior to the femoral nail can be successfully performed. In patients who initially had negative radiographs but continue to have hip pain following intramedullary nailing, an occult femoral neck fracture should be suspected and CT scans of the hip should be obtained.

Bilateral Femoral Shaft Fractures

Multiply injured patients with bilateral femoral shaft fracture have a higher rate of ARDS, mortality, and associated injuries. The increased risk seen in these patients is not caused by the femoral fractures but by the associated multiple organ system injuries that accompany these fractures.[38] If the patient is initially in shock, it may be appropriate to place external fixators on both femurs until the patient has been resuscitated and is in better condition for surgery. In the patient who can tolerate an early nailing of the femoral shaft or for those with femoral shaft fractures that can be nailed after removal of external fixators, retrograde nailing done sequentially or simultaneously is effective. Placing the patient supine eliminates the need for the fracture table or turning of the patient and is advantageous in patients who often have multiple injuries. This technique also significantly reduces the time required for the prepping and draping of one leg followed by the other as both limbs are prepared for surgery at the same time. The determination of limb length and rotation also can be easier with both limbs accessible; other fractures or wounds can be treated at the same time.

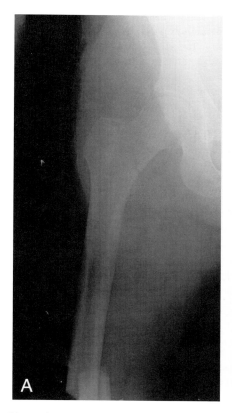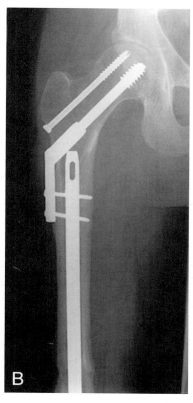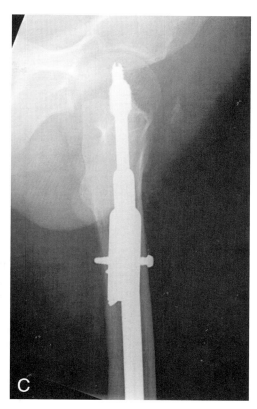

Figure 1 Radiographs of a 32-year-old man with multiple injuries, including a right basocervical femoral neck fracture and a femoral shaft fracture, from a motor vehicle crash **(A)**. **B,** Treatment consisted of open reduction and stabilization of the femoral neck fracture with a sliding hip screw and an antirotational screw. **C,** This treatment was followed by placement of a retrograde nail that terminated just distal to the barrel of the hip screw. The screws inserted through the side plate are bicortical screws directed around the retrograde nail.

Gunshot Wounds

Femoral diaphyseal fractures secondary to gunshot wounds should be treated with the same protocols that are used for open fractures. Injuries with small wounds caused by handguns can be treated without extensive débridement. Larger wounds may require débridement followed by insertion of a reamed intramedullary nail. For high-velocity wounds with greater soft-tissue damage, the administration of appropriate antibiotics and multiple débridements may be necessary after the placement of the intramedullary nail. Comminution at the fracture site should determine the placement and number of screws. External fixation should be used for the initial treatment of femoral fractures secondary to gunshot wounds that are associated with a vascular injury.

Annotated References

1. Johansen K, Lynch K, Paun M, Copass M: Noninvasive vascular tests reliably exclude occult arterial trauma in injured extremities. *J Trauma* 1991;31:515-519.

2. Gustilo RB, Mendoza RM, Williams DN: Problems in the management of type III (severe) open fractures: A new classification of type III open fractures. *J Trauma* 1984;24:742-746.

3. Nowotarski PJ, Turen CH, Brumback RJ, Scarboro JM: Conversion of external fixation to intramedullary nailing for fractures of the shaft of the femur in multiply injured patients. *J Bone Joint Surg Am* 2000;82:781-788.

   The outcomes of 59 fractures that were treated with temporary external fixation and later converted to fixation with intramedullary nailing were reported. Four patients had draining at the pin sites and required temporary traction before nail fixation. The overall union rate was 97%.

4. Pape HC, Hildebrand F, Pertschy S, et al: Changes in the management of femoral shaft fractures in polytrauma patients: From early total care to damage control orthopedic surgery. *J Trauma* 2002;53:452-462.

   In this retrospective review, the authors investigated the outcomes in multiple-trauma patients with associated femoral shaft fractures that were treated with early total care compared with DCO. The incidence of multiple organ failure and ARDS was significantly lower in the DCO group.

5. Krettek C, Muller M, Miclau T: Evolution of minimally invasive plate osteosynthesis (MIPO) in the femur. *Injury* 2001;32(suppl 3):SC14-SC23.

   In this tutorial review, the authors described the evolution and the technique of submuscular plating in the treatment of distal femoral shaft fractures.

6. Schutz M, Muller M, Krettek C, et al: Minimally invasive fracture stabilization of distal femoral fractures with the LISS: A prospective multicenter study: Results of a clinical study with special emphasis on difficult cases. *Injury* 2001;32(suppl 3):SC48-SC54.

   The authors treated 116 distal femoral fractures using the less invasive stabilization system-distal femur implant system. Twenty-three revision surgeries were necessary in 21 patients.

7. Ostrum RF, DiCicco J, Lakatos R, Poka A: Retrograde nailing of femoral diaphyseal fractures. *J Orthop Trauma* 1998;12:464-468.

8. Herscovici D Jr, Whiteman KW: Retrograde nailing of the femur using an intercondylar approach. *Clin Orthop* 1996;332:98-104.

9. Moed BR, Watson JT: Retrograde intramedullary nailing, without reaming, of fractures of the femoral shaft in multiply injured patients. *J Bone Joint Surg Am* 1995;77:1520-1527.

10. Moed BR, Watson JT, Cramer KE, Karges DE, Teefey JS: Unreamed retrograde intramedullary nailing of fractures of the femoral shaft. *J Orthop Trauma* 1998;12:334-342.

11. Ostrum RF, Agarwal A, Lakatos R, Poka A: Prospective comparison of retrograde and antegrade femoral intramedullary nailing. *J Orthop Trauma* 2000;14:496-501.

    In this study involving the use of 54 retrograde and 46 antegrade 10-mm nails, the authors showed that a greater number of the retrograde nails required dynamization compared with the antegrade group.

12. Ricci WM, Bellabarba C, Evanoff B, Herscovici D, DiPasquale T, Sanders R: Retrograde versus antegrade nailing of femoral shaft fractures. *J Orthop Trauma* 2001;15:161-169.

    The results of 104 retrograde and 94 antegrade intramedullary nailing procedures were reviewed. The nonunion rates were comparable in both groups (88% versus 89%). Patients in the retrograde group had a higher incidence of knee pain while the antegrade group had significantly more hip pain.

13. Tornetta P III, Tiburzi D: Antegrade or retrograde reamed femoral nailing: A prospective, randomised trial. *J Bone Joint Surg Br* 2000;82:652-654.

    This prospective comparison of 68 antegrade and 69 retrograde femoral nailing procedures showed no differences in surgery time, blood loss, and union rates between patients receiving the antegrade-inserted and retrograde-inserted nails. A greater incidence of limb shortening and malrotation was found in the group treated with retrograde nailing.

14. Tornetta P III, Tiburzi D: Reamed versus nonreamed anterograde femoral nailing. *J Orthop Trauma* 2000;14:15-19.

    The authors compared reamed versus unreamed femoral nailing. Time to union was 80 days for the reamed group and 109 days for the unreamed group ($P = 0.002$). The incidence of technical complications and delayed unions was higher in the unreamed group.

15. Weresh MJ, Hakanson R, Stover MD, Sims SH, Kellam JF, Bosse MJ: Failure of exchange reamed intramedullary nails for ununited femoral shaft fractures. *J Orthop Trauma* 2000;14:335-338.

16. Hak DJ, Lee SS, Goulet JA: Success of exchange reamed intramedullary nailing for femoral shaft nonunion or delayed union. *J Orthop Trauma* 2000;14:178-182.

17. Brumback RJ, Toal TR Jr, Murphy-Zane MS, Novak VP, Belkoff SM: Immediate weight-bearing after treatment of a comminuted fracture of the femoral shaft with a statically locked intramedullary nail. *J Bone Joint Surg Am* 1999;81:1538-1544.

18. Dodenhoff RM, Dainton JN, Hutchins PM: Proximal thigh pain after femoral nailing: Causes and treatment. *J Bone Joint Surg Br* 1997;79:738-741.

19. Delaney WM, Street DM: Fracture of the femoral shaft with fracture of neck of same femur: Treatment with medullary nail for shaft and Knowles pins for neck. *J Int Coll Surg* 1953;19:303.

20. Swiontkowski MF, Hansen ST, Kellam J: Ipsilateral fractures of the femoral neck and shaft: A treatment protocol. *J Bone Joint Surg Am* 1984;66:260-268.

21. Alho A: Concurrent ipsilateral fractures of the hip and shaft of the femur: A systematic review of 722 cases. *Ann Chir Gynaecol* 1997;86:326-336.

22. Shuler TE, Gruen GS, DiTano O, Riemer BL: Ipsilateral proximal and shaft femoral fractures: Spectrum of injury involving the femoral neck. *Injury* 1997;28:293-297.

23. Watson JT, Moed BR: Ipsilateral femoral neck and shaft fractures. *Clin Orthop* 2002;399:78-86.

The authors reviewed their database for patients who developed complications after fracture fixation of ipsilateral neck-shaft fractures. They reported that lag screw fixation of the femoral neck fracture and reamed intramedullary nailing were associated with the lowest complication rates.

24. Pape HC, Schmidt RE, Rice J, et al: Biomechanical changes after trauma and skeletal surgery of the lower extremity: Quantification of the operative burden. *Crit Care Med* 2000;28:3441-3448.

These authors quantified the surgical burden by measuring the intraoperative concentrations of interleukin-6, tumor necrosis factor, prothrombin fragments, and D-dimers. Multiply injured patients undergoing intramedullary femoral nailing had significantly higher interleukin-6 concentrations than patients with isolated femoral fractures and patients undergoing total hip arthroplasty.

25. Moore FA, Moore EE: Evolving concepts in the pathogenesis of postinjury multiple organ failure. *Surg Clin North Am* 1995;75:257-277.

26. Scalea TM, Boswell SA, Scott JD, et al: External fixation as a bridge to intramedullary nailing for patients with multiple injuries and femur fractures: Damage control orthopedics. *J Trauma* 2000;48:613-621.

The authors introduced the term damage control orthopedics into the literature. They reported favorable results and low complication rates in 43 patients who were treated with temporary external fixation for their femoral shaft fracture.

27. Rotondo MF, Schwab CW, McGonial MD, et al: Damage control: An approach for improved survival in exsanguinating penetrating abdominal injuries. *J Trauma* 1993;35:375-382.

28. Jaicks RR, Cohn SM, Moller BA: Early fracture fixation may be deleterious after head injury. *J Trauma* 1997;42:1-5.

29. Scalea TM, Scott JD, Brumback RJ, et al: Early fracture fixation may be "just fine" after head injury: No difference in central nervous system outcomes. *J Trauma* 1999;46:839-846.

30. Starr AJ, Hunt JL, Chason DP, Reinert CM, Walker J: Treatment of femur fracture with associated head injury. *J Orthop Trauma* 1998;12:38-45.

31. Pape HC, Regel G, Dwenger A, et al: Influences of different methods of intramedullary femoral nailing on lung function in patients with multiple trauma. *J Trauma* 1993;35:709-716.

32. Pape HC: Auf'm'Kolk M, Paffrath T, Regel G, Sturm JA, Tscherne H: Primary intramedullary femur fixation in multiple trauma patients with associated lung contusion: A cause of posttraumatic ARDS? *J Trauma* 1993;34:540-547.

33. Duwelius PJ, Huckfeldt R, Mullins RJ, et al: The effects of femoral intramedullary reaming on pulmonary function in a sheep lung model. *J Bone Joint Surg Am* 1997;79:194-202.

34. Wolinsky PR, Banit D, Parker RE, et al: Reamed intramedullary femoral nailing after induction of an "ARDS-like" state in sheep: Effect on clinically applicable markers of pulmonary function. *J Orthop Trauma* 1998;12:169-175.

35. Bosse MJ, MacKenzie EJ, Riemer BL, et al: Adult respiratory distress syndrome, pneumonia, and mortality following thoracic injury and a femoral fracture treated either with intramedullary nailing with reaming or with a plate: A comparative study. *J Bone Joint Surg Am* 1997;79:799-809.

36. Brundage SI, McGhan R, Jurkovich GJ, Mack CD, Maier RV: Timing of femur fracture fixation: Effect on outcome in patients with thoracic and head injuries. *J Trauma* 2002;52:299-307.

The outcomes of patients undergoing femoral fracture fixation within 24 hours after injury versus femoral fracture fixation between 2 and 5 days after injury were compared. In patients with associated head trauma, fixation between 2 and 5 days was associated with an increased incidence of ARDS, pneumonia, and fat embolization.

37. Johnson KD, Cadambi A, Seibert GB: Incidence of adult respiratory distress syndrome in patients with multiple musculoskeletal injuries: Effect of early operative stabilization of fractures. *J Trauma* 1985;25:375-384.

38. Copeland CE, Mitchell KA, Brumback RJ, Gens DR, Burgess AR: Mortality in patients with bilateral femoral fractures. *J Orthop Trauma* 1998;12:315-319.

The mortality and ARDS rates between patients with bilateral and unilateral femoral fractures were compared. Although the incidence of bilateral femoral fractures correlated with the incidence of mortality, the incidence of shock, closed head injury, and thoracic injury correlated more strongly with mortality.

Chapter 34

Fractures of the Distal Femur

Philip James Kregor, MD

Steven J. Morgan, MD

Introduction

Fractures of the distal femur, often the result of high-energy trauma, remain a vexing problem. The treatment of these fractures has progressed steadily over the past several decades, resulting in significant improvement in outcomes. Although techniques and implants have improved, the basic tenets of fracture care in the distal femur have remained the same. These include (1) visualization and precise reduction of the articular surface; (2) restoration of length, alignment, and rotation; (3) preservation of the soft-tissue envelope around the fracture; (4) stable internal fixation, and (5) early range of motion.

Early experience with traditional plating emphasized precise anatomic reduction of all cortical fragments in the metaphyseal region.[1] This technique provided stable, rigid fixation and improved eventual range of motion when compared with nonsurgical techniques. However, the fracture exposure and devitalization inherent in such a technique led to high rates of infection, nonunion, and need for bone grafting. Over the past decade, indirect reduction techniques have been popularized, and their use has proved efficacious in the treatment of fractures of the distal femur.[2] The major goal with such techniques in the treatment of fractures of the distal femur is to decrease the surgical trauma to the metaphyseal-diaphyseal component of the fracture. Indirect reduction techniques for the distal femur can include manual traction, supracondylar bumps, use of the femoral distractor, and use of the implant (such as a 95° angle blade plate or intramedullary nail) to allow the reduction. All techniques aid in the reduction of the fracture without direct fracture exposure. Indirect reduction techniques are essential for biologic plating of the distal femur.[2,3]

Further refinement of biologic plating evolved into submuscular plating techniques in which the plate is slid into the potential space beneath the vastus lateralis.[4,5] Such techniques may further diminish surgical insult to the fracture environment and allow for improved visualization of the joint surface (lateral parapatellar approach).

Plates with locked screws have obviated the need to place internal fixation on the medial aspect of the femur to prevent varus collapse. This fixation construct has been shown to be biomechanically superior in minimizing loss of fixation when tested in osteoporotic bone.[6] Clinically, it has also been advantageous in preventing varus collapse of the distal femur.[7,8]

Preoperative Assessment and Timing of Fixation

The prerequisites for surgical intervention for a distal femur fracture include a well-resuscitated patient without life-threatening injuries, a good understanding of the articular injury, and an appropriate surgical team. If these prerequisites are not met, the application of a unilateral external fixator to simply span the zone of injury is an excellent modality to restore length and provide temporary stability.

The type of articular injury determines the surgical approach and the type of implant to be used. As such, a complete understanding of the articular injury is vital. In every distal femur fracture, it is mandatory to obtain definitive answers to the following questions preoperatively: (1) Is there an intercondylar split? (2) If there is an intercondylar split, is it complex or simple? (Are there separate osteochondral fragments?) (3) Is there an associated Hoffa (frontal) plane fracture?

Oblique radiographs, and particularly supplemental AP and lateral traction views, usually allow for accurate diagnosis. Although not routinely necessary for all fractures, CT with sagittal and coronal reconstructions will delineate the articular pathology. Thus, if there is any question regarding the interpretation of plain and traction films, CT is indicated.

In patients with open distal femur fractures, urgent irrigation and débridement is performed. If the previously noted prerequisites are met and the surgeon is confident in the débridement of the fracture and wound, immediate fixation can ensue. If this is not the case, a spanning external fixator should be placed. Submuscular plating techniques may be helpful in minimizing the need

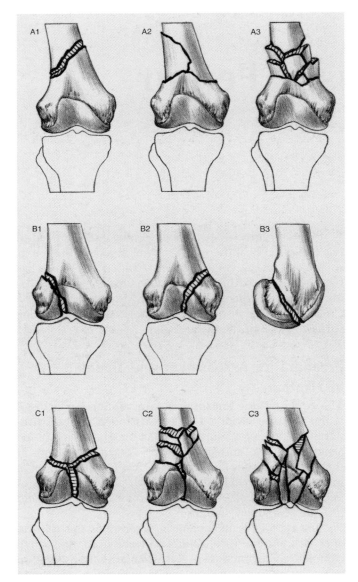

Figure 1 The AO/OTA classification of distal femur fractures. *(Reproduced with permission from Hansen ST, Swiontkowski MF (eds): Orthopaedic Trauma Protocols. New York, NY, Raven Press, 1993, p 296.)*

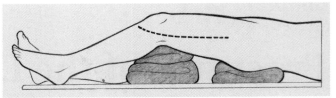

Figure 2 Skin incision *(dotted line)* for an anterolateral approach to the distal femur. This approach can be used for type A and C1/C2 injuries (simple articular split). It may be problematic when used for type C3 injuries. For example, a medial Hoffa fracture is difficult to reduce using this approach. *(Reproduced with permission from Hansen ST, Swiontkowski MF (eds): Orthopaedic Trauma Protocols. New York, NY, Raven Press, 1993, p 304.)*

for an additional large incision for plate application. A plate can often be slid in a submuscular manner through the open wound after irrigation and débridement.

Classification

The AO/Orthopaedic Trauma Association (OTA) classification for distal femur fractures aids in the choice of surgical approach and implant type (Figure 1). Type A fractures are extra-articular, type B fractures are partial articular (separating either the medial or lateral condyle from the shaft, but not both), and type C fractures are those with both condyles involved. A key differentiation is made in this classification system between a C1/C2 injury and a C3 injury. A C1/C2 injury is characterized by

a simple articular split, whereas a C3 injury is a complex articular injury characterized by either multiple fracture planes and/or frontal plane (Hoffa) involvement.

Surgical Approach and Technique

The classification of the distal femoral fracture will delineate the surgical approach. For an extra-articular injury (AO/OTA type A), no visualization of the joint via an arthrotomy is necessary, although it may be helpful to ensure proper positioning of a lateral plate. When using a retrograde intramedullary nail to treat an extra-articular fracture, the required visualization of the articular surface is minimal and can be limited to a percutaneous approach.

For supracondylar fractures with articular involvement, the differentiation between a C1/C2 and C3 injury will enable the surgeon to choose the appropriate approach. For a C1/C2 injury, the standard anterolateral approach to the distal femur is used. A curvilinear incision is made along the midlateral aspect of the femur and curves toward the tibial tubercle. A division in the iliotibial band then parallels the skin incision (Figure 2). The vastus lateralis is then lifted anteriorly, and the joint capsule is divided to the level of the meniscus. Exposure of the articular surface is aided by placement of a blunt retractor on the medial aspect of the femoral condyle.

If the surgeon uses the standard anterolateral approach to treat a C3 injury, however, visualization and reduction of separate osteochondral fragments and/or the Hoffa fracture may be difficult. For this reason, a lateral parapatellar approach may be a more appropriate surgical approach for this type of fracture (Figure 3). Comparable to the medial parapatellar approach used for total knee arthroplasty, the lateral parapatellar approach allows for eversion of the patella and complete visualization of the articular surface. To use the lateral parapatellar approach, however, the plate must be placed submuscularly.

The technique of articular reduction may be difficult. Complete visualization of the articular surface gives the surgeon the best opportunity to achieve the appropriate reduction and fixation. Tools that aid in reduction of the

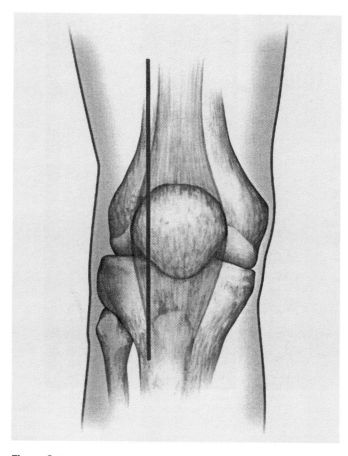

Figure 3 The lateral parapatellar approach to the knee (line indicates skin incision). This allows for eversion of the patella and excellent visualization of the distal femoral articular surface.

TABLE 1 | Possible Implants for Distal Femoral Fractures as Determined by AO/OTA Classification

Type A or C1/C2 Fractures
  Dynamic condylar screw
  95° blade plate
  Antegrade femoral nail
  Retrograde femoral nail
  Locked internal fixator (LISS, lateral plate with locked distal screws)
Type B Fractures
  Screw and/or plate fixation
Type C3 Fractures
  Standard condylar buttress plate
  Locked internal fixator (LISS, lateral plate with locked distal screws)

condylar blocks include pointed reduction clamps, large pelvic clamps, an external fixator pin in the medial femoral condyle to act as a joystick, and Kirschner wire fixation for provisional fixation. Lag screws, usually placed from lateral to medial, can then be used to address the articular surface. Although traditionally these lag screws have been 6.5-mm partially threaded lag screws, 3.5-mm cortical lag screws placed in the subchondral bone are more routinely being used.

Implant Choices

As with the choice of surgical approach, the choice of implant is guided by an understanding of the articular injury (Table 1). For extra-articular fractures and simple articular injuries, a variety of techniques have proven efficacy.

Intramedullary Nailing

Antegrade intramedullary nailing is generally reserved for treating extra-articular supracondylar fractures.[9] The main limitation of this technique is the proximity of the fracture to the joint surface. Sufficient distance between the fracture and the joint surface must exist to allow for the placement of two distal interlocking screws. Lack of two distal points of fixation in these fractures will lead to toggle around the distal aspect of the nail and eventual loss of reduction. In addition, placement of a relatively large intramedullary nail (such as a 13- to 15-mm nail) and distal (long) intramedullary nail will provide the best fixation of a distal femur fracture. Maintenance of the reduction before antegrade intramedullary nailing may require the use of a fracture table and skeletal traction. The unopposed pull of the gastrocnemius muscle on the distal femoral segment is the major deforming force. Correction of the common apex posterior deformity may be facilitated by the use of an auxiliary device placed at the apex of the deformity to eliminate the posterior sag of the fracture.

Retrograde intramedullary nailing has been used successfully in the treatment of distal femur fractures.[10-13] Retrograde insertion of an intramedullary nail has become a popular technique, especially for fixation of type A or C1/C2 distal femur fractures[14,15] (Figure 4). Although there are some reports of using retrograde intramedullary nail fixation to treat type C3 injuries,[11,12] it is not commonplace. There is considerable concern regarding disruption of the articular surface reduction when using this technique in patients with C3 injuries.

There are several advantages of retrograde nailing for distal femur fractures. Retrograde insertion obviates the need of a fracture table for reduction. Fracture reduction is obtained with minimal longitudinal traction and a wedge placed under the knee. Intramedullary nails designed for retrograde insertion have locking holes in close proximity to the distal aspect of the nail, allowing for distal interlocking in shorter supracondylar segments than can be obtained with antegrade nailing techniques. The intramedullary nails are also designed with an anterior to posterior locking hole in the proximal aspect of the nail to facilitate proximal interlocking in the upper portion of the femur. When using a retrograde intramed-

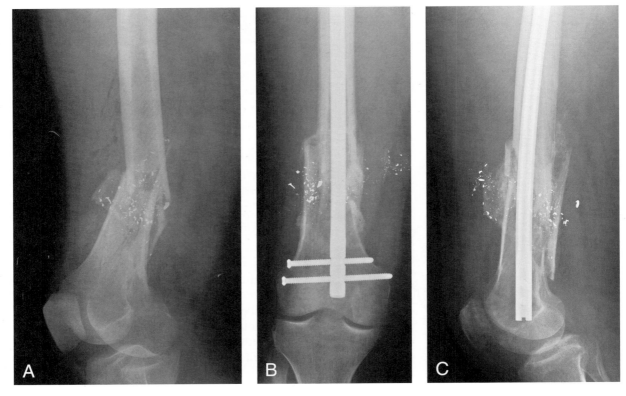

Figure 4 A, Injury radiograph of a patient with a distal femur fracture caused by a ballistic injury. AP **(B)** and lateral **(C)** radiographs at 2.5 months after injury shows rapid consolidation of the distal femur fracture.

ullary nail to treat a C1 or C2 injury, the articular injury must first be visualized, reduced, and fixed with traditional lag screws, which are placed outside the nail path. Retrograde intramedullary nailing can be performed via parapatellar arthrotomy (which allows for joint visualization) or a patellar tendon splitting approach. The entry site is located in line with the intramedullary femoral canal on the AP radiograph and 1 cm anterior to the posterior cruciate ligament or at the anterior aspect of the Blumensaat line on the lateral radiograph.

This technique of retrograde intramedullary nail insertion is not without controversy. Although the described insertion site is not thought to be an articulating surface, errant placement or nail prominence can result in altered contact pressures of the patellofemoral joint.[16,17] Reaming fragments generated during canal preparation are also deposited in the knee joint and require evacuation of the joint at the completion of the procedure, the long-term effects of which remain unknown. Retrograde intramedullary insertion in patients with open fractures is theoretically associated with the risk of delayed septic arthritis. When used to treat a fracture with articular extension, placement of the intramedullary nail may potentially result in displacement of the articular component of the fracture.

Standard Compression Plates

Standard compression plates (such as broad 4.5-mm compression plates) should be reserved for patients with simple supracondylar fracture patterns for whom direct fracture reduction and absolute stability is advantageous. The primary limiting factor is the presence of sufficient distal bone to allow a minimum of six cortices of fixation distal to the fracture segment. In comminuted fractures or fractures with insufficient distal bone stock, this fixation technique should be avoided because it often leads to varus collapse and malunion.

95° Angled Plates

The 95° angled blade plate and 95° dynamic condylar screw (DCS) plate (Synthes, West Chester, PA) have been the most commonly used plating options for the treatment of extra-articular or simple articular supracondylar femur fractures.[1,2,18-20] As with the retrograde intramedullary nail, these plates are not indicated for treatment of C3 injuries because either the blade or the condylar screw has a high likelihood of disrupting the frontal (Hoffa) plane fracture reduction. Both plates offer similar characteristics in terms of a fixed-angle device that will resist varus collapse or loss of distal fixation in comminuted fractures that would otherwise require the addition of a second medial plate. By design, both devices facilitate indirect reduction and restoration of the mechanical axis of the extremity when placed parallel to the distal femoral articular surface. Fracture reduction and plate application are achieved using the standard lateral approach to the distal femur. The application of either the 95° angled blade plate or DCS plate mandates a precise understanding of the distal femoral anatomy. In particular, the medial condylar surface slopes 20° to 25°, and the lateral condylar surface slopes 10° to 15°. Normal distal femoral valgus is 6° to 7° in males and 8° to 9° in females. The key in placement of either device is the correct placement of either the blade or DCS plate in the distal femoral block. In doing so, when the side plate is brought down to the lateral femoral cortex, correct axial alignment is ensured. With both devices, there must be adequate distal bone stock available. In some patients, a minimally invasive percutaneous approach can be used, exploiting the potential space deep to the vastus lateralis.[4,5] The DCS plate can be applied in this manner. The DCS plate, however, requires enough distal bone segment to place an additional screw to prevent rotation around the condylar screw once appropriate plate position is obtained. Blade plate fixation does not allow rotation of the distal segment around the blade, and this additional screw is not required, allowing for fixation of shorter distal segments. Imperfect placement of the blade, however, is more difficult to adjust afterward, and the reported malposition and subsequent malreduction rates are higher in inexperienced hands.[21,22]

Standard Condylar Buttress Plate

The standard condylar buttress plate historically has been used for the treatment of C3 distal femur fractures. Its advantages include relative ease of application and the ability to place multiple screws in the distal femoral block. Its disadvantage is that it can allow varus collapse because conventional screws tend to toggle, especially in osteoporotic bone. In the past, multiple modalities have been used to counteract the tendency of the standard condylar buttress plate to allow varus collapse, including medial plating, a diagonally placed screw into the medial femoral condyle, and medial external fixator placement.[3,23,24] Despite this concern, when the standard condylar buttress plate is used while taking care to preserve the soft-tissue envelope around the fracture, rapid consolidation of the fracture can be expected, and the risk of varus collapse is minimized.[2] However, with the advent of the newer locked internal fixators, the standard condylar buttress plate is less commonly used.

Locked Internal Fixators

Recently, two different plating systems have become commercially available with screws with threaded heads that lock into the plate: the less invasive stabilization system (LISS) and the locking condylar buttress plate (Figure 5). Both designs have screws that lock into the distal end of the plate, thereby providing multiple small blade plates into the distal femoral block. A variety of new implants are becoming available. Most can be inserted in a percutaneous manner and do not have to be in direct contact with the bone. Submuscular placement of a fixator has been shown to preserve blood supply to the distal femur in cadaver studies when compared with open plating.[25] These plates can be used to treat type A and type C fractures.[8,26,27] Because a variety of different implants can be used for the treatment of the type A and C1/C2 fractures (Table 1), it may be that the newer designs are most helpful in patients with type C3 injuries, especially in those with complex articular injuries, osteoporosis, and/or short distal segments. In patients with type C3 fractures, after the articular injury is addressed, a laterally based plate can be applied. Biomechanically, improved fixation of the distal femoral block can be achieved in patients with osteoporotic bone.[6] Early clinical series assessing the LISS have shown promise in the treatment of patients with distal femoral fractures with multiplane articular injuries, short distal femoral segments, osteoporosis, or large open wounds.[8] The LISS has also been used successfully in the treatment of supracondylar periprosthetic fractures.[28] These reports have established that locked distal screw fixation can maintain distal femoral fixation, even in patients with osteoporosis or a short distal femoral block.

The locking condylar buttress plate is characterized by distal screws that lock into the plate and proximal screws, which can be either locking or conventional. As such, it can be thought of as a hybrid of conventional plating systems and true internal fixators. With both systems, longer constructs rather than standard plating are typically used. Although the results of a few case series have been reported in the literature, the role of these implants in the treatment of type A and type C1/C2 fractures has yet to be defined. It appears that locked plating systems may be most useful in patients with multiplane articular involvement, osteoporosis, short distal segments, and/or fractures above total knee arthroplasties. In addition, their submuscular application may also make them helpful in the treatment of patients with open fractures.

Partial Articular Fractures

Isolated unicondylar fractures of the distal femur are uncommon. Fractures in the coronal plane (Hoffa fractures) can be easily missed on radiographic examination when minimally displaced. Most unicondylar injuries can be repaired with lag screw fixation alone. Traditional lag screw fixation in the past has relied on the placement of large fragment screws using a lag screw technique. Conical differential pitch screws without heads have gained

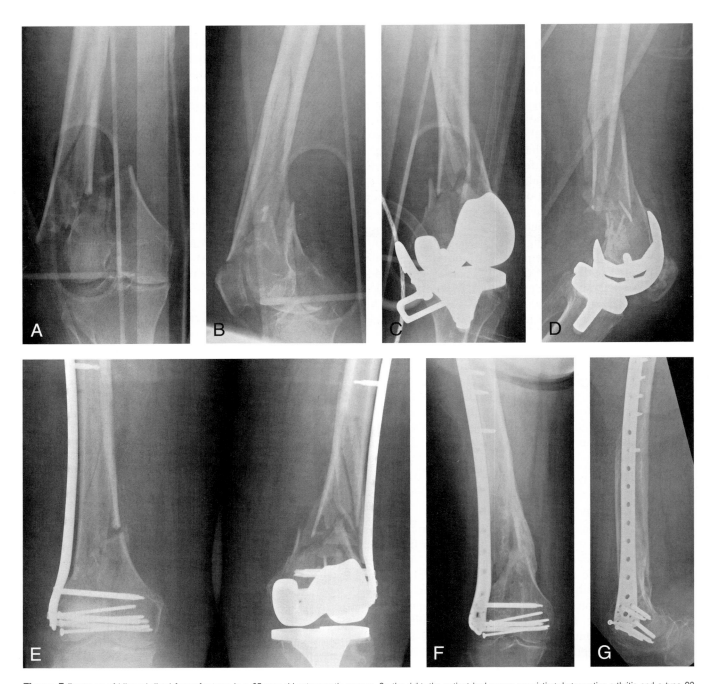

Figure 5 Treatment of bilateral distal femur fractures in a 65-year-old osteoporotic woman. On the right, the patient had severe preexisting degenerative arthritis and a type C2 injury. On the left, the patient had a distal femur fracture above a well-functioning total knee arthroplasty. Injury radiographs of the right (**A** and **B**) and left (**C** and **D**) femurs. **E,** Postoperative radiograph of the right and left femurs of the same patient. AP (**F**) and lateral (**G**) radiographs of the right femur at 1 year.

popularity. The absence of a head on the screw minimizes the hardware profile when used to treat sagittal splits, obviates the need to countersink traditional screws, minimizes additional cartilage damage, and helps to avoid prominent intra-articular hardware. Large diameter screws have fallen out of favor with most surgeons who use multiple smaller diameter screw fixation. In patients with condylar fractures that extend into the metaphysis, supplemental fixation with an antiglide or buttress plate provides additional fixation in conjunction with the lag screw fixation to resist shear forces (Figure 6).

Postoperative Care and Results

In most patients with extra-articular fractures, internal fixation is not sufficient to allow early weight bearing. Touchdown weight bearing should be initiated and main-

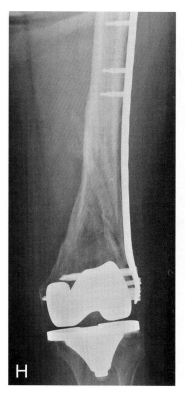
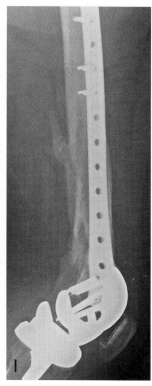

Figure 5, continued AP **(H)** and lateral **(I)** radiographs of the left femur at 1 year. The patient was fully ambulatory at 14 weeks after injury.

tained until sufficient callus formation is present to advance to full weight bearing. In patients with intra-articular fractures, touchdown weight bearing should be maintained for 8 to 10 weeks to protect the intra-articular portion of the repair. Early range-of-motion exercises should be instituted in the acute postoperative period if the condition of the soft tissue permits. Results are related to the severity of the initial injury, the quality of the articular reduction, and the care in which the soft tissues are handled at the time of fracture repair. More advanced indirect reduction techniques and percutaneous plate application appear to have decreased the time to union when compared with open techniques, but adequate data are not yet available to make a definitive statement. Overall, supracondylar fractures heal without the need for secondary surgical procedures because approximately 80% to 85% of fractures heal without complications[29] (Table 2).

Infection

Acute infection following surgical fixation of distal femur fractures ranges from 0 to 10% based on most recent reports.[29] The treatment of infection is straightforward. In the acute setting, the purulent material and necrotic tissue is evacuated. Stable fixation in the presence of infection is retained, systemic antibiotics are initiated, and a stable soft-tissue envelope is achieved either with

delayed closure or local or remote soft-tissue transfer. Later débridement and/or hardware removal after fracture union is then performed. In patients with unstable fixation or severe infection, temporary external fixation may be placed until the infection is controlled with débridement and appropriate antibiotic therapy. Refixation is then performed when the soft-tissue envelope allows.

Nonunion

The previously reported necessity of autologous bone grafting of comminuted fractures is of historical interest only because more advanced techniques of indirect reduction have yielded as high as 100% union rates in some reported series.[2,8,35,36] In patients with nonunion with stable fixation and no deformity or minimal deformity, direct bone grafting of the nonunion site is the preferred treatment method.

Nonunion with associated fixation failure and loss of reduction is more problematic. The short distal segment and concomitant disuse osteopenia limit fixation options. If significant bone stock remains in the distal segment, then blade plate fixation or locked plate fixation is preferred for secure distal segment fixation. In instances when distal fixation is suspect or a fixed-angle device cannot be used, medial plate augmentation may be required to achieve stable internal fixation.[37] In patients with significant medial cortical bone loss, an intramedullary strut to provide medial stability has been advocated.[38] Once the deformity has been corrected and secure fixation is achieved, then direct bone grafting of the nonunion site is performed.

In patients of advanced chronologic or physiologic age who have significant osteopenia, other reconstructive methods may be considered in the treatment algorithm. Augmentation of the fixation with polymethylmethacrylate can help facilitate secure fixation regardless of the device chosen by the surgeon. In patients with small distal articular segments, joint destruction, and preexisting arthritis, distal femoral replacement should be given serious consideration in the hope of restoring functional status.

Malunion

The most common malunion deformity is varus and extension of the distal fragment. Malunion (defined as > 5° of varus or valgus, 10° of angulation in the sagittal plane, and 15° of rotational deformity or 2 cm of shortening) requires removal of previous internal fixation if present, osteotomy, correction of mechanical axis, and application of stable internal fixation. A multitude of osteotomies have been described to correct deformity of the distal femur, including oblique single-cut and dome osteotomies. The oblique single-cut osteotomy performed in the plane of the deformity allows for simultaneous

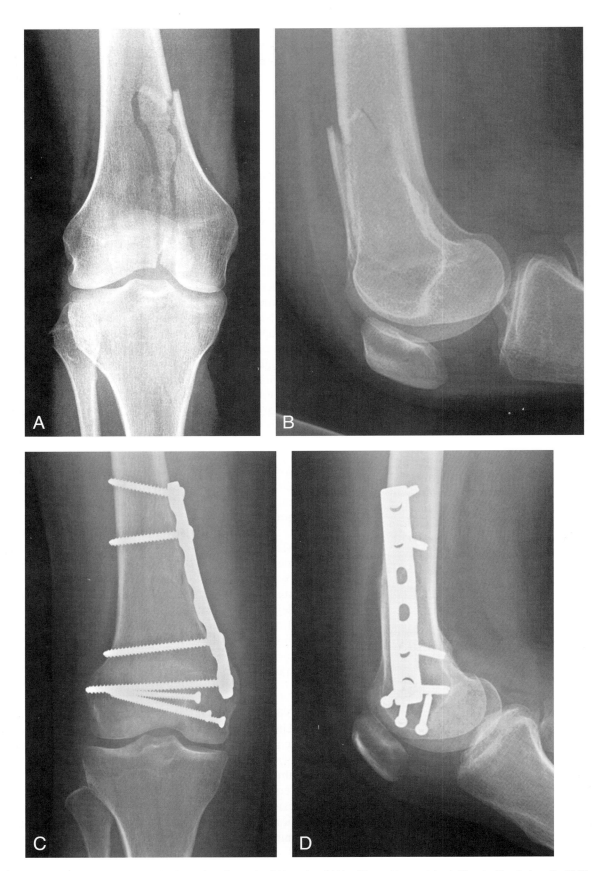

Figure 6 Injury AP **(A)** and lateral **(B)** radiographs of a B2 distal femur fracture (medial femoral condyle) in a 27-year-old woman injured while waterskiing. Postoperative AP **(C)** and lateral **(D)** radiographs show the injury was treated with direst visualization of the joint surface, 3.5-mm lag screws across the joint surface, and a neutralization plate on the distal medial femur.

TABLE 2 | Complications of Surgical Treatment of Supracondylar Femur Fractures: Case Series With > 40 Fractures (1989-2004)

Case Series	Year	No. of Fractures	Open (%)	Articular (%)	C3 (%)	Implant/ Technique	Nonunion Rate* (%)	Fixation Failure† (%)	Deep Infection Rate (%)	Secondary Surgical Procedures‡ (%)
Siliski et al[30]	1989	52	38	100	25	BP (81%), CBP (13%), Other (6%)	0	1.9	7.7	9.6
Yang et al[31]	1990	93	22	45	–	BP	12.9	2.2	11.8	15.1
Merchan et al[32]	1992	42	0	100	–	BP	7.1	0	4.8	28.6
Zehntner et al[22]	1992	59	29	68	17	BP (70%), CBP (14%), Other (26%)	8.4*	6.8*	8.5*	20.3
Iannacone et al[11]	1994	41	54	54	24	rIMN	19.5*	9.8	0	29.3
Bolhofner et al[2]	1996	57	19	61	16	BP (49%), CBP (51%)	0	0	1.8	0
Henry[14]	2000	111	–	–	–	rIMN	4.5	0	0	28.8
Ketterl et al[18]	1997	118	17	69	10	DCS	2.5*	2.5	1.7	8.5
Schütz et al[7]	2001	99	34	50	20	LISS	6.1	6.1	4	21.2
Seifert et al[15]	2003	45	21	23	–	rIMN	0	0	0	8.9
Kregor et al[8]	2004	103	34	57	36	LISS	6.8	4.9	2.9	17.5
Rademakers et al[33]	2004	67	30	100	7	Mainly CBP	1.5	0	10	11.5
Handolin et al[34]	2004	46	9	20	–	rIMN	4.3	6.5	0	8.7

BP = blade plate, DCS = dynamic condylar screw, rIMN = retrograde intramedullary nail, CBP = condylar buttress plate, LISS = less invasive stabilization system, C3 = comminuted articular injury type C3 according to the AO/OTA fracture classification.
*Including secondary surgical procedures for delayed unions, infected nonunions, and implant exchange before union. Note that fixation failures leading to an implant exchange are therefore included in the nonunion rate and the fixation failure rate. Also, deep infection leading to nonunion is included in the nonunion rate and the deep infection rate.
†Including clinically significant screw loosening, implant cutout/migration or breakage leading to a nonunion or malunion and fractures above the implant. (Clinically irrelevant screw/implant breakage or loosening was not included.)
‡Including partial (screws only) or complete implant removal and patient's refusal of an indicated reoperation as determined by the surgeon; does not include planned staged bone grafting in open fractures or planned irrigation and débridements.

correction of multiple deformities including length. The nature of the osteotomy provides a broad surface for lag screw fixation and subsequent consolidation of the osteotomy. Correction of the angular deformity will often restore adequate length, and some length can be obtained through the oblique osteotomy itself. In patients requiring greater length correction, distraction osteogenesis should be considered.

Intra-articular malunion may require an intra-articular osteotomy. In patients with articular loss or destruction, allograft reconstruction is an option. In these instances, careful evaluation of the opposing articular surface should be performed, and the patient should be appropriately counseled regarding the risk of future degenerative joint disease. In all patients undergoing malunion correction, careful preoperative planning cannot be overemphasized.

Joint Stiffness

Joint stiffness after surgical treatment of distal femoral fractures is problematic. Restriction in joint motion has many causes, ranging from intra-articular prominence of hardware to abundant scar tissue and hypertrophic callus formation. To avoid joint stiffness, early joint motion should be instituted once soft-tissue stabilization has oc-

curred. In patients with protracted joint stiffness despite aggressive therapy, surgical intervention is warranted. Joint manipulation has had minimal success in this patient population, and it has the inherent risk of periarticular fracture of the tibia. Quadricepsplasty, as first described by Judet, has been very successful in these patients, with an average reported increase in flexion of 53°.[39]

Summary

Distal femoral fractures are technically challenging injuries to treat. In more complex fractures, temporary stabilization of the distal femur with a unilateral external fixator allows the surgical team time to obtain traction films and CT scans to help determine fracture characteristics and develop a treatment plan. Careful handling of the soft tissues is paramount regardless of implant choice. Extra-articular fractures of the distal femur can be treated adequately with intramedullary nails or a variety of plates provided sufficient bone is intact in the periarticular area. Simple unicondylar intra-articular fractures can be treated with screw and/or plate fixation. Complex intra-articular fractures may be best treated with a lateral parapatellar approach and fixed-angle plating. Complications are best avoided by using adequate technique at the time of initial repair. When patients experience joint stiffness that is recalcitrant to aggressive therapy, Judet quadricepsplasty may restore functional range of motion, but is rarely necessary.

Annotated References

1. Schatzker J, Lambert DC: Supracondylar fractures of the femur. *Clin Orthop Relat Res* 1979;138:77-83.

2. Bolhofner BR, Carmen B, Clifford P: The results of open reduction and internal fixation of distal femur fractures using a biologic (indirect) reduction technique. *J Orthop Trauma* 1996;10:372-377.

3. Mast JW, Jakob R, Ganz R: *Planning and Reduction Technique in Fracture Surgery.* New York, NY, Springer-Verlag, 1989.

4. Krettek C, Schandelmaier P, Miclau T, Tscherne H: Minimally invasive percutaneous plate osteosynthesis (MIPPO) using the DCS in proximal and distal femoral fractures. *Injury* 1997;28(suppl 1):A20-A30.

5. Krettek C, Schandelmaier P, Miclau T, Bertram R, Holmes W, Tscherne H: Transarticular joint reconstruction and indirect plate osteosynthesis for complex distal supracondylar femoral fractures. *Injury* 1997;28(suppl 1):A31-A41.

   Fourteen patients with supracondylar or subtrochanteric fractures or osteotomies were stabilized with a DCS inserted with a submuscular technique. There were no infections, and 12 of 13 patients healed without a second procedure. There was one implant failure (plate screw breakage), which required repeat fracture fixation. At follow-up, there were two varus deformities greater than 5°, two shortenings greater than 20 mm, and one rotational deformity of 20°. The results of this technique compare favorably with those of other series of osteosynthesis of subtrochanteric or supracondylar femoral fractures treated with internal fixation without the added morbidity associated with an extensive approach or autogenous bone grafting.

6. Zlowodzki M, Williamson S, Cole PA, Zardiackas LD, Kregor PJ: Biomechanical evaluation of the less invasive stabilization system, angled blade plate, and retrograde intramedullary nail for the internal fixation of distal femur fractures. *J Orthop Trauma* 2004; 18:494-502.

   The stability of the retrograde intramedullary nail, angled blade plate, and a locked internal fixator (LISS) for internal fixation of distal femur fractures was evaluated using destructive biomechanical testing of matched pairs of fresh-frozen human cadaveric bone-implant constructs. A fracture model was created to simulate supracondylar femur fracture. Forty-eight matched pairs of specimens were used. Six groups of eight pairs each were tested to failure: LISS versus angled blade plate and LISS versus intramed-

   ullary nail (axial, torsional, and cyclical axial). The fixation strength (load/moment to failure) of the LISS constructs was 34% greater in axial loading ($P = 0.01$) and 32% less in torsional loading ($P = 0.05$) compared with angled blade plate constructs and 13% greater in axial loading ($P = 0.35$) and 45% less in torsional loading ($P < 0.01$) compared with intramedullary nail constructs. Loss of distal fixation in axial loading occurred in 1 of 16 cases with the LISS, in 3 of 8 cases with the angled blade plate, and in 8 of 8 cases with the intramedullary nail. Cyclical axial loading demonstrated significantly less plastic deformation for the LISS construct compared with angled blade plate constructs ($P < 0.01$) and similar plastic deformation compared with intramedullary nail constructs ($P = 0.98$). The authors concluded that all three fixation devices (LISS, angled blade plate, and intramedullary nail) offer sufficient torsional stability and sufficient proximal fixation that withstands axial loading without failing; the LISS provided improved distal fixation, especially in osteoporotic bone, at the expense of more elastic displacement at the fracture site.

7. Schütz M, Muller M, Krettek C, et al: Minimally invasive fracture stabilization of distal femoral fractures with the LISS: A prospective multicenter study. Results of a clinical study with special emphasis on difficult cases. *Injury* 2001;32:SC48-SC54.

   The LISS was applied to 112 patients with 116 distal femoral shaft or supracondylar femoral fractures. Ninety-six patients with 99 fractures were available for complete follow-up. Twenty-three revision operations were necessary in 21 patients. In two patients, implant failure occurred as the result of a pseudarthrosis. The complications can be attributed in nearly all patients to the severity of the trauma and/or lack of surgeon experience when applying the new type of implant to a wider range of indications. The authors concluded that there is generally no need for primary cancellous bone grafting in this patient population.

8. Kregor PJ, Stannard JA, Zlowodzki M, Cole PA: Treatment of distal femur fractures using the less invasive stabilization system: Surgical experience and early clinical results in 103 fractures. *J Orthop Trauma* 2004;18:509-520.

   One hundred nineteen consecutive patients with 123 distal femur fractures (OTA type 33 and distal type 32 fractures) were treated by three surgeons. One hundred three fractures (68 closed fractures and 35 open fractures) in 99 patients were followed-up at least until union. Ninety-six of 103 fractures (93%) healed without bone grafting. All fractures eventually healed with secondary procedures, including bone grafting (1 of 68 closed fractures and 6 of 35 open fractures). There were five losses of proximal fixation, two nonunions, and three acute infections. No instances of varus collapse or screw loosening in the distal femoral fragment were observed. Malreductions of the femoral fracture were seen in six fractures (6%). The mean range of knee motion was 1° to 109°. No loss of fixation in the distal femoral condyles was observed despite the treatment of 30 patients older than 65 years.

9. Leung KS, Shen WY, So WS, Mui LT, Grosse A: Interlocking intramedullary nailing for supracondylar and intercondylar fractures of the distal part of the femur. *J Bone Joint Surg Am* 1991;73:332-340.

10. Kumar A, Jasani V, Butt MS: Management of distal femoral fractures in elderly patients using retrograde titanium supracondylar nails. *Injury* 2000;31:169-173.

    In this study, 16 extra-articular fractures of the distal femur were treated with retrograde titanium supracondylar nails and outcomes were reviewed. Fifteen fractures (93.7%) united at an average duration of 3.6 months. The average range of motion achieved at the knee was 100.6°. There were no implant failures, knee sepsis, or wound healing problems. One nonunion and two stress fractures of the femur above the nail were the main complications in this series.

11. Iannacone WM, Bennett FS, DeLong WG Jr, Born CT, Dalsey RM: Initial experience with the treatment of supracondylar femoral fractures using the supracondylar intramedullary nail: A preliminary report. *J Orthop Trauma* 1994;8:322-327.

12. Lucas SE, Seligson D, Henry SL: Intramedullary supracondylar nailing of femoral fractures: A preliminary report of the GSH supracondylar nail. *Clin Orthop Relat Res* 1993;296:200-206.

13. Armstrong R, Milliren A, Schrantz W, Zeliger K: Retrograde interlocked intramedullary nailing of supracondylar distal femur fractures in an average 76-year-old patient population. *Orthopedics* 2003;26: 627-629.

14. Henry SL: Supracondylar femur fractures treated percutaneously. *Clin Orthop Relat Res* 2000;375:51-59.

15. Seifert J, Stengel D, Matthes G, Hinz P, Ekkernkamp A, Ostermann PA: Retrograde fixation of distal femoral fractures: Results using a new nail system. *J Orthop Trauma* 2003;17:488-495.

16. Morgan E, Ostrum RF, DiCicco J, McElroy J, Poka A: Effects of retrograde femoral intramedullary nailing on the patellofemoral articulation. *J Orthop Trauma* 1999;13:13-16.

17. Carmack DB, Moed BR, Kingston C, Zmurko M, Watson JT, Richardson M: Identification of the optimal intercondylar starting point for retrograde femoral nailing: An anatomic study. *J Trauma* 2003;55:692-695.

    In this cadaveric study, the optimal starting point for retrograde nailing of femoral shaft was evaluated. The starting holes averaged 6.21 mm anterior to the posterior cruciate ligament attachment and 2.67 mm medial to the intercondylar groove. In most femurs, the optimal entry portal for retrograde femoral nailing (in line with the long axis of the femur) is located in the expected safe position, anterior to the posterior cruciate ligament insertion and slightly medial to the center of the intercondylar groove. However, because of anatomic variability, the ideal starting position occasionally may be located in a patellofemoral contact area. Potential compromise of the patellofemoral contact area by the retrograde nail entry portal can and should be recognized before nailing, allowing the surgeon the option of altering the surgical technique.

18. Ketterl R, Kostler W, Wittwer W, Stubinger B: 5-year results of dia-/supracondylar femoral fractures, managed with the dynamic condylar screw. *Zentralbl Chir* 1997;122:1033-1039.

19. Ostrum RF, Geel C: Indirect reduction and internal fixation of supracondylar femur fractures without bone graft. *J Orthop Trauma* 1995;9:278-284.

20. Sanders R, Regazzoni P, Ruedi TP: Treatment of supracondylar-intracondylar fractures of the femur using the dynamic condylar screw. *J Orthop Trauma* 1989;3:214-222.

21. Schatzker J: Fractures of the distal femur revisited. *Clin Orthop Relat Res* 1998;347:43-56.

22. Zehntner MK, Marchesi DG, Burch H, Ganz R: Alignment of supracondylar/intercondylar fractures of the femur after internal fixation by AO/ASIF technique. *J Orthop Trauma* 1992;6:318-326.

23. Sanders R, Swiontkowski M, Rosen H, Helfet D: Double-plating of comminuted, unstable fractures of the distal part of the femur. *J Bone Joint Surg Am* 1991;73:341-346.

24. Simonian PT, Thompson GJ, Emley W, Harrington RM, Benirschke SK, Swiontkowski MF: Angulated screw placement in the lateral condylar buttress plate for supracondylar femoral fractures. *Injury* 1998;29:101-104.

25. Farouk O, Krettek C, Miclau T, Schandelmaier P, Tscherne H: Effects of percutaneous and conventional plating techniques on the blood supply to the femur. *Arch Orthop Trauma Surg* 1998;117:438-441.

26. Schütz M, Muller M, Regazzoni P, et al: Use of the less invasive stabilization system (LISS) in patients with distal femoral (AO33) fractures: A prospective multicenter study. *Arch Orthop Trauma Surg* 2005; 125:102-108.

27. Kregor PJ, Stannard J, Zlowodzki M, Cole PA, Alonso J: Distal femoral fracture fixation utilizing the Less Invasive Stabilization System (L.I.S.S.): The

technique and early results. *Injury* 2001;32(suppl 3): SC32-SC47.

28. Kregor PJ, Hughes JL, Cole PA: Fixation of distal femoral fractures above total knee arthroplasty utilizing the Less Invasive Stabilization System (L.I.S.S.). *Injury* 2001;32(suppl 3):SC64-SC75.

29. Zlowodzki M, Bhandari M, Marek DJ, Cole PA, Kregor PJ: Operative treatment of acute distal femur fractures: Systematic review of two comparative studies and 38 case series. *J Orthop Trauma* 2005. In press.

30. Siliski JM, Mahring M, Hofer HP: Supracondylar-intercondylar fractures of the femur: Treatment by internal fixation. *J Bone Joint Surg Am* 1989;71:95-104.

31. Yang RS, Liu HC, Liu TK: Supracondylar fractures of the femur. *J Trauma* 1990;30:315-319.

32. Merchan EC, Maestu PR, Blanco RP: Blade-plating of closed displaced supracondylar fractures of the distal femur with the AO system. *J Trauma* 1992;32: 174-178.

33. Rademakers MV, Kerkhoffs GM, Sierevelt IN, Raaymakers EL, Marti RK: Intra-articular fractures of the distal femur: A long-term follow-up study of surgically treated patients. *J Orthop Trauma* 2004;18: 213-219.

34. Handolin L, Pajarinen J, Lindahl J, Hirvensalo E: Retrograde intramedullary nailing in distal femoral fractures: Results in a series of 46 consecutive operations. *Injury* 2004;35:517-522.

35. Weight M, Collinge C: Early results of the less invasive stabilization system for mechanically unstable fractures of the distal femur (AO/OTA types A2, A3, C2, and C3). *J Orthop Trauma* 2004;18:503-508.

36. Ricci AR, Yue JJ, Taffet R, Catalano JB, DeFalco RA, Wilkens KJ: Less Invasive Stabilization System for treatment of distal femur fractures. *Am J Orthop* 2004;33:250-255.

37. Chapman MW, Finkemeier CG: Treatment of supracondylar nonunions of the femur with plate fixation and bone graft. *J Bone Joint Surg Am* 1999;81:1217-1228.
    This is a retrospective review of a single surgeon's experience in the treatment of the results of single- and double-plate fixation combined with autologous bone grafting in 18 patients with nonunion of supracondylar femur fractures. Union was achieved without repeat procedure in all but one patient. There were three complications, including one infection, one loss of motion, and one malunion. The average range of motion of the knee was 101°.

38. Matelic TM, Monroe MT, Mast JW: The use of endosteal substitution in the treatment of recalcitrant nonunions of the femur: Report of seven cases. *J Orthop Trauma* 1996;10:1-6.

39. Ebraheim NA, DeTroye RJ, Saddemi SR: Results of Judet quadricepsplasty. *J Orthop Trauma* 1993;7: 327-330.

Chapter 35

Knee Injuries

William J. Mills, MD

Craig S. Roberts, MD

Michael A. Miranda, MD

Knee Dislocation

Knee dislocation remains a potentially limb-threatening injury because of its common association with popliteal artery thrombosis or disruption. Even an isolated knee injury presents challenges in recovering stability, motion, and return to functional activities. Dislocations are commonly open and have associated vascular and peroneal nerve injuries, osteochondral fractures, meniscal tears, and/or extensor mechanism injuries. The definition of knee dislocation has undergone significant change in recent years. Several authors have expanded the definition to include not only patients presenting with frank dislocation, but also those patients with a knee that has undergone reduction and gross instability following multiligamentous disruption. Some have described patients with this latter type of injury as having dislocatable knees.[1] The significance of this more inclusive definition is in the equivalent risk of popliteal artery injury in patients with dislocated and dislocatable knees. No longer is there any question that the dislocated knee may have any variety of ligaments injured. Although historically it was thought to require tears of the anterior cruciate ligament (ACL) and the posterior cruciate ligament (PCL), it is now known that the dislocated knee may involve failure of only one cruciate ligament with associated collateral injury. A recent report described an anterior knee dislocation with osteochondral fracture of the femoral condyle but only ACL disruption.[2]

Classification

Knee dislocations are typically classified by the direction of the dislocation. Anterior and posterior dislocations are the most common, each comprising approximately 30% to 40% of all dislocations, with an equivalent risk of arterial injury. However, the constellation of ligamentous injuries cannot be predicted from the direction of dislocation. A classification system based on ligamentous injury ranging from two ligament (one collateral, one cruciate) injuries to four ligament injuries involving both collateral ligaments and both cruciate ligaments has been proposed.[3] A classification system that incorporates ligamentous injuries and associated soft-tissue injuries, such as meniscal tears, capsular disruption, and osteochondral fractures, would be too cumbersome for practical application and currently does not exist. However, these associated injuries, as with open knee dislocation, can impact patient treatment and long-term outcome.

History

Knee dislocation can occur from a variety of mechanisms, ranging from high-energy injuries in the multiply injured patient to ultra–low-energy isolated knee dislocation in obese patients, for whom knee dislocation has been reported to occur with a simple misstep.[4] The rate of vascular injury appears independent of the mechanism and should be the primary concern of the evaluating physician. The rate of vascular injury in obese patients with low-energy dislocations approaches 100%.[4] Because the rate of spontaneously reduced knee dislocation is comparable to the rate of frank dislocation, patients and emergency medical personnel should be carefully questioned regarding the presence of gross displacement and reduction that may have occurred in the field.[5]

Physical Evaluation

Evaluating the patient for vascular injury is the focus of the initial examination. Closed reduction is usually effective in the emergency department, generally requiring longitudinal traction and gentle manipulation. Dislocations are rarely irreducible. Open reduction may be required for posterolateral dislocations in which the medial femoral condyle is buttonholed through the capsule. The dislocated knee should be inspected circumferentially for open wounds because an open knee dislocation warrants rapid surgical débridement and irrigation. The reported incidence of vascular injury varies widely, ranging from 10% to 65%. A missed vascular injury or delay in surgical revascularization of a known vascular injury can lead to myonecrosis of the leg and above-knee amputation. Urgent arteriography was once considered routine in the evaluation of patients with a dislocated knee. Recently, however, some authors have questioned the need to perform arteriography on all patients.[6-9] These authors have suggested that hard findings on physical examination (active hemorrhage, expanding hematoma, absent pulses, distal ischemia, or bruit) are sufficient evidence for identifying arterial injury. Conversely, an absence of these findings in the presence of symmetric pedal pulses has been reported to effectively rule out the presence of significant vascular injury. Routine arteriography has been criticized for the delay it may cause in revascularization, its potential complications, and its high cost.[8] The most common finding in patients with vascular injury is diminished or absent pulse. Arteriography is indicated when abnormal physical examination findings suggest vascular injury, whereas patients with no hard signs of vascular injury are typically admitted for observation and regular reexamination to rule out the presence of progressive ischemia. The ankle-brachial index has been shown to be highly sensitive and specific in ruling out or diagnosing vascular injury after blunt and penetrating trauma and can be used as an adjunct in the physical examination of patients with acute knee dislocation.[9]

Peroneal nerve palsy has been reported to occur in 10% to 42% of patients with knee dislocations, with recovery rates of approximately 35%.[10] The etiology may be neurapraxia or frank disruption. A careful neurologic examination should be performed to identify peroneal nerve dysfunction. Ligamentous injury is typically assessed by examination in the emergency department, although ipsilateral limb injuries, guarding, and local swelling may limit the initial examination. An examination with the patient under anesthesia at the time of treatment for associated injuries can optimize the understanding of the constellation of ligamentous injuries. This includes an assessment of the cruciate ligaments, collateral ligaments, and capsular structures with varus, valgus, translational, and rotational stress in extension and 30° of flexion. Patellar tendon rupture and lateral patellar dislocation has been reported to occur in association with knee dislocation, and the status of the extensor mechanism should be assessed after reduction of the dislocation.[11] Ipsilateral patellar dislocation is usually associated with a complex medial soft-tissue injury, including disruption of the medial collateral ligament (MCL), medial capsule, and medial patellofemoral ligament.[11]

Diagnostic Imaging

Radiographic assessment of the dislocated knee includes AP and lateral radiographs to demonstrate the direction of the dislocation and then to confirm reduction. Plain radiographic findings can provide useful information regarding diagnosis and treatment. Femoral epicondylar fractures signify medial or lateral collateral avulsions, whereas marginal condylar fractures indicate medial or lateral capsular avulsions. Intercondylar eminence fractures are common and indicate ACL injury, whereas

tibial PCL avulsions are usually apparent on lateral radiographs but can also be seen as a central AP radiolucency. The lateral capsular avulsion or Segond sign is also associated with an ACL tear in patients with multiligament injuries. The "reverse Segond" sign has recently been described.[12] This medial capsular avulsion has been shown to be associated with the combination of MCL, PCL, and medial meniscus tears, to be the result of high-energy trauma, and to have an association with knee dislocation (Figure 1).

MRI has been found to be accurate for diagnosing most soft-tissue injuries in patients with knee dislocation, although it is less useful for identifying injury to lateral-sided structures.[1] It may provide information regarding meniscal and articular cartilage injuries that is unobtainable via physical examination or plain radiographs. MRI can also help confirm associated extensor mechanism injuries in multiply injured patients who are unable to comply with physical examination. Stress radiographs under anesthesia may also provide useful information, especially regarding collateral ligament injuries.

Surgical Management

There are few indications for nonsurgical treatment of ligamentous injuries following knee dislocation. Although there are no prospective studies comparing nonsurgical and surgical treatment for these injuries, a recent meta-analysis suggests that surgical treatment results in statistically significant improved range of motion, lesser flexion contracture, and improved functional knee scores.[13] Stability was not statistically different in this meta-analysis, nor was there a difference in return to preinjury employment or athletic activities. The authors emphasized that significant disability was still possible after surgical treatment. Indications for nonsurgical treatment include morbid obesity, a sedentary lifestyle, and elderly patients with low functional demands. The patient with knee dislocation and combined ACL and MCL injury but minimal posterior laxity may also be treated nonsurgically initially, with the expectation that the MCL will heal, at which time aggressive range-of-motion recovery exercises can be initiated.

Surgical treatment is always complex, and no two knee dislocations are identical. A fixed algorithm for treatment of all knee dislocations is impractical, but certain concepts can be outlined. Surgical timing, technique (open versus arthroscopic, ligament repair versus reconstruction), graft selection (allograft versus autograft), and whether to reconstruct one or both cruciates are common issues.

Surgical timing is generally divided into early (within 3 weeks of injury) or delayed (later than 6 weeks after injury). Early collateral ligament repair and cruciate ligament reconstruction has been advocated by many authors to provide a stable, congruous reduction allowing early motion recovery.[3,14-16] Although concerns have

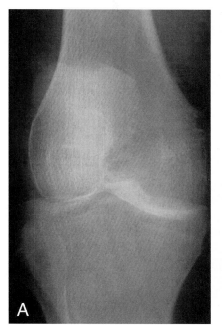
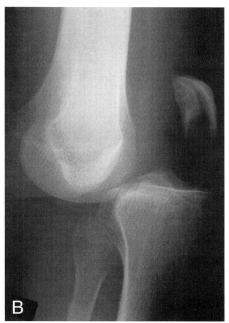
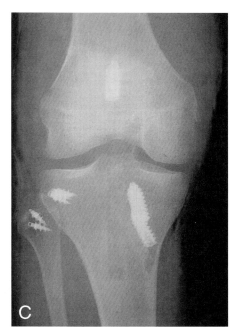
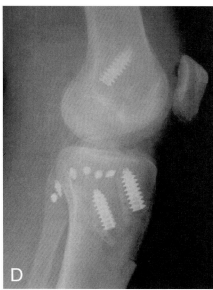

Figure 1 A, AP radiograph showing knee dislocation with ACL, PCL, and LCL tears and popliteus and biceps tendon ruptures in an 18-year-old man after a motorcycle accident. **B,** Lateral radiograph of the same patient before emergency department reduction. The patient had symmetrical lower extremity pulses after reduction and an ankle brachial index of 1.10. No disruption of the peroneal nerve was noted at surgery. Postoperative AP **(C)** and lateral **(D)** radiographs after ACL (with patellar tendon autograft) and PCL (with Achilles tendon allograft) reconstruction, LCL repair and reconstruction (with semitendinosus autograft), and popliteus and biceps tendon repair.

been raised in the past regarding the development of arthrofibrosis, recent studies emphasize that these motion concerns can be overcome with aggressive postoperative rehabilitation.[14,17] This early treatment can combine the surgical treatment of associated periarticular or osteochondral fractures, meniscal tears, and extensor mechanism injuries. The multiply injured patient with a knee dislocation presents a specific challenge. Heterotopic ossification about the knee after surgical treatment has been increasingly discussed and recently classified. The incidence of heterotopic ossification has been reported to range from 26% to 43% of patients, with the incidence of severe motion-limiting heterotopic ossification ranging from 12% to 17%.[15,18] A relationship be-

tween Injury Severity Score and the formation of severe, frequently ankylosing heterotopic ossification has been identified.[15]

Patients with open knee dislocation fall into a separate category. Although the open wounds may be small, these are frequently devastating soft-tissue injuries with marked soft-tissue loss and degloving, requiring multiple débridements and coverage procedures. These patients are best managed with temporary knee-spanning external fixation. Surgical wound extensions beyond those required for an adequate débridement are kept to a minimum. Although associated fractures and ligamentous avulsions are typically treated early, formal ligament reconstruction is delayed until the soft-tissue envelope is stable and the patient is able to participate in a rehabilitation program. Delayed reconstruction can be either open or arthroscopic, depending on the experience and preference of the surgeon. Arthroscopic reconstruction may minimize surgical trauma and incision volume and enhance rehabilitation.

Although no prospective studies have been done to compare early and delayed or open and arthroscopic reconstruction in patients with knee dislocation, there is general consensus that the multiligament injury that includes injury to the lateral structures requires early surgical treatment for optimal identification and repair. The lateral collateral ligament (LCL), popliteus tendon, popliteofibular ligament, and lateral capsule form a complex that is frequently injured in patients with dislocated knees. Anatomic repair of these structures is generally relatively straightforward within 2 weeks of injury, but it is quite challenging after 3 weeks because of the tendency for unidentifiable scar to form.

Reconstruction of both the ACL and PCL has been criticized in the past for increasing the risk of arthrofibrosis.[19] These criticisms are based on scant prospective data. Several authors have subsequently published the results of simultaneous ACL and PCL reconstructions as part of the acute treatment of patients with dislocated knees; when followed by a systematic, aggressive physical therapy protocol, patients were noted to achieve an acceptable range of motion and functional scores.[14,15,17]

A variety of graft options exist for reconstructing multiple ligament injuries. The tissue requirements can become prohibitive to only autograft use when three or four ligaments or ligament complexes require reconstruction. Furthermore, the dislocation produces marked soft-tissue injury about the knee that can be exacerbated by multiple local graft harvests. Many authors, therefore, advocate the liberal use of allograft.[14,16,17] Achilles tendon allografts are frequently recommended for PCL reconstruction (for both one- and two-bundle reconstruction). Options for ACL reconstruction include patellar tendon and hamstring tendon autografts or allografts. LCL disruptions are often difficult to repair primarily because of the small cross-sectional diameter of the LCL. Primary augmentation and/or reconstruction are often recommended with autograft or allograft. Residual PCL and posterolateral corner laxity remains the most common challenge to achieving preinjury stability, although most patients will tolerate mild laxity. Limiting early postoperative range of motion to a 70° arc may protect the PCL, but it can also result in stiffness, requiring manipulation with the patient under anesthesia or surgical release. The temporary use of a hinged external fixator has been proposed to allow aggressive physical therapy while protecting ligament grafts from undue stress.[20]

Peroneal Nerve Palsy

In patients with incomplete peroneal nerve palsy, complete functional recovery can be expected. Persistent, complete peroneal nerve palsy warrants surgical exploration independently or at the time of lateral ligament repair or reconstruction. Intact nerves may benefit from neurolysis. Reported recovery rates vary from 0 to 50%.[10] Physical therapy protocols should include maintaining ankle range of motion and use of an ankle-foot orthosis while anticipating recovery. Patients who do not recover likely have axonotmesis or neurotmesis. No recovery 3 months after injury should prompt electromyographic studies. For those nerves with no sign of recovery or those with known transection, the treatment options include continued use of an ankle-foot orthosis, tendon transfers for ankle dorsiflexion, or nerve grafting. Sural nerve grafting is gaining popularity, with reports of grade 3 to 4 strength recovery in 40% to 100% of patients, depending on graft length.[10]

Rehabilitation

Rehabilitation must be customized according to the constellation of ligaments injured and those requiring protection while healing spontaneously or after repair and/or reconstruction. Patients undergoing PCL reconstruction generally benefit from a range of motion that is limited to 70° of flexion for the first 6 weeks postoperatively. Limitation of active hamstring contractions for 8 to 12 weeks and use of a passive motion machine while the patient is hospitalized can help protect the PCL graft from undue stress. Collateral ligament repairs or reconstructions are protected in a removable splint or hinged knee brace for 8 to 12 weeks, and full weight bearing is limited for the same approximate duration to minimize graft loads. Hyperextension should be avoided for 3 to 6 months, although passive knee extension is encouraged early during the postoperative period.

Quadriceps Tendon Ruptures

Disruption of the quadriceps tendon, the proximal extensor mechanism of the knee, is a potentially disabling injury that can be missed initially. The stakes of treating quadriceps ruptures are high because the lack of a functioning extensor mechanism potentially requires knee fusion. Quadriceps tendon injuries can occur as isolated injuries or as a component of polytrauma. Injuries can be caused by noncontact (when an eccentric contraction of an abnormal tendon occurs in an attempt to catch oneself during a fall) or contact involving blunt or penetrating trauma. Penetrating injuries are often complex soft-tissue injuries with traumatic arthrotomies of the knee or mangled lower extremities. A range of clinical pathology exists including incomplete ruptures, acute unilateral ruptures, and bilateral ruptures.[21]

Epidemiology

Although quadriceps injuries generally occur in individuals younger than 40 years, the peak incidence in one study was reportedly during the sixth decade of life.[22] The average age of patients with bilateral ruptures has been reported to be 53 years versus 59 years for those with unilateral ruptures.[23] About 20% of patients with unilateral quadriceps tears and 33% of those with bilateral synchronous ruptures[24] have underlying medical conditions, including chronic renal failure, diabetes, rheumatoid arthritis, hyperparathyroidism, various connective tissue disorders, and conditions resulting from steroid use and intra-articular injection.[22,24,25] A workup for an underlying medical condition is warranted in any patient with bilateral spontaneous quadriceps ruptures.[21] Males have been reported to be affected more commonly, with a male-to-female ratio of 8:1 in one series.[22] The nondominant limb is twice as likely to be affected.

Biomechanics

Increased forces on the quadriceps tendon in relation to the patellar tendon at increasing flexion angles have been reported.[26] At 50% of flexion, forces are equal in the quadriceps and patellar tendon, whereas at 90% of flexion, the force in the quadriceps tendon is greater than the force in the patellar tendon.

Diagnostic Imaging

Radiographs are typically sufficient for diagnosing quadriceps tendon ruptures. Lateral radiographs may show a low-riding patella (patella infera). When additional diagnostic imaging is necessary, ultrasound is an efficient and accurate method of diagnosing a quadriceps tendon tear. Diagnosis can also be accurately made with MRI, but it is not a substitute for a careful history and physical examination. MRI is rarely indicated for this patient population, but it may be useful when there is a high index of suspicion of concomitant knee ligamentous or meniscal injuries.

Treatment

Incomplete Ruptures

Incomplete ruptures are usually managed nonsurgically. However, patients should be advised that partial ruptures might predispose them to future complete ruptures. The natural history of partial quadriceps ruptures is unknown. Aspiration of the hematoma may help the patient symptomatically, but the benefits of aspiration have not been scientifically studied.[21]

Acute Unilateral Rupture

Traditional methods of repair for the common pattern of rupture at the bone-tendon junction include primary repair of the tendon through osseous drill holes. The use of suture anchors for repair is becoming increasingly

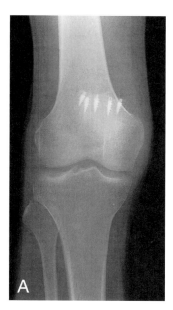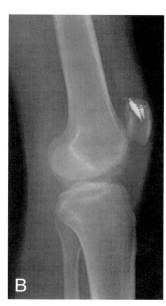

Figure 2 AP **(A)** and lateral **(B)** radiographs of a patient who underwent repair of a quadriceps tear with five metallic suture anchors.

popular and avoids having to pass intraosseous sutures[27,28] (Figure 2). Long-term follow-up of repairs using suture anchors has not been reported. In general, early rather than delayed repair appears to be associated with better clinical results; ruptures that are more than 2 weeks old may be retracted up to 5 cm.[29]

Bilateral Tendon Rupture

Identification of underlying disease is important when bilateral quadriceps injuries are encountered; orthopaedists should not assume that patients have already been evaluated for such underlying causes by another physician. Otherwise, bilateral ruptures should be treated in a manner similar to unilateral ruptures,[21] with the caveat that a period of nonambulation with thromboembolism prophylaxis may be necessary in order to avoid premature stressing of the repairs.

Chronic Tendon Rupture

The surgical treatment of chronic ruptures appears to be less successful than the treatment of acute ruptures.[23] Apposition of the tendon to the patella or apposition of two ends of the tendon may be impossible secondary to shortening and adhesions. In such instances, a Codivilla procedure or quadriceps tendon lengthening is recommended[21] (Figure 3). An inverted V-shaped full-thickness flap with a proximal apex is developed, with the distal base at least 1.3 to 2.0 cm from the site of disruption. The triangular flap is turned down distally, sutured, and the open proximal defect from the V-shaped full-thickness flap is then sutured side-to-side. The reconstruction of large deficits resulting from tumor excision has been reported using a gastrocnemius myotendinous flap, with

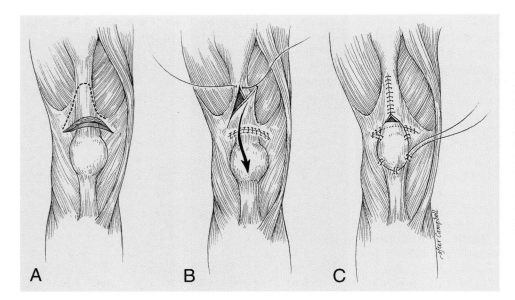

Figure 3 Codivilla method of quadriceps tendon lengthening and repair. **A,** Chronic quadriceps tendon tear exposed. Proximal retraction prevents direct apposition of the tear. Dotted lines represent inverted V cut (full thickness) to be made. **B,** The inverted V cut allows the tear to be approximated and repaired. **C,** The proximal aspect of the inverted V repaired side to side. A full-thickness or partial-thickness flap may be used to augment the repair, as in the Scuderi technique. *(Adapted with permission from Scuderi C: Ruptures of the quadriceps tendon: Study of twenty tendon ruptures.* Am J Surg *1958;95:626-635.)*

extension deficits of 5° to 15° at a minimum 2-year follow-up.[30]

Prognosis

One recent study reported that approximately one third of patients with a quadriceps tear had strength deficits at a mean follow-up of 22 months.[22] In another study, strength deficits were noted in 53% of patients with unilateral ruptures. Although more than 80% of patients returned to their preinjury occupation after surgical repair, 51% believed that they were unable to return to recreational activities at their former level of competitiveness.[24] There was less than 5° deficit in knee range of motion between affected and unaffected limbs, with no difference in quadriceps girth reported when comparing affected and unaffected limbs.[22] Therefore, the outcome of surgical repair of quadriceps tendon ruptures may be less satisfactory than previously assumed, and patients should be counseled accordingly.

Fractures of the Patella and Patellar Tendon Ruptures

Patellar fractures occur as a result of a direct mechanism (such as an impact with a dashboard during a motor vehicle accident) or indirect mechanism (such as distraction by knee hyperflexion). The modified tension band has been the mainstay in the treatment of fractures of the patella,[31] but recent investigative focus has been on improving the techniques for surgical treatment. Minimally invasive approaches have been used in the treatment of patellar fractures.

The patella is the largest human sesamoid bone. It has little periosteum and does not generate abundant callus during healing. Only the skin, a thin layer of subcutaneous tissue, and the prepatellar bursa overlie

the patella. This subcutaneous location makes the patella prone to injuries from direct blows and falls. Posteriorly, the proximal 75% of the surface of the patella is covered with articular cartilage that is among the thickest found anywhere in the body. The anterior bony surface contour only partially conforms to the posterior surface; therefore, it is not appropriate for indirect reduction techniques. The patella has three major facets: medial, lateral, and odd. Its vascular supply comes from branches of the geniculate arteries, which form a dorsal ring with a recurrent secondary supply through the posterior apex.[32]

The patella transmits tensile forces generated by the quadriceps to the tibia through the patellar ligament. The patella effectively increases the lever arm of the knee extension mechanism, thus increasing the knee extensor moment generated by contraction of the quadriceps. The contribution made by the patella increases with progressive extension of the knee, generating almost 30% of extensor power at full extension. Thus, total patellectomy should be avoided in the treatment of patellar injuries whenever possible. Forces on the patella change throughout its range of motion. With knee extension, it is loaded primarily in tension. In knee flexion, the articular surface contacts the distal femur and is subjected to a compressive force posteriorly and a distracting tension force anteriorly, creating a three-point bending configuration. This tension at the anterior surface of the patella is in addition to that generated by distraction from contraction of the quadriceps. The degree of flexion determines the bending forces of the knee, with maximum force at 45° of flexion.

Classification

Patellar fractures can be classified according to the mechanism of injury and/or the morphology. There are two major mechanisms of injury: direct and indirect trauma. A direct blow can cause considerable comminution associated with little displacement because of the small amount of prepatellar soft tissue. Direct blows to the patella damage the articular cartilage of the patella and femur. Early biochemical and histologic changes after such blows suggest the initiation of posttraumatic osteoarthrosis. Indirect trauma is frequently caused by unexpectedly rapid flexion of the knee against a fully contracted quadriceps. Fractures resulting from indirect injury tend to be transverse and displaced.

Patellar fractures can also be classified morphologically. Transverse fractures usually occur in the central or distal third of the patella. Although vertical fractures of the patella can occur, they rarely require surgical treatment. Marginal fractures can also occur, but they usually do not disrupt the extensor mechanism. Any of these fractures can have associated comminution. Severe comminution is characterized by stellate fracture patterns. More commonly, transverse fractures occur, with comminution of one or both poles. Displaced fractures are those with articular incongruity of more than 2 mm or separation of the fragments of more than 3 mm.

A direct blow or a patellar dislocation can create an osteochondral fracture consisting of articular cartilage, subchondral bone, and underlying trabecular bone. Another type of osteochondral fracture, a sleeve fracture, occurs when the inferior pole of the patella of a child or adolescent is avulsed together with articular cartilage.

Evaluation

Patients with patellar fractures typically present with pain, swelling, and an inability to extend the knee. These symptoms, along with a detailed history including the mechanism of injury, usually indicate extensor mechanism disruption. A history of a direct blow or unexpected, rapid knee flexion while the quadriceps was contracted together with localized pain and the inability to strongly extend the knee is nearly diagnostic.[33] AP and lateral radiographs are necessary for classification of the fracture. The patella is often difficult to see on AP radiographs. Lateral radiographs document the comminution and displacement of the fragments. A high-riding patella on the lateral radiograph indicates a patellar rupture; a low-riding patella on the lateral radiograph indicates a quadriceps tendon rupture.

Treatment

Recent studies have focused on improving the techniques of repairing fractured patellae. In a review of 51 patellar fractures, 22% of fractures treated with tension band wiring and early motion displaced 2 mm or more during the early postoperative period.[34] Catastrophic failure was associated with unprotected weight bearing, whereas loss of reduction was associated with technical

errors and noncompliance. Minor losses of reduction may or may not have long-term consequences. In tests of strength of the internal fixation constructs, including modified tension band screw fixation alone and cannulated screws with anterior tension band, screws plus anterior tension band was shown to be superior.[35] The results of another study that reported on the clinical use of tensioned anterior figure-of-8 wire placed through cannulated screws were comparable to historical results using modified tension band.[36] Proponents of this modification of the standard technique have cited the biomechanical finding that screws have the greatest resistance to tensile loads because of pure tension forces. Atrophy of interposed soft tissue has also been postulated to account for loss of reduction in the modified tension band technique. Also, use of cannulated screws may minimize the risk of patient discomfort because of prominent Kirschner wires. One cadaveric study found that 1-mm braided wire performs superiorly to 1-mm monofilament stainless steel wire in cyclic testing.[37] The cable appears more likely to conform and less likely to kink compared with 316L stainless steel wire. Another study used Instron mechanical testing and showed that stainless steel was superior to two Ethibond loops or one loop of Mersilene tape at load to failure for tension band constructs.[38] A recent study supports the use of arthroscopically assisted reduction and percutaneous placement of fixation in patients with compromised skin, a procedure that precludes the need for early open approaches.[39] A tibial tubercle osteotomy to aid in visualization and reduction of comminuted fractures of the patella can also be considered in certain instances.[40]

Patellar Tendon Rupture

Patellar tendon rupture is the most common cause of knee extensor mechanism disruption after patellar fracture and quadriceps tendon rupture. The injury most commonly occurs in patients younger than 40 years in whom the extensor mechanism is overloaded during athletic activity. It has been estimated that a force of 17.5 times body weight is required to cause rupture in healthy patients. Metabolic disorders, rheumatologic disease, renal failure, corticosteroid injection, and infection are associated with an increased risk of patellar tendon rupture. Patients with rupture of the patellar tendon typically present with pain, swelling, and inability to extend the knee. Radiographically, the patella is displaced superiorly (patella alta) on the lateral view. The Insall-Salvati ratio (greatest diagonal length of the patella to the length of the patellar tendon on lateral radiographs) is independent of knee flexion, and a ratio of less than 0.80 indicates patella alta. Frequently, there is a delay in diagnosis. In a series of 33 patients (36 patellar tendon ruptures), it was reported that 10 patellar tendon ruptures were misdiagnosed on initial examination and that 7 were repaired more than 2 weeks after injury.[41] MRI and ultrasound examination may help confirm the diagnosis. Repair is usually performed with an end-to-end repair using a Krakow stitch.[42] Late repairs may be supplemented with semitendinosus graft.[41]

Acknowledgment

Thanks to Dale Baker, MA, for his assistance with the images.

Annotated References

1. Twaddle BC, Hunter JC, Chapman JR, et al: MRI in acute knee dislocation: A prospective study of clinical, MRI, and surgical findings. *J Bone Joint Surg Br* 1996;78:573-579.

2. Toritsuka Y, Horibe S, Hiro-oka A: Knee dislocation following anterior cruciate ligament disruption without any other ligament tears. *Arthroscopy* 1999;15:522-526.

3. Schenck RC Jr: The dislocated knee. *Instr Course Lect* 1994;43:127-136.

4. Hagino RT, DeCaprio JD, Valentine RJ, Clagett GP: Spontaneous popliteal vascular injury in the morbidly obese. *J Vasc Surg* 1998;28:458-462.

5. Varnell RM, Coldwell DM, Sangeorzan BJ, Johansen KH: Arterial injury complicating knee disruption. *Am Surg* 1989;55:699-704.

6. Miranda FE, Dennis JW, Veldenz HC, et al: Confirmation of the safety and accuracy of physical examination in the evaluation of knee dislocation for injury of the popliteal artery: A prospective study. *J Trauma* 2002;52:247-251.

    In this study, 35 patients with knee dislocation were prospectively evaluated for possible vascular injury by physical examination alone. Patients with abnormal physical examination results (active hemorrhage, expanding hematoma, absent pulses, bruit, distal ischemia) underwent arteriography and surgical repair. Patients with normal physical examination results were admitted for observation and serial examination. No patient with normal physical examination results developed signs of limb ischemia acutely or at follow-up (negative predictive value, 100%). The sensitivity, specificity, and positive predictive value of abnormal physical examination results were 100%, 96%, and 88%, respectively.

7. Treiman GS, Yellin AE, Weaver FA, et al: Examination of the patient with knee dislocation: The case for selective arteriography. *Arch Surg* 1992;127:1056-1063.

8. Stannard JP, Sheils TM, Lopez-Ben RR, McGwin G, Robinson JT, Volgas DA: Vascular injuries in knee dislocations: The role of physical examination in determining the need for arteriography. *J Bone Joint Surg Am* 2004;86:910-915.

    The authors prospectively studied 126 patients with knee dislocation using an algorithm for selective arteriography based on physical examination findings. Patients with any decrease in pedal pulses, color, or lower extremity temperature, an expanding knee hematoma, or any history of abnormal physical examination before emergency department presentation underwent arteriography. Patients who did not meet these criteria were admitted for observation and serial examination of lower extremity perfusion. The prevalence of clinically significant arterial injury was 7%. Ten patients had abnormal findings on physical examination and underwent arteriography; nine of these patients had popliteal artery damage, and one patient had a false-positive result. Patients with normal physical examinations (N = 116) were followed for a minimum of 6 months. None developed any vascular complications. The authors concluded that routine arteriography is not indicated for knee dislocation, but should be used for patients with positive physical examination findings.

9. Mills WJ, Barei DP, McNair P: The value of the ankle brachial index for diagnosing arterial injury after knee dislocation: A prospective study. *J Trauma* 2004;56:1261-1265.

    In this study, 38 patients with knee dislocation were studied prospectively with physical examination and ankle brachial index (ABI). Patients with an ABI ≥ 0.90 (N = 27) were admitted for serial examinations of limb perfusion. Patients with an ABI < 0.90 (N = 11) underwent urgent arteriography and all had arterial injury requiring surgical treatment. No patients with an ABI ≥ 0.90 had any vascular compromise at an average 19-month follow-up. The sensitivity, specificity, and positive predictive value of an ABI < 0.90 was 100%.

10. Goitz RJ, Tomaino MM: Management of peroneal nerve injuries associated with knee dislocation. *Am J Orthop* 2003;32:14-16.

    This is a review of multiple articles describing the results of using grafting techniques to treat patients with peroneal nerve injuries. An aggressive treatment protocol for peroneal nerve injury is proposed. Patients with incomplete palsies can be observed, with expectation of functional recovery. Acute repair of partial or complete transection should be avoided unless tension-free repair is possible. In one report, 75% of patients with nerve injuries who underwent cable grafting ≤ 6 cm in length within 3 to 4 months from injury recovered at least grade 3 strength.

11. Mills WJ, Nowinski RJ: Dislocation of the knee with lateral dislocation of the patella: A report of four cases. *J Bone Joint Surg Br* 2001;83:530-532.

Lateral dislocation of the patella was reported in 16% of patients with knee dislocation. All had severe disruption of medial soft tissues, including deep and superficial MCL, medial capsule, and medial patellofemoral ligament injuries. Early reduction of the patella was recommended to avoid fixed contracture of lateral soft tissues. The severity of the MCL injury required reconstruction in two patients.

12. Escobedo EM, Mills WJ, Hunter JC: The "reverse Segond" fracture: Association with a tear of the posterior cruciate ligament and medial meniscus. *AJR Am J Roentgenol* 2002;178:979-983.

This is a retrospective review of the records of patients with plain radiographic findings of acute bony avulsion of the medial aspect of the proximal tibia after high-energy trauma. All patients had high-grade PCL and MCL injuries with associated tears of the medial meniscus; two thirds of patients had knee dislocation.

13. Dedmond BT, Almekinders LC: Operative versus non-operative treatment of knee dislocations: A meta-analysis. *Am J Knee Surg* 2001;14:33-38.

This meta-analysis identified 15 articles that addressed closed or surgical treatment for knee dislocation. Surgical treatment was associated with improved functional outcomes, range of motion, and knee extension. No difference in laxity or return to preinjury employment or athletics was found.

14. Noyes FR, Barber-Westin SD: Reconstruction of the anterior and posterior cruciate ligaments after knee dislocation: Use of early protected postoperative motion to decrease arthrofibrosis. *Am J Sports Med* 1997;25:769-778.

15. Mills WJ, Tejwani N: Heterotopic ossification after knee dislocation: The predictive value of the injury severity score. *J Orthop Trauma* 2003;17:338-345.

Heterotopic ossification occurred in 43% of patients with knee dislocation. An Injury Severity Score of ≥ 26 had a statistically significant risk of postoperative ankylosing heterotopic ossification formation, whereas those patients with an Injury Severity Score < 26 were spared this complication. The former group had a higher incidence of closed head injury. Patients with an Injury Severity Score < 26 who underwent surgery within 3 weeks of injury recovered an average range of motion of 126°. The authors concluded that the Injury Severity Score is a useful tool for determining which patients will benefit from early surgical treatment and which should have delayed formal reconstruction.

16. Wascher DC, Becker JR, Dexter JG, Blevins FT: Reconstruction of the anterior and posterior cruciate ligaments after knee dislocation: Results using fresh-frozen nonirradiated allografts. *Am J Sports Med* 1999;27:189-196.

17. Shapiro MS, Freedman EL: Allograft reconstruction of the anterior and posterior cruciate ligaments after traumatic knee dislocation. *Am J Sports Med* 1995;23:580-587.

18. Stannard JP, Wilson TC, Sheils TM, McGwin G, Volgas DA, Alonso JE: Heterotopic ossification associated with knee dislocation. *Arthroscopy* 2002;18:835-839.

This study combined prospective and retrospective data. Heterotopic ossification occurred in 26% of patients with knee dislocation; 12% had severe or motion-limiting heterotopic ossification. Patients with heterotopic ossification about the knee were more likely to have heterotopic ossification at other anatomic sites; however, periarticular fracture did not increase the risk of heterotopic ossification.

19. Shelbourne KD, Porter DA, Clingman JA, et al: Low-velocity knee dislocation. *Orthop Rev* 1991;20:995-1004.

20. Stannard JP, Sheils TM, McGwin G, Volgas DA, Alonso JE: Use of a hinged external knee fixator after surgery for knee dislocation. *Arthroscopy* 2003;19:626-631.

This prospective functional outcome study compared ligament reconstruction failure rates in patients treated with and without a hinged external knee fixator (compass knee hinge) after ligament reconstruction. Those patients treated with the hinged external knee fixator had statistically fewer failures of posterolateral reconstructions. No patient treated with a hinged external knee fixator developed more than 1+ PCL laxity.

21. Ilan DI, Tejwani N, Keschner M, Leibman M: Quadriceps tendon rupture. *J Am Acad Orthop Surg* 2003;11:192-200.

This article reviews the treatment of quadriceps ruptures.

22. O'Shea K, Kenny P, Donovan J, Condon F, McElwain JP: Outcomes following quadriceps tendon ruptures. *Injury* 2002;33:257-260.

These authors present functional outcome data for 27 patients who underwent surgical repair of quadriceps ruptures. Symptomatic outcome was excellent. No difference in thigh girth between affected and unaffected limbs was reported.

23. Rougraff BT, Reeck CC, Essenmacher J: Complete quadriceps tendon ruptures. *Orthopedics* 1996;19:509-514.

24. Konrath GA, Chen D, Lock T, et al: Outcomes following repair of quadriceps tendon ruptures. *J Orthop Trauma* 1998;12:273-279.

25. Lombardi LJ, Cleri DJ, Epstein E: Bilateral spontaneous quadriceps tendon rupture in a patient with renal failure. *Orthopedics* 1995;18:187-191.

26. Huberti HH, Hayes WC, Stone JL, Shybut GT: Force ratios in the quadriceps tendon and ligamentum patellae. *J Orthop Res* 1984;2:49-54.

27. Maniscalco P, Bertone C, Rivera F, Bocchi L: A new method of repair for quadriceps tendon ruptures: A case report. *Panminerva Med* 2000;42:223-225.

28. Richards DP, Barber FA: Repair of quadriceps tendon ruptures using suture anchors. *Arthroscopy* 2002;18:556-559.
    These authors present a brief technical note of two cases in which repair of a quadriceps tendon rupture was repaired with suture anchors.

29. Lhowe DW: Open fractures of the femoral shaft. *Orthop Clin North Am* 1994;25:573-580.

30. Rhomberg M, Schwabegger AH, Ninkovic M, Bauer T, Ninkovic M: Gastrocnemius myotendinous flap for patellar or quadriceps tendon repair, or both. *Clin Orthop* 2000;377:152-160.

31. Weber MJ, Janecki CJ, McLeod P, Nelson CL, Thompson JA: Efficacy of various forms of fixation of transverse fractures of the patella. *J Bone Joint Surg Am* 1980;62:215-220.

32. Scapinelli R: Blood supply to the human patella: Its relation to ischaemic necrosis after fracture. *J Bone Joint Surg Br* 1967;49:563-570.

33. Carpenter JE, Kasman R, Matthews LS: Fractures of the patella. *Instr Course Lect* 1994;43:97-108.

34. Smith ST, Cramer KE, Karges DE, Watson JT, Moed BR: Early complications in the operative treatment of patella fractures. *J Orthop Trauma* 1997;11:183-187.

35. Carpenter JE, Kasman RA, Patel N, Lee ML, Goldstein SA: Biomechanical evaluation of current patella fracture fixation techniques. *J Orthop Trauma* 1997;11:351-356.

36. Berg EE: Open reduction internal fixation of displaced transverse patella fractures with figure-eight wiring through parallel cannulated compression screws. *J Orthop Trauma* 1997;11:573-576.

37. Scilaris TA, Grantham JL, Prayson MJ, Marshall MP, Hamilton JJ, Williams JL: Biomechanical comparison of fixation methods in transverse patella fractures. *J Orthop Trauma* 1998;12:356-359.

38. Harrell RM, Tong J, Weinhold PS, Dahners LE: Comparison of the mechanical properties of different tension band materials and suture techniques. *J Orthop Trauma* 2003;17:119-122.

39. Turgut A, Gunal I, Acar S, Seber S, Gokturk E: Arthroscopic-assisted percutaneous stabilization of patellar fractures. *Clin Orthop* 2001;389:57-61.

40. Berg EE: Extensile exposure of comminuted patella fractures using a tibial tubercle osteotomy: Results of a new technique. *J Orthop Trauma* 1998;12:351-355.

41. Siwek CW, Rao JP: Ruptures of the extensor mechanism of the knee joint. *J Bone Joint Surg Am* 1981;63:932-937.

42. Krackow KA, Thomas SC, Jones LC: A new stitch for ligament-tendon fixation. Brief note. *J Bone Joint Surg Am* 1986;68:764-766.

Chapter 36

Fractures of the Tibial Plateau

J. L. Marsh, MD

Langdon Hartsock, MD, FACS

Introduction

Fractures of the tibial plateau comprise a diverse group of fracture patterns that range in severity from minor injuries that have predictably excellent outcomes after simple treatment to fractures at high risk for limb-threatening complications. These injuries include low-energy valgus loading fractures of the lateral plateau, high-energy knee dislocations with rim avulsions, and bumper injuries with severe soft-tissue injury and metaphyseal-diaphyseal disassociation. These diverse injuries require different assessment and management techniques to provide patients with optimal outcomes and minimal risks.

Advanced imaging techniques, which allow better assessment of fracture patterns and associated soft-tissue injuries, can assist in preoperative planning. Improved techniques of plate and screw fixation combined with better substances to fill the metaphyseal defects frequently created by compression injuries may better maintain reduction after surgical fixation. New data provide improved knowledge of patient outcomes, thereby allowing treatment choices that have the best chance of optimal results.

Incidence and Epidemiology

Tibial plateau fractures occur in adults, with the highest incidence in the fifth decade of life, with decreasing frequency during the fourth and sixth decades of life. Men have a higher incidence of tibial plateau fractures at a younger age, which reflects a high-energy mechanism of injury, whereas women have increasing incidence with advancing age, which peaks in the sixth and seventh decades of life and indicates fractures in osteopenic bone.

Classification

Although the AO/Orthopaedic Trauma Association classification system of proximal tibial fractures is now frequently used, it has not supplanted the Schatzker classification system for routine clinical fracture description (Figure 1). The descriptive terms in the Schatzker classification system provide information that is not easily conveyed by the alphanumeric system of the AO/Orthopaedic Trauma Association classification. Split (type I), split depression (type II), lateral compression (type III), medial condyle split (type IV), bicondylar (type V), and shaft disassociated from the condyles (type VI) describe most of the fracture patterns encountered by surgeons treating patients with tibial plateau fractures. These subgroups guide the choice of treatment techniques, determine the risk for complications, and influence patient outcomes.

Reliable classification of tibial plateau fractures depends on observer ability to make basic assessments about the presence and location of fracture lines and displacements. Unfortunately, these basic assessments are themselves not reliably made; one recent study showed that even measuring the degree of articular depression was subject to differences as great as 12 mm among observers.[1]

Examination

A careful physical examination of the knee and leg of a patient with a tibial plateau fracture is critically important to assess for associated injuries, indicate surgical versus nonsurgical treatment, diagnose and avoid severe complications, and determine optimal timing for surgical intervention.

Severe tibial plateau fractures may have communicating open wounds that would require urgent surgical treatment. Vascular injury to the popliteal artery with fracture-dislocation patterns and trifurcation injury with high-energy proximal tibial fractures and proximal joint extension are both well recognized associated injuries. Compartment syndrome may be more common after high-energy proximal tibia and tibial plateau fractures than any other lower extremity injury. Closed fractures may be associated with significant soft-tissue swelling, contusions of the skin and subcutaneous tissues, and serous or blood-filled fracture blisters. Accurately determining the initial severity of the closed soft-tissue injury

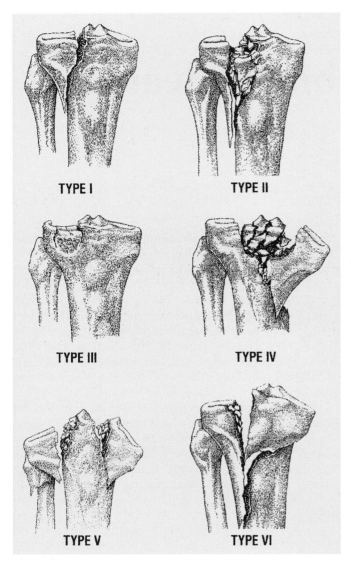

Figure 1 Schatzker classification of tibial plateau fractures: type I: lateral plateau split; type II: lateral split-depression; type III: lateral depression; type IV: medial plateau fracture; type V: bicondylar injury; and type VI: tibial plateau fracture with metaphyseal-diaphyseal dissociation. *(Reproduced from Beaty JH (ed): Orthopaedic Knowledge Update 6. Rosemont, IL, American Academy of Orthopaedic Surgeons, 1999, pp 521-532.)*

and assessing the recovery of the soft tissues are the most important factors for timing surgical intervention.

Examining for knee stability is an important step in assessing whether a fracture requires surgical intervention. A plateau fracture with knee instability requires surgical intervention to maximize the chances of healing with a well-aligned knee, which is an important predictor of patient outcome.

Imaging Studies

Routine radiographs are usually sufficient to make the diagnosis of a tibial plateau fracture. AP, lateral, and AP views in the plane of the plateau (10° caudal view) are standard. Occasionally, oblique views will enhance the assessment of fracture lines or degree of displacement, but they are not routinely obtained. In patients with severe fractures in which both condyles are displaced, radiographs with the patient in traction provide significantly more information than routine radiographs. A common way to apply traction in patients with severe fractures is by using a spanning external fixator.

An axial CT scan is another routine study and provides excellent detail of the fracture pathoanatomy. It is valuable as an aid to preoperative planning. The more limited the planned surgical approach, the more critical it is to understand the location of fracture lines and displacement. Typically, plain films underestimate the degree of articular injury compared with CT scans. Multislice CT now provides optimal visualization of the injured plateau in any two-dimensional plane or with high-quality three-dimensional images. In patients with complex fractures with significant displacement, provisional fracture realignment with a spanning fixator should be done before CT to enhance the value of the study and the quality of the scan.

MRI of the fractured plateau provides additional information about the periarticular soft-tissue structures that are frequently injured in association with tibial plateau fractures.[2] In one study, even patients with minimally displaced tibial plateau fractures for which conservative treatment was indicated were found to have a high percentage of associated soft-tissue injuries (meniscal injuries, 80%; ligament injuries, 40%); the clinical significance of these findings, however, is uncertain.[3] For these minimally displaced fractures, as for all tibial plateau fractures, it is difficult to know which soft-tissue injuries require surgical management to improve patient outcome. Some surgeons obtain an MRI study routinely to assess tibial plateau fractures, whereas others reserve MRI for patients for whom there is a particular concern about the status of the ligaments or the menisci that would not be otherwise assessed through the surgical approach.

Biomechanics of Fracture and Fixation Devices

Shearing and rotational forces typically produce knee ligament injuries. Tibial plateau fractures result from the addition of bending and axial load. Bending forces produce unicondylar fractures, and axial loads produce bicondylar fractures. The exact fracture pattern depends on the position of the knee and direction of the force.

In a cadaver study, increased displacement of a simulated split fracture of the lateral plateau led to increased contact pressure and valgus alignment, both of which were further increased by a lateral meniscectomy.[4] This study emphasizes the importance of maintaining joint alignment and preserving the meniscus. In another study in sheep, small displacements less than the full thickness of the articular cartilage led to remodeling, which supports clinical experience that residual articular displacement in the tibial plateau can result in good outcomes without posttraumatic arthritis if the knee remains well aligned.[5]

Fracture fixation devices must be designed and applied in a way to resist deforming forces. In simple split fractures, fixation with compression screws will suffice. In depression and split depression fractures, a plate typically functions as a buttress to prevent compression leading to redisplacement. Recent mechanical tests have shown that smaller plates used in conjunction with 3.5-mm screws may perform this function as well as or better than larger implants with 4.5-mm screws.[6] In particular, the 3.5-mm implants allow a raft of screws to be placed directly beneath elevated osteochondral fragments. In one cadaver study, four 3.5-mm subchondral screws provided better resistance to local depression loads in the lateral plateau than traditional L-buttress plates.[7]

In bicondylar fractures, the implants must resist deforming forces on both sides of the joint. When the shaft is disassociated from the condyles, axial and bending forces can be substantial. To prevent redisplacement, lateral plating has traditionally been augmented with a medial plate or external fixator. However, comparative testing has indicated that new designs of fixed-angle lateral plates appear to have the mechanical strength necessary to decrease the need for two-sided plating.[8]

Reduced lateral tibial plateau fractures leave a significant void in the area of joint depression. Filling this void has always been an integral part of surgically treating these fractures, and the material of choice has been cancellous autograft. Recent evidence, however, indicates that calcium phosphate cement can be used to replace cancellous autograft and that it is superior in preventing redisplacement in cadaver models.[9,10]

Indications for Nonsurgical Treatment

Nonsurgical treatment typically leads to predictably excellent outcomes in appropriately selected patients. Because obtaining and maintaining a closed reduction is difficult and in many fracture patterns impossible, nonsurgical techniques are reserved for patients with fractures that can be predicted to heal without significant deformity or for patients who are elderly, infirm, or have associated medical problems that make surgical intervention undesirable.

Predicting healing without deformity can be difficult. Surgeons must use information about the fracture pattern, examination of the patient, and knowledge of outcomes of various types of fractures to make this judgment. In a 20-year follow-up study, patients received nonsurgical treatment when they had less than 10° of coronal plane instability in full extension.[11] Good and

excellent results were achieved in 90% of patients, which indicates that lack of significant instability in full extension is a strong predictor of good results after conservative treatment. Although this information is helpful in clinical decision making, it is often difficult to reliably examine an acutely injured knee.

The type of fracture is a critical factor in achieving a good result after nonsurgical treatment. Patients with localized depressions of the lateral plateau of 5 mm or more may have stable knees and good outcomes with nonsurgical treatment. However, even nondisplaced fractures of the medial condyle tend to displace and lead to varus deformity, which is poorly tolerated over the long term. For this reason, treatment strategies based on an arbitrary number of millimeters of displacement are not sensible and do not provide a guideline for decision making across the range of tibial plateau fractures.

Most patients with tibial plateau fractures should not bear weight until early healing has begun; the duration depends on the fracture pattern, but is typically 4 to 8 weeks. Although patients with tibial plateau fractures can be treated with up to 6 weeks of cast immobilization, most surgeons prefer early mobilization with a hinged brace. Cast braces can be used to unload the injured side of the joint, but because fractures treated nonsurgically are generally considered to be stable, a removable lightweight hinged brace is usually sufficient.

Surgical Treatment
Planning
Surgical stabilization of tibial plateau fractures is indicated for displaced, unstable fractures. The treatment plan is based on the severity of the fracture, the soft-tissue status, and the overall condition of the patient. Plain radiographs must be critically reviewed before embarking on surgery. If the fracture cannot be adequately appreciated, then additional studies such as a CT or MRI should be performed.

A clear understanding of the severity of the fracture is essential to selecting the correct method of stabilization. Radiographs must be analyzed for fracture lines involving the lateral and medial condyles and the metaphysis. Coronal and sagittal fracture lines may require independent, specifically directed lag screws. Areas of joint depression need to be derotated, and the void needs to be filled with bone graft or a bone graft substitute. A separate tibial tubercle fragment mandates secure reattachment. Medial metaphyseal involvement requires fixation that can obviate varus collapse, such as a hybrid fixator, dual plates, or a locking plate.

The condition of the soft tissue is extremely important. Contusions, degloving, open wounds, abrasions, blisters, and edema can cause major problems in the postoperative period. The status of the soft tissues may

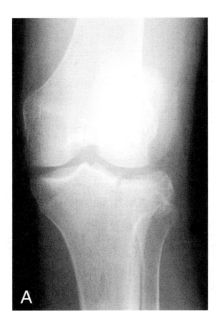 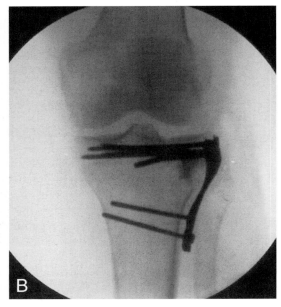

Figure 2 A, AP radiograph of a 30-year-old man with a split lateral depression tibial plateau fracture shows significant displacement and slight valgus alignment. **B,** Postoperative AP radiograph of the same patient shows reduction and fixation with a precontoured 3.5-mm plate and a raft of subchondral screws. Calcium phosphate cement was used as a void filler.

alter the surgical plan to minimize the risk of serious complications such as wound breakdown and infection.

The patient's overall condition must be recognized and considered in the treatment of the fracture. Multiple injuries, head injuries, and significant medical conditions (particularly diabetes, renal failure, and peripheral vascular disease) are examples of conditions that can affect the choice of treatment. As patients in their 40s and 50s continue to age, osteoporosis is more likely and will make stable fixation even more challenging.

Low-Energy Fractures

Low-energy fractures include simple split fractures of a condyle, depressions of the articular surface, or simple extra-articular fractures of the proximal tibia. These fractures can be stabilized by a variety of methods, depending on the experience of the surgeon and the needs of the patient.

Approaches

The classic technique is the direct surgical approach via a midline or anterolateral surgical incision. The fracture and joint surface are visualized directly. Usually a submeniscal arthrotomy is performed, and the meniscus is elevated to allow visualization of the joint surface. A joint distractor may be used. Detachment or incision of the meniscus should be avoided if possible. An open reduction is performed, depressed fragments are elevated, and provisional fixation is applied using Kirschner wires. The reduction is visually inspected, and internal fixation is applied.

In an attempt to minimize soft-tissue disruption, the classic approach has been altered by the use of fluoroscopy to take the place of direct visualization of the fracture and the reduction. This allows for a minimally invasive approach in which a smaller incision can be used to visualize the metaphyseal portion of the fracture line, remove soft tissue or hematoma, and then reduce the fracture. The overall reduction is then assessed with fluoroscopy without direct visualization of the joint. Many simple split-type fractures can be manipulated with closed reduction under the control of an image intensifier and then fixed with percutaneous lag screws.

Arthroscopy can be used as an aid to assess reduction of plateau fractures.[12,13] After lavage of the joint, the fracture reduction can be viewed through the arthroscope. Fixation is applied either during an open procedure or percutaneously. Arthroscopy is particularly useful for less complex joint depression fractures. A cortical window can be made in the proximal tibial metaphysis, and a bone tamp inserted. The tamp then elevates the metaphyseal bone underlying the depressed fragments. The extent of elevation can be monitored via arthroscopy until the joint surface has been reduced. There is a potential risk with arthroscopy of compartment syndrome if significant extravasation of fluid occurs.

Small Plates and 3.5-mm Screws

Low-energy tibial plateau fractures have been increasingly treated with smaller implants.[6,14-16] For example, 3.5-mm interfragmentary lag screws for the proximal tibia can be used instead of 6.5-mm or larger screws. Also, smaller, lower profile plates using 3.5-mm screws are as effective as larger plates and screws for many fracture patterns that do not extend into diaphyseal bone. A series of smaller subchondral screws can be used to support depressed fragments in a way that is not possible with larger implants. When combined with specially designed precontoured 3.5-mm plates, better buttressing of the reduced articular fracture can be achieved (Figure 2).

Void Fillers

There is an increasing number of bone graft substitutes and bone void fillers in the orthopaedic marketplace, including freeze-dried cancellous allograft, processed coral, processed collagen, demineralized bone matrix, calcium phosphates, and calcium sulfates as well as combinations of these products.[17-20] These products are gradually supplanting autologous iliac crest graft as a void filler in the treatment of patients with tibial plateau fractures. Calcium phosphate cement appears to be effective as a metaphyseal void filler because it provides increased resistance to compressive forces compared with autografts (Figure 2).

High-Energy Fractures

High-energy fractures are recognized radiographically by complex fracture patterns with significant comminution and multiple fracture lines. Both condyles are usually involved, and significant metaphyseal comminution may be noted. Severe articular surface crushing and depression with wide displacement is typical. In addition, there is usually serious soft-tissue injury, including swelling, bruising, degloving, laceration, open fractures, abrasions, and possibly compartment syndromes. These fractures can be challenging to treat, and complications can be frequent and severe.

Temporary Spanning: Rationale and Technique

A temporary spanning external fixator can be useful to treat patients with high-energy fractures for a variety of reasons. The fixator can be applied quickly with minimal blood loss and does not preclude other future interventions. Closed reduction can be performed, wounds débrided and irrigated, and overall alignment restored. Ongoing wound care is facilitated because no splint or brace is needed to augment the control provided by the external fixator. The fixator can also provide surgeons with valuable information about how the fracture responds to the simple application of traction (ligamentotaxis). Frequently, the major fragments of the condyles and the shaft will come back into alignment with traction through the use of the spanning external fixator. Better imaging studies can be obtained after the fracture is provisionally reduced.

The external fixator is easiest to apply if it has separate components to attach the pins to the bars. This construct allows for maximum modularity and control. Two half pins are usually applied to the mid and distal shaft of the femur and tibia. Traction is applied to the limb. The fluoroscope is used to check overall alignment, but its use is not critical if the patient is in an emergency situation. The connecting bars and clamps are applied to the pins, with care taken to keep the clamps away from

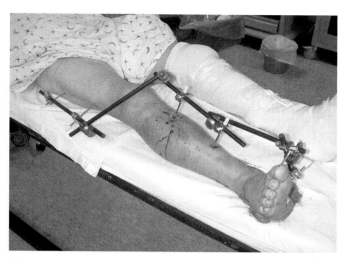

Figure 3 A clinical photograph showing a simple knee spanning pin bar external fixator placed for a high-energy tibial plateau fracture. The foot was included because of an additional, more distal injury.

the joint line where they can compromise postoperative radiographs. Any open wounds are also treated with excision of the traumatic wound and thorough irrigation. Definitive fixation can be performed on a delayed basis after imaging, soft-tissue recovery, and preoperative planning (Figure 3).

Definitive External Fixation

External fixation is useful for patients with severe soft-tissue injuries or patients with severe fracture patterns, such as bicondylar fractures or fractures with metaphyseal comminution. External fixation avoids the possible complications of surgical incisions to expose the fracture and apply plates. The disadvantages of external fixation include risk of pin site infection, soft-tissue irritation from the pins, the weight and bulk of the device, and the need for it to be kept in place until the fracture has completely healed. Use of a hybrid external fixator is frequently effective.[21,22] The condyles are usually stabilized with interfragmentary lag screws, and then the restored articular block is reduced and stabilized to the metaphysis and shaft with the external fixator.

Olive wires are placed to capture the proximal tibia. Care must be taken to place the wires approximately 10 to 14 mm below the joint surface to avoid placing the pin in an intra-articular position. A wire is applied posterolaterally to anteromedially, taking care to avoid the peroneal nerve. A second wire is applied posteromedially to anterolaterally. Additional wires or half pins can be useful. The wires are applied to a two-thirds ring or full ring, and tension is applied to the wires. The ring is then applied to a more traditional half-pin type unilateral frame constructed on the tibial shaft. The fluoroscope is used to confirm adequate reduction of the tibial plateau fracture and correct placement of the wires and pins.

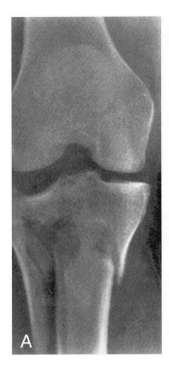
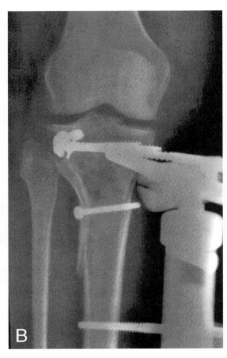
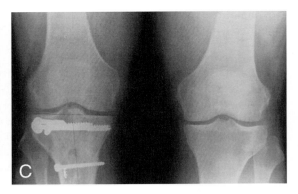

Figure 4 **A,** AP radiograph of a 28-year-old woman who was involved in a motor vehicle accident demonstrates the presence of a Schatzker type VI tibial plateau fracture. **B,** Postoperative AP radiograph of the same patient shows that she was treated with reduction screw fixation and an external fixator. **C,** Weight-bearing AP radiograph of both knees of the same patient obtained 6 years after injury shows no sign of posttraumatic joint narrowing.

Some surgeons prefer full ring fixators (such as an Ilizarov); however, others use traditional pin fixators. Similar principles apply when the fixator is used to reduce and fix a reconstructed articular segment to the diaphysis, spanning the metaphyseal injury (Figure 4).

Bicondylar Open Reduction and Internal Fixation Advances

The bicondylar tibial plateau fracture is the most challenging fracture pattern. The surgeon must create a smooth, anatomic joint surface from a comminuted proximal tibia, and then restore the head to the shaft with the correct length, rotation, and alignment. Intervention must minimize the complications of skin necrosis, wound breakdown, and infection. Incisions must be carefully planned to avoid creating thin skin bridges or ischemic tissue. Interfragmentary lag screws provide the best method for stable fixation of the two condyles. The fracture can be reduced through an open approach or a limited approach with the assistance of fluoroscopy and/or arthroscopy, or both. Whichever method is used, the additional soft-tissue injury created must be minimized.

Two incisions for placement of dual plates are safer than a single extensile approach. A straight posteromedial incision, which goes directly to bone without development of flaps, is safe. The interval is between the posterior margin of the pes tendons and the medial head of the gastrocnemius. A medial buttress (for example, a 3.5-mm plate acting in a buttress mode) plate can be applied with very little elevation of soft tissue from bone. This plate secures the medial tibial plateau to the shaft.[23]

A second incision is made anterolaterally, taking great care to make sure an adequate skin bridge is maintained between the two incisions. The anterolateral incision exposes the lateral aspect of the upper tibia, and a lateral plate can be applied to the lateral surface of the tibia. The wounds are closed with meticulous care.

Recent developments in the design of plates and screws have made the possibility of treating bicondylar fractures with a fixed-angle device a reality. This type of implant avoids the need for medial incision and the medial plate. The Less Invasive Stabilization System (Synthes USA, Paoli, PA) allows a plate to be applied on the lateral side of the tibia, and the screws are coupled to the plate via a threaded hole and matching threaded screw head (Figure 5). This creates a fixed-angle screwplate construct. This type of device is useful for treating patients with bicondylar tibial plateau fractures with significant metaphyseal comminution. The implant can be inserted through a limited incision on the proximal and lateral aspect of the tibia. The device functions as a bridging plate or as an internalized external fixator because all of the screws are fixed to the plate. A few clinical case series have been reported for use of this implant in proximal tibial fractures.[24] The Locking Proximal Tibial Plate (Synthes USA) is similar to the Less Invasive Stabilization System in that it has locking screws, but it can also use conventional screws and is inserted using an open technique. There are no comparative studies in the literature on the Locking Proximal Tibial Plate.

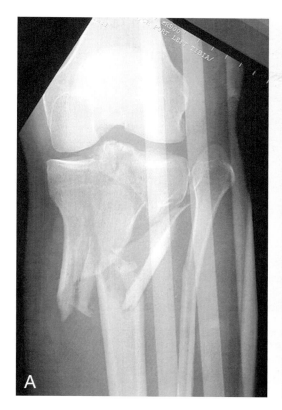

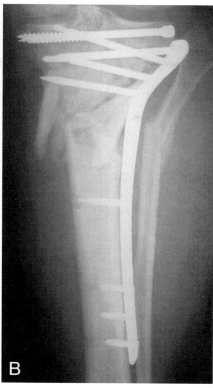

Figure 5 A, AP radiograph of a 57-year-old man with a high-energy proximal tibia fracture from a motorcycle accident shows a comminuted Schatzker type VI fracture pattern. The patient was initially treated with spanning external fixation; 10 days after injury, a locking plate was applied through limited approaches. **B,** Postoperative AP radiograph of the same patient shows satisfactory alignment. The plate was used to span the zone of the metaphyseal comminution.

Postoperative Care and Rehabilitation

Postoperative care includes monitoring for compartment syndrome, pain management, and deep venous thrombosis prophylaxis. The patient usually begins early passive and active range-of-motion exercises. Continuous passive motion exercises may be useful for multiple-trauma patients who are unable to participate in physical therapy because of other injuries. A postoperative brace is only needed for patients with residual ligamentous laxity. Patients may be foot-flat touchdown weight bearing for the first 6 weeks. Provided adequate progress is noted radiographically, patients can progress to partial weight bearing and then full weight bearing.

Complications

Low-energy tibial plateau fractures have a low risk for severe complications, but split, split depression, and local compression fractures of the lateral plateau, if untreated, have a high incidence of valgus alignment of the knee. Because optimal outcome requires good knee alignment, one of the goals of treatment is to prevent valgus deformity. Recent evidence indicates that surgical management of these fractures is frequently complicated by postoperative loss of reduction. In one study, 31% of knees had loss of position after surgical treatment, and in patients older than 60 years, this occurrence rose to 79%.[25] The clinical significance of loss of reduction is uncertain, but when it

leads to malalignment, patient outcome may be compromised (Figure 6). Improved methods of surgical fixation of low-energy fractures, such as smaller precontoured plates allowing numerous subchondral screws to raft under the reduced articular surface, may decrease the tendency for postoperative displacement.[7] Calcium phosphate cement used as void filler after reduction of the articular surface may be stronger than traditional techniques such as bone grafting.[10] Whether these new techniques will decrease the incidence of loss of reduction and thereby lead to improved patient outcome is uncertain, but given the tendency toward postoperative redisplacement, these refinements of technique seem warranted.

In patients with high-energy proximal tibial fractures, the injured soft-tissue envelope presents a considerable risk for complications during surgical management. The risk of wound breakdown, exposed hardware, and proximal tibial infection has decreased using current techniques such as delaying definitive surgery, using temporary spanning external fixation, avoiding extensile surgical approaches, and definitive fixation with external fixation. The use of definitive external fixation has presented its own complications. A small but persistent incidence of septic arthritis related to proximal external fixation wires or pins has been reported.[22] Studies have assessed the capsular reflections around the knee in an effort to define a safe zone for pins or wires. Unfortunately, in patients with high-energy fractures, some risk remains despite the use of careful technique. Current

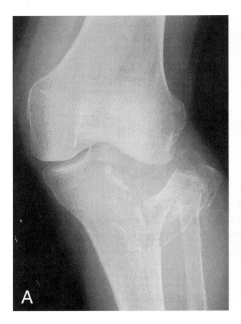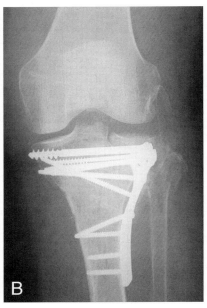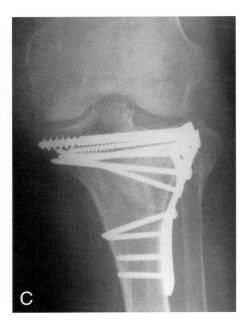

Figure 6 A, AP radiograph of a 72-year-old woman with a severe split depression lateral plateau fracture resulting from a fall shows a severe lateral side injury and osteopenic bone. **B,** Postoperative AP radiograph of the same patient shows reduction and fixation with a 3.5-mm plate and two 6.5-mm screws. **C,** AP radiograph of the same patient obtained 8 months postoperatively shows recurrent depression and valgus alignment.

recommendations are to place external fixation pins or wires as far from the articular surface as possible. In patients with severe comminution with multiple small fragments close to the joint, a prolonged period of cross-knee fixation may be preferable to risking joint sepsis in the early weeks after injury. Even patients with severely injured knees appear to tolerate cross-knee immobility for 6 weeks or longer, and they can still regain good motion and have reasonable function over the short and long term.[26]

Locked plating is a new treatment technique that is being investigated for high-energy proximal tibial fractures. Compared with other plating techniques, this device should decrease complications secondary to loss of position in patients with unstable bicondylar fractures because the fixed-angle screw plate device can resist common deforming forces. External screw targeting also allows the possibility of plate application through limited approaches. In combination, these advantages may decrease the incidence of wound complications. However, there is currently insufficient published data to determine the risks for complication compared with other techniques.

Patient Outcome

Most patients with tibial plateau fractures have good outcomes regardless of treatment technique. One recent study demonstrated that 5 to 11 years after injury even high-energy fractures treated with external fixation result in good knee function and a low rate of arthrosis and that the general health status of the patients equaled that of age-matched control subjects.[26] These generally favorable results emphasize the importance of avoiding complications during treatment of these complex fractures.

New evidence indicates that elderly patients have less favorable outcomes for all types of tibial plateau fractures.[27-29] In one study, only 12 of 21 patients older than 40 years equaled age-matched controls on patient-derived outcome measures at greater than 8-year follow-up.[27] These results were dramatically different than those found in patients younger than 40 years. Another study found that only 35% of patients (14 of 40) older than 50 years with tibial plateau fractures were satisfied with their results, regardless of fracture pattern or whether they underwent surgical or nonsurgical treatment.[28] The results of these two studies, when contrasted with those of the study of patients with high-energy fractures, suggest that younger patients with much higher-energy fractures have more favorable outcomes than older patients with less severe fractures.

Tibial plateau fractures do not frequently lead to total knee arthroplasty, indicating that satisfactory and long-lasting knee function is usually restored in most patients. Over an 11-year period at the Mayo Clinic, it was reported that only 62 knee arthroplasties were performed in patients with a previous fracture of the tibial plateau.[30] In another study, only 2 of 151 patients older than 60 years with a tibial plateau fracture required knee arthroplasty.[29]

It remains uncertain which treatment techniques most predictably lead to favorable versus unfavorable patient outcomes. A variety of techniques remains popular, and new techniques continue to be reported. Despite this support, there is little evidence that one technique is superior to others. For instance, currently acceptable techniques for visualizing the reduction of a split depression lateral plateau fracture include fluoroscopic, arthroscopic, and joint arthrotomy with meniscal incision or elevation. Fixation of the same fracture may be done with either small or large plates and screws, or screws alone. Numerous materials to fill the void created by the reduction are possible. It is difficult to ascertain which fractures and fracture patterns benefit from surgical versus nonsurgical management.

The quality of reduction of the displaced articular surface of the plateau has been considered by many surgeons to be an important predictor of patient outcome after surgical treatment. Others have believed that knee alignment and stability are more important. One recent study found that after open reduction and internal fixation (mean follow-up, > 8 years) neither the fracture pattern nor the quality of reduction affected patient outcome.[27] Two recent studies of high-energy fractures treated by external fixation highlight this controversy. One study found that knee scores were significantly better in patients with anatomic articular reductions, whereas the other found that good outcomes were predictable if alignment and stability were achieved.[22,26] In a recent review of articular fractures, it was noted that patients with tibial plateau fractures appear to have more tolerance for articular displacement than those with similar fractures of other lower extremity joints.[31] This may be because of the nature of the articulation, a load-sharing effect of the menisci, or other factors.

Reconstruction

Occasionally, reconstruction using osteotomy of intra-articular or extra-articular deformity in patients with malreduced tibial plateau fractures can improve knee function. The results of using fresh tibial osteochondral allografts to treat patients with tibial plateau fractures have been reported with long-term follow-up (mean, 12 years).[32] In this time interval, one third of the knees had been converted to prosthetic arthroplasty and 40% of remaining knees had moderate or severe degenerative changes. Despite these results, most surviving grafts continued to provide reasonable function. Tibial osteotomy to change alignment was a frequently associated procedure. There was a trend toward better results in patients who underwent concomitant meniscal transplantation.

Reconstruction using knee arthroplasty is a good option in elderly patients with painful posttraumatic arthritis or deformity after a tibial plateau fracture. Two recent case series have shown that although relief of pain and improved function are predictably achieved, there is a high incidence of postoperative complications and revisions including infection, component revisions, and knee manipulation.[30,33] In addition, these arthroplasties are often technically demanding because of hardware, proximal tibial deformity, scarred soft tissues, and stiffness. These results suggest that conversion of a symptomatic knee after a tibial plateau fracture to a knee arthroplasty should not be undertaken lightly.

Emerging Concepts

Long-term outcomes for the treatment of tibial plateau fractures correlate with preventing axis deformity and avoiding complications, and are improved in younger patients. For these reasons, further advances will require better methods to control limb alignment and minimize complications. Recent innovations in locked plating and buttressing with small-fragment specially contoured plates indicate that further hardware improvements will continue to emerge. The most promising area for future advances is in the development of new materials to fill metaphyseal voids that can prevent postoperative settling while avoiding the morbidity of iliac crest grafts.

As the population ages, better methods to restore function in elderly patients will need to be developed, and clinical research will need to define the reasons for poorer outcome in this patient population. Only in this way will treatment advances be directed toward improving the poor results that typically occur in these patients.

Summary

The evaluation of tibial plateau fractures is more frequently assisted by obtaining complex imaging studies such as CT or MRI, which are of most value as an aid to preoperative planning. Surgical indications have not changed for patients with this type of fracture and should be based on preserving alignment and stability. Because small degrees of valgus are better tolerated than varus in this patient population, patients with medial plateau fractures and those with bicondylar fractures with medial tilt have much tighter surgical thresholds.

High-energy fractures are frequently managed initially by using spanning external fixation to provisionally restore alignment and length before definitive fixation. This technique facilitates soft-tissue recovery and decreases complications in patients with severe fractures. Locked plating is a new method for stabilizing bicondylar fractures, and it has mechanical advantages over traditional single-side plating and biologic advantages over dual plating. Additional research is needed to assess the relative advantages of this technique compared with external fixation; currently, both methods are used for similar indications.

Low-energy fractures have a high incidence of loss of position after reduction and fixation. To minimize settling, buttress plating of lateral fractures is now frequently accomplished using small fragment precontoured plates that permit multiple screws to be rafted under the reduced articular surface. New void fillers have decreased the need for iliac crest grafts, and phase-changing calcium phosphate cements have proved to be mechanically superior to grafts.

Treatment outcomes are good for most patients with tibial plateau fractures, regardless of treatment technique. Elderly patients are an exception to this generally favorable outlook because they have a high incidence of pain and poor function. Although total knee replacement in patients with tibial plateau fractures is not commonly required, it can improve function and decrease pain; however, total knee replacement has a high complication rate in this patient population.

Annotated References

1. Martin J, Marsh JL, Nepola JV, Dirschl DR, Hurwitz S, DeCoster TA: Radiographic fracture assessments: Which ones can we reliably make? *J Orthop Trauma* 2000;14:379-385.

2. Yacoubian SC, Nevins RT, Sallis JG, Potter HG, Lorich DG: Impact of MRI on treatment plan and fracture classification of tibial plateau fractures. *J Orthop Trauma* 2002;16:632-637.

3. Shepard L, Abdollahi K, Lee J, Vangsness CT Jr: The prevalence of soft tissue injuries in nonoperative tibial plateau fractures as determined by magnetic resonance imaging. *J Orthop Trauma* 2002;16:628-631.

4. Bai B, Kummer FJ, Sala DA, Koval KJ, Wolinsky PR: Effect of articular step-off and meniscectomy on joint alignment and contact pressures for fractures of the lateral tibial plateau. *J Orthop Trauma* 2001;15:101-106.

5. Trumble T, Allan Ch, Miyano J, et al: A preliminary study of joint surface changes after an intraarticular fracture: A sheep model of a tibia fracture with weight bearing after internal fixation. *J Orthop Trauma* 2001;15:326-332.

6. Westmoreland GL, McLaurin TM, Hutton WC: Screw pullout strength: A biomechanical comparison of large-fragment and small-fragment fixation in the tibial plateau. *J Orthop Trauma* 2002;16:178-181.

7. Karunakar MA, Egol KA, Peindl R, Harrow ME, Bosse MJ, Kellam JL: Split depression tibial plateau fractures: A biomechanical study. *J Orthop Trauma* 2002;16:172-177.

   This cadaver study compared 3.5-mm subchondral raft screws to traditional L-buttress plating for experimental split depression of tibial plateau fractures. A raft of 3.5-mm subchondral screws was reported to be more resistant to local compression loads than traditional L-buttress plating.

8. Mueller KL, Karunakar MA, Frankenburg EP, Scott DS: Bicondylar tibial plateau fractures: A biomechanical study. *Clin Orthop* 2003;412:189-195.

9. Welch RD, Zhang H, Bronson DG: Experimental tibial plateau fractures augmented with calcium phosphate cement or autologous bone graft. *J Bone Joint Surg Am* 2003;85-A:222-231.

   In an animal model assessing the treatment of lateral tibial plateau fractures with autograft or calcium phosphate cement, calcium phosphate cement was reported to be better at preventing subsidence of the articular fracture fragment.

10. Yetkinler DN, McClellan RT, Reindel ES, Carter D, Poser RD: Biomechanical comparison of conventional open reduction and internal fixation versus calcium phosphate cement fixation of a central depressed tibial plateau fracture. *J Orthop Trauma* 2001;15:197-206.

11. Lansinger O, Bergman B, Korner L, Andersson GBJ: Tibial condylar fractures: Twenty-year follow-up. *J Bone Joint Surg Am* 1986;68:13-19.

12. Hung SS, Chao EK, Chan YS, et al: Arthroscopically assisted osteosynthesis for tibial plateau fractures. *J Trauma* 2003;54:356-363.

13. Roerdink WH, Oskam J, Vierhout PA: Arthroscopically assisted osteosynthesis of tibial plateau fractures in patients older than 55 years. *Arthroscopy* 2001;17:826-831.

14. Cooper HJ, Kummer FJ, Egol KA, Koval KJ: The effect of screw type on the fixation of depressed fragments in tibial plateau fractures. *Bull Hosp Jt Dis* 2001-2002;60:72-75.

15. Kankate RK, Singh P, Elliott DS: Percutaneous plating of low energy unstable tibial plateau fractures: A new technique. *Injury* 2001;32:229-232.

16. Ballmer FT, Hertel R, Notzli HP: Treatment of tibial plateau fractures with small fragment internal fixation: A preliminary report. *J Orthop Trauma* 2000;14:467-474.

17. Keating JF, Hajducka CL, Harper J: Minimal internal fixation and calcium phosphate cement in the treatment of fractures of the tibial plateau. A pilot study. *J Bone Joint Surg Br* 2003;85:68-73.

   In this review of 49 fractures that were treated with minimal internal fixation and calcium phosphate cement, 38 fractures had an anatomic reduction. Sixteen percent of patients had some loss of reduction. At 1-year follow-up, 42 of 44 patients had excellent or good results.

18. Horstmann WG, Verheyen CC, Leemans R: An injectable calcium phosphate cement as a bone graft

substitute in the treatment of displaced lateral tibial plateau fractures. *Injury* 2003;34:141-144.

19. Larsson S, Bauer TW: Use of injectable calcium phosphate cement for fracture fixation: A review. *Clin Orthop* 2002;395:23-32.

20. Lobenhoffer P, Gerich T, Witte F, Tscherne H: Use of an injectable calcium phosphate cement in the treatment of tibial plateau fractures: A prospective study of twenty-six cases with twenty-month follow up. *J Orthop Trauma* 2002;16:143-149.

21. Watson JT, Ripple S, Hoshaw SJ, Fhyrie D: Hybrid external fixation for tibial plateau fractures: Clinical and biomechanical correlation. *Orthop Clin North Am* 2002;33:199-209.

22. Kumar A, Whittle AP: Treatment of complex (Schatzker type VI) fractures of the tibial plateau with circular wire external fixation: Retrospective case review. *J Orthop Trauma* 2000;14:339-344.

    This is a retrospective review of 57 fractures (35 closed fractures and 22 open fractures). Closed indirect reduction was done in all patients and limited open reduction was done in seven patients. Forty-five patients with anatomic reductions had an average knee score of 83 and nine patients without anatomic reduction had an average knee score of 52. The authors concluded that although the results may have been better with more frequent open reduction, bone grafting, and internal fixation with severely depressed fractures, circular fixators were indicated for patients with complex fractures with soft-tissue injury.

23. Ballmer FT, Hertel R, Notzli HP: Treatment of tibial plateau fractures with small fragment internal fixation: A preliminary report. *J Orthop Trauma* 2000; 14:467-474.

24. Cole PA, Ziowodsku M, Kregor PJ: Less Invasive Stabilization System (LISS) for fractures of the proximal tibia: Indications, surgical technique and preliminary results of the UMC Clinical Trial. *Injury* 2003;34(suppl 1):A16-A19.

25. Ali AM, El-Shafie M, Willett KM: Failure of fixation of tibial plateau fractures. *J Orthop Trauma* 2002;16: 323-329.

    In this study, loss of reduction was identified in 31% of 42 patients who underwent surgical treatment of tibial plateau fractures. In those older than 60 years, the authors reported that 79% of patients lost reduction.

26. Weigel DP, Marsh JL: High-energy fractures of the tibial plateau: Knee function after longer follow-up. *J Bone Joint Surg Am* 2002;84-A:1541-1551.

    The authors of this study assessed 20 patients with high-energy bicondylar tibial plateau fractures who were treated with external fixation at 5- to 11-year follow-up. They found that 17 knees had minimal or no arthrosis, and the Iowa Knee Score averaged 90 on a 100-point scale. Most knees had good outcomes in the second 5 years after surgery.

27. Stevens DG, Beharry R, McKee MD, Waddell JP, Schmeitsch EH: The long-term functional outcome of operatively treated tibial plateau fractures. *J Orthop Trauma* 2001;15:312-320.

    In this study, 47 fractures were reviewed a minimum of 5 years after open reduction and internal fixation. The most important association with outcome was the age of the patient; only 12 of 21 patients older than 40 years achieved outcome scores equivalent to those of age-matched control subjects. The authors reported that fracture classification and quality of reduction were not important predictors of outcome.

28. Schwartsman R, Brinker MR, Beaver R, Cox DD: Patient self-assessment of tibial plateau fractures in 40 older adults. *Am J Orthop* 1998;27:512-519.

29. Keating JF: Tibial plateau fractures in the older patient. *Bull Hosp Jt Dis* 1999;58:19-23.

30. Weiss NG, Parvizi J, Trousdale RT, Bryce RD, Lewallen DG: Total knee arthroplasty in patients with prior fracture of the tibial plateau. *J Bone Joint Surg Am* 2003;85-A:218-221.

31. Marsh JL, Buckwalter J, Gelberman R, et al: Articular fractures: Does an anatomic reduction really change the result? *J Bone Joint Surg Am* 2002;84-A: 1259-1271.

32. Shasha N, Krywulak S, Backstein D, Pressman A, Gross AE: Long-term follow-up of fresh tibial osteochondral allografts for failed tibial plateau fractures. *J Bone Joint Surg Am* 2003;85-A(suppl 2):33-39.

33. Saleh KJ, Sherman P, Katkin P, et al: Total knee arthroplasty after open reduction and internal fixation of fractures of the tibial plateau: A minimum five-year follow-up study. *J Bone Joint Surg Am* 2001;83-A:1144-1148.

Chapter 37

Fractures of the Tibial Diaphysis

Thomas Higgins, MD

David Templeman, MD

Introduction

Fractures of the tibial shaft are the most common long bone fracture and are responsible for a significant loss of productivity and health care expenditures. The National Center for Health Statistics reports that this injury accounts for 77,000 hospitalizations and 569,000 hospital days per year. Because fractures of the tibial diaphysis represent a large spectrum of injuries, a single treatment method is not appropriate for all the varieties of soft-tissue and bony injuries.

Epidemiology

Most published studies regarding fractures of the tibial diaphysis focus on specific treatments chosen for specific injuries; therefore, a good understanding of the epidemiology of tibial fractures does not exist. A recent study indicated that most tibial fractures are the result of low-energy injuries.[1] There is an increasing tendency for elderly patients to experience tibial fractures during falls, and this population subset has a higher rate of type III open fractures and comminuted injuries. In younger age groups, the most common mechanism of injury is a motor vehicle accident. Several classification systems describe bony injury and categorize soft-tissue injuries for both closed and open fractures. The AO/Orthopaedic Trauma Association (OTA) classification system identifies bony injuries as simple (type A), wedge (type B), or complex (type C) fractures. Soft-tissue injuries in closed fractures are classified by the system of Tscherne in which a grade 0 injury has minimal soft-tissue damage and minimal displacement of the fractures secondary to a low-energy injury, a grade I injury has abrasions with moderate swelling, a grade II injury has deep abrasions with significant soft-tissue swelling and a potential impending compartment syndrome, and a grade III injury is a decompensated compartment syndrome requiring fasciotomy (Table 1 and Figure 1).

Classification

The most widely used system for classifying open tibial fractures was developed by Gustilo and later modified. This system ranges from type I minor open injuries to type III major open fractures. Type III open fractures are subsequently divided into type IIIA (fractures with a soft-tissue envelope that can be closed with local soft tissue), type IIIB (fractures requiring flap coverage), or type IIIC (fractures that have a vascular disruption requiring revascularization for limb survival). Because of the subjective nature of the classification systems, as well as the inherent difficulty in trying to categorize a continuous spectrum of injuries, the intraobserver agreement of the Gustilo classification has been noted to be relatively low (60%).[2] Because tibial fractures are a marker of significant injury, the initial management of patients should follow advanced trauma life support protocols. As many as 75% of patients with open fractures have associated injuries. Treatment of a tibial fracture begins with appropriate evaluation of the skin and soft-tissue injury and a detailed documentation of the circulation and motor and sensory examination findings. Compartments are palpated to assess the risk of subsequent compartment syndrome. Both open and closed fractures should be immediately splinted to protect the soft tissues and neurovascular structures. The immediate care of open fractures requires administration of intravenous antibiotics, tetanus toxoid booster, and placement of a sterile dressing. Recent studies have been unable to definitively quantitate the relationship of time to immediate irrigation and débridement and subsequent development of infection. However, it is unlikely that prolonged delays are beneficial to patients. Interpretation of any open fracture studies must consider that the most crucial variable is likely to be the quality of the initial surgical débridement performed, irrespective of timing.

Patient Evaluation

All patients with tibial shaft fractures must be assessed for the development of the signs and symptoms of compartment syndrome both at presentation and after surgical or nonsurgical treatment. This assessment is especially challenging in patients with altered consciousness, but it must be part of the standard treatment of patients with these injuries.

TABLE 1 | Oestern and Tscherne Classification of Closed-Fracture Soft-Tissue Injury

Grade	Description
0	Injuries from indirect forces with negligible soft-tissue damage
I	Superficial contusion/abrasion, simple fractures
II	Deep abrasions, muscle/skin contusion; direct trauma, impending compartment syndrome
III	Excessive skin contusion; crushed skin or destruction of muscle, subcutaneous degloving, acute compartment syndrome, and rupture of major blood vessel or nerve

(Reproduced with permission from Oestern HJ, Tscherne H: Pathophysiology and classification of soft tissue injuries associated with fractures, in Tscherne H, Gotzen L (eds): Fractures With Soft Tissue Injuries. Berlin, Germany, Springer-Verlag, 1984, pp 1-9.)

No data support the need for immediate fracture fixation or the benefits of a prolonged delay. Clinical judgment is required to determine when the soft tissues are suitable for the surgical incisions that are required for fixation. No evidence suggests the risk of fat embolism syndrome is increased by early or late fixation with intramedullary nailing. Once the decision is made to perform fracture stabilization, there seems to be little benefit to patients in prolonged delays.

Treatment

The choice of fixation for tibial fractures includes intramedullary techniques (with and without reaming), plate fixation, and various forms of external fixation. There are numerous indications for stabilization of tibial fractures and numerous devices available for their fixation. Although the precise indications for fracture stabilization remain unclear, one study found that when patients with fractures with greater than 50% displacement at the fracture site and greater than 10° angulation were treated with intramedullary nailing, results were superior to those achieved with closed reduction and immobilization with cast.[3] Most authorities recommend fracture fixation for displaced and unstable fractures of the tibia.

Several meta-analyses have assessed a large number of comparative trials, uncontrolled studies, and published series regarding tibial fractures. These comparisons showed that treatment with a cast is associated with a lower rate of superficial infection compared with open reduction and internal fixation, but open reduction and internal fixation is associated with a higher rate of union (by 20 weeks) compared with treatment with a cast.[4] Critical review of these meta-analyses suggests that data available in the literature may be inadequate for decision making regarding the treatment of closed tibial fractures. However, a recent study suggests that there is no association between fracture malalignment and subsequent knee/ankle arthritis in 30-year follow-up after closed treatment of tibial fractures.[5] Another study indicates that there is a preference among orthopaedic surgeons to stabilize the tibial shaft by intramedullary nailing and wide differences in the techniques of intramedullary nailing, including duration of antibiotic use, timing of wound closure in open fracture care, and use of reaming.[6] Multiple studies confirm the high success and reproducibility of using intramedullary nails for stabilizing tibial shaft fractures.[7-12]

Contraindications to the use of intramedullary nailing to treat tibial shaft fractures include (1) a very narrow canal (less than 6 cm diameter), (2) gross contamination of the intramedullary canal, (3) deformity of the intramedullary nail canal from preexisting injury or growth disturbance, and (4) the presence of a total knee replacement implant or knee arthrodesis that prevents obtaining an adequate entry portal.

Because of the success of intramedullary nailing, many traumatologists have expanded the indications beyond the diaphysis and are treating fractures of the proximal and distal fourths of the tibia. However, with the reduced contact between the intramedullary nail and the endosteal surface of the metaphysis, these fracture constructs are more difficult to align and stabilize compared with intramedullary nailing of fractures within the true diaphysis. The literature demonstrates a higher rate of malunion with nailing proximal metaphyseal fractures than distal metaphyseal fractures, but technical challenges are presented at both sites when using intramedullary nails.

Proximal tibial fractures are frequently secondary to high-energy trauma; many of these are the result of pedestrians being struck by motor vehicles. Many proximal tibial fractures may be comminuted and associated with more severe soft-tissue injuries that further complicate treatment. The proximal metaphyseal bony comminution also results in increased osseous instability. The treatment alternatives for proximal tibial fractures include intramedullary nails, standard external fixators, plates, combinations of nails and plates, and multiplanar external fixators. Open reduction and plate fixation can obviate most of the alignment problems seen with intramedullary nailing, and it allows for the use of rigid fixation with intrafragmentary lag screws. Recent advances in locking plate technology have expanded the indications for plating. Locking plate technology is also associated with the use of plates that have been specifically designed for use in the treatment of fractures of the proximal tibia, allowing fracture reduction and stabilization with smaller incisions.

Intramedullary nailing of proximal tibia fractures has been associated with a high incidence of malunion and nonunion. In contrast to the tibial diaphysis where intramedullary nails can effectively reduce most fractures, the unique anatomy of the proximal tibia has led to

Groups:

Tibia/Fibula, diaphyseal, simple (42-A)
1. Spiral (42-A1)

Tibia/Fibula, diaphyseal, wedge (42-B)
1. Spiral wedge (42-B1)

Tibia/Fibula, diaphyseal, complex (42-C)
1. Spiral (42-C1)

2. Oblique (≥ 30°) (42-A2)

2. Bending wedge (42-B2)

2. Segmented (42-C2)

3. Transverse (< 30°) (42-A3)

3. Fragmented wedge (42-B3)

3. Irregular (42-C3)

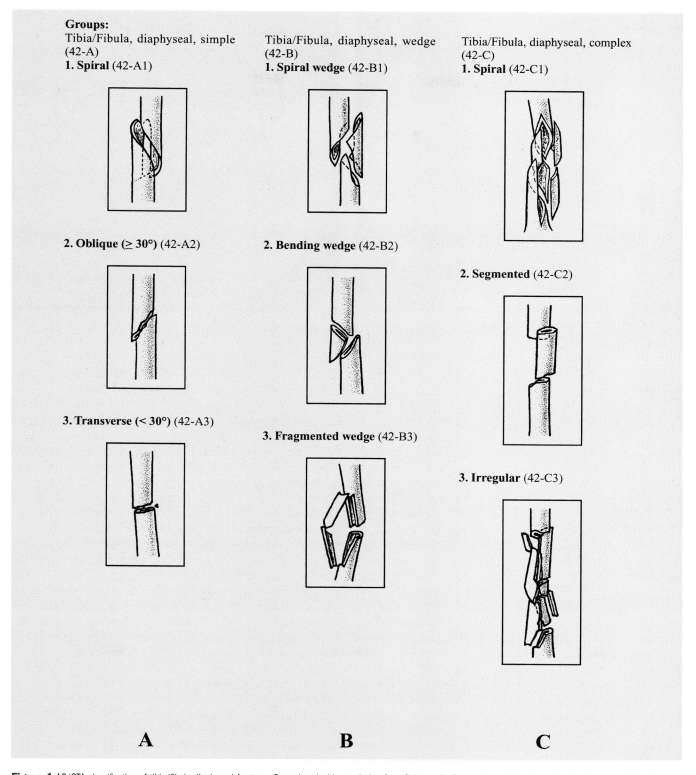

A   B   C

Figure 1 AO/OTA classification of tibia/fibula diaphyseal fracture. *(Reproduced with permission from Orthopaedic Trauma Association Committee for Coding and Classification: Fracture and dislocation compendium. J Orthop Trauma 1996;10(suppl 1):1-155.)*

malunion rates as high as 84% in the treatment of these fractures with intramedullary nails. Patients with proximal tibial fractures are susceptible to valgus displace-ment as a result of (1) greater space laterally than medially in the intramedullary area of the proximal metaphysis, (2) a nail starting point that is too medial,

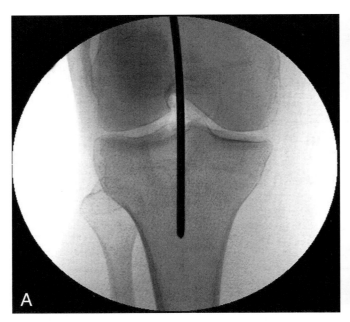
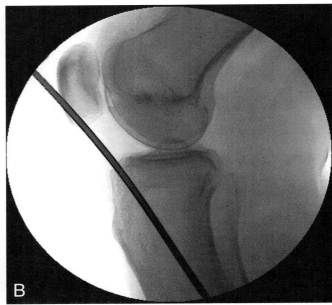

Figure 2 The correct starting point for intramedullary nailing is demonstrated on true AP (**A**) and lateral (**B**) fluoroscopy projections. For a very proximal fracture (*not shown*), the guidewire must hug the anterior cortex.

(3) tension on the proximal fragment from the pes anserinus, and (4) eccentric reaming in the proximal metaphyseal segment.

The standard entry portal medial to the patellar tendon is medial to the intramedullary canal. Insertion of an intramedullary nail through this portal causes a predictable valgus angulation and apex anterior angulation. Valgus can be avoided by using a more lateral entry point. Radiographically, this site is located slightly medial to the lateral tibial spine on the AP radiograph and adjacent to the anterior articular surface on a true lateral radiograph. The entry portal should be confirmed fluoroscopically to be in an ideal location to prevent malalignment and avoid injury to intra-articular structures (Figure 2).

Flexion deformity (apex anterior angulation of the tibia) is caused by (1) flexion of the knee during intramedullary nail insertion, which exacerbates proximal fragment displacement caused by extensor mechanism insertional tension on the tibial tubercle; (2) the shape and location of the sagittal bend in the nail; and (3) the eccentric starting point and entrance angle of the nail. Placement of the knee in a semiextended position during intramedullary nail insertion helps to avoid flexion deformity by reducing the pull of the extensor mechanism on the proximal fragment. The semiextended position requires subluxation of the patella that may necessitate proximal extension of the surgical approach. Alternatively, a stout pin can be inserted sagittally, just lateral to the entrance site to flex the proximal fragment and counteract the pull of the patellar ligament. A starting awl is directed to remain near the anterior part of the tibia so that the intramedullary nail subsequently follows an an-

terior path. This prevents the nail from causing apex anterior angulation and anterior translation of the proximal segment relative to the diaphysis. The bends of intramedullary nails used to treat proximal tibial fractures should be as proximal as possible to avoid a posterior translation of the tibia during intramedullary nail insertion. Recent biomechanical testing data also suggest that oblique proximal locking screws may enhance stability of nailed proximal metaphyseal fractures.[13] Modifications of entry site, the careful use of fluoroscopy, and greater attention to the technique of intramedullary nail insertion provide reliable and reproducible methods for successfully stabilizing proximal tibial fractures with intramedullary nailing.

An additional technique for proximal tibial metaphyseal fracture reduction is the use of blocking screws (Poller screws.) This method uses independently inserted bicortical screws placed just outside the intended path of the intramedullary nail that deflect the reamer and intramedullary nail into the correct path. In simpler terms, the blocking screws must be placed to prevent intramedullary nail passage into the portion of the bone that the intramedullary nail must not occupy. This technique may be used to facilitate and hold reduction in any intramedullary fixation (particularly metaphyseal), but it is especially helpful in treating fractures of the proximal tibia. Given the propensity of these fractures to malalign into valgus and flexion, blocking screws would be placed in the lateral and posterior metaphysis (Figure 3).

Fractures of the distal third of the tibia are similar to proximal third fractures in that the insertion of the tibial intramedullary nail does not automatically correct any angulatory deformity. However, the rates of malalign-

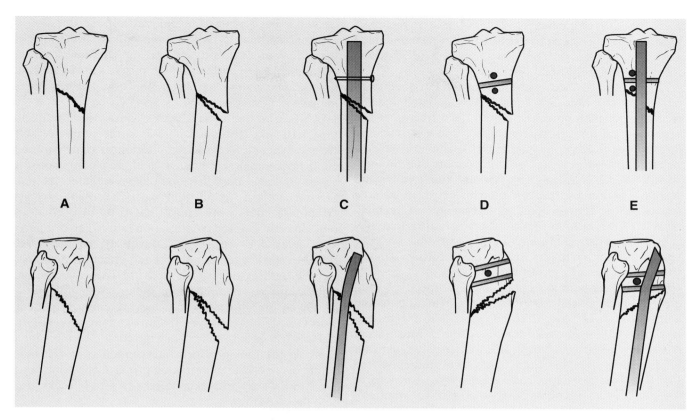

Figure 3 Illustration of blocking screws used to assist in intramedullary nailing of proximal metaphyseal tibial fracture. Fracture pattern **(A)** and characteristic deformity **(B)** on AP and lateral views. **C**, Nailing without blocking screws reinforces valgus and flexion deformities. **D**, Nail removed, blocking screws are placed to redirect the path of the reamer and nail. Poller screws placed laterally and posteriorly occupy the space that the nail must not occupy. **E**, After re-reaming, the re-placed nail now helps to maintain correct reduction and alignment. (Illustration courtesy of TF Higgins, MD.)

ment after intramedullary nailing have been less than those in patients with proximal tibial fractures. There are several intramedullary nails available with two to three multiplanar holes positioned beginning within 1.5 cm of the nail tip. The multiplanar nature of the distal interlocking screws and very distal seating of the intramedullary nail allows many distal fractures to be treated by closed intramedullary nailing. The major technical challenge is to avoid valgus angulation, and this may be addressed in several ways. The first of these is fixation of the fibula to align the distal tibial block before the insertion of the intramedullary nail. Other surgeons have relied on the use of either calcaneal traction or a femoral distractor to achieve correction of angulation of the distal fracture. The most important technical aspect is placement of the guidewire in the center of the distal fragment perpendicular to the ankle plafond. The insertion of a smooth transfixation pin across the distal tibia parallel to the joint may also aid in reduction of the fracture.

Some fractures involving the distal quarter of the tibia will also feature articular involvement. If the articular fractures consist of simple splits amenable to lag screw fixation, or a tibial fracture occurs in combination with a noncontiguous ankle fracture, then tibial in-

tramedullary nailing may still be a compatible solution. However, absolute articular congruity is the primary objective of reduction and fixation, and this goal should ultimately guide surgical treatment.

Because the intramedullary nail does not contact the endosteal surface of the distal metaphysis fracture site, instability is more problematic than with the intramedullary nailing of diaphyseal fractures. This instability likely produces a slightly higher rate of delayed union and nonunion. Recently, exchange intramedullary nailing has been recommended instead of dynamization for these distal fractures with incomplete healing because dynamization further increases fracture site instability and has led to shortening in some instances.[14]

Fractures of the diaphysis are generally treated with proximally and distally locked intramedullary nails. The indications for primary dynamic intramedullary nailing of diaphyseal injuries are few and are based on fracture patterns. Diaphyseal fractures with a short oblique pattern and no comminution may be nailed without proximal interlocking screws. Simple transverse diaphyseal patterns with no comminution may be locked proximally with a single screw placed in a longitudinal slotted locking hole proximally to allow fracture site compression with weight bearing while maintaining rotational alignment. Because of the increased loads borne by the interlocking screws, early weight bearing is not recommended after static locked intramedullary nailing of proximal third or distal third tibial fractures.

The role of reamed versus nonreamed intramedullary nailing of the tibia has been widely debated for the treatment of both open and closed tibial fractures. The presumed advantages of reaming are that it permits the insertion of a larger diameter intramedullary nail for better interference fit and greater stability and the possibility of bone grafting the fracture site locally with reamings and intramedullary contents extruded into the fracture site. The accepted disadvantages of reaming include elevation of intraosseous temperatures that may contribute to thermal osseous necrosis, possible systemic episodes of fat embolism, and potential further damage to already traumatized soft tissues.

Multiple authors have performed prospectively randomized clinical trials to evaluate the healing potential and outcomes of reamed versus unreamed intramedullary tibial nailing of closed fractures.[8,11,15,16] Most recent trials have failed to demonstrate a statistically significant difference in ultimate healing rates. One study reported that a reamed technique had a higher rate of healing at 4 months, with no difference at 6 and 12 months.[15] Multiple studies have shown a higher rate of broken locking screws with unreamed technique, which was likely caused by a looser fitting nail and smaller locking bolts used with unreamed techniques.[8,11,17]

Reamed nailing of open tibial fractures was initially considered dangerous, given the possibility of exacerbating damage to already insulted soft-tissue injuries, especially in patients with Gustilo type III injuries. Researchers have attempted to model the osseous and soft-tissue damage of reaming in sheep, demonstrating an early insult to cortical bone, but ultimately having no effect on callus vascularity or strength of united bone.[18] Attempts to quantify the perfusion and oxygenation of the soft tissues in human subjects during randomized reamed and unreamed intramedullary tibial nailing have not demonstrated any differences that could be attributed to technique.[19] Many authors now suggest using a reamed technique for treating open fractures up to and including Gustilo type IIIB. A limited reaming technique may be used, passing power reamers over a guidewire, but not without aggressively cutting the inner cortical surface with the reamers.

Several authors suggest a separate protocol for treating Gustilo type IIIB injuries and have advocated aggressive débridement and initial external fixator stabilization, followed by delayed definitive intramedullary tibial nailing. An early study using this treatment algorithm reported unacceptably high infection and nonunion rates after an average time in external fixation of 8.5 weeks.[20] Subsequent studies showed only a 5% deep infection rate in patients with Gustilo type IIIB injuries who were treated using a reamed technique (average duration of external fixation, 17 days). A pin holiday (time interval between fixator removal and nail implantation) has been recommended to ensure that the pin sites are healed and do not appear to be harboring infection, but this staged management may be unnecessary.

Critical to the management of patients with Gustilo type IIIB and IIIC open injuries is the timing of soft-tissue coverage. Skeletal stabilization in some form accompanies initial débridement, and the planning of soft-tissue coverage must be initiated immediately as well. Several authors found that early free-flap coverage (within 72 hours from injury) had a positive effect on outcome and lowered complication rates when compared with delayed coverage.[21,22] Conversely, another study failed to show a temporally related effect on outcomes, but the authors did concur that free-flap coverage had significantly less complications than rotational flaps.[23]

Given the difficulties in achieving union in patients with Gustilo type III open fractures, many surgeons endorse early prophylactic bone grafting. Recommendations on the timing of this intervention vary, but most protocols advocate undertaking prophylactic bone grafting 2 to 6 weeks after skin closure or 4 to 6 weeks after free-flap coverage.

In addition to intramedullary nailing, surgical choices for the fixation of diaphyseal tibial injuries include plating and external fixation. Plating has been recommended primarily for patients with metaphyseal tibial fractures. Plating of shaft fractures has been associated with an unacceptably high rate of soft-tissue breakdown and infectious complications.[9] The recent introduction of more percutaneous and submuscular plating techniques and fixed-angle screw-plate constructs has led to a resurgence in tibial plating, but the long-term success of these techniques has yet to be demonstrated. These devices appear to offer technical advantages, particularly in patients with tibial fractures with long diaphyseal fracture extensions.

External fixation may be used for temporary fixation or definitive treatment. Severe soft-tissue wounds, hemodynamic instability, and questionable limb viability are all indications for provisional external fixation and future conversion to more definitive treatment. Diaphyseal injuries may be treated definitively with unilateral external fixation. Several series report an 85% to 95% union rate using this technique.[24,25] Other indications for definitive treatment with external fixation include extensive metaphyseal and diaphyseal comminution, open physes, and complex combined articular and diaphyseal fractures, the latter often managed with ring fixator constructs. Pin loosening and pin tract infection have been reported to be the most common complications of definitive treatment with external fixation (50% of patients in some series).[26]

The definition of a delayed union and the most appropriate intervention for delayed healing remain points of discussion. The anticipated time to union, ranging from 2 to 18 weeks, increases with the severity of soft-tissue injury in patients with closed or open tibial fractures. However, so many variables affect union estimates that setting a firm deadline is somewhat arbitrary. The treating surgeon must assess clinical and radiographic data and take into account the initial degree of soft-tissue damage when determining how early to intervene in the healing process.

The algorithm and timing for the treatment of delayed union in patients with closed injuries or lower grade open injuries are controversial issues. Dynamization of a statically locked nail (the removal of locking screws to allow more compression and mechanical stimulation of the fracture site) is a simple step in fracture treatment in which enough healing has occurred that excessive shortening and rotational instability are not anticipated. Although dynamization is straightforward, its results are unimpressive. Exchange nailing, which entails nail removal, intramedullary reaming, and placement of a larger diameter nail, is a more invasive option, but one that is associated with excellent results. This procedure has a success rate of 88% to 100%, but is associated with a wound infection rate of 11% to 12%.

Cancellous autograft placed through a posterolateral approach is a proven treatment of tibial nonunion. Graft material may be inserted via an anteromedial or posterolateral interval, but the latter approach exploits the superior muscle coverage and vascularity of the posterior border of the tibia. In particularly resistant nonunions, tibiofibular synostosis may also be achieved through this approach if deemed desirable.

Other options for treatment of delayed union or nonunion include partial fibulectomy (to permit axial compression of the fracture site), secondary plating, and the use of ring fixator systems. Several reports have demonstrated favorable results with the use of capacitive-coupled electrical stimulation or low intensity ultrasound for treatment of nonunion, but independent randomized comparison data remain scarce. The indications for these noninvasive modalities and other bone stimulation techniques in clinical treatment is discussed in chapter 12.

Complications of tibial nailing include knee pain, infection, malunion, and nonunion. In one study, a 56% incidence of anterior knee pain after nailing of tibial fractures was reported.[17] Careful handling of soft tissue at the insertion site (particularly the patellar tendon), and the precise placement of the starting point and nail may help to reduce this problem. Most knee pain after nailing did respond to hardware removal in this series. The infection rate for nailing of closed tibial fractures ranges from 0 to 5%, with the rate for open fractures varying with fracture type. Malunion has already been discussed and is particularly prevalent in metaphyseal injuries treated with intramedullary nails.

Summary

A thorough review of the literature reveals many modalities for successful treatment of tibial fractures. Regardless of the method chosen, success likely depends on technique and attention to detail. Despite the extensive coverage of tibial fracture care in the literature, many treatment questions have not yet been definitively answered.

Annotated References

1. Court-Brown CM, McBirnie J: The epidemiology of tibial fractures. *J Bone Joint Surg Br* 1995;77:417-421.

2. Brumback RJ, Jones AL: Interobserver agreement in the classification of open fractures of the tibia: The results of a survey of two hundred and forty-five orthopaedic surgeons. *J Bone Joint Surg Am* 1994; 76:1162-1166.

3. Hooper GJ, Keddell RG, Penny ID: Conservative management or closed nailing for tibial shaft fractures: A randomised prospective trial. *J Bone Joint Surg Br* 1991;73:83-85.

4. Littenberg B, Weinstein LP, McCarren M, et al: Closed fractures of the tibial shaft: A meta-analysis of three methods of treatment. *J Bone Joint Surg Am* 1998;80:174-183.

5. Milner SA, Davis TR, Muir KR, Greenwood DC, Doherty M: Long-term outcome after tibial shaft fracture: Is malunion important? *J Bone Joint Surg Am* 2002;84-A(6):971-980.
   Twenty to 43 year follow-up on 164 tibial shaft fractures treated by closed means demonstrated that the occurrence of knee, ankle, or subtalar arthritis appeared unrelated to occurrence of malunion.

6. Bhandari M, Guyatt GH, Tornetta P III, et al: Current practice in the intramedullary nailing of tibial shaft fractures: An international survey. *J Trauma* 2002;53:725-732.
   The authors of this study concluded that consensus among orthopaedic surgeons exists regarding the use of irrigation and intravenous antibiotics in the treatment of open tibial shaft fractures; however, considerable variability was noted regarding the surgical technique of intramedullary nailing, duration of antibiotic therapy, and the timing of wound closure.

7. Bhandari M, Guyatt GH, Tong D, Adili A, Shaughnessy SG: Reamed versus nonreamed intramedullary

nailing of lower extremity long bone fractures: A systemic overview and meta-analysis. *J Orthop Trauma* 2000;14:2-9.

The authors of this study concluded that pooled analysis of randomized trial data indicates that reamed intramedullary nailing of lower extremity long bone fractures significantly reduces rates of implant failures and nonunion when compared with nonreamed intramedullary nailing.

8. Finkemeier CG, Schmidt AH, Kyle RF, Templeman DC, Varecka TF: A prospective, randomized study of intramedullary nails inserted with and without reaming for the treatment of open and closed fractures of the tibial shaft. *J Orthop Trauma* 2000;14: 187-193.

In this prospective, "surgeon-randomized" trial, no significant differences were reported between two groups of patients who underwent intramedullary nail insertion with and without reaming for the treatment of open and closed fractures. More broken screws were reported in the unreamed group.

9. Schmidt AH, Finkemeier CG, Tornetta P: Treatment of closed tibial fracture. *Instr Course Lect* 2003; 52:607-622.

This is a review of the surgical and nonsurgical treatment of closed tibial shaft fractures.

10. Bone LB, Sucato D, Stegemann PM, Rohrbacher BJ: Displaced isolated fractures of the tibial shaft treated with either cast or intramedullary nailing: An outcome analysis of matched pairs of patients. *J Bone Joint Surg Am* 1997;79:1336-1341.

11. Keating JF, O'Brien PJ, Blachut PA, Meek RN, Broekhuyse HM: Locking intramedullary nailing with and without reaming for open fractures of the tibial shaft: A prospective, randomized study. *J Bone Joint Surg Am* 1997;79(3):334-341.

12. Blachut PA, O'Brien PJ, Meek RN, Broekhuyse HM: Interlocking intramedullary nailing with and without reaming for the treatment of closed fractures of the tibial shaft: A prospective randomized study. *J Bone Joint Surg Am* 1997;79(5):640-646.

13. Laflamme GY, Heimlich D, Stephen D, et al: Proximal tibial fracture stability with intramedullary nail fixation using oblique interlocking screws. *J Orthop Trauma* 2003;17:496-502.

Authors of this cadaveric study showed that the addition of oblique proximal locking screws to a nailed proximal tibia fracture enhanced flexion/extension and varus/valgus stability approximately 50%.

14. Templeman D, Larson C, Varecka T, Kyle RF: Decision making errors in the use of interlocking tibial nails. *Clin Orthop* 1997;339:65-70.

15. Keating JF, O'Brien PI, Blachut PA, et al: Reamed interlocking intramedullary nailing of open fractures of the tibia. *Clin Orthop* 1997;338:182-191.

16. Court-Brown CM, Will E, Christie J, McQueen MM: Reamed or unreamed nailing for closed tibial fractures: A prospective study in Tscherne C1 fractures. *J Bone Joint Surg Br* 1996;78:580-583.

17. Greitbauer M, Heinz T, Gaebler C: Unreamed nailing of tibial fractures with the solid tibial nail. *Clin Orthop* 1998;350:105-114.

18. Schemitsch EH, Kowalski MJ, Swiontkowski MF, Harrington RM: Comparison of the effect of reamed and unreamed locked intramedullary nailing on blood flow in the callus and strength of union following fracture of the sheep tibia. *J Orthop Res* 1995; 13(3):382-389.

19. Lindström T, Gullichsen E, Lertola K, Niinikoski J: Leg tissue perfusion in simple tibial shaft fractures treated with unreamed and reamed nailing. *J Trauma* 1997;43(4):636-639.

20. McGraw JM, Lim EV: Treatment of open tibial-shaft fractures: External fixation and secondary intramedullary nailing. *J Bone Joint Surg Am* 1988; 70(6):900-911.

21. Godina M: Early microsurgical reconstruction of complex trauma of the extremities. *Plast Reconstr Surg* 1986;78(3):285-292.

This is the classic landmark series demonstrating the benefits of early flap coverage of open extremity trauma.

22. Gopal S, Majumder S, Batchelor AG, Knight SL, De Boer P, Smith RM: Fix and flap: The radical orthopaedic and plastic treatment of severe open fractures of the tibia. *J Bone Joint Surg Br* 2000;82(7):959-966.

This was a retrospective review of 84 grade IIIB and IIIC injuries. The authors recommend open reduction and internal fixation and free flap coverage within 72 hours of injury.

23. Pollak AN, McCarthy ML, Burgess AR: Short-term wound complications after application of flaps for coverage of traumatic soft-tissue defects about the tibia: The Lower Extremity Assessment Project (LEAP) Study Group. *J Bone Joint Surg Am* 2000; 82-A(12):1681-1691.

Study data on 195 flap-covered lower extremities showed a 27% overall complication rate. AO/OTA type C fractures had significantly fewer complications with free flap coverage than with rotational flaps. The findings failed to show a relationship between flap timing and complication rate.

24. Kenwright J, Richardson JB, Cunningham JL, et al: Axial movement and tibial fractures: A controlled randomised trial of treatment. *J Bone Joint Surg Br* 1991;73:654-659.

25. Helland P, Boe A, Molster AO, Solheim E, Hordvik M: Open tibial fractures treated with the Ex-fi-re external fixation system. *Clin Orthop* 1996;326:209-220.

26. Henley MB, Chapman JR, Agel J, et al: Treatment of Type II, IIIA, and IIIB open fractures of the tibial shaft: A prospective comparison of unreamed interlocking intramedullary nails and half-pin external fixators. *J Orthop Trauma* 1998;12(1):1-7.

Chapter 38

Fractures of the Ankle and Distal Tibial Pilon

David A. Sanders, MD

Michael Sirkin, MD

Fractures of the Ankle

Introduction

Fractures of the ankle are among the most common injuries requiring orthopaedic care. Ankle fractures comprise a heterogeneous group of injuries, ranging from simple injuries with minimal long-term effects to complex injuries with severe long-term sequelae. The goal of treatment is to minimize both short- and long-term disability. This goal is accomplished by adherence to the basic principles of fracture care, including restoration of normal anatomy and early functional treatment.

Normal Anatomy and Biomechanics

In the fractured ankle, loss of the bone and ligamentous support can render the ankle unstable.[1] Instability is problematic because any abnormal translation between the talus and tibia results in abnormal joint loading patterns and can lead to premature arthritic degeneration. Instability can be obvious following a fracture; typically, in this situation, routine radiographs document lateral shift of the talus. In other situations, instability is more difficult to diagnose and plain films may not demonstrate shift of the talus. In these situations, physical examination, stress radiographs, and other imaging modalities may be required to document instability.

Injuries to the Ankle Syndesmosis

Injuries to the ankle syndesmosis comprise a wide spectrum of injuries. Presentation can vary from an apparent ankle sprain that seems to have a prolonged recovery time to a wide tibiofibular diastasis with associated fractures and ligamentous injuries. Subtle syndesmotic injuries can be difficult to diagnose. Typical symptoms include anterolateral ankle pain and mild swelling above the lateral ankle. Several physical examination maneuvers exist to better assess the syndesmotic ligaments. These include the squeeze test, the external rotation stress test, and direct palpation of the syndesmosis for tenderness. In the squeeze test, the tibia and fibula are compressed together at the midcalf level. Pain at the anterior ankle region is considered a positive test. The external rotation test is performed with the knee flexed to 90°, the tibia position stabilized, and the ankle dorsiflexed to neutral. Pain at the ankle when an external rotation ankle stress is applied is indicative of a positive test. Although the physical examination is helpful, sensitivity of the examination depends on time from injury and other factors, and interobserver reliability is low.[2] Therefore, other diagnostic methods are frequently necessary.

Bone scintigraphy has a reported sensitivity of 100% to detect syndesmosis injury. A positive scan detects increased uptake in the region of the syndesmosis. Because of low specificity, bone scintigraphy is rarely the primary diagnostic test. Alternatively, stress radiographs can be performed to confirm a syndesmosis injury. The tibia is stabilized at neutral rotation, and an external rotational force is applied to the ankle. An increase in the tibiofibular clear space or decrease in tibiofibular overlap can be used to diagnose instability (Figure 1). Stress examination for syndesmotic instability is simple and inexpensive and is a useful functional test[2] (Figure 2). Other useful examinations include CT, which has improved sensitivity compared with plain radiography. Findings consistent with syndesmotic instability include syndesmotic widening and anterior or posterior fibular displacement. Additionally, CT may detect a shallow incisura fibularis or retained bone and cartilage fragments.[3] MRI has also become increasingly important in difficult or equivocal instances of syndesmosis injury. MRI has high sensitivity to detect tears of the anterior or posterior tibiofibular ligaments as well as fluid in the syndesmosis, and it can also be used to determine extent of interosseous membrane injury in ankle fractures.

Treatment of syndesmosis injuries can be determined by the degree of instability. In general, patients with no static instability and small degrees of dynamic instability can be treated with a short period of immobilization followed by functional rehabilitation. These injuries usually correspond to isolated tears of the anteroinferior tibiofibular ligament or limited tears of the interosseous membrane. Recovery is prolonged compared with that for routine ankle sprains, but overall functional treat-

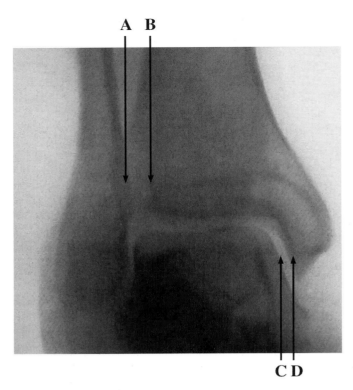

Figure 1 Radiographic measurements of the lateral tibiofibular clear space (A to B) and medial clear space (C to D).

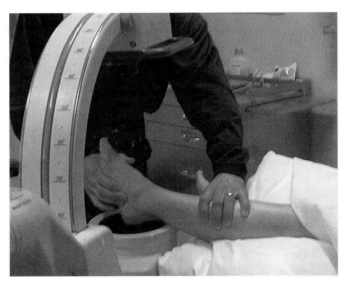

Figure 2 Photograph showing external rotation stress examination. The patient is positioned supine with a bolster under the knee and proximal tibia. The knee is slightly flexed to facilitate relaxation. The examiner stabilizes the tibia with one hand and gently externally rotates the ankle with the contralateral hand.

ment results in a high rate of good and excellent results. In some patients, heterotopic ossification is noted within the interosseous membrane. The clinical significance of this finding is unknown. Patients with static instability, and some patients with pronounced dynamic instability,

require surgical reduction and stabilization of the syndesmosis.

Surgical stabilization of syndesmotic injuries requires an anatomic reduction of the distal fibula to the tibial incisura. Most failures of syndesmotic repair can be ascribed to inaccurate reduction of fibular length, translation, and rotation. Reduction can be accomplished with closed, percutaneous, or open techniques. Closed and percutaneous techniques rely on an accurate interpretation of radiographic parameters, including fibular length, translation, and rotation. Open reduction of the syndesmosis is frequently necessary to ensure an anatomic reduction. Ligament remnants and bone or cartilage debris is often noted within the syndesmosis at the time of open reduction and should be removed.

Techniques of syndesmotic stabilization vary. Several fixation techniques have been advocated for syndesmosis reconstruction, including metallic or bioabsorbable screws of varying sizes and number and various soft-tissue fixation devices.[4,5] From a mechanical standpoint, there may be an advantage to increasing screw number and size. However, there is no compelling clinical evidence to define one fixation technique as the gold standard for syndesmotic stabilization. Because of the high incidence of fatigue failure, stainless steel screws with a core diameter of less than 2.4 mm should not be used. Recently, it has been reported that dorsiflexion of the ankle during syndesmosis stabilization is probably unnecessary.[6] Cadaveric tests confirmed that overtightening of the syndesmosis, which is thought to occur when the ankle was plantar flexed during stabilization, does not occur. Furthermore, range of motion of the ankle following screw insertion is not affected by the position of the ankle at the time of screw insertion.

Malleolar Ankle Fractures

Malleolar ankle fractures occur through a rotational mechanism. These injuries are typically the result of a lower energy mechanism than that of tibial plafond fractures. Commonly used fracture classifications include the Weber and the Lauge-Hansen systems. Treatment decisions, including surgical versus nonsurgical care, are based fracture displacement and ankle stability.

Weber A Ankle Fractures

Weber A ankle fractures involve a fracture of the fibula distal to the tibiofibular syndesmosis. Injury occurs with an inversion mechanism, or supination and adduction according to the Lauge-Hansen fracture classification system. Because of the infrasyndesmotic location, Weber A fractures are less likely to result in instability than other ankle fractures. Indications for surgery are therefore more dependent on the status of the medial side of the ankle.

In many patients, the fibular fracture is an isolated avulsion injury. No surgery is required, and excellent results are often achieved with early functional rehabilitation. However, if an associated medial fracture is present, it may be related to a shearing mechanism. Large vertical medial malleolar fractures occur and can be associated with an impaction injury to the tibial plafond adjacent to the fracture site. These chondral fractures frequently require disimpaction, reduction, and bone grafting to restore articular congruity. A recent study noted that the prevalence of these articular impaction injuries was 42% in patients with supination adduction injuries with vertical medial malleolus fractures.[7]

Weber B Ankle Fractures

The most common ankle fractures are Weber B injuries, which usually result from a supination/external rotation mechanism. The pattern includes a fibular fracture, beginning at the level of the ankle syndesmosis and extending from the region of the anteroinferior tibiofibular ligament in a proximal and posterior direction. Despite their frequency, management of these injuries remains controversial.

Surgery is clearly indicated when patients with Weber B fractures have a shift of the talus within the ankle mortise. Classic biomechanical studies have demonstrated that slight lateral displacement of the talus (as little as 1 mm) causes a marked increase in the contact force and a decrease in contact area between the tibia and talus.[8] As a result, an anatomic reduction of the talus within the ankle mortise is a critical feature of any treatment regimen. Closed treatment of Weber B fractures with talar shift is usually contraindicated because of the high frequency of loss of reduction.

In patients without displacement of the talus within the ankle mortise, the decision to operate or not is more difficult. Indications for surgery depend on the degree of ankle instability. If the deltoid ligament remains competent, the ankle remains relatively stable, and late talar displacement is unlikely to occur even with early functional treatment. Conversely, if the deltoid ligament is ruptured, there is a significant risk of late displacement such that treatment should be directed toward maintaining ankle stability. Previously, surgeons relied on the absence of medial ankle tenderness and swelling to indicate an intact deltoid ligament. Physical signs of medial injury were thought to indicate deltoid ligament rupture and the need for a treatment approach designed to carefully maintain ankle reduction. Recent studies, however, have suggested that medial tenderness and swelling are not reliable physical signs of ankle instability.[6] As a result, other investigations such as a radiographic ankle stress test, which is performed by obtaining a mortise radiograph while applying an external rotation force to the foot with the ankle fixed, have been advocated as a better measure of dynamic ankle instability. The external

rotation stress test is easy to apply, generally well tolerated by the patient, and seems to be a reliable predictor of deltoid ligament injury.[6,9] Although the external rotation stress test demonstrates potential instability, the risk of loss of reduction and talar shift with cast treatment is unknown.

Other indications for surgery have included the degree of fibular displacement. In general, isolated fibular displacement does not affect ankle mechanics. The amount of fibular displacement seen is usually reflective of internal rotation of the proximal fragment, with the talus and distal fibular fragment remaining aligned and congruent. If the relationship between the talus and fibula is disrupted, an uncommon injury pattern results and reduction and stabilization should be performed.

When surgery is indicated for patients with unstable or displaced Weber B ankle fractures, several treatment options exist. The mainstay of treatment is open reduction and internal fixation. The fibula is usually approached first. An anatomic reduction is essential. Soft-tissue stripping should be minimized. Open reduction techniques are preferred to percutaneous techniques to achieve an anatomic reduction. Once the fibula is exposed and reduced, stable fixation can be achieved with several techniques. Traditionally, a lag screw directed from anterior to posterior is placed first and supplemented with a lateral neutralization plate. Other options include the use of an antiglide plate applied to the posterolateral cortex of the fibula. This technique has the biomechanical advantage of improved resistance to an external rotation moment. There may also be less skin irritation and perhaps less need for hardware removal when the plate is applied to the posterior surface of the fibula.[7,10] However, the plate must be carefully applied to avoid irritation of the peroneal tendons. A third option that may be useful in certain patients is the use of lag screw fixation alone to stabilize the ankle fracture, but this technique should be restricted to patients with oblique or spiral, noncomminuted fracture patterns in which at least two lag screws can be applied 1 cm apart.[11] Associated fracture fragments, such as tibiofibular ligament avulsion fragments, can also be reduced and stabilized concurrently with the primary fibular fracture. Syndesmotic instability occurs in approximately 30% of patients with Weber B fracture patterns and frequently requires stabilization.

The nature of the medial injury in patients with unstable Weber B fracture patterns is variable. In some patients, the medial injury is purely ligamentous. Healing of the deltoid ligament is usually sufficient to prevent late valgus instability without direct surgical repair. Medial bone injuries may involve only the anterior colliculus or the entirety of the malleolus. Anterior colliculus injuries are indicative of a combined bone and ligamentous injury. Because the origin of the deep deltoid ligament is posterior to the anterior colliculus, the deep deltoid ligament may be completely torn in conjunction with an anterior colliculus fracture.[12] Stabilization of the anterior colliculus alone in this situation may not restore medial stability. If the malleolus fracture is supracollicular, stabilization is more likely to restore ankle stability.

Weber C Ankle Fractures

Weber C ankle fractures are associated with fibular fractures above the level of the ankle syndesmosis. These injuries occur with an external rotation mechanism. Weber C fractures require stabilization because of the substantial ankle instability incurred.

In addition to fixation of the lateral and medial malleoli, the ankle syndesmosis frequently requires internal fixation. Although biomechanical criteria have been established to determine the need for syndesmotic fixation, these should be applied cautiously. Preferable techniques of intraoperative determination of syndesmotic integrity include dynamic manipulation of the fibula relative to the tibia. For example, a sharp hook or a periosteal elevator may be used to stress the tibiofibular syndesmosis in conjunction with intraoperative fluoroscopy. The external rotation stress test may also be used. Decrease in the tibiofibular overlap or increase in medial clear space as noted with these examinations may be more accurate than biomechanical criteria to detect syndesmotic instability in conjunction with fibular fractures.

Fractures of the Posterior Malleolus

Injuries to the posterior malleolus have been the subject of some recent studies. The posterior malleolus is typically an associated injury with bimalleolar ankle fractures. In Weber B injuries, the posterolateral tibia may be avulsed with the posterior inferior tibiofibular ligament. The size of the posterolateral fragment varies. Traditionally, fractures of the posterior malleolus measuring less than 25% can be treated without internal fixation. However, fractures larger than 25% and all fractures associated with posterior subluxation of the talus require reduction and stabilization.

Techniques to address the posterior malleolus vary. In many patients, reduction of the fibula will reduce the posterior malleolus itself, especially if the interosseous membrane and tibiofibular ligaments are intact and the fracture plane of the posterior malleolus has been débrided. For large fragments, application of anterior to posterior lag screws may be sufficient to stabilize the posterior malleolus. If partial threaded screws are used, caution is required to ensure that the threads of the screw completely pass the fracture site. Alternatively, overdrilling of the near side of the fracture before reduction and use of a fully threaded screw is an excellent means of achieving compression.

When the posterior malleolar fragment does not reduce with fibular reduction, several techniques exist to stabilize the posterior malleolus, including open reduction through a posterolateral approach or percutaneous clamp reduction and stabilization with anterior-to-posterior lag screws. When the posterior approach is used, a buttress plate can be used to enhance stability. In addition, any loose fragments can be extracted. Some higher-energy ankle fractures, in which the posterior malleolus fracture is large or more comminuted, can be addressed from the posterior approach as well. This approach has also been applied successfully to the treatment of certain tibial plafond fractures with a large posterior fragment.

Rehabilitation After Ankle Fracture

Rehabilitation for patients with ankle fractures continues to evolve. Patients with stable fracture patterns, such as isolated fibula fractures without talar shift or instability to stress examination, can generally be safely treated with early functional rehabilitation. Because these injuries are stable, immediate motion and early weight bearing is reasonable. Similarly, patients with ankle fractures that are treated with open reduction and internal fixation can often be treated with early motion and potentially early weight bearing. It may be best to delay early mobilization until wound healing has occurred. In a recent report, patients treated with immediate mobilization in a removable ankle brace had a higher incidence of wound complications compared with those treated with a period of immobilization.[13] Overall, although early mobilization is theoretically appealing, the data comparing early motion and cast treatment are thus far inconclusive. Early functional outcome may be improved with immediate mobilization, but the differences between the two rehabilitation techniques have not been shown to persist beyond 1 year after the injury.[13,14]

When ankle fractures are associated with syndesmotic instability, weight bearing and mobilization are delayed. Appropriate treatment of the associated syndesmotic injury may require reduction and stabilization of the tibiofibular syndesmosis or delayed weight bearing and a longer period of immobilization.

Outcome and Complications

Recent studies have demonstrated that functional outcome is variable after ankle fracture.[15,16] For example, although weight bearing is usually initiated within 6 to 8 weeks after malleolar fractures, functional deficits can persist. Sequential measurement of functional outcomes after ankle fracture has shown that recovery is still expected up to 2 years after injury.[17]

Nonetheless, most patients with ankle fractures that are treated appropriately will achieve a gradual restoration of normal function. Many patients have specific concerns after fracture of the ankle, such as anticipated return to work, athletic, and other activities. A recent study considered restoration of driving function after ankle fracture and noted that patients regain functional ability to drive within 9 to 12 weeks after injury.[18]

The most important factor that can be influenced by the surgeon is the ability to maintain an anatomic reduction of the ankle mortise. Whether a fracture is treated with open reduction and internal fixation or nonsurgical management, the maintenance of a stable anatomic reduction is critical to achieving a successful outcome.

Complications with nonsurgical management of ankle fractures include loss of reduction, malunion, and late arthrosis. Loss of reduction is particularly common when unstable ankle fractures are treated with closed reduction and casting. For this reason, the potential for instability should be considered in all patients with ankle fractures. Patients treated with immobilization require frequent reassessment to rule out loss of reduction. If a malunion occurs, fibular osteotomy can successfully restore ankle function, even many years after the original injury.

Following surgery, complications may include infection, wound healing problems, loss of fixation, stiffness, and thromboembolism. Complications are particularly common in elderly patients, or those with systemic disease such as diabetes. In elderly patients, surgical treatment may be preferable to nonsurgical management of unstable displaced ankle fractures. In one randomized controlled trial, elderly patients with displaced ankle fractures were randomized to receive surgical or nonsurgical treatment.[19] Overall, patients who received surgical management had better maintenance of reduction, range of motion, and functional outcome scores than those in the nonsurgically treated group. However, the risk of surgical complications is also greater in elderly patients.

Many patients with osteoporosis also have an ankle fracture. The diagnosis of osteoporosis should be considered, particularly in perimenopausal women, smokers, and patients with a low body mass index. In many patients, an ankle fracture is a symptom of osteoporosis. Osteoporosis diagnosis and intervention may help to prevent the occurrence of additional fractures.

Patients with fractures with associated soft-tissue injury, such as open fractures or fracture-dislocations, are more likely to develop complications. Patients with diabetes and open fractures constitute perhaps the worst possible scenario. In general, patients with significant soft-tissue injury benefit from early reduction and stabilization. The incidence of wound complications following fracture-dislocations is lower when surgery is performed within 24 hours of the injury.

The development of osteoarthrosis after ankle fracture may be more common than previously thought. In some patients, results may be affected by associated injuries. For example, ankle fractures accompanied by chondral injuries to the distal tibia or talus are associated with worse results. In one study of surgically treated

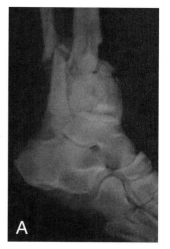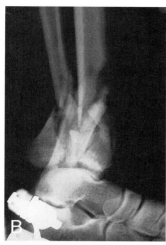

Figure 3 A, Injury radiograph showing sagittal plane malalignment and articular incongruity before external fixation. **B,** Lateral radiograph after external fixation. Note articular incongruity but realignment.

ankle fractures with a minimum 10-year follow-up, radiographic signs of arthritis were found in more than half of patients.[15] Additional long-term follow-up studies will help determine which factors influence the development of arthrosis after ankle fractures.

Ankle fractures are some of the most commonly treated and among the most controversial orthopaedic injuries. The goals of treatment are simple: obtain and maintain an anatomic reduction of the ankle mortise and facilitate early return to normal activities. Recent studies have documented that not all ankle fractures heal well; recovery is often slow and incomplete. Improved diagnosis and treatment of associated ligament injuries and improved rehabilitation strategies offer promise for better outcomes.

Fractures of the Distal Tibial Pilon
Introduction
Distal tibial pilon or plafond fractures involve the weight-bearing articular surface of the tibia. These injuries are typically the result of high-energy falls or motor vehicle accidents. Current treatment algorithms attempt to maximize function and minimize complications. However, even patients who receive optimum management have a guarded prognosis with regard to functional outcome.

Radiographic Evaluation
Initial radiographs should include AP and lateral radiographs that are centered on the ankle joint. The AP view provides a guide to the amount of articular impaction and shortening. The lateral view shows articular incongruity[20] and demonstrates whether the posterior articular segment is disconnected from the intact shaft (Figure 3, *A*). In addition, plain films of the entire tibia should be

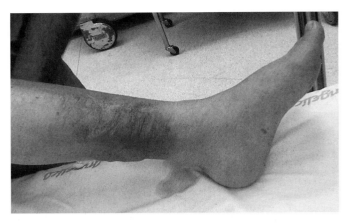

Figure 4 Photograph of a Tscherne grade CIII soft-tissue injury.

obtained to assess the extent of metaphyseal and diaphyseal involvement.

CT is indicated for all complex distal tibial pilon fractures to aid in the identification of fracture fragments, to analyze the extent of articular involvement and comminution, and to plan surgery and guide approaches.[21] CT helps determine whether a fracture can be reduced by percutaneous means or whether an open approach will be required. If temporizing external fixation is planned, CT provides more information when performed after the limb has been realigned and brought out to length.

The Rüedi and Allgöwer classification system divides the fractures into three types based on increasing articular comminution and displacement. The AO/ASIF fracture classification system is based on the convention that the tibia has the designation of 4 and the distal end has a designation of 3; therefore, all tibial plafond fractures are identified by the number 43. Subdivision of this fracture category into 43A, 43B, or 43C depends on whether fractures are extra-articular, partial articular, or complete articular. Further subdivision occurs based on comminution and fracture pattern. Because this classification system has only moderate to fair reliability, its use in interpreting research results remains limited.

The most common soft-tissue classification system used to categorize distal tibial injuries is that devised by Tscherne. Grade C0 and grade CI soft-tissue injuries are more typically the result of indirect mechanisms associated with ankle fractures, whereas grade CII and grade CIII soft-tissue injuries are often the result of high-energy mechanisms associated with pilon fractures (Figure 4). Most treatments are predicated on safely managing the soft-tissue envelope.

Evolution of Treatment

Initial reports of open reduction and internal fixation as described by Rüedi and Allgöwer found 74% good to

excellent long-term results. The classic principles of treatment include (1) restoration of lateral column length by reducing and fixing the fibula, (2) anatomic reduction of the articular surface of the tibia, (3) bone grafting of metaphyseal defects, and (4) using a buttress plate medially to prevent varus collapse. Higher-energy injures were found to follow a more malignant course. When treated in a classic fashion, disastrous soft-tissue complications occurred. These vexing results led to the increased use of external fixation and delayed treatment protocols. These different strategies have returned the rate of complications to a more acceptable level, even when treating patients with the most severe injuries.[22-26]

Treatment Options

Treatment for pilon fractures is either surgical or nonsurgical. Nonsurgical treatment applies only to patients with fractures that are axially stable and nondisplaced at the articular surface or nonambulatory patients. Nonsurgical treatment of unstable or displaced fractures has generally yielded poor results.

Surgical treatment generally involves definitive external fixation or definitive plating. Definitive external fixation uses limited approaches to obtain articular reduction with minimal internal fixation at the joint surface. Both ankle bridging and nonbridging methods have been successfully used.[27] Plating techniques use staged protocols that involve temporizing external fixation with delayed definitive plate reconstruction.

The treatment goal is the same for all methods of stabilization: a well-aligned limb with pain-free joint motion. The joint should be reduced as anatomically as possible, whether an open approach or a percutaneous technique is used. The mechanical axes of the limb must be restored and maintained. Complications must be minimized because unexpected problems will almost certainly guarantee poor results. The most successful outcome will be achieved when goals are maximized and complications are avoided. A substantial benefit of temporary external fixation is that it provides time to gather information and determine a patient's needs and expectations.

Definitive External Fixation

Definitive external fixation may or may not span the ankle joint, depending on several variables. The main benefit of definitive external fixation is the potential reduction of soft-tissue complications. However, joint reduction may be more difficult with these limited approaches.[28] Fibular fixation may or may not be performed, and no clear advantage has been demonstrated for either protocol.

The ankle bridging technique typically involves placing distal pins in the calcaneus and talar neck while the proximal pins are placed medially in the tibia.[28,29] The transarticular fixator is placed, and the articular surface is provisionally reduced with ligamentotaxis (Figure 3, *B*). Percutaneously placed clamps directly over fracture lines and displaced fragments are used to gain reduction. Lag screws are placed to hold articular fragments rigidly. The external fixator maintains the length, rotation, and alignment of the extremity and serves as a buttress for the articular surface while protecting the joint as fracture healing occurs. This technique prioritizes soft-tissue presentation. The fixator should initially be placed in the setting of acute injury. When the soft-tissue envelope allows, articular reduction performed early facilitates manipulation of the fragments before consolidation and early callus formation. The tendency to do the articular reduction early must be tempered by the potential risks of soft-tissue complications. Even though reductions may become more difficult to obtain, surgical delay is indicated when the soft-tissue envelope is severely injured.

Nonspanning hybrid fixation uses a combination of half pins, thin wires, circular rings, and unilateral bars.[30-33] The technique has evolved to become a staged protocol[26,30] that consists of initial spanning fixation accompanied by definitive articular reconstruction and conversion to a nonbridging frame.[28] The articular reconstruction may occur at the time of initial external fixation or at conversion to a nonbridging construct. Timing depends on the amount of articular displacement, the condition of the soft tissue, and whether an open or a percutaneous technique will be used. Hybrid fixation for the distal tibia uses no pins or wires distal to the ankle joint and typically relies on metaphyseal fixation with thin tensioned wires connected to more proximal half pins via rings, bars, and clamps. Even when using safe corridors, these thin wires across the distal tibia frequently impale a tendon or a neurovascular structure. Wires within 20 mm of the anterior joint line or 30 mm of the tip of the medial malleolus can be intracapsular[34] (Figure 5). These small tolerances demonstrate the attention to detail required for this technique.

Definitive Plate Fixation

Definitive plate fixation of high-energy injuries should only be done using a staged protocol.[24,25] In patients who have undergone early single-stage reconstruction, wound-related complication rates as high as 33%, infection rates as high as 28%, and amputation rates as high as 17% have been reported.[35] Phase one may include immediate fibular plating to regain and maintain lateral column length and transarticular external fixation followed by a typical delay of 14 to 24 days. Phase two is a formal open reduction and internal fixation. This approach appears to reduce previously reported high complications rates for early single-stage management.

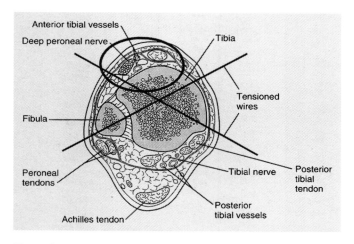

Figure 5 Illustration of the safe zone position for placement of thin wires in the distal tibia. Anterior compartments are structures at risk (circle). *(Reproduced with permission from Tornetta P III, Weiner L, Bergman M, et al: Pilon fractures: Treatment with combined internal and external fixation. J Orthop Trauma 1993;7:489-496.)*

Initially, a simple realignment should be done as the extremity is splinted. This reduction minimizes further soft-tissue injury. After medical stabilization, the patient is immediately brought to the operating room. Fibular fixation is done only if an anatomic reduction can be achieved. If malreduced, anatomic articular reconstruction of the tibia will be inhibited. Care should be taken when making this lateral incision to attempt to maximize the skin bridge. Transarticular external fixation is then performed.

Temporizing external fixation is a technique of portable traction that should typically be applied within hours of the injury. Distraction and ligamentotaxis aid in the reduction of displaced fragments and realignment of the limb. By maintaining the length, alignment, and rotation of the extremity, the injured soft tissues are stabilized and swelling is allowed to resolve.

Simple frames are often used for this stage, but any external fixator can be used. Stability can be safely achieved by placing a centrally threaded 5- or 6-mm transfixation pin through the calcaneus and two half pins in the anterior tibia. Sagittal plane stability and alignment are maintained using this frame (Figure 6). Any displacement should be corrected to reduce direct pressure on the soft tissue from underlying bony fragments and to prevent axial shortening (Figure 7). It is critical not to neglect the forefoot at this stage, which can stiffen in fixed midfoot equinus if not splinted effectively. Alternatively, one or two small half pins can be placed in the metatarsal bases and connected to the fixator. Patients are typically discharged and subsequently undergo surgery within 10 to 24 days after injury.

After soft-tissue swelling resolves, definitive plating may be done. Current treatment uses smaller implants[23] that may be precontoured and placed through a partial or completely percutaneous method.[36] Nonetheless, an

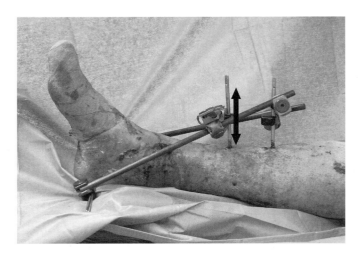

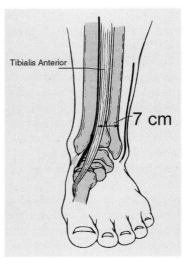

Figure 6 Photograph showing a temporizing transarticular fixator. The distal pin in the tibia controls the position of the foot in the sagittal plane. By sliding the frame up or down on this pin (*arrow*), the ankle can be translated anteriorly or posteriorly in relation to the tibial shaft. After locking this clamp, the alignment will be maintained, even when an anterior-directed force is put on the distal segment by resting the foot on the bed.

Figure 8 Illustration of the incision used for the medial approach to the pilon. Superficial dissection stays lateral to the tibial crest and deep dissection stays medial to the tendon of the tibialis anterior. *(Reproduced with permission from Sirkin M, Sanders R: The treatment of pilon fractures. Orthop Clin North Am 2001;32(1):91-102.)*

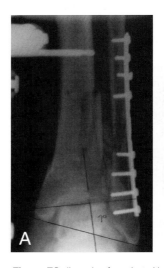
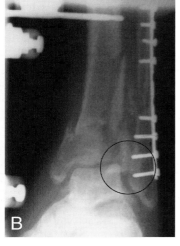

Figure 7 Radiographs of a patient with transarticular fixation. **A,** The talus has been left shortened and limb length not realigned. **B,** Note position of Chaput fragment as the guide to length. The normal talocrural angle should be 84°. In this patient, it is 70° because the medial malleolus has not been reduced to the appropriate length.

exposure that is large enough to anatomically reduce the articular surface is required. Larger incisions are sometimes required, but periosteal stripping is only performed at or near the ends of the fracture to preserve blood supply and diminish potential soft-tissue problems.

The typical incision is a modified anteromedial incision[25] (Figure 8), which is extended to the foot over the talus. The anterolateral approach has been successfully used recently with plates specifically designed for anterolateral placement. The tibia and fibula may be stabilized through this singular anterolateral incision.[37] Posteromedioanterior[38] and posterolateral[39] approaches have recently been described for treating patients with pilon fractures.

Surgical Timing

Although it was previously thought that early surgery may be well tolerated when swelling occurs from hematoma rather than edema, no data exist to show this to be true. Large, open, early procedures undertaken at a time when the soft tissue has not had time to stabilize have been shown to be associated with a significant incidence of infection, wound dehiscence, and amputation.[35] Delaying surgical intervention, therefore, makes surgery safer and decreases the incidence of these complications.[23-25,40] The use of minimally invasive techniques or staged protocols has also helped to reduce the overall complication rates.[22,23] Although reduction may be easier when definitive fracture fixation is performed earlier, open procedures must be avoided in most patients with fractures of the distal tibia in the acute phase. Percutaneous techniques may be used, but care must be exercised not to exceed the limits of tolerance of the soft-tissue envelope.

Early treatment of these injuries should be limited to realignment of the limb with a splint and compressive dressing, appropriate trauma workup, and usually some sort of bridging external fixation to maintain length, rotation, and alignment while the soft-tissue envelope is allowed to heal. Patients are followed in the office (if their condition is stable for discharge) or while in the hospital. They are only taken for definitive stabilization when wrinkles have appeared in the overlying soft tissue and blisters have reepithelialized, which typically occurs 14 to 24 days after injury.[24,37]

Comparison of Treatment Methods

Comparison of treatment methods is difficult because there are conflicting data in the literature. One study reviewed 107 fractures of the distal tibial articular surface, all of which were initially stabilized with calcaneal traction.[26] Tscherne grade C0 and CI injuries were treated with open reduction and internal fixation, whereas those with more severe soft-tissue injuries were managed with hybrid external fixation. Patients treated with external fixation had fewer complications, even though the limbs of these patients had the more severe soft-tissue injuries. All AO/ASIF type C fractures had significantly poorer results than type AO/ASIF type A and B injuries. Another study reported on the treatment of 63 fractures with either hybrid fixation or definitive internal fixation using a staged protocol.[30] Hybrid fixation was used in patients with more comminuted fracture patterns as well as those with poorer soft tissue. Better range of motion and clinical ankle scores and a lower complication rate were noted in those patients whose ankles were treated with open reduction and internal fixation. These two studies show the inherent difficulty in understanding different treatment methods and outcomes.

The only direct prospective comparison compared hybrid fixation with open reduction and internal fixation and found significantly more soft-tissue complications in the internal fixation group and a 17% rate of amputation.[35] This study clearly demonstrated the dangers of performing one-stage reconstruction at 3 to 5 days when the soft tissue is not adequately prepared for a surgical insult. Modern treatment with a delayed staged reconstruction has decreased these complications to rates comparable to those noted using external fixation protocols.[23,24,30,33,41]

Several series have reviewed results of various management protocols.[22,28,30-33,42] Some results favor external fixation for definitive management, especially in patients with severe soft-tissue injury. Other assessments support two-stage protocols of initial bridging external fixation followed by definitive open reduction and internal fixation. The individual choice must take into account the personality of the fracture and the experience of the surgeon.

Complications

The underlying goal of all treatment regimens includes the minimization of complications, but soft-tissue problems continue to be a major complication regardless of management protocol. Wound dehiscence should be treated aggressively to try to prevent deep infection. Local wound care, immobilization, and free-tissue transfer should be used to treat surgical wound breakdown.

Deep infection is most commonly seen as a complication of local wound problems. Treatment should consist of extensive débridement. Some patients will require hardware removal, placement of bridging external fixation, and local or intravenous antibiotics. Soft-tissue defects require free-tissue transfer, whereas bony defects can be managed with either delayed bone grafting or bone transport.

Nonunion of the articular surface is rare, but it occurs frequently in the metaphyseal area, especially in patients

who have been treated with external fixation. Treatment of the nonunion must also correct any deformity. The bone must be stabilized, and bone graft should be used for bony defects and to promote union. Recent reports have shown the 90° blade plate to be an excellent method of fixation to accomplish this goal.[43,44] Often soft-tissue coverage is precarious and free-flap coverage may be warranted. The use of a fibula-pro-tibia technique may also be useful in obtaining healing in patients with these complex nonunions.[45]

Posttraumatic Arthrosis

Arthritis continues to be a major problem in patients with distal tibial fractures because most experience some degree of arthrosis following treatment.[46] Intra-articular malunion is associated with an increased incidence of late degeneration, but even those with anatomically reconstructed cartilage may develop arthrosis. Ankle fusion is an excellent method for treating pain associated with this late complication. Screws, plating, and external fixation are accepted methods of achieving fusion. The angled blade plate can be an invaluable implant for this purpose.[43]

Outcomes

One study assessed 31 patients (35 ankles) who were treated with monolateral hinged external fixation coupled with screw fixation of the articular surface.[46] These patients were followed for 5 to 12 years. Five ankles required arthrodesis, and two required screw removal; there were no other surgeries performed. Most patients had radiographic evidence of arthrosis, and 20 patients had evidence of grade 2 arthrosis). The average Iowa Ankle Score was 78, and the Medical Outcomes Study Short Form 36-Item Health Survey Questionnaire (SF-36) scores showed the injury's long-term negative effect. Most patients had some limitation in performing recreational activities and were unable to run. About half of the patients changed jobs because of ankle injuries. The average patient felt that they had improved for a 2.4-year period. Another study also showed a significant decrease in the SF-36 scores compared with those of age-matched control subjects.[47] Patients were found to have stiffness (35%), swelling (29%), and ongoing pain (33%). Thirty percent of the patients who were previously employed were unemployed as a result of their ankle injuries. The presence of two or more comorbidities, including being married, low income, not having attained a high school diploma, and having been treated with external fixation related to worse outcomes.

Summary

The treatment of tibial pilon fractures remains challenging. Successful treatment requires skill, judgment, and experience. Patients with high-energy injuries have a high risk of complications. By adhering to the principles of careful soft-tissue handling and delayed surgical tactics, these problems can be minimized with the use of temporizing external fixation. Modern surgical techniques including indirect reduction, minimizing implant size, and minimal soft-tissue stripping must be used to help diminish these problems. The goals of treatment are similar for all articular fractures: anatomic reduction of the articular surface and restoration of limb alignment and length. These goals can be attained by internal fixation, external fixation, or a combination of both. Multiple techniques may be needed for different fractures and not one method will be applicable to all injuries. Experience with different procedures will aid in the successful treatment of this devastating injury. It is important for treating physicians to understand what can be expected as well as their own limitations in performing each technique.

Annotated References

1. Michelson JD, Hamel AJ, Buczek FL, Sharkey NA: Kinematic behavior of the ankle following malleolar fracture repair in a high-fidelity cadaver model. *J Bone Joint Surg Am* 2002;84-A:2029-2038.

2. McConnell T, Creevy W, Tornetta P III: Stress examination of supination external rotation-type fibular fractures. *J Bone Joint Surg Am* 2004;86-A:2171-2178.

   In this study, 138 patients with Weber B ankle fractures were examined for associated deltoid ligament incompetence using physical examination (medial tenderness, ecchymosis, and swelling) and stress radiographs. Physical examination was not predictive of deltoid incompetence. Stress radiographs of the injured ankle improved the diagnosis of instability compared with physical examination in patients with Weber type B fibular fractures.

3. Ebraheim NA, Elgafy H, Padanilam T: Syndesmotic disruption in low fibular fractures associated with deltoid ligament injury. *Clin Orthop* 2003;409:260-267.

4. Hovis WD, Kaiser BW, Watson JT, Bucholz RW: Treatment of syndesmotic disruptions of the ankle with bioabsorbable screw fixation. *J Bone Joint Surg Am* 2002;84-A:26-31.

5. Thordarson DB, Samuelson M, Shepherd LE, Merkle PF, Lee J: Bioabsorbable versus stainless steel screw fixation of the syndesmosis in pronation-lateral rotation ankle fractures: A prospective randomized trial. *Foot Ankle Int* 2001;22:335-338.

6. Tornetta P III, Spoo JE, Reynolds FA, Lee C: Overtightening of the ankle syndesmosis: Is it really possible? *J Bone Joint Surg Am* 2001;83-A:489-492.

7. McConnell T, Tornetta P III: Marginal plafond impaction in association with supination-adduction ankle fractures: A report of eight cases. *J Orthop Trauma* 2001;15:447-449.

8. Ramsey PL, Hamilton W: Changes in tibiotalar area of contact caused by lateral talar shift. *J Bone Joint Surg Am* 1976;58:356-357.

9. Michelson JD, Varner KE, Checcone M: Diagnosing deltoid injury in ankle fractures: The gravity stress view. *Clin Orthop* 2001;387:178-182.

10. Lamontagne J, Blachut PA, Broekhuyse HM, O'Brien PJ, Meek RN: Surgical treatment of a displaced lateral malleolus fracture: The antiglide technique versus lateral plate fixation. *J Orthop Trauma* 2002;16:498-502.

11. Tornetta P III, Creevy W: Lag screw only fixation of the lateral malleolus. *J Orthop Trauma* 2001;15:119-121.

12. Tornetta P III: Competence of the deltoid ligament in bimalleolar ankle fractures after medial malleolar fixation. *J Bone Joint Surg Am* 2000;82:843-848.

13. Lehtonen H, Jarvinen TL, Honkonen S, Nyman M, Vihtonen K, Jarvinen M: Use of a cast compared with a functional ankle brace after operative treatment of an ankle fracture: A prospective, randomized study. *J Bone Joint Surg Am* 2003;85-A:205-211.

    This prospective randomized trial of patients with ankle fractures treated with open reduction and internal fixation compared the use of a cast with functional bracing for postoperative management. The authors studied 100 patients and noted a higher incidence of wound complications in the brace group. Functional outcomes at 2-year follow-up did not differ between the groups.

14. Egol KA, Dolan R, Koval KJ: Functional outcome of surgery for fractures of the ankle: A prospective, randomised comparison of management in a cast or a functional brace. *J Bone Joint Surg Br* 2000;82:246-249.

    This prospective randomized trial of patients with ankle fractures treated with open reduction and internal fixation also compared the use of a cast with functional bracing for postoperative management. The authors studied 60 patients and noted advanced improvement in functional outcome at early follow-up and earlier return to work in the patients treated with a brace. The differences in functional outcome did not differ between the groups after 1 year.

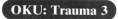

15. Day GA, Swanson CE, Hulcombe BG: Operative treatment of ankle fractures: A minimum ten-year follow-up. *Foot Ankle Int* 2001;22:102-106.

16. Pagliaro AJ, Michelson JD, Mizel MS: Results of operative fixation of unstable ankle fractures in geriatric patients. *Foot Ankle Int* 2001;22:399-402.

17. Obremskey WT, Dirschl DR, Crowther JD, Craig WL III, Driver RE, LeCroy CM: Change over time of SF-36 functional outcomes for operatively treated unstable ankle fractures. *J Orthop Trauma* 2002;16:30-33.

18. Egol KA, Sheikhazadeh A, Mogatederi S, Barnett A, Koval KJ: Lower-extremity function for driving an automobile after operative treatment of ankle fracture. *J Bone Joint Surg Am* 2003;85-A:1185-1189.

19. Makwana NK, Bhowal B, Harper WM, Hui AW: Conservative versus operative treatment for displaced ankle fractures in patients over 55 years of age: A prospective, randomised study. *J Bone Joint Surg Br* 2001;83:525-529.

20. Ebraheim N, Sabry FF, Mehalik JN: Intraoperative imaging of the tibial plafond fracture: A potential pitfall. *Foot Ankle Int* 2000;21:67-72.

21. Tornetta P III, Gorup J: Axial computed tomography of pilon fractures. *Clin Orthop* 1996;323:273-276.

22. Blauth M, Bastian L, Krettek C, Knop C, Evans S: Surgical options for the treatment of severe tibial pilon fractures: A study of three techniques. *J Orthop Trauma* 2001;15:153-160.

23. Helfet DL, Shonnard PY, Levine D, Borrelli J Jr: Minimally invasive plate osteosynthesis of distal fractures of the tibia. *Injury* 1997;28(suppl 1):A42-A47.

24. Patterson MJ, Cole JD: Two-staged delayed open reduction and internal fixation of severe pilon fractures. *J Orthop Trauma* 1999;13:85-91.

25. Sirkin M, Sanders R, DiPasquale T, Herscovici D Jr: A staged protocol for soft tissue management in the treatment of complex pilon fractures. *J Orthop Trauma* 1999;13:78-84.

26. Watson JT, Moed BR, Karges DE, Cramer KE: Pilon fractures: Treatment protocol based on severity of soft tissue injury. *Clin Orthop* 2000;375:78-90.

27. Bonar SK, Marsh JL: Tibial plafond fractures: Changing principles of treatment. *J Am Acad Orthop Surg* 1994;2:297-305.

28. El-Shazly M, Dalby-Ball J, Burton M, Saleh M: The use of trans-articular and extra-articular external fixation for management of distal tibial intra-articular fractures. *Injury* 2001;32(suppl 4):SD99-SD106.

29. Mitkovic MB, Bumbasirevic MZ, Lesic A, Golubovic Z: Dynamic external fixation of comminuted intra-articular fractures of the distal tibia (type C pilon fractures). *Acta Orthop Belg* 2002;68:508-514.

30. Anglen JO: Early outcome of hybrid external fixation for fracture of the distal tibia. *J Orthop Trauma* 1999;13:92-97.

31. French B, Tornetta P III: Hybrid external fixation of tibial pilon fractures. *Foot Ankle Clin* 2000;5:853-871.

32. Manca M, Marchetti S, Restuccia G, Faldini A, Faldini C, Giannini S: Combined percutaneous internal and external fixation of type-C tibial plafond fractures: A review of twenty-two cases. *J Bone Joint Surg Am* 2002;84-A(suppl 2):109-115.

33. Pugh KJ, Wolinsky PR, McAndrew MP, Johnson KD: Tibial pilon fractures: A comparison of treatment methods. *J Trauma* 1999;47:937-941.

34. Vives MJ, Abidi NA, Ishikawa SN, Taliwal RV, Sharkey PF: Soft tissue injuries with the use of safe corridors for transfixion wire placement during external fixation of distal tibia fractures: An anatomic study. *J Orthop Trauma* 2001;15:555-559.

35. Wyrsch B, McFerran MA, McAndrew M, et al: Operative treatment of fractures of the tibial plafond: A randomized, prospective study. *J Bone Joint Surg Am* 1996;78:1646-1657.

36. Khoury A, Liebergall M, London E, Mosheiff R: Percutaneous plating of distal tibial fractures. *Foot Ankle Int* 2002;23:818-824.

37. Shantharam SS, Naeni F, Wilson EP: Single-incision technique for internal fixation of distal tibia and fibula fractures. *Orthopedics* 2000;23:429-431.

38. Kao KF, Huang PJ, Chen YW, Cheng YM, Lin SY, Ko SH: Postero-medio-anterior approach of the ankle for the pilon fracture. *Injury* 2000;31:71-74.
    The authors of this study assessed 45 patients who underwent the "postero-medio-anterior" approach for the

treatment of pilon fractures. Minimal complications were reported.

39. Konrath GA, Hopkins G II: Posterolateral approach for tibial pilon fractures: A report of two cases. *J Orthop Trauma* 1999;13:586-589.

40. Thordarson DB: Complications after treatment of tibial pilon fractures: Prevention and management strategies. *J Am Acad Orthop Surg* 2000;8:253-265.

41. Sirkin M, Sanders R: The treatment of pilon fractures. *Orthop Clin North Am* 2001;32:91-102.

42. Marsh JL, Bonar S, Nepola JV, Decoster TA, Hurwitz SR: Use of an articulated external fixator for fractures of the tibial plafond. *J Bone Joint Surg Am* 1995;77:1498-1509.

43. Chin KR, Nagarkatti DG, Miranda MA, Santoro VM, Baumgaertner MR, Jupiter JB: Salvage of distal tibia metaphyseal nonunions with the 90 degrees cannulated blade plate. *Clin Orthop* 2003;409:241-249.

    This study assessed 13 patients with nonunions of the distal tibia that were treated with a 90° blade plate. Three patients also had ankle fusion performed. All patients healed at an average of 15.6 weeks. All patients ambulated without supportive devices.

44. Reed LK, Mormino MA: Functional outcome after blade plate reconstruction of distal tibia metaphyseal nonunions: A study of 11 cases. *J Orthop Trauma* 2004;18:81-86.

    This is a prospective case series of 11 patients with a metaphyseal nonunion of the distal tibia who were treated with a 90° blade plate that was contoured and placed via a posteromedial approach. All patients healed at an average of 16 weeks and were able to bear full weight at an average of 12 weeks. The average Orthopaedic Foot and Ankle Society Ankle Hindfoot score increased from 29 preoperatively to 80 postoperatively. One infection was reported.

45. DeOrio JK, Ware AW: Salvage technique for treatment of periplafond tibial fractures: The modified fibula-pro-tibia procedure. *Foot Ankle Int* 2003;24:228-232.

46. Marsh JL, Weigel DP, Dirschl DR: Tibial plafond fractures: How do these ankles function over time? *J Bone Joint Surg Am* 2003;85-A(suppl 2):287-295.

    The authors of this study evaluated the intermediate outcomes of 35 fractures of the tibial plafond between 5 and 12 years after injury. There were five ankle fusions and other than two prominent screw removals, there were no other procedures performed. The average ankle score was 78. The authors reported a long-term negative effect of the injury on general health and ankle pain and function. Recreational activities were most commonly limited, with the inability to run occurring in 27 of 31 patients. Fourteen patients changed jobs. There were 25 patients with good to excellent results, 7 with fair results, and 1 with a poor result. Nine patients had improvement of their ankle scores, and patients reported that their ankles had improved for an average 2.4 years.

47. Pollak AN, McCarthy ML, Bess RS, Agel J, Swiontkowski MF: Outcomes after treatment of high-energy tibial plafond fractures. *J Bone Joint Surg Am* 2003;85-A:1893-1900.

    This is a retrospective intermediate review of the health, function, and impairment of 80 patients who underwent treatment for injury to the tibial plafond. At an average follow-up of 3.2 years, the general health of these patients was reported to be significantly poorer than that of age-matched control subjects. Thirty-five percent of patients had ankle stiffness, 29% had persistent swelling, and 33% had ongoing pain. Forty-three percent of the patients who had been previously employed reported being unemployed. Poor results were associated with the presence of two or more of the following factors: being married, annual income less than $25,000, no high school diploma, and treatment with external fixation.

Chapter 39

Foot Injuries

Alexandra K. Schwartz, MD

Michael E. Brage, MD

Richard T. Laughlin, MD

David Stephen, MD, FRCSC

Calcaneal Fractures

Mechanism of Injury and Pathoanatomy

The calcaneus is the most frequently fractured tarsal bone. A combination of compression, shear, and angulation forces results in a variety of fractures that can be simple or comminuted and may extend to the adjacent articulations. Motor vehicle accidents and falls from heights remain the most common mechanisms of injury. The talus acts as a wedge, and two consistent fracture lines develop. One fracture line results from shear forces and runs obliquely, dividing the calcaneus into the sustentacular medial fragment and the tuberosity lateral fragment. Both of these elements may contain a variable portion of the posterior facet. The sustentacular fragment typically remains aligned with the talus, whereas the tuberosity piece is shortened and rotated. Distally, the fracture may enter the calcaneocuboid joint and may divide the anterior facet. The other fracture line results from compression forces and divides the calcaneus into anterior and posterior portions, starting from the angle of Gissane and running medially. In higher-energy injuries, secondary fracture lines develop, resulting in higher degrees of facet joint comminution. The lateral cortex is frequently comminuted and poorly defined, resulting in lateral wall blowout, which may impinge on the fibulocalcaneal space and predispose the peroneal tendons to entrapment or dislocation. The intact Achilles tendon pulls the tuberosity fragment proximally, whereas the talus settles into a more horizontal alignment, predisposing patients to tibiotalar impingement.

Open fractures of the calcaneus may be caused by low-velocity, high-velocity, or blast injuries. Low-velocity open fractures often present with a medial skin split caused by the sustentaculum fragment. The fracture of the sustentaculum tali results from an axial load on the heel combined with eversion of the foot. In these injuries, lateral soft-tissue swelling is minimal because of the immediate evacuation of fracture hematoma through the medial wound. Open fractures of the calcaneus caused by high-velocity or blast injuries are more severe and result in complex bony and soft-tissue injuries.

Initial Management

Patients should be placed into a bulky dressing and splint to prevent equinus contracture. A foot pump may also be used to expedite resolution of swelling. Patients should be instructed to elevate the affected extremity above the level of the heart. Fracture blisters appear when there is a cleavage at the dermal/epidermal junction (Figure 1). If the dermis retains some epidermal cells, the fluid is clear. If the dermis is completely devoid of epidermal cells, the fluid is bloody. Although no difference has been demonstrated between protocols that recommend leaving blisters intact, débridement, and application of silver sulfadiazine cream and protocols that recommend débridement and application of a nonadherent dressing, an increased risk of wound complications exists when surgery is performed through blood-filled blisters. Surgical treatment is best delayed until blisters have reepithelialized and the skin shows wrinkles at the lateral aspect of the heel with dorsiflexion and eversion of the foot.

Open fractures of the calcaneus are uncommon, representing approximately 10% of all calcaneal fractures. These fractures require immediate and thorough irrigation and débridement. Low-energy open fractures can be treated by serial irrigation and débridement of the open wound, followed by definitive fixation once the soft tissues permit. High-energy open fractures may require temporary placement of antibiotic beads, provisional external fixation, and/or free-tissue transfer.

Patients with prominently displaced avulsion/tongue type fractures should be considered for urgent intervention to prevent skin necrosis at the posterior heel (Figure 2). Such displaced fractures cause significant pressure to this precarious skin region and can lead to rapid full-thickness necrosis if not addressed immediately.

Diagnostic Imaging

All patients with calcaneal fractures should have a standard set of radiographs, including a lateral view of the hindfoot, an AP view of the foot, a mortise view of the ankle, and an axial view of the heel. The lateral view confirms the presence of a fracture and can be used to

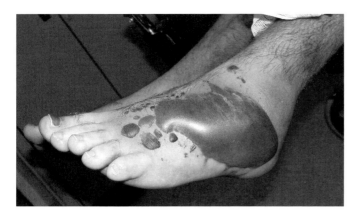

Figure 1 Photograph showing severe blistering of a foot after a motorcycle accident.

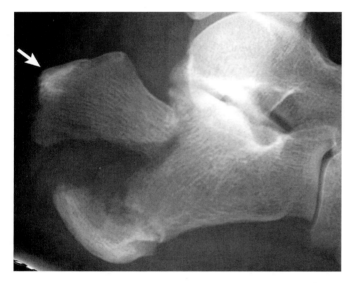

Figure 2 Radiograph showing a large avulsion fracture of the calcaneal tuberosity (*arrow*).

assess the Böhler angle and the crucial angle of Gissane. Displacement of the posterior facet and calcaneal body comminution may decrease this angle. Significant loss of the Böhler angle has been shown to correlate with poorer outcome.[1] The angle of Gissane or crucial angle is formed by a line along the posterior facet and a line from the inferior aspect of the posterior facet to the beak of the calcaneus. The lateral view shows the posterior facet as well as the fracture pattern. A joint depression fracture has dissociation of the posterior facet fragment from the tuberosity, whereas a tongue-type fracture demonstrates continuity between the posterior facet and the tuberosity.

An AP view of the foot is important to evaluate the calcaneocuboid joint, the amount of lateral wall blowout, and any subluxation at the talonavicular articulation. A mortise view of the ankle allows further assessment of the posterior facet. Up to 8.7% of intra-articular calcaneal fractures have associated lateral subluxation or dis-

location of the posterior facet, peroneal tendon subluxation, lateral ankle ligament disruption, and/or fibula fractures. Therefore, varus talar tilt in conjunction with a displaced intra-articular calcaneal fracture warrants further examination of ankle stability. Avulsion of a thin shell of distal fibula, which represents retinacular damage and/or peroneal tendon subluxation, is another typical finding on the mortise view.

The Harris axial view of the heel is obtained with the foot in maximal dorsiflexion and the beam angled 45° cephalad. This view shows the tuberosity, sustentaculum tali, posterior facet, loss of length, and increase in width and angulation of the calcaneal tuberosity. Broden's views allow better visualization of the posterior facet.

CT has become a routine preoperative tool for assessment of intra-articular calcaneal fractures. Because of the oblique nature of the facets with the foot in neutral, a 30° oblique coronal plane is needed to obtain coronal sections perpendicular to the facets. Coronal images allow visualization of the number of fragments, amount of intra-articular displacement, sustentaculum, degree of varus and widening, and peroneal and flexor hallucis tendons. The transverse view is 90° to the coronal view and is parallel to the long axis of the foot. These axial images allow for assessment of the calcaneocuboid joint, anteroinferior aspect of the posterior facet, and lateral wall.

The most common CT classification is the Sanders classification, which relies on the coronal section that shows the widest surface of the inferior facet of the talus. The posterior facet of the calcaneus is divided by three lines (A, B, and C) into four potential fracture fragments: lateral, central, medial, and sustentacular. There are four types of calcaneal fracture patterns based on the Sanders classification. Type I fractures are nondisplaced, regardless of the number of fracture lines. Type II fractures are two-part fractures of the posterior facet and are subdivided into type IIA, IIB, or IIC based on the location of the fracture line (Figure 3). Type III fractures are three-part fractures, created by two fracture lines and subdivided according to fracture line location. This results in possible combinations of type IIIAB, IIIAC, and IIIBC fractures. Type IV fractures are four-part (or more) articular fractures with severe comminution. In some series, this classification system has been found to be prognostic for outcome after surgical treatment via a lateral approach.[2,3]

Treatment Options

The decision to begin surgical or nonsurgical treatment of patients with calcaneal fractures is based on several factors. Important variables include predicted compliance with treatment and concomitant comorbidities. Untreated drug or alcohol addictions may compromise the ability to comply with treatment; older patients with early organic brain disease may also have difficulty com-

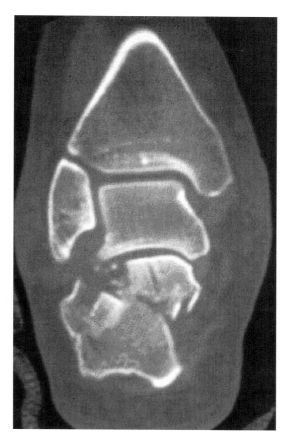

Figure 3 CT scan of a Sanders type II fracture.

plying with treatment. Factors that may significantly increase the risk of wound dehiscence or infection should be considered contraindications to surgery. These factors include type 1 diabetes mellitus with advanced neuropathy, significant peripheral vascular disease, venous stasis disease, or active dermatitis in the surgical area. Patients who smoke must be counseled regarding the significantly increased risk of postoperative wound complications, and smoking cessation should be strongly encouraged.

Nondisplaced fractures are treated without surgery. Treatment should consist of early range-of-motion exercises, with weight bearing commencing after healing.

Displaced fractures with simple patterns of posterior facet injury typically have better outcomes than fractures with comminuted posterior facets. Excellence of the reduction is an important factor in attaining successful results; however, an anatomic reduction does not guarantee a good clinical outcome. The surgeon's ability to anatomically reduce the fracture diminishes as early fracture healing progresses. Thus, patients who begin treatment 3 weeks or more after injury may have more problematic wound closure if the fracture had marked shortening and flattening. After restoration of height and length, the flap may not be as pliable as desired to achieve tension-free closure.[4] Surgical repair of the calcaneus has a well-documented learning curve. The com-

plexity of the fracture should be weighed against the surgeon's experience.

Young, active patients with nondisplaced calcaneal fractures may be treated nonsurgically with early range-of-motion exercises. Cast immobilization is not required and may add to stiffness. Patients who are smokers or noncompliant with initial treatment are not good surgical candidates. However, young, healthy patients with displaced intra-articular calcaneal fractures most often warrant surgical treatment. Surgery is delayed until soft-tissue swelling has significantly subsided and the wrinkle sign is present; this often takes 3 weeks. While awaiting surgery, the patient should be placed in a bulky Jones splint with the ankle at neutral. The affected extremity must be strictly elevated to expedite resolution of soft-tissue swelling. The preferred approach is the extensile lateral approach. Studies support that an anatomic or near-anatomic reduction provides a positive effect on outcome.[2] Postoperative treatment includes immobilization with a bulky Jones splint until the wound is healed, followed by active and passive range of motion. The usual time to weight bearing is 3 months.

Surgical Approaches

The current surgical options for treating displaced calcaneal fractures can be divided into medial, lateral, and minimally invasive approaches; external fixation; and primary arthrodesis.

Medial

The medial approach allows for direct visualization of the sustentacular fragment and avoids the need for an incision through the tenuous lateral skin. However, this approach requires meticulous dissection near the neurovascular structures, and it is associated with up to a 20% incidence of injury to the medial calcaneal sensory branch. This approach allows reduction of the tuberosity by direct exposure of the medial wall, but the articular reduction must be done indirectly. In addition, the lateral wall blowout cannot be addressed through this approach, nor can any fracture involving the calcaneocuboid joint. Therefore, this approach is indicated primarily for patients with isolated fractures of the sustentaculum tali.

Combined limited medial and lateral approaches may address some of the limitations of the isolated medial approach. The medial approach is used to reduce the tuberosity fragment. A small direct lateral incision is used to reduce the posterior facet and/or anterior process fragments. The combined technique has the advantages of medial and lateral visualization, but it adds significant surgical time and risk.

Lateral

The extensile lateral surgical approach is most commonly used for the treatment of displaced calcaneal fractures. It permits direct visualization of the joint injuries and al-

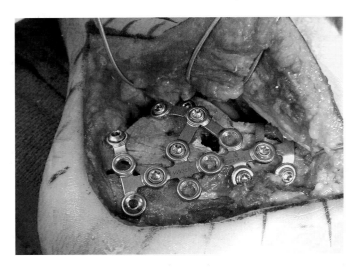

Figure 4 Photograph showing how the lateral extensile approach exposes the lateral calcaneus completely. The hardware shown is a lateral plate.

lows indirect reduction of the medial wall. Although wound breakdown is the most concerning complication associated with this approach, it can be minimized with perioperative antibiotics, cessation of smoking, allowing soft-tissue swelling to subside, and careful soft-tissue technique.[4-7] An extensile L-shaped incision is made 2 to 3 cm proximal to the tip of the fibula just anterior and parallel to the Achilles tendon, and it is extended plantarward to the junction of glabrous and nonglabrous skin. The incision then curves 90° and is extended distally approximately 3 cm. The incision curves slightly dorsal at the base of the fifth metatarsal. A full-thickness flap is created containing the peroneal tendons, sural nerve, and calcaneofibular ligament. Subperiosteal dissection is performed until the subtalar joint is reached (Figure 4). This approach allows visualization of the lateral wall, posterior facet, and calcaneocuboid joint. Comminution of the calcaneocuboid joint may preclude adequate fixation in the anterolateral fragment and may require temporary spanning of this joint with a plate. For bilateral fractures, the extensile lateral approach can be performed with the patient in the prone position.

Autograft bone has not been shown to improve functional outcome. Allograft bone or graft substitutes such as injectable cement may be used to fill the void created once the fracture fragments are elevated and reduced, but their efficacy and necessity have not been proved. Intraoperative fluoroscopy is used to assess the reduction and placement of hardware. The wound is closed in a layered fashion over a drain. The periosteum is closed by sequentially tying the sutures, beginning at the wound apex. This technique allows for reduced tension on the wound edges. The skin is then closed with modified Donati sutures.

Postoperatively, patients are placed into a compressive bulky Jones dressing and splint. Range-of-motion exercises begin once the wound edges are secure and dry.

Sutures are removed approximately 3 weeks after surgery. Patients should not bear weight for 3 months or sometimes longer in patients with severe comminution.

A large, prospective, randomized study of 309 patients with 371 fractures compared the outcomes of surgical versus nonsurgical treatment of patients with displaced intra-articular calcaneal fractures.[2] This study included 14 surgeons from seven medical centers. All surgeons used a lateral approach with rigid internal fixation for surgical treatment. Nonsurgical treatment involved no attempt at closed reduction, and patients were treated with only ice, elevation, and rest. Validated outcomes instruments were used at a minimum 2-year follow-up. Without stratification of the groups, the outcomes of nonsurgical treatment were not significantly different from those of surgical treatment. However, statistical analysis verified that women, patients who were not receiving workers' compensation, younger males, patients with a larger Böhler angle, patients with a lighter workload, and those with a single, simple displaced intra-articular calcaneal fracture have superior outcomes after surgical treatment. The findings of smaller studies support these findings and confirm the prognostic value of the Böhler angle and the poorer outcomes achieved in patients receiving workers' compensation.[1,8]

Minimally Invasive

Minimally invasive or percutaneous techniques offer an alternative approach for the treatment of certain calcaneus fracture types, especially in patients for whom the risk of open reduction is too great and nonsurgical treatment is insufficient. This technique was originally described as the Essex-Lopresti procedure and has since evolved to include fixation of simple displaced intra-articular fractures. Fractures must be treated early because organized hematoma cannot be removed percutaneously. Advantages of using this technique include less postoperative swelling, less periarticular scarring, and a greater ease of early postoperative motion. Ideally, this technique reduces postoperative wound complications, especially in patients with diabetes, peripheral vascular disease, or in those who smoke.

The fracture pattern most amenable to percutaneous techniques is the tongue type fracture in which the posterior facet is in continuity with the tuberosity. With surgeon experience, two-part joint depression fractures can be approached this way. However, in most patients, a true anatomic reduction of the articular surfaces will not be achieved. The ideal fracture pattern for this approach is a Sanders type 2C fracture in which the posterior facet is virtually intact but separated from the sustentaculum fragment.[9] Simultaneous subtalar joint arthroscopy as an adjunct to percutaneous techniques offers an exact assessment of the repair of the articular surface.[10]

External Fixation

Although infrequently used to treat calcaneal fractures, external fixation may be helpful in patients with open fractures and severe soft-tissue injury. In one study, 21 patients with 22 severe calcaneal fractures with bony defects resulting from land mine explosions were treated using a circular external fixator and osteogenic distraction.[11] A plantigrade foot was achieved in all patients, and no amputations were recorded. Fifteen patients had good to excellent results.

Primary Arthrodesis

Primary arthrodesis of the subtalar joint is recommended for some patients, primarily those with Sanders type IV highly comminuted intra-articular fractures. During the surgery, the calcaneal fracture is repaired and stabilized to reestablish the extra-articular dimensions of the calcaneus. Then the remaining cartilage is removed from both sides of the posterior facet, the surfaces are co-apted, and the bony defects are grafted. Cannulated screws are inserted using a lag technique from the posterior tuberosity of the calcaneus into the talus. Postoperatively, patients are immobilized and avoid bearing weight for 3 months. No consensus yet exists regarding which patients, if any, benefit from primary arthrodesis, but support for using fusion to treat patients with Sanders type IV fractures can be found.[3]

Whether treated nonsurgically or surgically, patients with displaced calcaneal fractures who do medium and heavy labor activities generally take longer to return to full-time work and have a larger decrease in work capability. These patients require more recovery time and a better outcome to resume heavy labor activities. More timely return to work can be facilitated by surgical management.

Complications

Compartment syndrome occurs in up to 10% of patients with displaced calcaneal fractures. Long-term sequelae of compartment syndrome of the foot include clawing of lesser toes, pain, dysesthesias, and atrophy.[12] The central compartment containing the intrinsic toe flexors is most commonly involved. A high index of suspicion and prompt fasciotomies are required to minimize chronic problems. A longitudinal, medial incision over the abductor hallucis is used to perform the fasciotomy.

The subcutaneous nature of the calcaneus renders fracture fixation problematic. Cadaveric injection studies have shown that the lateral calcaneal artery is responsible for the majority of blood flow to the surgical flap and that inaccurate incisions can add insult to this injury by rendering the flap hypoxic.[13] Wound dehiscence and necrosis occur most often at the apex of the incision. Cultures should be obtained if the wound drains for prolonged periods and patients should be treated with appropriate antibiotics, dressing changes, and surgical débridement if needed. Risk factors for wound complications include single-layered closure, high body mass index, open fractures, diabetes, and smoking.[5,7]

If an infection is superficial in patients with osteomyelitis, hardware may be kept in place to allow fracture healing. However, if an infection is deep, not treated early, and extensive, all hardware and necrotic tissue must be removed. This is a devastating complication and may result in the need for coverage or even amputation.

The axial loading mechanism of calcaneal fractures may cause damage to the septae within the heel pad. Modified shoe wear with firm heel counters and cushioned soles are used to reduce the severity of painful symptoms. Despite various attempts at treatment, no single treatment has been shown to be successful at relieving pain reproducibly. Heel pain can also occur as a result of plantar exostoses that form as a sequelae of unreduced plantar fracture fragments. These fragments may be surgically removed if nonsurgical measures fail.

Common deformities include varus malalignment, shortening with subsequent Achilles tendon contracture, and widening. Nonsurgical treatment of these deformities includes modified shoe wear and orthotic devices. If these modalities fail, surgical treatment includes corrective osteotomy with or without fusion.

In patients with subtalar arthritis, a diagnostic subtalar injection can help verify the source of pain. Initial conservative treatment modalities include orthotic devices, anti-inflammatory medications, and ambulatory aids. If these measures fail, patients may be candidates for subtalar arthrodesis. Patients with fractures with high initial energy reflected by initial Böhler angle ≤ 0,[1] those with highly comminuted fracture patterns, those receiving workers' compensation, and those with displaced intra-articular fractures that were treated nonsurgically[8] have a higher likelihood of requiring subtalar arthrodesis.

Lateral impingement and peroneal tendinitis can occur with the nonsurgical treatment of patients with calcaneal fractures with lateral wall blowout. In such patients, the fracture typically heals in this position and results in a wide heel. Lateral impingement and peroneal tendinitis can also occur after surgical treatment, but the incidence is lower with the extensile lateral approach, which maintains the tendons in a full-thickness flap.[14-16]

The sural nerve is the most common nerve to be symptomatic after a lateral approach. Damage to this nerve may result in complete loss of sensation or may lead to a painful neuroma. A neuroma can be assessed with diagnostic injections or electromyography. If patients with a painful neuroma do not respond to nonsurgical treatment, the neuroma may be resected and the remaining stump buried deep into tissue.

The posterior tibial nerve may become trapped medially, most often after nonsurgical treatment and a subsequent malunion. This can result in pain after prolonged walking or standing. A trial diagnostic injection into the tarsal tunnel or electrodiagnostic studies can help make a diagnosis.

Painful hardware occurs less commonly in patients who undergo surgical treatment for calcaneal fractures because of advancements in periarticular plating systems that use low-profile screws and plates. If irritation is caused solely by a prominent screw head, the screw can be removed percutaneously. If the patient has symptoms of cold intolerance, the hardware may be removed in its entirety, but pain relief is inconsistent.

Talar Fractures

Sixty percent of the talus is covered by articular cartilage. Vascular supply is derived from the artery of the tarsal canal, the deltoid artery, and the sinus tarsi artery. The trabecular content of the neck is substantially less and oriented in a different direction than the bone of the talar body and head. The low-density bone in the talar neck is most likely to fracture. Also, because of decreased density in this area, it is important not to excessively compress fractures and risk malreduction.

Talar Neck Fractures

More than 50% of talar fractures involve the talar neck. Comminution of the dorsal and medial regions commonly occurs. As the energy of the injury increases, the talar body may displace and dislocate out of the mortise. Talar neck fractures are classified according to the degree of displacement and attendant risk of osteonecrosis. Type I fractures are nondisplaced. Type II fractures are displaced, producing subluxation or dislocation of the subtalar joint. Type III fractures are displaced with subluxation or dislocation of the subtalar and ankle joints. Type IV fractures are displaced with subluxation or dislocation of the subtalar and ankle joints and subluxation or dislocation of the talar head from the talonavicular joint.

Displaced talar neck fractures require aggressive treatment. Shortening or malalignment significantly affect the alignment of the hindfoot and function of the subtalar joint complex. Displaced fractures must be reduced through a two-incision technique to ensure anatomic reduction and avoid malrotation. In patients with high-energy fractures, comminution at the fracture site presents challenges to maintaining reduction. Isolated screw fixation does not always prevent shortening. Plate application on the side of the talus with the most comminution (usually medially) appears to prevent varus collapse. Despite the theoretic advantages of emergent reduction, no decrease in osteonecrosis has been demonstrated with early surgery. However, frankly dislocated injuries often place the overlying skin at risk and mandate immediate realignment.

Talar Body Fractures

Talar body fractures may carry a higher rate of morbidity than talar neck fractures. Because of the location of the talar body within the mortise, surgical exposure is more difficult. Additionally, because almost the entire surface is covered by articular cartilage, fixation with hardware that can be buried into subchondral bone is required. CT helps surgeons plan screw fixation and anticipate the need for malleolar osteotomy. When osteotomy is required for access to the fracture, the medial malleolus is typically chosen because it allows preservation of the deltoid ligament attachments and vasculature to the talar body.[17] The posteromedial approach allows access to the posterior aspect of the talar body. Treatment requires lag screw fixation to allow early motion. Primary fusion can be used to treat patients with severe comminution.

Several series have recently been published describing rates of union and osteonecrosis[18-25] (Table 1). With modern fixation techniques, rates of osteonecrosis are lower than those previously reported. Subtalar and ankle posttraumatic arthrosis are the most common long-term sequelae. In short-term follow-up, relatively few patients progress to hindfoot fusions.

Open Fractures

Open fractures occur in up to 25% of patients with talar fractures. Up to 50% of Hawkins III injuries are open. Infection rates have been reported to be as high as 38%, which correlates with poor functional outcome. Despite meticulous adherence to modern techniques in soft-tissue débridement and early coverage, infection remains a risk. No consensus exists on the management of patients with a completely extruded talus. Because of high infection rates, some authors have advocated excision and early tibiocalcaneal fusion;[26] however, there are case reports in the literature that describe successful reinsertion of the extruded talus. In patients in whom stable soft-tissue coverage can be obtained and the talus is not grossly contaminated, it appears reasonable to reinsert the talar body with the awareness that there is a relatively high failure rate.

Complications

Delayed union and nonunion are more common in patients with fractures that were treated without internal fixation. Delayed union for the talus can be defined as no healing at 6 months and nonunion can be defined as no healing at 12 months. Treatment includes cancellous bone grafting and rigid fixation to maintain alignment. When alignment is satisfactory, cancellous bone graft can be inserted into the site of the defect (medial or lateral). It is rare to have a nonunion with no deformity because the neck will collapse on the side of the comminution (for example, medial comminution leads to varus collapse). When there is deformity, a corticocancellous au-

TABLE 1 | Rates of Union and Nonunion in Patients With Talar Fractures

Authors	Fracture Type	No. of Fractures	Results	Osteonecrosis	Arthritis
Fleuriau Chateau et al[18]	Neck	23	100% Union 8% Malunion	17%	9% Ankle 4% Subtalar
Jones et al[19]	Neck	47	100% Union	8.5%	21%
Schulze et al[20]	All talus	80	44% Good/very good	11%	68%
Rosati et al[21]	Neck Body		56% Good/excellent	37.5%	50%
Elgafy et al[22]	Neck	27	79 (American Orthopaedic Foot and Ankle Society score)	16% Overall 26% Body/neck	53% Subtalar 25% Ankle
	Lateral Process	22	85 (Hindfoot score)		
	Body	11	58		
Pajenda et al[23]	Neck	50	Hawkins I, II: 95% Good/excellent Hawkins III: 70% Good/excellent Hawkins IV: 10% Good/excellent	8%	48% Ankle 8% Subtalar
Low et al[24]	Neck	22	82% Good/excellent	9%	
Meinberg et al[25]	Neck	84		6%	12%

togenous graft is used to restore alignment and provide structural support. In both instances, rigid internal fixation must be used to restore or maintain alignment. Many patients with talar fractures develop posttraumatic arthritis. Both the ankle and subtalar joints can be involved, and progression appears dependent on the amount of initial cartilage damage and the quality of the reduction.

Varus and dorsiflexion are the most common deformities in patients with talar neck fractures, which can have a significant effect on hindfoot mechanics and lead to hindfoot varus and forefoot adduction. Historically, the salvage option for this problem has been triple arthrodesis; however, osteotomy of the talar neck may be attempted when the ankle and subtalar joints are still mobile and salvageable.

Osteonecrosis occurs commonly after talar neck and body fracture because of the tenuous blood supply of the talar body. Reported incidences of osteonecrosis in patients with talar neck fractures are 0 to 13% for those with Hawkins I fractures, 20% to 50% for those with Hawkins II, 20% to 100% for those with Hawkins III, and 100% for those with Hawkins IV.[22] The incidence of osteonecrosis seems to be lower in more recent series that use rigid, anatomic fixation to treat patients with talar neck fractures. Although radiographic signs of osteonecrosis may be present in this patient population, a relatively small percentage progresses to collapse of the talar neck, and revascularization can take up to 36 months.[27] The natural history of osteonecrosis is not well defined, and no evidence has yet been reported that indicates outcome is improved with prolonged periods of no weight bearing. In a recently published series of patients with talar body fractures, 38% developed osteonecrosis, 50% of whom went on to collapse of the talar

body.[27] When collapse occurred, it did so within 10 months of the injury. Patients who develop arthritis of the ankle or subtalar joint or osteonecrosis with talar body collapse have significantly worse functional outcome scores. Treatment of this complication can be challenging. The necrotic portion of the talus is débrided and a tibiocalcaneal fusion is done. If the talar head is viable, it should be preserved to save the function of the talonavicular joint. The classic Blair technique uses a sliding corticocancellous graft from the anterior tibia to the remaining talar head. This procedure can be combined with iliac crest tricortical grafts to restore height and to bridge the gap between the tibia and the calcaneus. Alternatively, the tibia can be directly fused to the calcaneus, with the subsequent limb-length discrepancy managed by tibial lengthening using the methods of Ilizarov.

Lateral Process Fractures

The proposed mechanism of injury for lateral process fractures includes dorsiflexion with inversion and an axial load; this type of injury most commonly occurs while snowboarding.[28,29] Fractures of the lateral process of the talus frequently can be missed or underestimated because of inadequate diagnostic imaging. Lateral process injuries can often be detected on AP and mortise views of the ankle. CT should be done to delineate comminution and subtalar joint involvement and to assess the size of the fragments, which can be larger than suggested by plain radiographs. Nondisplaced fractures can be treated with immobilization and protected weight bearing. Displaced fractures should be reduced and surgically fixed when the fragment is large enough. Small or comminuted fractures that are displaced can be excised. Treatment outcome seems to depend on the amount of subtalar joint involvement and the ability to reconstruct the articular surface. Late débridement typically yields less predictable results. Patients with lateral process fractures and subtalar arthrosis generally require subtalar fusion.

Tubercle Fractures

Medial tubercle fractures, which are caused by inversion and axial load on the hindfoot, are difficult to diagnose and require a high index of suspicion. They can also be associated with subtalar dislocation and detected at the time of reduction or on a postreduction CT scan. Management and outcome are similar to that for lateral process fractures; however, in tubercle fractures that are not surgically stabilized, the hindfoot must be carefully observed to ensure that a gradual drift into varus does not occur. Posterior process fractures arise from plantar flexion injuries. Again, the major difficulty in management lies in making a timely diagnosis. Posterior ankle pain and pain with forced plantar flexion are hallmarks of this injury. The fracture fragment can frequently be palpated on the medial side of the ankle at the level of the neurovascular bundle. These tubercle injuries seldom cause instability or deformity, but they can lead to chronic pain when left untreated. Smaller, minimally displaced fragments can be treated with a short course of immobilization. Displaced, small fragments can be excised. Open reduction and internal fixation has been used to treat patients with large fragments and acceptable results have been achieved.[30]

Navicular Fractures

Navicular fractures present a treatment challenge because function of the talonavicular joint is a crucial component of hindfoot motion. Fractures can be simple dorsal lip avulsions, tuberosity avulsions, body fractures, or stress fractures. All treatment decisions are predicated on maintaining talonavicular joint alignment and function.

The mechanism of injury for dorsal lip avulsions is an acute plantar flexion force with inversion. Small extraarticular fragments are commonly treated symptomatically. Patients with this type of injury must be examined closely for a concomitant midtarsal joint injury. When the fragment contains a portion of the articular surface or when there is any midtarsal instability or malalignment, open reduction and internal fixation of the fragment should be done. Transarticular screw fixation of ligamentous injuries should be done to restore stability and to preserve the alignment of the medial column.[31]

A tuberosity fracture can be an acute fracture or, more commonly, a disruption of a fibrous union of an os navicular. In both instances, the cause is an eversion force on the foot that places tension on the posterior tibialis tendon. Any displacement or involvement of the

articular surface will compromise the integrity of the posterior tibialis muscle and should be repaired. Large fragments can be addressed with lag screw fixation. Small fragments can be excised; however, if this is done, the posterior tibial tendon must be advanced and reattached to the navicular. In patients with chronic symptoms or those in whom the posterior tibial tendon will not reach the defect, transfer of the flexor digitorum longus augments the repair.

Intra-articular body fractures must be treated aggressively because of the important function of the talonavicular articulation in hindfoot motion. These fractures have been classified into three types. Type 1 fractures occur in the coronal plane with no malalignment of the remaining midfoot. Type 2 fractures occur with a dorsolateral to plantar medial fracture line, and the main fragment is usually displaced and the medial column adducted. Type 3 fractures have central or lateral comminution with abduction of the medial column and are frequently accompanied by compression injury to the lateral column. Lag screw or small plate fixation should be performed when displacement is present or when fracture location may prevent early motion. In patients with type 2 and 3 fractures, treatment focuses on restoring the talar articular surface of the navicular and maintaining the proper lengths of the medial and lateral columns of the foot. Transarticular screw fixation may be necessary to hold the navicular reduced. Fixation may be directed distally into the cuneiforms to achieve stability. In patients with severe comminution or joint instability, bridge plating may be used to maintain the length of the column until healing occurs, at which time the plate should be removed. Transarticular screws may be removed at 16 to 20 weeks or shortly after the patient has progressed to full weight bearing. In general, patients are allowed to do range-of-motion exercises once wounds are stable. They are kept on protected touchdown weight bearing for 12 weeks, at which time weight bearing is progressed. Transarticular screws and bridge plates should be removed to avoid hardware breakage. A general guideline is to remove transarticular fixation at 16 to 20 weeks. This is extrapolated from recommendations on tarsometatarsal dislocations, but no hard data exist on the optimal time for hardware removal. Once weight bearing is started, patients may benefit from using a rigid University of California Biomechanics Laboratory-type orthotic device to help support the arch. This orthotic device should be used for 6 months after injury and continued if symptoms warrant. Comminuted navicular fractures often result in long-term posttraumatic arthritis and disability. The loss of motion that accompanies many of these injuries highlights the importance of restoring proper length and alignments of the columns so a plantigrade foot can be maintained.

Stress fractures of the navicular typically occur in athletes or patients who participate in repetitive activities. Cavovarus and other more subtle malalignments may predispose patients to stress fractures of the navicular. Diagnosis of these fractures is often delayed. Physical examination usually reveals arch pain, no change in alignment, and pain with activity. Point tenderness over the navicular necessitates additional assessment, usually with nuclear medicine bone scanning followed by CT.[32] Treatment includes immobilization with strict instructions to not bear weight for 6 weeks. A gradual return to activity may be initiated when no tenderness remains at the fracture site. These patients are frequently protected by using a University of California Biomechanics Laboratory orthotic device. Healing is assessed by plain films and CT, but solid union (as identified on CT) may take many months. In patients who do not respond to nonsurgical management, surgery is indicated. Lag screw fixation is performed with the screws directed lateral to medial. The stress fracture/nonunion generally occurs in the central third, is oriented in the sagittal plane, and should be grafted with autologous bone. Patients with recurrent fracture or those who fail to heal may require evaluation of the overall alignment of the foot.

Cuboid Fractures

Most cuboid fractures are avulsions that can be seen as flakes of bone in the region of the calcaneocuboid joint on oblique radiographs of the foot. These injuries can be treated symptomatically, but as with the navicular, particular attention must be paid to alignment and length of the lateral column. Compression injuries to the cuboid (nutcracker fractures) result in shortening of the lateral column and an obligate pes planus deformity with abduction through the midfoot. The lateral column length must be restored with distraction and fixation of the cuboid and supplemented with bone graft if needed.[33] The repair often must be protected with a bridge plate or external fixator if the soft tissues are compromised.

Tarsometatarsal Fracture-Dislocations (Lisfranc Injuries)

Tarsometatarsal fracture-dislocations (Lisfranc injuries) occur in many patterns. As many as 95% of patients with tarsometatarsal injuries have associated metatarsal fractures and 39% have tarsal fractures.[34] Diagnosis of the injury is critical. Subtle disruptions can easily be missed.[35] When the mechanism of injury includes direct impact of the midfoot, crushing, or an axial load through a hyperplantarflexed foot, there should be a high index of suspicion for a tarsometatarsal fracture-dislocation. Physical examination may reveal plantar bruising, swelling through the midfoot, and tenderness across the tarsometatarsal articulation.

The anatomy of the tarsometatarsal articulation is complex. Little motion occurs in these articulations, which are predominantly flat joints. Lack of depth at the mortise joint at the base of the second metatarsal may

	No. of	
Author	**Patients**	**Results**
O'Connor et al[39]	16	Four excellent, seven good, three fair, and two poor.
Teng et al[40]	11	Despite anatomic reduction in 10 of 11 patients, normal dynamic walking patterns, American Orthopaedic Foot and Ankle Society midfoot scores averaged 71 (range, 30 to 95).
Mulier et al[41]	28	Twelve patients treated with primary arthrodesis had poorer outcomes than those with open reduction and internal fixation alone.
Vertullo et al[42]	12	Used dorsal transverse and T incisions. One wound had complications. Transverse incisions should not be used in patients that require lengthening through the tarsometatarsal joint.
Kuo et al[43]	48	52-month follow-up. Average American Orthopaedic Foot and Ankle Society score, 77. Average Musculoskeletal Functional Assessment score, 19. Six patients required late arthrodesis.

TABLE 2 | Results of Treatment of Tarsometatarsal Fracture-Dislocations

predispose patients to Lisfranc injuries.[36] The ligamentous restraints to dislocation are the dorsal tarsometatarsal ligaments, plantar tarsometatarsal ligaments, and the Lisfranc ligament from the base of the second metatarsal to the base of the medial cuneiform. The plantar and Lisfranc ligaments are significantly stronger and stiffer than the dorsal ligaments;[37] however, the dorsal cuneometatarsal ligament provides important stabilization to the base of the second metatarsal.[38]

The treatment of these injuries has evolved from closed reduction with percutaneous pinning to the open reduction and rigid internal fixation. There is now nearly universal agreement that these injuries require anatomic reduction and stable fixation to achieve a good result. Table 2 summarizes the results of recent clinical studies.[39-43] Despite anatomic reduction and restoration of normal gait mechanics, many patients can still have long-term symptoms, which are presumably related primarily to arthrosis of the involved joints.

Fractures and Dislocations of the Metatarsals

During the stance phase, each of the lesser metatarsals supports an equal load, with the first metatarsal supporting twice this amount.[44] Significant displacement alters the loading patterns of the foot, leading to metatarsalgia or transfer metatarsalgia.[44] A direct force or crush mech-

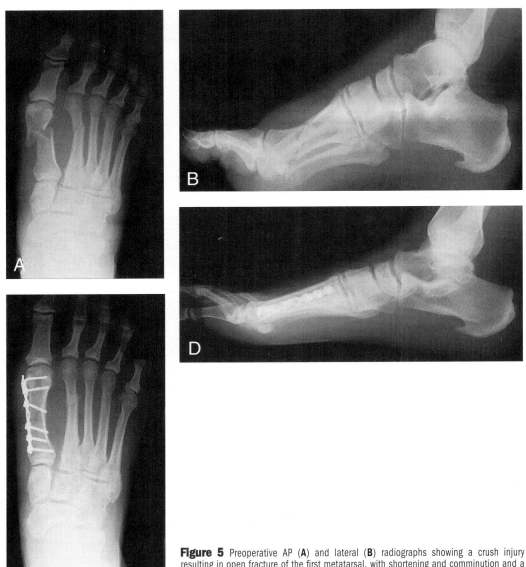

Figure 5 Preoperative AP (**A**) and lateral (**B**) radiographs showing a crush injury resulting in open fracture of the first metatarsal, with shortening and comminution and a second metatarsal fracture. Postoperative AP (**C**) and lateral (**D**) radiographs at 3 months show healed fractures. Treatment included irrigation, débridement, and internal fixation with a mini-fragment blade plate. *(Reproduced with permission from Stephen DJG: Injuries of the midfoot and forefoot, in Schatzker J, Tile M (eds): The Rationale of Operative Fracture Care, ed 3. New York, NY, Springer-Verlag, 2005.)*

anism is usually responsible for fractures of the second, third, and fourth metatarsals and often causes multiple fractures. An indirect force, such as twisting of the foot (inversion), often causes fractures of the fifth metatarsal. Patients with multiple injuries may have missed or neglected metatarsal fractures. Care must be taken to evaluate swelling, pain, and/or deformity in the region of the forefoot. Radiologic evaluation includes anteroposterior, lateral, and oblique views centered over the forefoot. Nondisplaced fractures of the metatarsal shaft or neck can be treated functionally to allow early weight bearing. Fractures of the diaphysis of the first metatarsal require correction of dorsal or plantar displacement. Comminuted fractures of the first metatarsal may result in a

shortened first ray and lead to second ray transfer metatarsalgia. The length of the first ray must be restored, either by closed means (finger traps) and percutaneous Kirschner wire fixation to the second metatarsal or by open reduction and internal fixation via a dorsomedial incision using wires or low-profile plates and screws[45] (Figure 5). Intra-articular fractures of the first metatarsocuneiform joint must be reduced anatomically, with either closed or open reduction. In patients with comminuted fractures of this joint, primary fusion may be indicated. Displaced fractures of the lesser metatarsals that are amenable to closed reduction require percutaneous intramedullary Kirschner wire fixation or cross fixation to an adjacent metatarsal. Persistent plantar prominence of the head of the fractured metatarsal resulting from plantar or dorsal fracture displacement mandates open reduction via a dorsal incision with intramedullary Kirschner wire or plate fixation. Depending on the severity and number of injuries, weight bearing is initiated at approximately 4 to 6 weeks, at which time Kirschner wires are typically removed. A custom-molded arch support may be beneficial when casting or bracing is discontinued.

Metatarsal head fractures usually require functional management directed at regaining unrestricted metatarsophalangeal joint motion for gait. If closed reduction is successful, the injured toe is buddy taped to an adjacent toe. Persistent displacement necessitates open reduction via a dorsal incision to prevent late metatarsalgia. Sesamoid views often help determine whether this procedure is necessary. The dorsal capsule is split longitudinally, with care taken to protect both neurovascular bundles. A Kirschner wire is inserted through the metatarsal head and out of the plantar surface of the foot. The fracture is then reduced, and the Kirschner wire is advanced retrograde into the metatarsal shaft. A well-molded weight-bearing cast or a postoperative shoe is applied, and the Kirschner wires are removed 3 weeks after injury. Mini-fragment and/or mini-Herbert screws can be used.

Dislocations of the metatarsophalangeal joints usually can be treated with closed reduction and buddy taping. In patients who do not seek treatment immediately after injury or in those with irreducible or unstable dislocations, open reduction and Kirschner wire fixation may be required. In patients with irreducible dislocations of the metatarsophalangeal joints, the plantar plate or the sesamoids can be incarcerated in the joint.[46] For the irreducible first metatarsophalangeal joint, a medial incision allows access to the sesamoids and plantar plate (Figure 6).

A fractured sesamoid must be differentiated from a bipartite sesamoid and osteochondritis dissecans of the sesamoid. The former has smooth, sclerotic edges, whereas the latter has fragmentation and irregularity. The initial treatment of a sesamoid fracture involves a short leg weight-bearing cast, followed by a metatarsal pad behind the head of the first metatarsal. Symptoms may persist for 4 to 6 months; therefore, patients must be aware of the possibility of prolonged disability. If significant pain and disability persist for more than 6 months, partial excision of the fractured sesamoid is indicated. Total sesamoid excision should be avoided.

Fractures of the Proximal Fifth Metatarsal

The proximal fifth metatarsal has been divided into three zones[47] (Figure 7, *A*). Zone 1 fractures begin laterally on the tuberosity and extend proximally entering the metatarsocuboid joint. This area is made up of cancellous bone and has an excellent blood supply.[48] The mechanism of injury is inversion causing an avulsion by the peroneus brevis tendon and/or the lateral portion of the plantar aponeurosis. Most of these fractures heal with only symptomatic treatment with a postoperative firm sole shoe and weight bearing as tolerated. A persistent radiolucent line, which suggests a delayed union or a nonunion, is rarely symptomatic. Patients with chronic pain that is refractory to conservative measures may require excision of small fragments or fixation of larger fragments (Figure 7, *B*).

Zone 2 fractures begin more distal on the tuberosity, entering the articulation between the fourth and fifth metatarsals.[49] These injuries are more symptomatic and often require treatment with a short leg weight-bearing cast. There is often more comminution of the fracture. The recovery period for these fractures is often prolonged and patients may remain symptomatic for several months.

Zone 3 fractures occur in the metadiaphysis distal to the strong intermetatarsal ligaments. Fractures in this zone are usually stress fractures and typically occur in competitive athletes involved in running or jumping and pivoting activities. These fractures have a high risk of delayed union and nonunion, especially in patients who continue moderate activity.[49] Patients with zone 3 fractures often have a history of 2 to 3 weeks of ankle or foot pain. Radiologic evaluation during this prodrome period reveals subperiosteal reaction with new bone formation at the area of maximal tenderness. When no changes are seen on plain films, technetium bone scanning may show increased uptake in this region. At this stage before fracture, modification of activity and symptomatic treatment are usually successful. If there is an obvious fracture and patients need to resume athletic or employment activities quickly, surgical management may be relatively indicated. If there is no urgency, patients can be treated with a short leg weight-bearing cast. Although controversial, there is no evidence to indicate that refraining from bearing weight improves the outcome in patients with zone 3 fractures.[49]

The fifth metatarsal shaft is triangular and often bowed, which makes percutaneous placement of a screw difficult. Patients are placed either in the lateral decubitus position or with the affected limb internally rotated approximately 45°. A 2- to 3-cm dorsolateral incision is made, with retraction of the peroneus brevis tendon.[49] Image intensification and the use of a cannulated system can help place the cancellous compression screw. It is recommended that the fracture site be explored if there is any preexisting sclerosis, in which instance the fixation should be supplemented with bone graft. Patients should not bear weight for approximately 2 to 3 weeks, followed by the use of a weight-bearing cast for 4 to 6 weeks. The decision whether to continue immobilization or return to graduated activities is based on the results of clinical and radiologic evaluations. A functional wrap-around thermoplastic brace may be used for 4 to 6 weeks after the

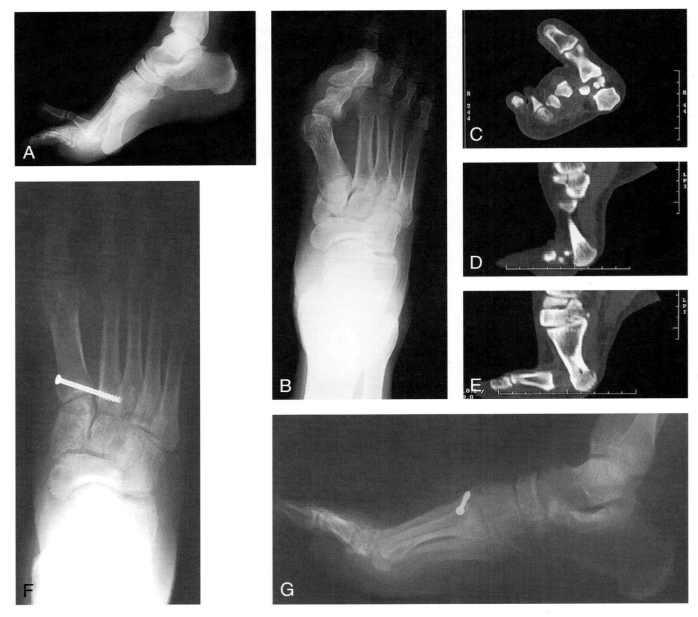

Figure 6 A and **B**, Radiographs showing an irreducible dislocation of the first metatarsophalangeal joint in a 50-year-old male patient who was involved in a motor vehicle collision. This dislocation was irreducible. **C** through **E**, Transverse and sagittal CT scans demonstrate incarcerated sesamoids. Open reduction was carried out via a medial approach, and partial excision of the medial sesamoid was required as a result of comminution. The first metatarsocuneiform joint was unstable during stress examination and was stabilized with a single cancellous screw (**F** and **G**). *(Reproduced with permission from Stephen DJG: Injuries of the midfoot and forefoot, in Schatzker J, Tile M (eds): The Rationale of Operative Fracture Care, ed 3. New York, NY, Springer Verlag, 2005.)*

cast is removed, especially in patients returning to high-risk activities. For patients with acute fractures treated without fixation, there is a 38% incidence of delayed union and a 14% incidence of nonunion.[50] Supplemental bone graft is indicated for patients with a persistent gap at a nonunion site despite screw compression or in those in whom the site is opened.

Compartment Syndromes of the Foot
Crush injuries, forefoot and midfoot fractures (and/or dislocations), and fractures of the calcaneus can increase the risk of compartment syndrome in the foot.[51,52] The typical clinical findings found with compartment syndromes in the lower leg and forearm are less reliable than those in the foot. Although extreme swelling may increase suspicion of compartment syndrome, invasive measures are often required for definitive diagnosis. At least nine compartments exist in the foot[53] (Table 3). Three incisions (two dorsal and one medial) usually are used to gain access to the foot compartments.[53] A 6-cm incision is made medially, approximately 4 cm from the posterior aspect of the heel and 3 cm from the plantar

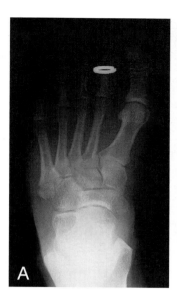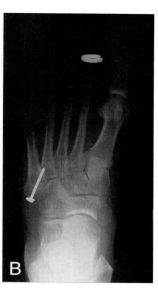

Figure 7 A, Radiograph showing an inversion injury resulting in an open (< 1 cm) fracture of the proximal fifth metatarsal tuberosity in a 35-year-old patient. Zones 1 through 3 of the proximal fifth metatarsal are shown. **B**, Treatment consisted of irrigation and débridement, followed by internal fixation with a 2.7-mm lag screw. *(Reproduced with permission from Stephen DJG: Injuries of the midfoot and forefoot, in Schatzker J, Tile M (eds): The Rationale of Operative Fracture Care, ed 3. New York, NY, Springer Verlag, 2005.)*

TABLE 3	Compartments of the Foot

Hindfoot (one compartment)

Calcaneal

  Muscle:

    Quadratus plantae

  Neurovascular structures:

    Posterior tibial nerve, artery, vein (site of communication with deep posterior leg compartment)

    Lateral plantar nerve, artery, vein

    +/− medial plantar nerve

Forefoot (five compartments)

Interosseous (×4)

  Interossei

Adductor

  Adductor

Full length (three compartments)

Medial

  Flexor hallucis

  Abductor hallucis

Lateral

  Abductor digiti quinti

  Flexor digiti minimi

Superficial

  Flexor digitorum brevis

  Lumbricals (4)

  Flexor digitorum longus

  +/− medial plantar nerve

(Adapted with permission from Fulkerson E, Razi A, Tejwani N: Review: Acute compartment syndrome of the foot. *Foot Ankle Int* 2003;24:180-187.)

surface, and is slightly concave plantar to follow the contour of the plantar surface of the foot.[52] The fascia over the abductor hallucis is released (medial compartment), and this muscle is reflected plantar or dorsal to expose the medial intermuscular septum. This structure is opened to expose the lateral plantar nerve and vessels in the region of the quadratus plantae muscle, which is in the calcaneal compartment. This compartment has been shown to communicate with the deep posterior compartment of the lower leg.[53] The superficial central compartment containing the flexor digitorum brevis is opened by staying superficial to the abductor hallucis fascia. Then the lateral compartment (abductor digiti quinti) is released by retracting the flexor digitorum brevis plantarward. Two dorsal incisions are made, over to the second and fourth metatarsals, allowing release of the four interosseous compartments. The adductor hallucis compartment is released by dissecting along the medial border of the second metatarsal in a subperiosteal fashion. If the patient has underlying fractures, the incisions may be modified depending on the exposure required for internal fixation. The wounds are left open and closed or grafted, usually within 7 days.

The most common deformity observed in patients with untreated compartment syndrome is claw toes. A cavus foot has also been reported. Ischemic injury to the intrinsic musculature is thought to be the cause of these deformities. As a result of the communication between the compartments in the foot and leg, a compartment syndrome of the deep compartment of the leg can result in claw toes. Late correction of claw toes can be done using either proximal interphalangeal joint excision arthroplasties or a flexor-to-extensor tendon transfer in patients with flexible claw toes.

Annotated References

1. Loucks C, Buckley R: Bohler's angle: Correlation with outcome in displaced intra-articular calcaneal fractures. *J Orthop Trauma* 1999;13:554-558.

2. Buckley R, Tough S, McCormack R, et al: Operative compared with nonoperative treatment of displaced intra-articular calcaneal fractures: A prospective, randomized, controlled multicenter trial. *J Bone Joint Surg Am* 2002;84:1733-1744.

   The authors of this study report that although overall outcomes were similar in surgically treated and nonsurgically treated fractures, surgical treatment produced significantly better results in women, patients not receiving workers' compensation, men younger than 29 years, and those with a lower Böhler angle (0° to 14°), a comminuted fracture, a light workload, or an anatomic reduction.

3. Sanders R: Displaced intra-articular fractures of the calcaneus. *J Bone Joint Surg Am* 2000;82:225-250.
   The author of this article discusses the mechanism, treatment, and complications of calcaneal fractures.

4. Barei D, Bellabarba C, Sangeorzan B, Benirschke S: Fractures of the calcaneus. *Orthop Clin North Am* 2002;33:263-285.

5. Abidi N, Dhawan S, Gruen G, Vogt M, Conti S: Wound-healing risk factors after open reduction and internal fixation of calcaneal fractures. *Foot Ankle Int* 1998;19:856-861.

6. Assous M, Bhamra M: Should os calcis fractures in smokers be fixed? A review of 40 patients. *Injury* 2001;32:631-632.

7. Ebraheim N, Elgafy H, Sabry F, Tao S: Calcaneus fractures with subluxation of the posterior facet: A surgical indication. *Clin Orthop* 2000;377:210-216.

8. Csizy M, Buckley R, Tough S, et al: Displaced intra-articular calcaneal fractures: Variables predicting late subtalar fusion. *J Orthop Trauma* 2003;17:106-112.
   In this study, subtalar distraction bone-block arthrodesis with tricortical bone graft was used to treat 45 displaced intra-articular calcaneal fractures. The authors found that the amount of initial injury involved with the calcaneal fracture was the primary prognostic determinant of long-term patient outcome.

9. Tornetta P III: Percutaneous treatment of calcaneal fractures. *Clin Orthop* 2000;375:91-96.
   The author of this study assessed 46 patients with 41 successful closed reductions of 36 type IIC and 5 type IIB tongue-type fractures of the calcaneus. The surgical technique described is a modification of the original Essex-Lopresti maneuver. The Maryland Foot Score and radiographs were used to evaluate patients. At a mean follow-up of 3.4 years, 85% of patients reported good to excellent results; no poor results were reported.

10. Gavlik J, Rammelt S, Zwipp H: Percutaneous, arthroscopically-assisted osteosynthesis of calcaneus fractures. *Arch Orthop Trauma Surg* 2002;122:424-428.
    Fifteen patients with Sanders 2A and 2B fractures were managed with subtalar arthroscopy and percutaneous reduction techniques. Anatomic joint position was achieved in 13 patients.

11. Ebraheim N, Elgafy H, Sabry F, Freih M, Abou-Chakra I: Sinus tarsi approach with transarticular fixation for displaced intra-articular fractures of the calcaneus. *Foot Ankle Int* 2000;21:105-113.

12. Myerson M, Manoli A: Compartment syndromes of the foot after calcaneal fractures. *Clin Orthop* 1993; 290:142-150.

13. Borrelli J Jr, Lashgari C: Vascularity of the lateral calcaneal flap: A cadaveric injection study. *J Orthop Trauma* 1999;13:73-77.

14. Isbister JF: Calcaneo-fibular abutment following crush fracture of the calcaneus. *J Bone Joint Surg Br* 1974;56:274-278.

15. Gould N: Lateral approach to the os calcis. *Foot Ankle* 1984;4:218-220.

16. Zwipp H, Tscherne H, Thermann H, Weber T: Osteosynthesis of displaced intraarticular fractures of the calcaneus: Results in 123 cases. *Clin Orthop* 1993; 290:76-86.

17. Ziran BH, Abidi NA, Scheel MJ: Medial malleolar osteotomy for exposure of complex talar body fractures. *J Orthop Trauma* 2001;15:513-518.
    The authors of this article used a technique of medial malleolar osteotomy in a small series of patients to gain access to the talar body because traditional approaches did not provide adequate exposure.

18. Fleuriau Chateau PB, Brokaw DS, Jelen BA, Scheid DK, Weber TG: Plate fixation of talar neck fractures: Preliminary review of a new technique in twenty-three patients. *J Orthop Trauma* 2002;16:213-219.
    In this study, 23 displaced fractures were managed with small plate stabilization. The authors report healing without varus collapse.

19. Jones CB, Zietz PM, Ringler JR, Endres TJ, Anderson JJ, Bohay DR: Technique and results of mini-fragment plate fixation of talar neck fractures. *Proceedings of the Orthopaedic Trauma Association 19th Annual Meeting, Salt Lake City, UT, November 11, 2003.* Rosemont, IL. Orthopaedic Trauma Association, 2003. Available at: http://www.hwbf.org/ota/am/ota03/otapa/OTA03746.htm. Accessed February 16, 2005.

20. Schulze W, Richter J, Russe O, Ingelfinger P, Muhr G: Surgical treatment of talus fractures: A retrospective study of 80 cases followed for 1-15 years. *Acta Orthop Scand* 2002;73:344-351.

21. Rosati M, Longo G, Nesti C, Lisanti M: Our experience in treatment of fractures of the astragalus. *Chir Organi Mov* 2001;86:45-53.

22. Elgafy H, Ebraheim NA, Tile M, Stephen D, Kase J: Fractures of the talus: Experience of two-level one trauma centers. *Foot Ankle Int* 2000;21:1023-1029.

23. Pajenda G, Vecsei V, Reddy B, Heinz T: Treatment of talar neck fractures: Clinical results of 50 patients. *J Foot Ankle Surg* 2000;39:365-375.

24. Low CK, Chong CK, Wong HP, Low YP: Operative treatment of displaced talar neck fractures. *Ann Acad Med Singapore* 1998;27:763-766.

25. Meinberg EG, Kellam JF, Bosse MT, Obremskey WT: Timing of surgical fixation of talar neck fractures. *Proceedings of the Orthopaedic Trauma Association 19th Annual Meeting, Salt Lake City, UT, November 11, 2003.* Rosemont, IL, Orthopaedic Trauma Association, 2003. Available at: http://www.hwbf.org/ota/am/ota03/otapa/OTA03745.htm. Accessed February 16, 2005.

26. Marsh JL, Saltzman CL, Iverson M, Shapiro DS: Major open injuries of the talus. *J Orthop Trauma* 1995;9:371-376.

27. Vallier HA, Nork SE, Benirschke SK, Sangeorzan BJ: Surgical treatment of talar body fractures. *J Bone Joint Surg Am* 2003;85-A:1716-1724.

28. Chan GM, Yoshida D: Fracture of the lateral process of the talus associated with snowboarding. *Ann Emerg Med* 2003;41:854-858.

29. Boon AJ, Smith J, Zobitz ME, Amrami KM: Snowboarders talus fracture: Mechanism of injury. *Am J Sports Med* 2001;29:333-338.

30. Nadim Y, Tosic A, Ebrahein N: Open reduction and internal fixation of fracture of the posterior process of the talus: A case report and review of the literature. *Foot Ankle Int* 1999;20:50-52.

31. Schildhauer TA, Nork SE, Sangeorzan BJ: Temporary bridge plating of the medial column in severe midfoot injuries. *J Orthop Trauma* 2003;17:513-520.

32. Boden BP, Osbahn DC: High risk stress fractures: Evaluation and treatment. *J Am Acad Orthop Surg* 2000;8:344-353.

33. Weber M, Lochner S: Reconstruction of the cuboid in compression fractures: Short to midterm results in 12 patients. *Foot Ankle Int* 2002;23:1008-1013.

34. Vuori JP, Aro HT: Lisfranc joint injuries: Trauma mechanisms and associated injuries. *J Trauma* 1993;35:40-45.

35. Philbin T, Rosenberg G, Sterra JJ: Complications of missed or untreated Lisfranc injuries. *Foot Ankle Clin* 2003;8:61-71.

36. Peicha G, Labovitz J, Seibert FJ, et al: The anatomy of the joint as a risk factor for Lisfranc dislocation and fracture dislocation: An anatomical and radiological case control study. *J Bone Joint Surg Br* 2002;84:981-985.

37. Solan MC, Moorman CT III, Miyamato RG, Jasper LE, Belkoff SM: Ligamentous restraints of the second tarsometatarsal joint: A biomechanical evaluation. *Foot Ankle Int* 2001;22:637-641.

38. Kura H, Luo ZP, Kitawla HB, Snutz WP, An KN: Mechanical behavior of the Lisfranc and dorsal cuneometatarsal ligaments: In vitro biomechanical study. *J Orthop Trauma* 2001;15:107-110.

39. O'Connor PA, Yeap S, Noel J, et al: Lisfranc injuries: Patient- and physician-based functional outcomes. *Int Orthop* 2003;27:98-102.

40. Teng AL, Pinzur MS, Lomasney L, Mahoney L, Harvey R: Functional outcome following anatomic restoration of tarsometatarsal fracture dislocation. *Foot Ankle Int* 2002;23:922-926.

41. Mulier T, Reynders P, Dereymaeker G, Zroor P: Severe Lisfranc injuries: Primary arthrodesis or ORIF? *Foot Ankle Int* 2002;23:902-905.

42. Vertullo CJ, Easley ME, Nunley JA: The transverse dorsal approach to the Lisfranc joint. *Foot Ankle Int* 2002;23:420-426.

43. Kuo RS, Tejwani NC, Digiovanni CW, et al: Outcome after open reduction and internal fixation of Lisfranc joint injuries. *J Bone Joint Surg Am* 2000;82:1609-1618.

    The authors of this study report that at 52-month follow-up, 48 patients with purely ligamentous injuries had worse outcomes than patients with ligamentous and osseous injuries. Anatomic reduction was the major determinant of good results.

44. Shereff MJ: Fractures of the forefoot. *Instr Course Lect* 1990;39:133-140.

45. DeLee JG: Fractures and dislocations of the foot, in Mann RA, Coughlin MJ (eds): *Surgery of the Foot and Ankle*, ed 6. St. Louis, MO, Mosby, 1986.

46. Jahss MH: Traumatic dislocations of the first metatarsophalangeal joint. *Foot Ankle* 1980;1:15-21.

47. Lawrence SJ, Botte MJ: Jones fractures and related fractures of the proximal fifth metatarsal. *Foot Ankle* 1993;14:358-365.

48. Smith JW, Arnoczky SP, Hersh A: The intraosseous blood supply of the fifth metatarsal: Implications for proximal fracture healing. *Foot Ankle* 1992;13:143-152.

49. Dameron TB: Fractures of the proximal fifth metatarsal: Selecting the best treatment option. *J Am Acad Orthop Surg* 1995;3:110-114.

50. Arangio GA: Proximal diaphyseal fractures of the fifth metatarsal (Jones' fractures): Two cases treated by cross pinning with review of 106 cases. *Foot Ankle* 1983;3:293-296.

51. Myerson MS: Experimental decompression of the fascial compartments of the foot: The basis for fasciotomy in acute compartment syndromes. *Foot Ankle* 1988;8:308-314.

52. Manoli A II: Foot fellows review: Compartment syndromes of the foot. *Foot Ankle* 1990;10:340-344.

53. Manoli A II, Weber TG: Fasciotomy of the foot: An anatomical study with special reference to release of the calcaneal compartment. *Foot Ankle* 1990;10:267-275.

Section 6

Geriatric and Pediatric Trauma

Section Editor:
Kenneth J. Koval, MD

Chapter 40

Perioperative and Postoperative Considerations in the Geriatric Patient

Kenneth A. Egol, MD

Indications for Surgery

There is near-universal agreement that optimum recovery can best be accomplished surgically in patients with hip fractures. Historically, nonsurgical management has resulted in high rates of medical morbidity and mortality, as well as malunion and nonunion. Nonsurgical management is appropriate only in selected nonambulatory patients who experience minimal discomfort from their injuries. Certainly, other lower extremity fracture patterns require surgical intervention in the elderly population. Most subtrochanteric and femoral shaft fractures require surgical stabilization to promote early mobilization, pain control, and prevention of further soft-tissue damage. Other lower extremity fractures in the elderly population are treated either surgically or nonsurgically depending on several patient factors, such as comorbid medical conditions, preinjury level of function, and bone quality. If nonsurgical treatment of a lower extremity fracture is chosen, these patients should be rapidly mobilized to avoid the complications of prolonged recumbency, which can include decubiti, atelectasis, urinary tract infection, and thrombophlebitis.

The indications for surgical treatment of upper extremity fractures in the elderly population follow those for younger patients and include fracture displacement that is not amenable to closed treatment, significant intra-articular displacement, multiple fractures, and open wounds. In patients with these types of injuries, medical contraindications and the possibility of permanent functional limitations must be considered. Nonsurgical treatment of such patients will cause less impairment of ambulatory ability.[1]

Timing of Surgery

In general, lower extremity fracture surgery should be performed as soon as possible after optimization of treatable comorbid medical conditions; in this respect, particular attention must be paid to cardiopulmonary problems and fluid and electrolyte imbalances. In one series of 399 patients with hip fractures, it was reported that a surgical delay of less than 1 week to stabilize medical problems was not associated with increased mortality.[2] Interestingly, the authors found that even healthy patients who underwent surgery within 24 hours of hospital admission had a 34% rate of mortality at 1-year follow-up versus 5.8% for those who underwent surgery between the second and fifth days. Another study found that relatively healthy patients with hip fractures (those with up to two comorbid conditions) who had surgery within 24 hours after admission had a higher survival rate than similar patients who had surgery after 24 hours.[3] However, patients with three or more comorbid conditions had a poorer survival rate when they underwent surgical treatment within 24 hours than those who underwent surgical treatment after 24 hours. A more recent prospectively followed series of 367 elderly patients with hip fractures reported that a surgical delay of more than 2 calendar days from hospital admission approximately doubled the risk of the patient dying before the end of the first postoperative year.[4] This relationship was significant when the patient age, sex, and the number of comorbidities were controlled.

Medical Evaluation

Although advanced age is not an independent risk factor for complication after surgery, older people tend to have more coexisting medical conditions that affect surgical risk. These factors must be evaluated to optimize the patient's outcome. Many elderly patients have pulmonary, renal, cardiovascular, or neurologic disorders that are concurrent with the normal aging process, and they may be taking multiple medications. The anesthesiologist frequently assumes care for chronically ill patients who have recently experienced an acute traumatic episode with associated pain, anemia, and hypovolemia.

Comorbid conditions that can affect surgical risk are listed in Table 1. The mortality rate in patients with these comorbid conditions in the first year after a hip fracture can range from 14% to 36%.[2] The outcome of patients with fractured hips has been studied in relation to comorbidity.[5,6] In patients with four to six comorbidities, the mortality rate was significantly greater than in pa-

TABLE 1 | Comorbid Conditions Affecting Surgical Risk

Hypertension
Diabetes
Cardiac disease
Chronic obstructive pulmonary disease
Neurologic disorders
Gastrointestinal disorders
Genitourinary disorders

tients with zero to three comorbidities. In determining morbidity and mortality rates based on the American Society of Anesthesiologists' classification of surgical risk, another study noted that patients identified as American Society of Anesthesiologists' grade I or II were at no greater risk of mortality than age- and sex-matched control subjects (mortality rate, 8% per year). However, patients identified as American Society of Anesthesiologists' grade III or IV had significantly higher mortality rates than control subjects (49% or 6.3 times that of the control group).[1]

One study reported that comorbidity is a predictor of postoperative death in patients undergoing noncardiac surgery.[7] Decreased renal function (low creatinine clearance), history of hypertension or use of antihypertensive agents, and severely limited activity were associated with increased mortality rates. There was a 20% mortality rate when two or more factors were present, which was eight times the mortality rate of patients with no or one risk factor.

Cardiac Evaluation

The American College of Cardiology and the American Heart Association have recently published guidelines on the perioperative cardiac evaluation of patients undergoing noncardiac surgery. In summary, these guidelines suggest that the need for further cardiac workup is identical whether or not the patient requires surgical intervention. A perioperative stress test should be considered in patients who have an unstable cardiac profile and in those patients who have new onset angina or a change in their anginal pattern. Patients with fractures of the proximal femur should have a dipyridamole thallium stress test or a dobutamine echocardiogram stress test. Additionally, a cardiac stress test should be considered in patients in whom the mechanism of injury suggests a cardiac event. An echocardiogram may also be useful in patients with a history of angina; for patients with decreased left ventricular function, a more aggressive medical approach should be taken.

Pulmonary Evaluation

Multiple studies seem to suggest that the most important factor in determining risk of pulmonary complication in the perioperative period is a prior history of smoking and a low oxygen level as determined by arterial blood gas monitoring. Incentive spirometry has not been shown to be particularly useful in the prevention of pulmonary complications. Controversy exists whether preoperative treatment and optimization of patients with chronic obstructive pulmonary disease are useful in the prevention of postoperative pulmonary complications.

Diabetes

Diabetes mellitus is a comorbid condition that is common in the elderly population. For these patients, oral hypoglycemic agents are usually stopped the morning of surgery. Serum glucose levels are checked every 4 to 6 hours, and sliding scale low-dose regular insulin is administered to blunt the onset of severe hyperglycemia. Intravenous fluids should not contain glucose. Oral hypoglycemic agents are resumed when the patient is eating well. For the patient who requires insulin, a general rule of thumb is to give one third to one half of the usual dose of long-acting insulin on the morning of surgery, with an intravenous drip containing dextrose. A sliding scale of insulin coverage is also required.

Anemia

Elderly patients are frequently anemic secondary to coexisting medical conditions or bleeding at the fracture site. A reasonable rule of thumb is that otherwise healthy elderly patients can tolerate a hemoglobin level as low as 8.0 g/dL, whereas those with cardiac or pulmonary disease should maintain a hemoglobin level above 9.0 to 10.0 g/dL. The temptation to perform automatic transfusion in elderly patients should be resisted. In addition to direct transmission of infectious diseases such as hepatitis and acquired immunodeficiency syndrome, there is evidence that allogeneic blood transfusion is associated with immunosuppression. A prospective study of 687 community dwelling, geriatric patients with hip fractures reported that allogeneic red blood cell transfusion was associated with an increased incidence of postoperative infection.[8] There are no known studies that define an acceptable hematocrit level before surgery; the accepted preoperative hemoglobin level should be based on the expected blood loss.

Deep Venous Thrombosis Prophylaxis

Patients who have sustained a lower extremity fracture are at increased risk for thrombophlebitis.[9] The reported incidence of deep venous thrombosis after hip fracture is 36% to 60% of patients, whereas the incidence of thrombi involving the proximal venous system ranges between 17% and 36%.[10,11] A review of the medical literature revealed that the overall reported incidence of pulmonary embolus after hip fracture ranges from 4.3% to 24% of patients, whereas overall the incidence of fatal pulmonary embolus ranges from 3.6% to 12.9%. Thrombi limited to the veins in the lower leg are rarely associated with pulmonary emboli. Popliteal and more proximal venous thrombi carry a much higher risk of pulmonary emboli. However, most deep venous thrombi that occur above the knee represent extensions of thrombi from the venous system in the lower leg. Some authors recommend duplex screening for all patients with hip fractures during the postoperative period.[12]

Additional clinical risk factors for deep venous thrombosis include advanced patient age, previous venous thromboembolism, malignant disease, congestive heart failure, prolonged immobility or paralysis, obesity, and deep system venous disease. In a recent prospective study of 133 hip fracture patients who underwent venography upon hospital admission, 13 (9.8%) had evidence of deep venous thrombosis; patients for whom hospital presentation was delayed more than 2 days from injury were at significantly increased risk for deep venous thrombosis (55% versus 6%).[13] The two approaches that can be used to prevent fatal pulmonary embolism are (1) early detection of subclinical venous thrombosis by screening high-risk patients and (2) primary prophylaxis using either drugs or physical methods that are effective for preventing deep venous thrombosis and pulmonary embolism. Several prophylactic measures have been recommended, including subcutaneous heparin, low-molecular-weight heparin, intravenous dextran, warfarin sodium, aspirin, intermittent pneumatic compression of the foot or leg, and various combined modalities.[14,15]

The use of some of these regimens in elderly patients with fractures has been extrapolated from their use in patients undergoing total hip replacement. Aspirin is effective and has the advantages of low cost and easy administration. However, its effectiveness has been demonstrated primarily in men. Although warfarin (Coumadin) has been shown to be effective in preventing fatal pulmonary embolism, it results in an increased incidence of bleeding problems (hematoma), particularly when the prothrombin time of patients exceeds 1.5 times that of control subjects. Dextran alone or in combination with dihydroergotamine has also been shown to be effective. However, dextran requires a large fluid administration that increases the risk of fluid overload. Low-dose intravenous heparin or heparin in combination with dihydroergotamine has been effective specifically in patients with hip fracture, whereas low-dose subcutaneous heparin has not been shown to be effective. The subcutaneous injection of low-molecular-weight heparin has been shown to be an effective prophylaxis in patients undergoing total joint arthroplasty and hip fracture surgery. Intermittent external pneumatic compression may also be of value, but the cost of specialized equipment and the need for recumbency limit its usefulness.

Pain Issues

Issues of pain control in elderly patients undergoing orthopaedic fracture surgery involve more than deciding which opiate to administer. Elderly patients are frequently either undermedicated, which can lead to increased morbidity, or overmedicated, which can lead to respiratory depression or delirium.

Most guidelines for the assessment and treatment of acute pain in the elderly population involve a baseline pain assessment. This is accomplished by obtaining a pain history if possible, determining the mental status of the patient, degree of family involvement, and selection of a pain intensity tool to be used repeatedly throughout the course of treatment. The pain history should include previous use of analgesic medications, including those that relieved pain as well as those that did not.

In confused or noncommunicative patients, nonverbal cues should be assessed. These include behavioral cues such as restlessness, agitation, guarding, splinting, rocking, or rapid blinking. Verbal cues such as moaning, groaning, crying, grunting, or the use of profanity can signal the presence of acute pain. Facial expressions such as brow lowering, jaw dropping, clenched teeth, or wincing can alert the physician to untreated pain problems. Finally, physiologic changes such as changes in pulse rate or blood pressure in the absence of a medical cause are signs of increased pain in these patients.[16]

Elderly patients and especially cognitively impaired elderly patients generally receive substantially less pain medication that younger adults.[17] Furthermore, many elderly patients have medical comorbidities that may influence the choice as well as dosage of selected analgesics. Drug interactions and potential complications must be considered when choosing an analgesic. With regard to dosing, elderly patients generally receive greater peak and longer duration of analgesic action than younger patients because of slower clearance in elderly patients. Thus, elderly patients should be started at lower doses of analgesics than younger patients and the dosage slowly increased based on pain reduction ratings.[18]

Route of administration should be the least invasive and safest. Oral administration should be considered first in these patients. Postsurgical analgesia is best accomplished via intravenous or epidural access. Medications include both opioid and nonopioids. Morphine sulfate, hydromorphone, oxycodone, and intravenous fentanyl (all opioid medications) are acceptable for use in the elderly population. Demerol should be avoided because its use is associated with the development of delirium. Nonsteroidal anti-inflammatory medications and acetaminophen are the mainstays of the nonopioid medications. Nephrotoxicity, bleeding, and confusion are the adverse effects that can be associated with the use of nonsteroidal anti-inflammatory medications.

TABLE 2 | Multidisciplinary Care

An acute care evaluation should be performed by an orthopaedist that includes a review of the patient's diagnosis, surgical procedure, and weight-bearing status.

The patient's current medical status should be assessed by a geriatrician for factors that can affect the rehabilitation process.

Range of joint motion, muscle strength, and flexibility should be assessed and recorded by a physical therapist or physiatrist, with special attention given to the involved extremity and to the upper extremities if they will be needed for assistive devices.

Selected neurologic, balance, and functional assessments can also be made by a physical therapist or orthopaedist.

The patient's social and living situation should be elicited and evaluated by a social worker.

A physical therapy treatment plan is then formulated by a physical therapist or physiatrist based on this initial evaluation and the physical therapy orders of the orthopaedic surgeon.

Multidisciplinary Approach

The surgical treatment of fractures in elderly patients is often successful in terms of fracture union; however, such patients are often unable to achieve their preinjury levels of function. In the mid 1990s, the American Academy of Orthopaedic Surgeons developed a task force to serve elderly orthopaedic patients. This task force developed several recommendations, including the use of collaborative practice.

Collaborative practice or the multidisciplinary approach involves the coordination of multiple services within an institution to address certain nonsurgical patient care issues that affect outcome (Table 2). These programs involve the orthopaedist, geriatricians, physiatrists, therapists, pharmacists, nutritionists, pain specialists, and nurses, with each acting on specific issues to reduce comorbidities and complications in the perioperative period. By reducing these potential problems, physicians, patients, and hospitals have benefited with improved functional outcomes, decreased costs per admission, and reduced lengths of stay and appropriate discharges.

Anesthesia

The preoperative placement of intravenous monitors (such as central venous or pulmonary artery catheters) can help provide better understanding of a patient's hemodynamic status and can be advantageous when preoperative evaluation shows that invasive monitoring techniques are indicated. Elevated pulmonary artery pressures can be treated with diuretics. With a pulmonary artery catheter in place, transfusions can be administered while ensuring that a patient with a history of congestive heart failure does not become overloaded with fluids. Urinary output can be monitored with a

bladder catheter, and the results used to assess hydration status.

Recent evaluations of anesthetic techniques do not demonstrate that any one technique is superior. Two studies demonstrated that there was no significant difference between spinal and general anesthesia in patient outcome.[19,20] These results suggest that anesthetic technique is less important than the physical status of the patient. Patients who undergo surgery and receive regional anesthesia seem to "look" better to many anesthesiologists, surgeons, and internists; however, no difference in postoperative mental status has been found between patients who underwent surgery with regional versus general anesthesia. Studies have demonstrated the efficacy of regional anesthesia (spinal and epidural) in preventing deep venous thrombosis and pulmonary embolism. For this reason, regional anesthesia may be preferable, especially when other factors prevent the institution of thromboembolism prophylaxis.

General Anesthesia

During induction of general anesthesia, slow circulation time may result in overdose, low intravascular volume can lead to hypotension, and cardiac disease can present as ischemic electrocardiographic changes or arrhythmias. Hyperventilation from high tidal volumes can cause hypotension as can airway obstruction during mask ventilation that blocks venous return to the central circulation. The incidence of loss of consciousness and abolition of eyelash reflex when using thiopental was demonstrated to be 44% lower in patients older than 65 years than for a control group of comparably premedicated younger patients.[21]

Vasodilation and myocardial depression as well as hypotension and cardiac arrhythmias may result from the use of halogenated inhalation agents. A narcotic-relaxant technique can be used in patients with coronary artery disease. Nitrous oxide can be used, but it may cause some myocardial depression, especially in patients with coronary artery disease and angina.

Regional Anesthesia

Hypotension is a common adverse effect noted with the use of intrathecal and epidural anesthesia, although the blood pressure decrease associated with epidural anesthesia may be slower in onset than that seen with spinal anesthesia. The infusion of a large volume of fluid to compensate for a decrease in blood pressure should be avoided. Unfortunately, after the spinal anesthetic recedes, fluid overload may occur and cause congestive heart failure. An intermittent bolus of a vasopressor such as neosynephrine or a continuous infusion may help maintain adequate blood pressure. Bradycardia, nausea, vomiting, and hypotension may result if the spinal level is high and the cardioaccelerator fibers are blocked. Atropine or glycopyrrolate can help reverse the bradycardia, nausea, or vomiting. Because the regional anesthetic usually has not receded before arrival in the postanesthesia care unit, the anesthesiologist and nursing personnel must be aware that hemodynamic changes still occur. These changes will become especially apparent as the anesthetic recedes and the intravascular volume shrinks. For patients with a significant history of congestive heart failure, it is prudent to administer a small amount of diuretic at this time. If a pulmonary artery catheter is present, the pulmonary arterial pressures can be used as a guide for management.

Peripheral Nerve Blocks

Other techniques that can be used to provide anesthesia to repair upper and lower extremities include brachial and lumbar plexus blocks or peripheral nerve blocks.[22] Lumbar plexus blocks have been used successfully for patients undergoing surgical treatment of fractured hips and other lower extremity procedures. A modification of this technique using a nerve stimulator and insulated needle has been advantageous in patients in whom neither general anesthesia nor spinal anesthesia is indicated.

Rehabilitation

Physical therapy for patients who undergo surgery for a lower extremity fracture should begin on the first day after surgery. The prescription for unrestricted weight bearing may be modified if construct instability is noted at surgery. Older patients with hip fractures and long bone fractures that are stabilized with intramedullary implants are allowed to bear weight as tolerated regardless of fracture pattern or implant selection. Fractures about the knee and ankle are treated with restricted weight bearing until there is radiographic evidence of healing.

Although ambulation and transfer training occur during physical therapy, patients are given instruction regarding activities of daily living. By helping patients learn bathing and toileting skills as well as how to dress and cook, the therapist contributes to recovery. A visit to the patient's home is ideal, although not always practical; if a home visit is not possible, the rehabilitation and social work team should obtain pertinent information regarding the home environment from the patient, family, and friends. Useful information that can aid in the rehabilitation and training of the patient includes the number and placement of staircases, access to rooms (including kitchen and bathroom), home furnishings, placement of rugs, and resources or support available to the patient at home. Based on this information, the rehabilitation team can devise safety precautions that should be taken to prevent further patient falls and injury and determine specifications for special equipment to help facilitate independence.

Discharge Disposition

During the early postoperative period, a social worker should meet with the patient and family to assess the patient's needs and resources for hospital discharge. The goal of treatment is to return patients to their preinjury level of independence. Depending on each patient's ambulatory ability, social support network, and financial resources, discharge disposition can include return to community dwelling, transfer to an inpatient rehabilitation facility, or placement in a skilled nursing facility.

A variety of other settings are available in which the elderly may receive therapy, each of which should be considered when planning hospital discharge. Skilled nursing facilities offer various degrees of rehabilitation, ranging from little or no therapy to 3 hours of therapy per day. The elderly often benefit from less intense rehabilitation programs in skilled nursing facilities or subacute units; patients may be placed in this type of facility either to build strength before beginning a more intense acute inpatient rehabilitation program or to improve skills learned in an acute rehabilitation program before discharge home.

Day hospitals allow individuals with good social support systems to receive a full day of therapeutic activity in a hospital setting while being able to return home at night. Although outpatient facilities generally offer less comprehensive interdisciplinary therapeutic programs than may be provided on an inpatient basis, they are ideal for patients requiring limited rehabilitative intervention. Finally, physical and occupational therapy can be provided in the home environment where patients have the opportunity to make functional gains in familiar surroundings. In making discharge and therapy decisions, the financial resources and social support systems of the patient should be considered.

Annotated References

1. Koval KJ, Meek R, Schemitsch E, Liporace F, Strauss E, Zuckerman JD: An AOA critical issue: Geriatric trauma. Young ideas. *J Bone Joint Surg Am* 2003;85:1380-1388.

2. Kenzora JE, McCarthy RE, Lowell JD, Sledge CB: Hip fracture mortality: Relation to age, treatment, preoperative illness, time of surgery, and complications. *Clin Orthop* 1984;186:45-56.

3. Sexson SB, Lehner JT: Factors affecting hip fracture mortality. *J Orthop Trauma* 1987;1:298-305.

4. Zuckerman JD, Skovron ML, Koval KJ, Aharonoff G, Frankel VH: Postoperative complications and mortality associated with operative delay in older

patients who have a fracture of the hip. *J Bone Joint Surg Am* 1995;77:1551-1556.

5. Richmond J, Aharonoff GB, Zuckerman JD, Koval KJ: Mortality risk after hip fracture. *J Orthop Trauma* 2003;17:53-56.

   In this study, 836 patients older than 65 years were followed over a 2-year period. The mortality rate was highest in the first 3 months. Patients age 65 to 84 years had higher mortality risks than those older than 85 years.

6. Su H, Aharonoff GB, Hiebert R, Zuckerman JD, Koval KJ: In-hospital mortality after femoral neck fracture: Do internal fixation and hemiarthroplasty differ? *Am J Orthop* 2003;32:151-155.

   In this study, 51,003 patients age 65 years or older who were treated for femoral neck fractures between 1985 and 1996 were reviewed. The incidence of in-hospital mortality was 5.1% overall, whereas it was 3.9% for the open reduction and internal fixation group and 5.6% for the hemiarthroplasty group.

7. Browner WS, Li J, Mangano DT: In-hospital and long-term mortality in male veterans following non-cardiac surgery: The Study of Perioperative Ischemia Research Group. *JAMA* 1992;268:228-232.

8. Koval KJ, Rosenberg AD, Zuckerman JD, et al: Does blood transfusion increase the risk of infection after hip fracture? *J Orthop Trauma* 1997;11:260-265.

9. Snook GA, Chrisman OD, Wilson TC: Thromboembolism after surgical treatment of hip fractures. *Clin Orthop* 1981;155:21-24.

10. Powers PJ, Gent M, Jay RM, et al: A randomized trial of less intense postoperative warfarin or aspirin therapy in the prevention of venous thromboembolism after surgery for fractured hip. *Arch Intern Med* 1989;149:771-774.

11. Agnelli G, Volpato R, Radicchia S, et al: Detection of asymptomatic deep vein thrombosis by real-time B-mode ultrasonography in hip surgery patients. *Thromb Haemost* 1992;68:257-260.

12. Lieberman DV, Lieberman D: Proximal deep vein thrombosis after hip fracture surgery in elderly patients despite thromboprophylaxis. *Am J Phys Med Rehabil* 2002;81:745-750.

   This interventional prospective study included 644 elderly patients undergoing rehabilitation after undergoing surgery for hip fracture. Thromboprophylaxis included graduated compression stockings and subcutaneous low-molecular-weight heparin, and all patients underwent Doppler ultrasonography to identify proximal deep venous thrombosis.

The authors reported that 39 patients developed proximal deep venous thrombosis despite thromboprophylaxis, which led them to concluded that despite thromboprophylaxis, screening Doppler sonography should be performed on this patient population to identify deep venous thrombosis.

13. Mantoni M, Strandberg C, Neergaard K, et al: Triplex US in the diagnosis of asymptomatic deep venous thrombosis. *Acta Radiol* 1997;38:327-331.

14. Jorgensen LN, Rasmussen LS, Wille-Jorgensen PA, Wiberg-Jorgensen F: Lumbar regional analgesia in patients during antithrombotic treatment. Procedures used at the Danish anesthesiologic departments illustrated by a questionnaire study. *Ugeskr Laeger* 1991;153:346-348.

15. Eriksson BI, Lassen MR: Duration of prophylaxis against venous thromboembolism with fondaparinux after hip fracture surgery: A multicenter, randomized, placebo-controlled, double-blind study. *Arch Intern Med* 2003;163:1337-1342.

   In this double-blind multicenter trial, 656 patients undergoing hip fracture surgery were randomly assigned to receive prophylaxis with a once-daily subcutaneous injection of either 2.5 mg of fondaparinux sodium or placebo for 19 to 23 days. Before randomization, all patients had received fondaparinux for 6 to 8 days. The authors reported that extended prophylaxis with fondaparinux for 3 weeks after hip fracture surgery reduced the risk of venous thromboembolism by 96% and was well tolerated.

16. Wynne CF, Ling SM, Remsburg R: Comparison of pain assessment instruments in cognitively intact and cognitively impaired nursing home residents. *Geriatr Nurs* 2000;21:20-23.

   This study of 37 patients in a restorative rehabilitation program was conducted to determine which pain severity and location instruments were most useful in the nursing home setting. The authors concluded that new strategies are needed for pain assessment in the elderly, especially the cognitively impaired elderly, and a combination of instruments to assess pain in the latter group may be required.

17. Horgas AL, Tsai PF: Analgesic drug prescription and use in cognitively impaired nursing home residents. *Nurs Res* 1998;47:235-242.

18. Morrison RS, Magaziner J, McLaughlin MA, et al: The impact of post-operative pain on outcomes following hip fracture. *Pain* 2003;103:303-311.

   This prospective cohort study was conducted to assess the impact of pain on outcomes following hip fracture in

411 older adults. Patients were interviewed daily using standardized pain assessments. The authors found that postoperative pain was associated with increased hospital length of stay, delayed ambulation, and long-term functional impairment and concluded that improved pain control may decrease length of stay, enhance functional recovery, and improve long-term functional outcomes.

19. Valentin N, Lomholt B, Jensen JS, Hejgaard N, Kreiner S: Spinal or general anaesthesia for surgery of the fractured hip? A prospective study of mortality in 578 patients. *Br J Anaesth* 1986;58:284-291.

20. Davis FM, Laurenson VG, Gillespie WJ, Foate J, Seagar AD: Leg blood flow during total hip replacement under spinal or general anaesthesia. *Anaesth Intensive Care* 1989;17:136-143.

21. Koval KJ, Aharonoff GB, Rosenberg AD, Bernstein RL, Zuckerman JD: Functional outcome after hip fracture: Effect of general versus regional anesthesia. *Clin Orthop* 1998;348:37-41.

22. Chayen D, Nathan H, Chayen M: The psoas compartment block. *Anesthesiology* 1976;45:95-99.

Chapter 41

Hip Fractures in the Geriatric Population

George J. Haidukewych, MD

Clifford B. Jones, MD

Geriatric Femoral Neck Fractures

Intracapsular hip fractures are among the most common and potentially devastating injuries that orthopaedists encounter. The number of femoral neck fractures continues to increase proportionately with the growing elderly population. These fractures typically occur after low-energy falls in older patients with poor bone quality. Although there is general consensus that in the younger patient all treatment efforts should be focused on preservation of the host femoral head, the optimal treatment of intracapsular hip fractures in the elderly population remains highly controversial. Treatment options for elderly patients include internal fixation, hemiarthroplasty, and total hip arthroplasty.

Preoperative Evaluation

For any patient with a fracture, attention to other potentially life-threatening injuries is important. For example, frail, elderly patients may have a subdural hematoma caused by a seemingly minor associated head injury from a fall, and this should be carefully ruled out. Associated injuries to the ipsilateral upper extremity are probably the most common orthopaedic injuries associated with a hip fracture.[1] Thorough medical clearance before surgery is important (specifically, electrolyte imbalances, anemia, and/or hydration deficits should be corrected). In general, elderly patients should be brought to surgery as soon as possible. This allows earlier mobilization postoperatively and may potentially improve the patient's chances of successful rehabilitation and independent living. Medical management in concert with a geriatrician may decrease length of hospital stay, decrease complication rates, and provide excellent general medical care.

Patients with femoral neck fractures will typically present with groin pain after a low-energy fall. Patients with displaced fractures may hold the affected leg in a shortened, flexed, and externally rotated position. A patient with a nondisplaced or impacted fracture may have groin pain on internal rotation of the limb without limb deformity. Proper AP and lateral radiographs are important to adequately evaluate the fracture. The lateral view will often demonstrate displacements that would otherwise be undetected.[2] Occasionally, however, patients present with a more indolent course of hip pain. Plain films may be completely normal. In this situation, MRI or bone scanning should be performed to rule out occult hip fracture. MRI can provide a rapid diagnosis and rule out other potential causes of hip pain such as osteonecrosis, pubic ramus stress fracture, and neoplasm. Although bone scanning may be useful for claustrophobic patients or for those whose symptoms have been apparent for several days, it cannot provide information as quickly as MRI.

Indications for Surgery

Essentially all patients with a femoral neck fracture should be treated surgically. The very rare exception for which nonsurgical treatment is considered would be a nonambulatory patient with dementia and either an acute or a neglected fracture, significant prohibitive medical comorbidity, and minimal pain from the injury. Although in the past nonsurgical treatment for nondisplaced and so-called stable valgus impacted injuries has been considered, a recent series demonstrated a nonunion rate of 39% in this cohort.[3] Typically, nonsurgical treatment for such stable injuries would involve a short period of bed rest. The benefits of early mobilization in this patient population should not be underestimated. The negative effects of recumbency on ultimate rehabilitation, medical complications, and decubiti have been well documented. Fracture displacement increases the risk of nonunion and osteonecrosis and usually necessitates a more extensive surgical procedure; therefore, surgical treatment of nondisplaced femoral neck fractures is typically indicated.

In general, for the geriatric patient, decision making is based on whether the fracture is (1) displaced or (2) nondisplaced or valgus impacted. Although the Garden classification system has classically grouped fractures into four subtypes (stages I through IV), it is more practical to consider fractures in these two general categories.[2] The Orthopaedic Trauma Association classification system is more comprehensive in that it distinguishes subcapital, transcervical, and basicervical fractures[4] (Figure 1). Nondisplaced

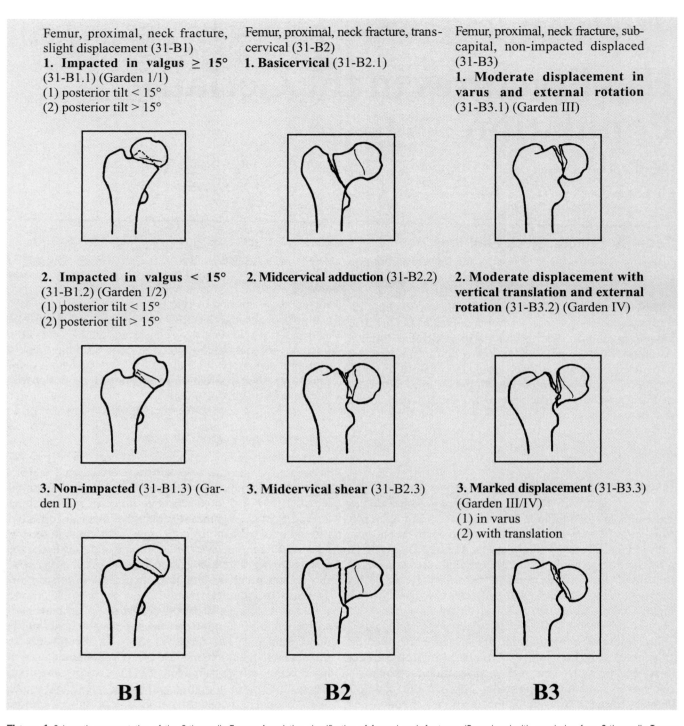

Femur, proximal, neck fracture, slight displacement (31-B1)
1. Impacted in valgus ≥ 15° (31-B1.1) (Garden 1/1)
(1) posterior tilt < 15°
(2) posterior tilt > 15°

2. Impacted in valgus < 15° (31-B1.2) (Garden 1/2)
(1) posterior tilt < 15°
(2) posterior tilt > 15°

3. Non-impacted (31-B1.3) (Garden II)

B1

Femur, proximal, neck fracture, trans-cervical (31-B2)
1. Basicervical (31-B2.1)

2. Midcervical adduction (31-B2.2)

3. Midcervical shear (31-B2.3)

B2

Femur, proximal, neck fracture, sub-capital, non-impacted displaced (31-B3)
1. Moderate displacement in varus and external rotation (31-B3.1) (Garden III)

2. Moderate displacement with vertical translation and external rotation (31-B3.2) (Garden IV)

3. Marked displacement (31-B3.3) (Garden III/IV)
(1) in varus
(2) with translation

B3

Figure 1 Schematic representation of the Orthopaedic Trauma Association classification of femoral neck fractures. *(Reproduced with permission from Orthopaedic Trauma Association Committee for Coding and Classification: Fracture and dislocation compendium. J Orthop Trauma 1996;10(suppl 1):1-155.)*

or valgus impacted fractures are typically treated with in situ cancellous screw fixation, whereas displaced fractures are treated with arthroplasty or an attempt at internal fixation in certain patients.

Although most surgeons agree on the preferred treatment of nondisplaced and valgus impacted fractures, the ideal treatment of a displaced femoral neck fracture in the elderly patient remains controversial. For the general purposes of this chapter, elderly patients include those age 65 years and older; however, no clear published data exist regarding a specific age at which arthroplasty is preferred. The treatment of choice for these fractures in patients younger than 65 years is open reduction and internal fixation in an attempt to preserve the host fem-

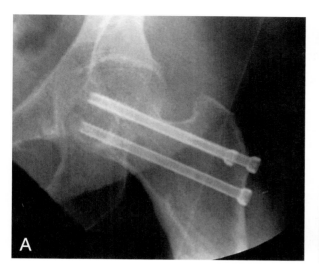
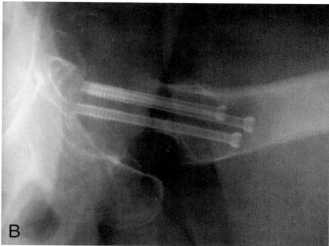

Figure 2 AP (**A**) and lateral (**B**) radiographs of a valgus impacted fracture treated with cannulated cancellous screws.

oral head. In this patient population, nonunion rates of less than 10% and osteonecrosis rates of approximately 25% have been consistently reported with open reduction and internal fixation.[5-8] In older patients with displaced fractures, however, nonunion remains more problematic than osteonecrosis. Nonunion rates in the 30% range have been reported, which likely reflect the difficulty in achieving stable fixation of the proximal osteopenic fragment.[6,9-11] This has led many surgeons to embrace prosthetic replacement as the primary treatment for displaced femoral neck fracture in elderly patients. Multiple series have documented excellent durability, predictable pain relief, reasonable clinical function, and importantly, a low revision surgery rate for elderly patients who cannot tolerate the prolonged convalescence and multiple surgeries associated with fixation failure.[1,6,9-11] In Europe, however, many centers continue to treat patients with displaced femoral neck fractures with reduction and internal fixation and perform arthroplasty when fixation fails. In a recent series, however, acute arthroplasty provided better results and fewer complications than arthroplasty performed when fixation failed.[12]

Role of Internal Fixation

Nondisplaced and valgus impacted femoral neck fractures (Garden stages I and II) can be treated successfully with in situ cannulated cancellous screw fixation. Nonunion rates of approximately 5% and osteonecrosis rates as low as 15% have been reported with this technique.[5,8] It is important to realize that the positioning of the screws in the femoral head and neck fragment are essential to optimize treatment.[13,14] The three-point principle has been described.[14] Because the center of the femoral neck in an elderly patient is typically hollow and lacks the cancellous support that a younger patient's cancel-

lous bone may provide, the shafts of the cancellous screws should be placed as near the femoral neck cortex as possible. Typically, one screw is placed distally along the medial neck region, a second screw is placed posteriorly along the posterior femoral neck cortex, and a third screw is placed anteriorly, completing a triangular pattern. A cadaver study demonstrated significantly improved stability when such cortical support was compared with more central screw placement in the femoral-neck[13] (Figure 2). The insertion of screws below the level of the lesser trochanter or the use of an inverted V pattern should be avoided to minimize the chance of later subtrochanteric fracture (Figure 3). Screws should be placed as parallel as possible to allow uniform fracture compression. Data from a more recent cadaver study demonstrate less fracture displacement with loading into the typical varus, shortening, and external rotation position when three screws are used instead of two[15] (Figure 4). Although the addition of a fourth screw has shown some benefit when posterior comminution exists, three screws are usually adequate.[16,17]

Additional factors must be considered when choosing the appropriate internal fixation device for the treatment of a displaced femoral neck fracture. Although most femoral neck fractures in elderly patients are relatively horizontal, in some, especially in those with better bone quality and higher-energy injuries, the fracture patterns are more vertical. These vertical fractures will have higher shear forces imparted across the fracture site and may be inadequately stabilized by cannulated screws alone. One study reported a higher incidence of fixation failure in patients with such transcervical shear fractures treated with cannulated screws alone, which has led some authors to recommend fixation with a fixed-angle device such as an angled blade plate or a dynamic hip screw in fractures that exhibit a tendency to shear.[18-20]

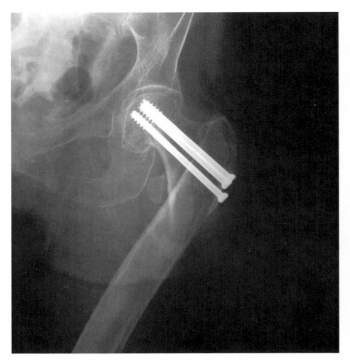

Figure 3 Radiograph showing a subtrochanteric fracture 2 months after internal fixation of a nondisplaced femoral neck fracture.

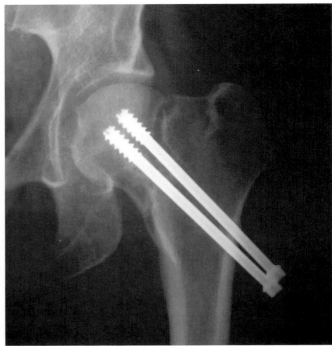

Figure 4 Radiograph showing failure of a cannulated screw internal fixation. Then two narrowly spaced screws were placed centrally in the femoral neck and, lacking cortical support, the fracture collapsed.

One study demonstrated a higher rate of fracture redisplacement when cancellous screws were used to stabilize higher angled fractures (Pauwels angle > 50°).[21] It should be noted that most femoral neck fractures can be treated successfully with parallel cancellous screws; however, surgeons should be cognizant of the increased failure rate and the potential need for an alternative method of internal fixation when such high shear fractures are encountered.

Additionally, the so-called basicervical fracture should be treated differently from a transcervical or subcapital fracture. This fracture, in all likelihood, behaves more like an intertrochanteric fracture and should be stabilized by a sliding hip screw device, with the use of a proximal derotation screw as indicated. Multiple cancellous screws alone should not be used to stabilize this type of fracture.[22]

There is a substantial cohort of patients older than 65 years who could benefit from an attempt at open reduction and internal fixation of a displaced femoral neck fracture. For example, extremely active patients in their 70s with excellent bone stock, a displaced femoral neck fracture, and no medical comorbidity may be reasonable candidates for an attempt at internal fixation.[23] Even though approximately 40% of patients undergoing internal fixation in this setting will experience failure caused by osteonecrosis or nonunion, 60% will not. Therefore, elderly patients with excellent bone stock who can and are willing to tolerate a fixation failure should it occur may be ideal candidates for internal fixation. One study

recommended the use of a physiologic score when treating elderly patients with displaced femoral neck fractures.[8] According to the study protocol, patients younger than 65 years or those with a nondisplaced fracture were all treated with cannulated cancellous screw fixation. All patients older than 80 years were treated with hemiarthroplasty. Patients between the age of 65 and 80 years were treated based on the results of a physiologic score that took into account bone quality, medical comorbidity, activity level, and cognitive status. Only 5% of the entire cohort required revision surgery. These findings underscore the importance of not using chronologic age alone when determining appropriate treatment. For patients in the gray zone, consideration of other physiologic variables is important because many of these patients would benefit from an attempt at preservation of their native femoral head. Although the nebulous and subjective term physiologic age is sometimes used to help in decision making in this setting, one study showed that the success of internal fixation was related to the quality of reduction and the surgeon's perceived ease of reduction.[24] For example, a displaced femoral neck fracture that reduces nicely with slight internal rotation may heal reasonably well with internal fixation; however, a widely displaced fracture that is either irreducible closed or aligned in varus when closed reduction is attempted will likely not heal well and may be best treated with prosthetic replacement.[25] Quality of reduction has been shown to have a significant effect on outcome in multiple studies. Overall, it is probably unwise to automatically rule out internal fixation for the treatment of a displaced femoral neck fracture because the patient is older than 65 years. With the growing elderly population, a substantial subset of these surprisingly healthy and active patients heal without osteonecrosis and are able to return to relatively high physical demand activities that may not be possible with arthroplasty.

Role of Arthroplasty

There are several reasons why arthroplasty is considered by many in the United States to be the treatment of choice for elderly patients with displaced femoral neck fractures. First and foremost, arthroplasty provides a durable, predictable treatment method with an acceptably low complication rate.[1,6-12] Patients can typically be mobilized, and can bear weight as tolerated immediately after surgery without the risk of loss of fixation. Additionally, the functional results of arthroplasty have been generally favorable in patients who are not physically active. Considerable controversy exists regarding prosthesis selection; whether to use unipolar, bipolar, or total hip arthroplasty; and which method of fixation to use, cemented or uncemented.

It is recommended that the use of an uncemented monoblock unipolar prosthesis (Austin-Moore prosthesis) be reserved for the most minimally ambulatory or nonambulatory demented patients confined to assisted-living facilities. These outdated designs have been shown to result in a significant rate of residual pain and revision surgery when implanted into active, ambulatory patients.[1,26] If these devices are used, it is important to seat the prosthesis accurately on the calcar and avoid undersizing the acetabular component because both of these factors have been associated with residual pain and the need for revision surgery.[26] Newer modular uncemented "low-demand" designs offer a variety of metaphyseal and diaphyseal geometries to provide better fit and fill and rotational stability in the proximal femur and various modular neck lengths to allow restoration of leg lengths to offset hip stability. Despite these design improvements, however, if the patient is ambulatory, a cemented stem is usually a better choice.[1,9]

Unipolar Versus Bipolar Arthroplasty

Several retrospective and prospective randomized studies have been conducted to compare unipolar and bipolar bearings. Overall, a bipolar bearing does not appear to provide any advantage in short-term to midterm follow-up.[27] However, a meta-analysis in which patients were followed longer than 7 years reported a lower revision surgery rate when patients were treated with a bipolar prostheses compared with those treated with unipolar prostheses.[9] This is not surprising because patients who survived longer than 7 years were likely more active and placed more physical demands on the hip.

Acetabular wear is a time-dependent phenomenon. Surgeons, therefore, are faced with the challenge of trying to predict how active a patient is and will be, estimating their life-expectancy, and demand-matching the prosthesis accordingly. Uncemented Austin-Moore type arthroplasties are typically reserved for demented, essentially nonambulatory patients with major medical comorbidity.

Cemented Versus Uncemented Fixation

Several studies have documented improved outcomes when hemiarthroplasties were cemented.[1,9] The femoral canals in these patients are typically osteopenic and capacious and do not lend themselves well to uncemented fixation. Cement also offers the advantage of secure prosthetic fixation that will allow immediate full postoperative weight bearing. There is concern, of course, that a medical complication or intraoperative death can occur during the cementation process as a result of embolization of marrow contents when using cement to treat a patient population with diminished cardiopulmonary reserve. One study assessed the risk of sudden death for patients undergoing hip arthroplasty and reported an incidence of approximately 1 in 500 for patients undergoing cemented hip arthroplasty for a displaced femoral neck fracture.[28] With improvements in canal lavage and drying techniques over time, the mortality rate was reduced. A more recent study demonstrated a decreased embolic load as well when careful preparation of the femoral canal and lavage, drying, and venting are performed.[29] Little, if any, cement pressurization should be performed, and the femoral canal should be thoroughly lavaged and dried when treating patients with diminished cardiopulmonary reserve. Overall, cement appears to provide better results based on the available data, but it should be used with caution.

Role of Total Hip Arthroplasty

Historically, total hip arthroplasty has been indicated for patients with displaced femoral neck fractures and severe preexisting, symptomatic, ipsilateral degenerative joint disease of the hip. This combination of pathologies, however, is extremely rare. There has been a recent trend to expand the indications for acute total hip arthroplasty to include the treatment of elderly patients with displaced femoral neck fractures. In a recent report, patients were randomized to either internal fixation, hemiarthroplasty, or total hip arthroplasty.[10] Total hip arthroplasty provided the most complete pain relief and the best functional outcome. Morbidity and mortality did not differ in these three subgroups. Two other recent randomized controlled studies have also reported that in elderly patients with displaced femoral neck fractures, total hip arthroplasty provides a better outcome than internal fixation for relatively healthy, lucid patients.[30,31] Although total hip arthroplasty does appear to provide the best functional outcome, the primary complication when performing an acute total hip arthroplasty in the setting of a displaced femoral neck fracture is prosthetic dislocation.[32] These arthroplasties typically will not fail because of aseptic loosening, but because of dislocation. Dislocation rates averaging 10% have been reported across multiple series, even when the procedures were performed by experienced arthroplasty surgeons. Approximately 25% of patients who experience dislocation in this setting become recurrent dislocators. Considering the enormous number of femoral neck fractures treated worldwide, the potential economic and societal impact of such recurrent dislocations is substantial. If total hip arthroplasty is undertaken in this setting, therefore, the use of approaches that have historically been associated with a lower dislocation rate, such as the anterolateral approach, and the selected use of elevated lipped liners and larger diameter femoral heads may be justified. There are no data to substantiate the theory that these interventions will decrease the dislocation rate in this patient population.

Several explanations have been proposed for the increased dislocation rate. Patients with femoral neck fractures are typically frail and do not have the stiff, thick hip capsules commonly associated with degenerative joint disease. It is possible that they regain motion quickly, and the prosthesis may impinge and dislocate. Additionally, these patients may have mild dementia and adduction and flexion contractures as well as difficulty following hip precautions. Regardless of the etiology, surgeons and patients should be cognizant of the increased dislocation rate.

Economic Factors in Implant Selection

Increasingly, orthopaedic surgeons are faced with reimbursement pressures and pressures from the institution that employs them to provide the most cost-effective care of elderly patients with femoral neck fractures. In a study comparing the total costs of care for patients with displaced femoral neck fractures who underwent internal fixation, cemented total hip arthroplasty, or hemiarthroplasty, the most cost-effective treatment option for these patients was cemented total hip arthroplasty when the cost of revision surgeries, complications, and failed internal fixations were considered.[33] Fracture stems without costly features such as distal centralizers, forged fabrication, and multiple offset options are commercially available. Patient-specific demand issues should be taken into consideration when selecting the appropriate femoral component. It is important to note, however, that the primary mode of failure for a cemented bipolar hemiarthroplasty, for example, is aseptic femoral loosening, not acetabular wear.[1] Multiple variables of cemented stem design such as cross-sectional geometry, surface roughness, and precoating have had both a positive and negative effect on cemented femoral component durability. The use of a cemented stem with a good record of clinical performance is therefore recommended. The use of a

bipolar bearing will add additional cost over that of a unipolar bearing, and this must be considered when selecting the appropriate components.[27] Hip fracture implant costs, in general, account for a small proportion of the overall cost of care of elderly patients. Most costs are associated with a prolonged hospital stay, typically as a result of difficulties with assisted-living placement.

Intertrochanteric and Pertrochanteric Femoral Fractures

With the current annual incidence of hip fracture being 63 per 100,000 elderly females and 34 per 100,000 elderly males, it can be estimated that the annual incidence of intertrochanteric hip fractures will increase from approximately 125,000 annually to approximately 250,000 annually by 2040.[34] In contradistinction to patients with femoral neck fractures, patients with trochanteric hip fractures tend to be older and have more medical comorbidities. The term pertrochanteric femoral fracture is often used when describing intertrochanteric and distal extensions of the intertrochanteric fracture. Although elderly patients usually develop pertrochanteric fractures as the result of a low-energy fall, the existence of osteoporosis and/or balance abnormalities create an environment in which the fracture pattern can be consistent with that caused by a complex high-energy injury (such as comminution, multiplanar, or severe displacement). Accurate fracture reduction and appropriate implant insertion can improve healing rates and lower the risk of complications.

Preoperative Evaluation

Initial radiographs should include AP pelvis and lateral hip views. The anatomy of the contralateral hip is important to determine normal anatomic alignment. The lateral hip view will help determine potentially problematic fracture displacement (flexion, external rotation, and abduction) and greater trochanteric quality (coronal shear fracture or multiplanar fractures). The initial pelvic radiograph will help determine if the patient has osteoporosis (trabecular quality) or a history of falls (healed fractures, contralateral fracture). A gentle initial traction radiograph in the emergency department will determine fracture alignment, the result of ligamentotaxis, and help determine stability. Furthermore, if insertion of an intramedullary nail is being considered, the presence of a distal femoral implant (stemmed knee arthroplasty, plate, or intramedullary nail fixation) and the femoral radius of curvature (associated with Paget's disease, normal bowing associated with aging or osteoporosis, or diaphyseal medullary abnormality from a previous fracture) must be assessed with femoral shaft radiographs. If a coronal shear fracture of the proximal femur is suspected, a preoperative CT scan is useful. If a patient has hip pain that was or was not preceded by a fall, an initial internal rotation AP hip radiograph may reveal the fracture line. If radiographs are inconclusive, MRI is more helpful than bone scanning in diagnosing hip pathology. Except for a minority of patients with severe medical comorbidities, pertrochanteric hip fractures in the elderly population require surgical intervention to reduce the risk of death, pulmonary problems, pressure sores, deep venous thrombosis, and pulmonary embolism by restoring ambulatory status. Treatment for nonambulatory patients is debatable.

Classification

Pertrochanteric fractures were first classified more than 50 years ago.[35] The number and orientation of fracture fragments determined the likelihood of achieving and maintaining a reduction. Five basic fracture configurations were noted. To simplify the evaluation, surgeons typically predict the likelihood of a fracture being stable or unstable based on initial radiographic findings. Stable fractures have a simple fracture pattern that realigns anatomically with traction or ligamentotaxis. Stable fractures, therefore, have appropriate soft-tissue attachments, stable compressive medial anatomy, and heal without deformity or shortening. Unstable fractures typically have comminution along the trochanteric line or in the medial compressive zone, behave unpredictably with traction, and are associated with an increased rate of complications such as fracture shortening, fixation failure, and hardware failure. Stable fractures have a predictably better treatment outcome, whereas unstable fractures treatment outcomes are less predictable.

In 1990, the Müller/AO fracture classification system was formulated to better evaluate fracture comminution, location, and stability.[4] Pertrochanteric fractures fall into the 31-A1 fracture classification section using this system. The A1 fracture (classic intertrochanteric) is an oblique stable two-part fracture. The A2 fracture (classic unstable intertrochanteric) has comminution within the trochanteric area without violation of the lateral cortical column. The A3 fracture (classic pertrochanteric) has extension into the lateral column with more involvement distal to the trochanteric line. The A3.1 fracture constitutes the reverse oblique pattern. Lesser trochanteric involvement with the iliopsoas pull can help predict fracture stability, shortening, and displacement during and after fracture reduction. Stable fracture patterns are typically Evans type 1 and Müller/AO types A1 and A2, whereas unstable fractures are typically Evans type II and AO types A2.2, A2.3, and A3. With or without the use of a classification system, stability must be determined. Reverse fracture line obliquity, posteromedial fracture displacement, or subtrochanteric extension are patterns of instability.

Fracture Reduction

Most pertrochanteric fractures are best reduced with foot traction; a boot is placed onto the injured foot. Supine patient positioning is preferred over lateral positioning. The peroneal post should be wide and well padded. Fluoroscopy AP, lateral, and oblique views are obtained to determine fracture reduction alignment and rotation. If the lesser trochanter remains attached to the proximal fragment, an external rotation and abduction deformity can be present. A tenaculum clamp inserted through the incision or percutaneously will assist in reduction of the deformity. A temporary crutch or bone hook can improve posterior sag deformities until the implant is inserted. Although anatomic alignment is optimal, it has been reported that posterior sag of up to 30° was not associated with increased failure.[36]

Treatment Options
Sliding Hip Screws
Sliding hip screws allow for controlled dynamic compression across the fracture site. An incision large enough for submuscular or open plate insertion is placed laterally over the proximal portion of the femur. In patients with stable fractures, sliding hip screws have been characterized as a tension band construct. The force is transmitted through the intact stable medial cortex. In patients with unstable fractures, the lag screw will compress and the lever arm will shorten until a stable buttress is found or healing occurs. If the sliding component shortens enough to allow bottoming out on the barrel, the device becomes a fixed-length construct, a structure that has been reported to have high failure rates.[37] The average shortening of stable and unstable fractures is 5.3 mm and 15.7 mm, respectively. Although medial displacement osteotomies have been attempted to improve osseous contact and healing, the osteotomies did not improve clinical outcomes. Overall, excessive fracture compression and limb shortening led to pain and immobility.[38,39] Recent plate adjuncts and advances have attempted to further control fracture healing.

Regardless of implant choice, the lag screw must be correctly positioned. In an analysis of screw placement, it was noted that screw placement was the most important indicator of fixation failure.[40] Optimal screw placement is deep within the center of the femoral head on both AP and lateral radiographic views (center-center position). The tip-apex distance is used to measure screw placement and outcome. No implants with tip-apex distance measuring less than 25 mm had screw cutout. If tip-apex distance was greater than 35 mm, screw cutout was likely. With sliding hip screws, the primary cause of implant failure was reported to be screw cutout.[40] Even though two-hole implants are biomechanically and clinically acceptable,[41,42] implant length should be determined by intraoperative screw purchase. Mechanical failures have been reported to range from 4% to 12.5% of patients.[43] With unstable fracture patterns, failure rates of 25% have been reported.[44]

Recent Plate Advances

The Medoff sliding plate is a system that administers biaxial compression to the fracture site. The dynamic lag screw is inserted routinely through the barrel of the side plate. The second dynamic component is placed in the vertical direction. The inner portion of the plate allows for axial compression, whereas the outer portion is attached to the proximal femoral diaphysis. One study noted a lower rate of cutout at the cost of increased axial impaction (15 mm), blood loss, and surgical time using this device to treat patients with intertrochanteric fractures.[45] The Medoff sliding plate is recommended for the treatment of patients with unstable fracture patterns only. When compared with the proximal femoral nail and other dynamic hip screw systems, similar outcomes were noted.[46]

The trochanteric buttress plate is an adjunctive plate that attaches to a standard sliding hip screw. One study noted that the laterally and proximally based plate buttresses against excessive fracture site impaction and limb shortening in 90% of patients with unstable fracture patterns.[47] When compared with dynamic hip screw and intramedullary hip screw applications, the dynamic hip screw/trochanteric stabilizing plate combination had less failures and fracture site displacement.[48]

The Gotfried percutaneous compression plate (Efratgo Ltd, Hitech Biosurgical, Kiryat Bailik, Israel) is a percutaneously inserted side plate that has two 9.3-mm sliding screws inserted at a 120° angle. For patients with unstable fractures, percutaneous compression plating was reported to be two to three times stronger than the Gamma intramedullary hip screw implant (Stryker Orthopaedics, Mahwah, NJ).[49] This system has the potential to reduce infection rates and blood loss because of the small percutaneous incisions required for insertion. The clinical results are similar when compared with standard sliding hip screws. The percutaneous insertion has an associated learning curve.[50]

The variable angle hip screw (Vari-Angle, Biomet, Warsaw, IN) is a system that allows for anatomic fracture reduction and freehand lag screw insertion. The plate can be dialed into the corresponding angle to accept the lag screw. Therefore, the center-center lag screw position is optimized with the potential for fewer failures. Advantages include potential percutaneous insertion and inventory reduction. A disadvantage is the added cost per implant.

The Talon hip compression screw (Talon CHS, Orthopaedic Designs, St. Petersburg, FL) is a lag screw with retractable talons at the base of the screw threads. Ideally, these deploy along the calcar femorale portion of the femoral neck to improve screw interference. In bio-

mechanical testing, the Talon hip compression screw had two times the compression and three times the rotatory stability compared with the standard lag screw.[51] Improved torsion and fracture impaction occurs only when the talons engage or penetrate the medial cortical bone of the neck.

Intramedullary Hip Screws

Intramedullary hip screws are implants that rely on insertion through the gluteus medius. With a 16- or 17-mm entrance insertion, the correct nail insertion site is the tip of the greater trochanter. If inserted too laterally, it can lead to a varus reduction and a cephalad lag screw position. The average amount of gluteus medius disruption with nail insertion has been measured at 27%.[52] The amount of disruption may lead to postoperative morbidity. The appropriate depth of the nail is determined by the correct placement of the lag screw through the nail into the femoral head. Whether to use short or long intramedullary nails is debatable. Intramedullary hip screws are relatively difficult to insert in patients with hip contractures, femoral diaphyseal pathoanatomy, and stemmed total knee arthroplasties.

The intramedullary hip screw implant is a load-sharing device. The lag screw allows for compression at the fracture site. If dynamic or no interlocking is performed, added compression through the diaphysis can occur. The two most commonly used intramedullary hip screw implants are the Gamma nail and the IMHS (Smith & Nephew, Memphis, TN). The stiff load sharing of these implants dissipates stress to the tip of the implant. Intraoperative complications using these implants consist of fracture site extension, proximal blowout, iatrogenic femoral fracture, malalignment, distal interlocking, and geometric mismatch. Postoperative complications include femoral fracture at the tip (2% to 12% of patients), lag cutout, malunion, prominent hardware, thigh pain, and total knee arthroplasty alignment difficulties; tip-apex distance measurements are important in predicting lag screw success.[53] Lag screw cutout ranges from 2.5% to 8.3%.[43] Thigh pain, which is thought to be caused by the stiff intramedullary implant, has been reported to occur in 0 to 14% of patients.[54,55]

Several implant changes have improved intramedullary hip screw fixation. The proximal nail valgus offset has changed from approximately 10° to 4°, which has decreased nail breakage. Percutaneous nail insertion systems, such as the ITST system (Zimmer, Warsaw, IN), have been developed. The percutaneous system uses a cannula to accurately insert a terminally threaded guide pin at the tip of the trochanter. The incision is much smaller (2.5 to 3.0 cm) and more proximal (closer to the iliac crest) than the standard incisions. Furthermore, some intramedullary nails have a shortened transition zone, which decreases the tendency of the nail to jam within the lesser trochanteric zone. Premature jamming can impede complete intramedullary nail insertion into the femur. The development of more aggressive lag screw designs has improved lag screw insertion into the deeper dense subchondral bone. The "J" design in the ITST system (J Lag, Zimmer) has clinically improved lag screw insertion. Some intramedullary hip screw implants allow for a temporary or permanent antirotational lag screw. This antirotational screw can assist in stabilization of fractures with an unstable neck component; however, the two screws increase tip-apex distance of the second or both screws, potentially increasing the risk of failure or cutout. The failure of dual screws in osteoporotic bone has been attributed to the so-called Z-effect. The Z-effect occurs when the cephalad screw fails by penetrating the joint while the caudad screw fails by backing out. This is thought to occur by differing tension versus compression forces on the two screws. Additional clinical and biomechanical investigation will be required before two screws can be successfully placed in all intramedullary nails. Another intramedullary hip screw implant advancement involves decreasing the radius of curvature (from 108 inches to 75 inches) for full-length nails. The change approaches the anatomic curvature for the femur (49 inches). Insertion into the distal femur becomes more central instead of into the anterior portion of the distal femur.

Sliding Hip Screws Versus Intramedullary Hip Screws

In a biomechanical evaluation, no difference between sliding hip screw implants and intramedullary hip screw implants was noted when used to treat patients with stable fractures.[56,57] By distributing the force distally, improved stability is noted with intramedullary hip screw implants over sliding hip screw implants when treating unstable fracture patterns. In evaluations of initiation of lag screw sliding, the IMHS was reported to be least resistant to lag shortening when compared with the Gamma nail (Stryker Orthopaedics).[58,59] In addition, a lower angle of lag screw insertion and more barrel overlap provided more resistance to sliding. One large or two smaller lag screws were reported to not change sliding characteristics.[60]

In clinical comparisons, cutout, blood loss, wound complications, hospital stay, patient mortality, and surgical time were reported to be similar for the two types of implants.[53-55,61-64] The technical learning curve, complications, and revision surgery rates are higher with intramedullary hip screws than sliding hip screws. A uniquely consistent complication associated with early reports of intramedullary hip screws was femoral fractures. In one study, sliding hip screw implants with a trochanteric stabilizing plate had an increased incidence of return to prefracture independence when compared with sliding hip screw or intramedullary hip screw implants.[48] In two other studies that compared the Medoff sliding plates and sliding hip screws, the surgical time was

shorter for intramedullary hip screw implants than for dynamic hip screw implants.[65,66] The Medoff plate had less fixation failures than the sliding hip screws. Greater limb shortening was noted with the Medoff sliding plates than sliding hip screws.

With reverse oblique fracture patterns (AO type A3.1), intramedullary hip screw implants were shown to be biomechanically superior to both fixed-angle and sliding hip screw devices. Two separate clinical studies evaluated this particular fracture pattern and reported that the intramedullary hip screw device was superior to a fixed-angle device, which in turn was superior to a sliding hip screw device.[45,67] Predictably high failure rates have been noted when treating reverse oblique fracture patterns with sliding hip screws; therefore, intramedullary hip screw implants are recommended to treat this type of injury.

Economic Factors in Implant Selection

The cost of an intramedullary hip screw implant ranges from about three to four times the cost of a sliding hip screw implant. The cost of the Medoff sliding plate, percutaneous compression plating, or variable angle hip screw device is more than a sliding hip screw implant, but the smaller necessary implant volume of the variable hip screw devices may offset the higher implant costs. With annual intertrochanteric hip fracture treatment costs estimated to be $5 billion, implant selection is important; however, a less expensive device (such as the sliding hip screw implant) should not be inserted inappropriately (for example, using a sliding hip screw implant instead of an intramedullary hip screw implant to treat a reverse oblique pattern) to offset the higher cost of revision surgery and patient outcome.

Biologics

Injectable polymethylmethacrylate and calcium phosphate cement pastes harden within the bone. These materials are used to improve implant purchase and implant stability and to substitute for posteromedial comminution. By improving screw purchase and implant bone interphase, polymethylmethacrylate can be inserted into the femoral head. A new compound, bisphenol-a-glycidyl dimethacrylate-based composite, has been reported to decrease screw cutout.[68] Calcium phosphate cement (Norian Skeletal Repair System, Synthes, Paoli, PA) is resorbable and osteoinductive. Once hardened, calcium phosphate cement has an improved compressive strength over cancellous bone, but it is biomechanically weaker in shear and tension.[69] Although early results are encouraging, more research is required to improve delivery and containment of the compounds.

Surgical Complications

With most sliding hip screw implant complications associated with screw cutout, the rates of cutout range from

1.2% to 6.3%.[43] Unstable fracture patterns have been noted to increase screw failure rates.[39] Placing the screw within 5 mm of the subchondral bone reduces failure rates in patients with unstable fracture patterns. A tip-apex distance of less than 25 mm has been reported to significantly reduce failure rates.[40] Sliding hip screw implants used to treat patients with unstable fracture patterns can lead to limb-length discrepancies.[58,66] Extremity shortening of > 18.7 mm has been reported to be related to decreased postoperative mobility, and the need for an ambulatory aid doubled from 36% to 70% in patients with axial shortening compared with patients with lesser axial shortening.[61] Osteonecrosis has been shown to occur in fewer than 1% of patients.[70]

With decreased offset, smaller diameter, and increased radius of curvature (increased radius of curvature refers to the osteoporotic femur, whereas the relative decreased radius of curvature refers to the intramedullary nail), second-generation intramedullary hip screw implants have lower complication rates compared with early reports on the Gamma nail device. Cutout rates still range from 2.5% to 8.3% of patients.[43] In two studies, rates for postoperative mobility and the need for an ambulatory aid were noted to be less than those reported for patients with sliding hip screw implants.[54,55] Secondary to the double curvature, revision surgery may be complicated by difficult intramedullary nail removal.[63]

Salvage of Failed Fixation

Salvage of failed internal fixation requires an understanding of failure etiology, failed implant type, and patient comorbidities. If the patient has multiple comorbidities and severe osteopenia, a single-step conversion to an implant allowing immediate weight bearing should be performed. For most patients, a calcar replacing hemiarthroplasty with a long stem is used. Implant survivability has been reported to be excellent.[45] If the failure is associated with acetabular erosion from the lag screw, a total hip arthroplasty may be required. For patients with better bone quality, a high-angle blade plate and bone grafting can usually result in healing.[45,71]

Summary

Intertrochanteric hip fractures are common. The costs to stabilize the fracture, rehabilitate the patient, and institutionalize patients if necessary continues to rise. Efficient and meticulous surgical intervention should be provided to these patients to optimize care. The sliding hip screw implant remains the gold standard for the treatment of patients with stable fracture patterns. Intramedullary hip screw implants, which are more costly than sliding hip screw implants, seem to improve outcomes in patients with unstable fracture patterns. Either treatment should permit full weight bearing and mobilization.

Appropriate center-center lag screw positioning deep within the subchondral bone (tip-apex distance) of the head can help to reduce implant failure.

Annotated References

1. Haidukewych GJ, Israel TA, Berry DJ: Long-term survivorship of cemented bipolar hemiarthroplasty for fracture of the femoral neck. *Clin Orthop* 2002; 403:118-126.

   The authors of this study report the results of 212 patients older than 60 years who were treated with cemented bipolar hemiarthroplasty. Overall, the 10-year survivorship rate (free of reoperation for any reason) was 94%. Only one patient underwent revision surgery for acetabular cartilage wear. More than 90% of patients had no pain or minimal pain at follow-up, and the overall dislocation rate was less than 2%. Aseptic femoral loosening was the most common reason for revision surgery.

2. Oakes DA, Jackson KR, Davies MR, et al: The impact of the Garden classification on proposed operative treatment. *Clin Orthop* 2003;409:232-240.

   To improve the reliability and usefulness of the Garden classification, the authors suggest that the classification system should be modified to only two stages (nondisplaced or valgus impacted and displaced). The authors also recommend the use of a lateral radiograph to identify these injuries.

3. Tanaka J, Seki N, Tokimura F, Hayashi Y: Conservative treatment of Garden stage I femoral neck fracture in elderly patients. *Arch Orthop Trauma Surg* 2002;122:24-28.

   Nonsurgical treatment of nondisplaced or valgus impacted (Garden stage 1) femoral neck fractures demonstrated a 39% nonunion rate.

4. Orthopaedic Trauma Association Committee for Coding and Classification. Fracture and dislocation compendium. *J Orthop Trauma* 1996;10(suppl 1):1-154.

5. Asnis SE, Wanek-Sgaglione L: Intracapsular fractures of the femoral neck: Results of cannulated screw fixation. *J Bone Joint Surg Am* 1994;76:1793-1803.

6. Bhandari M, Devereax PJ, Swiontkowski MF, et al: Internal fixation compared with arthroplasty for displaced fractures of the femoral neck: A meta-analysis. *J Bone Joint Surg Am* 2003;85-A:1673-1681.

   The authors evaluated published trials between 1969 and 2002 regarding the treatment of displaced femoral neck fractures in patients age 65 years or older. Arthroplasty provided a significantly lower rate of revision surgery (*P* = 0.0003), but it was associated with greater blood loss, longer surgical time, and a trend toward a higher mortality rate in the first 4 months.

7. Hudson JI, Kenzora JE, Hebel JR, et al: Eight year outcome associated with clinical options in the management of femoral neck fractures. *Clin Orthop* 1998;348:59-66.

8. Robinson CM, Saran D, Annan IH: Intracapsular hip fractures: Results of management adopting a treatment protocol. *Clin Orthop* 1994;302:83-91.

9. Lu-Yao GL, Keller RB, Littenberg B, Wennberg JE: Outcomes after displaced fractures of the femoral neck: A meta-analysis of one hundred and six published reports. *J Bone Joint Surg Am* 1994;76:15-25.

10. Keating JF, Mzasson M, Scott N, et al: Randomized trial of reduction and fixation versus bipolar hemiarthroplasty versus total hip arthroplasty for displaced subcapital fractures in the fit older patient, in *70th Annual Meeting Proceedings*. Rosemont, IL, American Academy of Orthopaedic Surgeons, 2003, pp 582-583.

  The authors report superior functional outcomes for patients with fractures treated with total hip arthroplasty compared with open reduction and internal fixation or hemiarthroplasty.

11. Rogmark C, Carlsson Å, Johnell O, Sernbo I: Primary hemiarthroplasty in old patients with displaced femoral neck fracture: A 1-year follow-up of 103 patients aged 80 years or more. *Acta Orthop Scand* 2002;73:605-610.

  The authors of this study report that patients treated with primary hemiarthroplasty demonstrated a lower failure rate than those treated with internal fixation. There was no difference in length of hospital stay or mortality rates.

12. McKinley JC, Robinson CM: Treatment of displaced intracapsular hip fractures with total hip arthroplasty: Comparison of primary arthroplasty with early salvage arthroplasty after failed internal fixation. *J Bone Joint Surg Am* 2002;84-A:2010-2015.

  In this matched-pair, case-controlled study, the authors report better outcomes and fewer complications with primary arthroplasty than when arthroplasty is performed after internal fixation fails.

13. Booth KC, Donaldson TK, Dai QG: Femoral neck fracture fixation: A biomechanical study of two cannulated screw placement techniques. *Orthopedics* 1998;21:1173-1176.

14. Bout CA, Cannegieter DM, Juttmann JW: Percutaneous cannulated screw fixation of femoral neck fractures: The three point principle. *Injury* 1997;28:135-139.

15. Maurer SG, Wright KE, Kummer FJ, Zuckerman JD, Koval KJ: Two or three screws for fixation of femoral neck fractures? *Am J Orthop* 2003;32:438-442.

  The authors of this study reported that the use of three screws resulted in less fracture displacement than two screws during axial loading in embalmed cadaver specimens with subcapital osteotomies.

16. Kauffman JI, Simon JA, Kummer FJ, Pearlman CJ, Zuckerman JD, Koval KJ: Internal fixation of femoral neck fractures with posterior comminution: A biomechanical study. *J Orthop Trauma* 1999;13:155-159.

17. Parker MJ, Blundell C: Choice of implant for internal fixation of femoral neck fractures: Meta-analysis of 25 randomised trials including 4,925 patients. *Acta Orthop Scand* 1998;69:138-143.

18. Hammer AJ: Nonunion of the subcapital femoral neck fracture. *J Orthop Trauma* 1992;6:73-77.

19. Broos PL, Vercruysse R, Fourneau I, Driesen R, Stappaerts KH: Unstable femoral neck fractures in young adults: Treatment with the AO 130-degree blade plate. *J Orthop Trauma* 1998;12:235-240.

20. Heyse-Moore GH: Fixation of intracapsular femoral neck fractures with a one-hole plate dynamic hip screw. *Injury* 1996;27:181-183.

21. Weinrobe M, Stankewich CJ, Mueller B, Tencer AF: Predicting the mechanical outcome of femoral neck fractures fixed with cancellous screws: An in vivo study. *J Orthop Trauma* 1998;12:27-37.

22. Deneka DA, Simonian PT, Stankewich CJ, Eckert D, Chapman JR, Tencer AF: Biomechanical comparison of internal fixation techniques for the treatment of unstable basicervical femoral neck fractures. *J Orthop Trauma* 1997;11:337-343.

23. Jain R, Koo M, Kreder HJ, Schemitsch EH, Davey JR, Mahomed NN: Comparison of early and delayed fixation of subcapital hip fractures in patients sixty years of age or less. *J Bone Joint Surg Am* 2002;84-A:1605-1612.

  In this study, the authors reported that delayed treatment of subcapital fractures was associated with a higher rate of osteonecrosis; however, this complication did not significantly affect functional outcome at follow-up.

24. Chua D, Jaglal SB, Schatzker J: Predictors of early failure of fixation in the treatment of displaced subcapital hip fractures. *J Orthop Trauma* 1998;12:230-234.

25. Alho A, Benterud JG, Solovieva S: Internally fixed femoral neck fractures: Early prediction of failure in 203 elderly patients with displaced fractures. *Acta Orthop Scand* 1999;70:141-144.

26. Sharif KM, Parker MJ: Austin Moore hemiarthroplasty: Technical aspects and their effects on outcome, in patients with fractures of the neck of femur. *Injury* 2002;33:419-422.

    This retrospective study compared radiographic findings with outcomes and revision rates for 243 patients (mean age, 81 years) who were treated with Austin-Moore hemiarthroplasty. The authors report that undersizing of the prosthetic head and poor seating of the prosthesis on the calcar were associated with loosening and residual pain.

27. Ong BC, Maurer SG, Aharonoff GB, Zuckerman JD, Koval KJ: Unipolar versus bipolar hemiarthroplasty: Functional outcome after femoral neck fracture at a minimum of thirty-six months of follow-up. *J Orthop Trauma* 2002;16:317-322.

    The authors of this study report that no difference in functional outcome at midterm follow-up was noted when comparing patients who underwent unipolar or bipolar cemented hemiarthroplasties.

28. Parvizi J, Holiday AD, Ereth MH, Lewallen DG: Sudden death during primary hip arthroplasty. *Clin Orthop* 1999;369:39-48.

29. Pitto RP, Blunk J, Kößler M: Transesophageal echocardiography and clinical features of fat embolism during cemented total hip arthroplasty: A randomized study in patients with a femoral neck fracture. *Arch Orthop Trauma Surg* 2000;120:53-58.

30. Tidermark J, Ponzer S, Svensson O, Soderqvist A, Tornkvist H: Internal fixation compared with total hip replacement for displaced femoral neck fractures in the elderly: A randomised, controlled trial. *J Bone Joint Surg Br* 2003;85:380-388.

    In this study, 102 patients (mean age, 80 years) with an acute displaced fracture of the femoral neck were randomized to undergo either internal fixation with two cannulated screws or total hip replacement and followed up at 4, 12, and 24 months after surgery. Outcome measures included hip complications, revision surgery, hip function, and the health-related quality of life. The failure rate after 24 months was higher in the internal fixation group than in the total hip replacement group with regard to hip complications (36% and 4%, respectively; *P* < 0.001) and the number of revision procedures (42% and 4%, *P* < 0.001). The authors concluded that total hip replacement provides a better outcome than internal fixation for elderly, relatively healthy, lucid patients with a displaced fracture of the femoral neck.

31. Rogmark C, Carlsson A, Johnell O: A prospective randomised trial of internal fixation versus arthroplasty for displaced fractures of the neck of the femur: Functional outcome for 450 patients at two years. *J Bone Joint Surg Br* 2002;84:183-188.

    In this 2-year prospective multicenter study, the authors randomized 409 patients (age, 70 years and older) with subcapital fractures (Garden grade 3 or 4) to undergo internal fixation or arthroplasty. At 2-year follow-up, the rate of failure was 43% in the internal fixation group and 6% in the arthroplasty group (*P* < 0.001), which led the authors to recommend primary arthroplasty to treat displaced fractures of the neck of the femur in this patient population.

32. Lee BP, Berry DJ, Harmsen WS, Sim FH: Total hip arthroplasty for the treatment of an acute fracture of the femoral neck: Long term results. *J Bone Joint Surg Am* 1998;80:70-75.

33. Iorio R, Healy WL, Lemos DW, Appleby D, Lucchesi CA, Saleh KJ: Displaced femoral neck fractures in the elderly: outcomes and cost effectiveness. *Clin Orthop* 2001;383:229-242.

34. Cummings SR, Rubin SM, Black D: The future of hip fractures in the United States: Numbers, costs, and potential effects of postmenopausal estrogen. *Clin Orthop* 1990;252:163-166.

35. Evans EM: The treatment of trochanteric fractures of the femur. *J Bone Joint Surg Br* 1949;31:190-203.

36. Joseph TN, Chen AL, Kummer FJ, Koval KJ: The effect of posterior sag on the fixation stability of intertrochanteric hip fractures. *J Trauma* 2002;52:544-547.

37. Simpson AH, Varty K: Dodd CA: Sliding hip screws: Modes of failure. *Injury* 1989;20:227-231.

38. Baixauli F, Vicent V, Vaixauli E, et al: A reinforced rigid fixation device for unstable introchanteric fractures. *Clin Orthop* 1999;361:205-215.

39. Kim WY, Han CH, Park JI, Kim JY: Failure of intertrochanteric fracture fixation with a dynamic hip screw in relation to preoperative fracture stability and osteoporosis. *Int Orthop* 2001;25:360-362.

40. Baumgaertner MR, Curtin SL, Lindskog DM, Keggi JM: The value of the tip-apex distance in predicting

failure of fixation of peritrochanteric fractures of the hip. *J Bone Joint Surg Am* 1995;77:1058-1064.

41. Bolhofner BR, Russo PR, Carmen B: Results of intertrochanteric femur fractures treated with a 135-degree sliding screw with a two-hole side plate. *J Orthop Trauma* 1999;13:5-8.

42. McLoughlin SW, Wheeler DL, Rider J, Bolhofner B: Biomechanical evaluation of the dynamic hip screw with two- and four-hole side plates. *J Orthop Trauma* 2000;14:318-323.

43. Lorich DG, Geller DS, Nielson JH: Osteoporotic pertrochanteric hip fractures: Management and current controversies. *Instr Course Lect* 2004;53:441-454.

44. Ellis TJ, Kyle RF: The results of open reduction internal fixation of a highly unstable intertrochanteric hip fracture with a dynamic hip screw, in *67th Annual Meeting Proceedings.* Rosemont, IL, American Academy of Orthopaedic Surgeons, 2000, p 467.

45. Haidukewych GJ, Berry DJ: Salvage of failed internal fixation of intertrochanteric hip fractures. *Clin Orthop* 2003;412:184-188.

46. Lunsjö K, Ceder L, Skytting B, Sernbo I, Norberg S, Hjalmars K: A randomized multicenter trial of the Medoff sliding plate vs three screw-plate systems for the fixation of unstable intertrochanteric fractures in 569 elderly patients, in *67th Annual Meeting Proceedings.* Rosemont, IL, American Academy of Orthopaedic Surgeons, 2000, p 546.

47. Babst R, Renner N, Biedermann M, et al: Clinical results using the trochanter stabilizing plate (TSP): the modular extension of the dynamic hip screws (DHS) for internal fixation of selected unstable intertrochanteric fractures. *J Orthop Trauma* 1998;12: 392-399.

48. Madsen JE, Naess L, Aune AK, Alho A, Ekeland A, Stromsoe K: Dynamic hip screw with trochanteric stabilizing plate in the treatment of unstable proximal femoral fractures: A comparative study with the Gamma nail and compression hip screw. *J Orthop Trauma* 1998;12:241-248.

49. Gotfried Y: Percutaneous compression plating fro intertrochanteric hip fractures: Treatment rationale. *Orthopedics* 2002;25:647-652.

50. Kosygan KP, Mohan R, Newman RJ: The Gotfried percutaneous compression plate compared with the conventional classic hip screw for the fixation of intertrochanteric fractures of the hip. *J Bone Joint Surg Br* 2002;84:19-22.

51. Bramlet DG, Wheeler D: Use of the talon hip compression screw in intertrochanteric fractures of the hip. *J Orthop Trauma* 2003;17:618-624.

52. McConnell T, Tornetta P III, Benson E, Manuel J: Gluteus medius tendon injury during reaming for gamma nail insertion. *Clin Orthop* 2003;407:199-202.

53. Adams CI, Robinson CM, Court-Brown CM, McQueen MM: Prospective randomized controlled trial of an intramedullary nail versus dynamic screw and plate for intertrochanteric fractures of the femur. *J Orthop Trauma* 2001;15:394-400.

54. Baumgaertner MR, Curtin SL, Lindskog DM: Intramedullary versus extramedullary fixation for the treatment of intertrochanteric hip fractures. *Clin Orthop* 1998;348:87-94.

55. Hardy DC, Descamps PY, Krallis P, et al: Use of an intramedullary hip-screw with a plate for intertrochanteric femoral fractures: A prospective, randomized study of one hundred patients. *J Bone Joint Surg Am* 1998;80:618-630.

56. Sim E, Freimuller W, Teiter TH: Finite element analysis of the stress distributions in the proximal end of the femur after stabilization of a pertrochanteric model fracture: A comparison of two implants. *Injury* 1995;26:445-449.

57. Curtis MJ, Jinnah FH, Wilson V, Cunningham BW: Proximal femoral fractures: A biomechanical study to compare intramedullary and extramedullary fixation. *Injury* 1994;25:99-104.

58. Kyle RF, Cabanela ME, Russell TA, et al: Fractures of the proximal part of the femur. *Instr Course Lect* 1995;44:227-253.

59. Loch DA, Kyle RF, Bechtold JE, Kane M, Anderson K, Sherman RE: Forces required to initiate sliding in second-generation intramedullary nails. *J Bone Joint Surg Am* 1998;80:1626-1631.

60. Kubiak EN, Bong M, Park SS, Kummer F, Egol K, Koval KJ: Intramedullary fixation of unstable intertrochanteric hip fractures: One or two lag screws. *J Orthop Trauma* 2004;18:12-17.

61. Ahrengart L, Tornkvist H, Fornander P, et al: A randomized study of the comparison hip screw and Gamma nail in 426 fractures. *Clin Orthop* 2002;401: 209-222.

62. Herrera A, Domingo LJ, Calvo A, Martinez A, Cuenca J: A comparative study of trochanteric fractures treated with the Gamma nail or the proximal femoral nail. *Int Orthop* 2002;26:365-369.

63. Parker MJ, Handoll HH: Pre-operative traction for fractures of the proximal femur. *Cochrane Database Syst Rev* 2003;3:CD000168.

64. Saudan M, Lubbeke A, Sadowski C, Riand N, Stern R, Hoffmeyer P: Pertrochanteric fractures: Is there an advantage to an intramedullary nail? A randomized, prospective study of 206 patients comparing the dynamic hip screw and proximal femoral nail. *J Orthop Trauma* 2002;16:386-393.

65. Leung KS, So WS, Shen WY, Hui PW: Gamma nails and dynamic hip screws for peritrochanteric fractures: A randomized prospective study in elderly patients. *J Bone Joint Surg Br* 1992;74:345-351.

66. Watson JT, Moed BR, Karges DE, Cramer KE: Comparison of the compression hip screw with the Medoff sliding plate for intertrochanteric fractures. *Clin Orthop* 1998;348:79-86.

67. Sadowski C, Lubbeke A, Saudan M, Riand N, Stern R, Hoffmeyer P: Treatment of reverse oblique and transverse intertrochanteric fractures with use of an intramedullary nail or a 95 degrees screw-plate: A prospective, randomized study. *J Bone Joint Surg Am* 2002;84-A:372-381.

68. Szpalski M, Descamps PY, Hayez JP, et al: Prevention of hip lag screw cut-out by cement augmentation: Description of a new technique and preliminary clinical results. *J Orthop Trauma* 2004;18:34-40.

69. Goodman SB, Bauer TW, Carter D, et al: Norian SRS cement augmentation in hip fracture treatment: Laboratory and initial clinical results. *Clin Orthop* 1998;348:42-50.

70. Mattan Y, Mimant A, Mosheiff R, Peyser A, Mendelson S, Liebergall M: Avascular necrosis and related complications following healed osteoporotic intertrochanteric fractures. *Isr Med Assoc J* 2002;4:434-437.

71. Haidukewych GJ, Berry DJ: Hip arthroplasty for salvage of failed treatment of intertrochanteric hip fractures. *J Bone Joint Surg Am* 2003;85-A:899-904.

Chapter 42

Osteoporosis and Pathologic Bone

Charles N. Cornell, MD

John T. Gorczyca, MD

Management of Fractures in Osteoporotic and Pathologic Bone

Introduction

Osteoporosis currently affects 28 million Americans, 80% of whom are women. Osteoporosis is a systemic disease characterized by decreased bone mass and a deteriorated bone microarchitecture that results in an increased fracture risk. Metaphyseal regions of the skeleton are composed of primarily cancellous bone, which has a greater surface area for bone turnover compared with the compact cortical bone of the diaphysis. As a result, the metaphyseal regions lose bone more profoundly early after the onset of osteoporosis. Fractures resulting from osteoporosis generally involve the metaphyseal regions of the skeleton and are caused by low-energy falls. Osteoporosis is associated with 75% of the fractures that occur in the elderly population. It has been estimated that 50% of women and 18% of men older than 50 years will sustain a fracture related to osteoporosis. In the United States, 1.5 million fractures are reported annually. Of these there are 300,000 fractures of the proximal femur, 250,000 are fractures of the distal radius, and 300,000 are other fractures that occur through regions of the skeleton affected by osteoporosis. Each year $13.8 billion in health care costs is used to treat these fractures. However, fewer than 50% of patients with hip fractures recover fully after injury and treatment.[1,2]

These statistics emphasize the need for skilled fracture care in these patients. A reasonable return of function after fracture treatment in elderly patients often requires aggressive internal fixation and rapid rehabilitation. Conversely, prolonged immobilization of the patient through nonsurgical care increases the risk of thromboembolic disease, pulmonary compromise, decubitus ulceration, and further generalized musculoskeletal deterioration from which complete recovery is unlikely. Because the need for stable internal fixation in patients with osteoporotic bone is paramount, it is important that physicians understand the strategies for achieving this goal.

General Principles of Fracture Management in Patients With Osteoporosis

Elderly patients are best served by rapid, definitive fracture care aimed at early restoration of function. These patients are commonly healthiest on the day of injury and are usually in the best condition to undergo surgery within the first 48 hours of injury. Nevertheless, many concurrent illnesses are often present and should be thoroughly evaluated before surgery. In some patients, judicious preoperative medical management to reverse medical decompensations causing or resulting from the injury benefits survival. Similarly, surgical procedures should be kept simple to minimize surgical time, blood loss, and physiologic stress.

The aim of surgical intervention is to achieve stable fracture fixation that permits early return of function. In patients with fractures of the lower extremity, this implies early weight bearing. Although anatomic restoration is important for patients with intra-articular fractures, metaphyseal and diaphyseal fractures are best managed by efforts to primarily achieve stability rather than anatomic reduction.

Appropriate treatment of fractures that occur secondary to osteoporosis requires an understanding of the effect of this disease on the material and structural properties of bone as well as any effect on the process of fracture healing. An age-related decline in the capacity for fracture repair has been reported. A disturbance of the development of strength within the fracture callus has been reported in experimental models in the rat; however, little is known regarding the effect of osteoporosis and its causes on the process of fracture repair in humans.[3-5] Nonetheless, surgeons can assume that fracture healing in patients with osteoporosis is impaired. Whenever possible, the principles of biologic fracture repair should be applied. These principles include careful handling of the surrounding soft tissues and avoiding unnecessary stripping of fracture fragments to preserve blood supply to the fracture site. In addition to minimizing the surgical exposure of the fracture, preservation of the fracture hematoma may speed the development of the fracture callus. Adherence to these principles improves the speed of healing and improves the chances for successful fixation.

The primary mode of failure of internal fixation in osteoporotic bone results from bone failure rather than implant breakage. Because bone mineral density correlates linearly with the holding power of screws, osteoporotic bone often lacks the strength to hold plates and screws securely. Furthermore, comminution can be severe in patients with osteoporotic fractures. Surgical treatment of fractures of the proximal humerus, proximal and distal femur, and the proximal tibia has historically yielded a high incidence of poor results in elderly patients with osteoporosis. For example, plate fixation of proximal humerus fractures in an elderly patient group resulted in fair to poor results in more than 50% of patients, with screw loosening and pullout from the humeral head occurring in at least 20%.[6,7] In 10% of patients with intertrochanteric fractures of the proximal femur, internal fixation is typically unsuccessful, with the mode of failure being cutout of the lag screw from the cancellous bone of the femoral head.[8] Although open reduction and internal fixation yields superior results to nonsurgical management in supracondylar fractures of the femur, 25% of fractures treated with the angle-blade plate resulted in fair to poor results because of loss of reduction from loosening of the implant in the osteoporotic bone of the femoral condyles. Traditional techniques of internal fixation must be modified to achieve satisfactory results in patients with osteoporotic bone. Internal fixation devices that allow load sharing with host bone should be chosen to minimize stress at the bone-implant interface. For these reasons, sliding nail plate devices, intramedullary nails, antiglide plates, and tension band constructs are ideal for osteoporotic bone. Combined with surgical tactics that adhere to the principles of biologic fracture repair, these devices can achieve excellent results.[9,10]

Biomechanics of Implant Fixation in Osteoporotic Bone

Internal Fixation Using Screws

Resistance to pullout of a screw placed in bone depends on the length of the screw purchase, the thread diameter of the screw, and the quality of the bone into which it is inserted. Recent studies have also indicated that the trabecular orientation within the bone is also important.[11] Bone is highly anisotropic (it has physical properties that are different in different directions). Screws placed parallel to the trabecular pattern have greater pullout strength than those placed across the trabeculae. In osteoporotic bone, the variable of bone quality becomes the primary determinant of screw holding power. When bone mineral content falls below 0.4 g/cm^2, the effect of varying thread diameter is lost. Therefore, a

surgical plan to place screws into osteoporotic bone should be designed to place screws as parallel to the cancellous trabeculae as possible and should use the largest screw thread diameter that is compatible with the scale of the fracture being fixed. Most importantly, screws should be placed to secure fixation into cortical bone, if possible. Cortical bone always has greater mineral density and therefore resistance to screw pullout than adjacent trabecular bone. As a result, in bone of poor quality, a smaller diameter cortical screw may be a superior choice over a larger diameter cancellous screw, which cannot secure cortical purchase.

In patients with severe osteoporosis, the surgeon should be ready to augment screw fixation with cement. Polymethylmethacrylate cement has historically been used most commonly for this purpose. Polymethylmethacrylate cement has poor adhesion to bone, but its intrusion into the cancellous structure results in a vastly stronger composite after the cement sets. The technique used begins with removal of any screws that have inadequate purchase or have stripped with tightening. The methylmethacrylate powder and liquid should be cooled to slow polymerization; once mixed, the liquid cement is placed into a 10-mL syringe with the tip widened by drilling it out with a 3.5-mm drill. Alternatively, a catheter-tipped syringe can be used. The cement is then injected with pressure into the stripped screw holes, and the screws are replaced but incompletely tightened. Care should be taken to avoid intrusion of the cement into the fracture site or into the intra-articular space in epiphyseal fractures. Once the cement has hardened, a final tightening of the screw can be performed. Manipulation of the screw while the cement is setting loosens the bond between the cement, bone, and screw, lowering the pullout strength. Cement can also be used in a manner similar to cement techniques used for fixation of an intramedullary prosthesis. In this method, the medullary canal is blocked proximal and/or distal to the fracture site, and the entire medullary cavity is filled with cement. The fracture is reduced, and the cement is allowed to cure. The screws are then inserted by drilling and tapping the cement if it is fully cured or adhering to the principle of only tightening the screws after the cement is hardened if the screws are placed during the curing process. This technique is very useful for situations in which poor screw fixation is combined with significant bone loss. Additional studies have proposed other strategies for using cement to improve fixation.[12]

Internal Fixation Using Plates

The security of plate fixation is affected primarily by the degree of comminution and the resulting size of any gap at the fracture site. In addition, the pattern of screw placement influences the strains experienced within the plate and its screws. The most important factor, which reduces strain in plated fractures, is the degree to which cortical contact at the fracture site can be achieved. Experimental fractures stabilized by plates spanning a gap experience three times the strain as fractures stabilized with secure cortical contact. In addition, for a given fracture pattern the spacing of screws is more important than the number of screws used for fixation. Strain within a plated construct is least when screws are placed as close to and as far away from the fracture site as possible. In two-part fractures or those with solid cortical contact and no gap, the farther the screws are placed from the fracture, the lower the strain within the plate. Therefore, the longer the plate, the better it is to place screws as close to and as far away from the fracture site as possible. Intervening screws add little to the overall strength of fixation. In comminuted fractures or those with a gap, the longer plate retains its advantage, but an increased number of screws adjacent to the fracture site reduces the strain within the plate. Experimental data suggest that three screws should be placed in the plate holes that are closest to either side of the fracture gap as well as the most distant hole of the plate.[13] Again, additional intervening screws add little to the load experienced by the plate.

These principles become extremely important when treating patients with osteoporotic bone. In patients with osteoporotic bone, longer plates with widely spaced screws should be used. When using plate and screw fixation in patients with osteoporotic bone, the surgeon must try to achieve cortical contact at the fracture site. If moderate areas of comminution exist, then the fracture should be shortened to achieve contact, especially in the cortex opposite the plate. In essence, this principle suggests that plates should not be used to bridge gaps in patients with osteoporotic bone; instead, plates should be used as tension bands that require an intact, load-sharing cortex opposite the plate. In patients in whom comminution is extensive and prevents stable contact opposite the plate, then the surgeon must consider double plating to secure stability. In addition, the surgeon should try to place the plates to act as antiglide plates whenever possible. Antiglide plates are especially useful in the treatment of short oblique or spiral oblique fracture patterns. In these types of fractures, the plate can be positioned to create an axilla with the cortex at the apex of the oblique tongue of the fracture (Figure 1). This position of the plate acts to prevent fracture displacement and places less importance on screw fixation within the weak, adjacent metaphyseal bone and positions the plate nicely for insertion of lag screws, which are important for the oblique fracture pattern.

A major advance in the treatment of osteoporotic fractures has been realized with the introduction of fixed-angle screw plates.[14] These plates, also referred to as locking buttress plates, are designed with threaded screw holes. The locking screws have heads with threads that engage the plate holes and rigidly thread into place, creating a fixed-angle screw. These devices confer all the

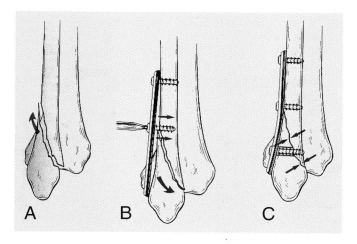

Figure 1 A through **C,** Schematic representations demonstrating the antiglide principle. The plate is positioned to create an axilla at the apex of the fracture. The distal fragment reduces into the axilla. The plate then prevents the tendency for displacement and achieves compression along the fracture line.

advantages of fixed-angle blade plates, but offer several other advantages. The insertion of these devices is simple. The complexity of inserting a femoral blade plate is avoided. The pattern of screw insertion also captures a greater area of metaphyseal bone, leading to more stable fixation and the ability to withstand a greater load to failure. These plates typically fail because of an all or nothing phenomenon, with all screws pulling out within a region of bone from the metaphysis. Also, because stability does not rely upon plate-bone contact and the screws cannot toggle or loosen within the plate, these plates confer far greater stability when they are used to bridge gaps. This allows much more limited exposure and surgical manipulation of comminuted metaphyseal fractures. This design feature has permitted methods of less invasive surgical stabilization to be developed. Using the less invasive surgical stabilization type of plates, small exposure of the intra-articular components of metaphyseal fractures can be performed to reduce intra-articular incongruities, followed by percutaneous, submuscular plate placement for stabilization of the metaphysis to the diaphysis. Early clinical experience has demonstrated the exceptional effectiveness of this new technology in the treatment of fractures of the proximal and distal tibia, supracondylar fractures of the femur[15-17] (Figure 2), and fractures of the proximal humerus[18] (Figure 3). Many of the older techniques that were successful in treatment of osteoporotic fractures, such as the angle-blade plate and tension band wiring, are likely to be used less often in the wake of this new technology.

Intramedullary Nails
Intramedullary nail fixation is nicely suited for treating patients with osteoporotic bone, especially for those with diaphyseal fractures. Intramedullary nails provide a broad area of purchase, allow load sharing, and provide

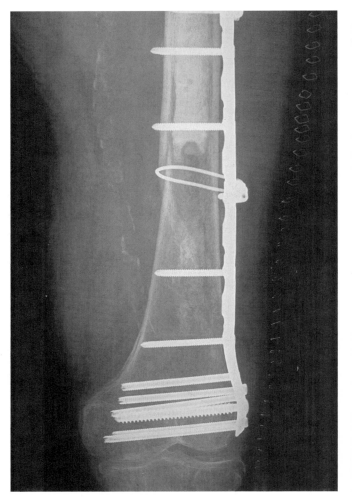

Figure 2 Radiograph demonstrating fixation of a supracondylar fracture of the femur using the locking 95° condylar buttress plate.

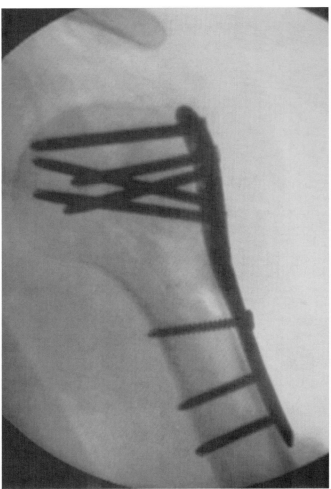

Figure 3 Radiograph demonstrating the use of a locking proximal humeral plate in the repair of a two-part proximal humerus fracture.

secure fixation to allow immediate weight bearing in some patients. Intramedullary nailing is the treatment of choice for the treatment of diaphyseal fractures of the femur and tibia.[19,20] The development of interlocking nails has extended the indications for intramedullary nailing to include metaphyseal fractures as well. Intramedullary nails are positioned closer to the mechanical axis of the bones in which they are placed; as a result, they are subject to smaller bending forces than plated constructs placed on the external surface of the bone. Intramedullary nails are less likely to experience fatigue failure than plate constructs. Mechanically locked intramedullary nails provide greater strength in axial loading than condylar blade plates, but they are significantly less stable in bending and torsion when applied to the distal femur.

The major weakness of locked intramedullary nails is the security of the locking screws. The locking screws can easily loosen, especially within the bone of the distal femur leading to loss of control of the distal fragment. This may result in rotational and varus/valgus malalignment. There are many recently published studies that report successful outcomes using retrograde femoral nails that have been modified to improve fixation in the elderly patient population.[21-24] Locking screw fixation can be improved by using different planes of screw orientation (AP and transverse placement), osteoporotic nuts and washers on the medial side of the femur where the locking bolts emerge, or cement to improve fixation.

Tension Band Wiring

Tension band wiring as a fixation technique is most often used to treat transverse fractures, which are distracted by the pull of attached tendons and ligaments. Tension band wiring provides strong, secure and biologically friendly fixation and allows for immediate mobilization of involved joints. Fractures of the olecranon and patella have been successfully treated using this technique. In patients with osteoporotic bone, the tension band wire has additional advantages. In metaphyseal locations such as the proximal humerus or medial malleolus, tendon and ligament insertions to bone can provide better strength for fixation than the bone itself. In these areas,

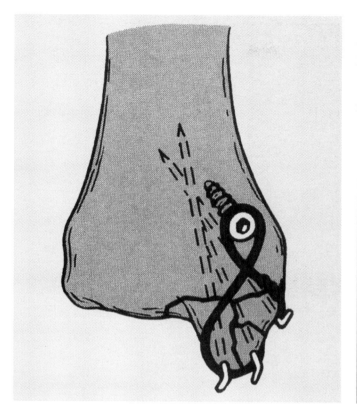

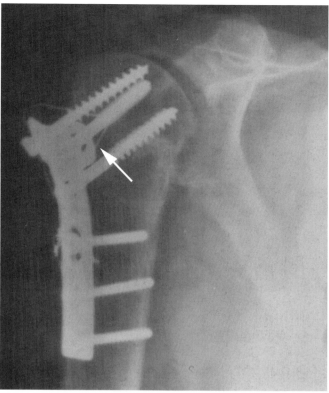

Figure 4 Schematic representation of tension band wiring. Kirschner wires are placed to hold the medial malleolus fracture reduced. A wire is then passed in a figure-of-8 fashion distal to the wires through the substance of the deltoid ligament and anchored to a screw placed proximal to the fracture.

Figure 5 AP radiograph of a tension band wire augmenting plate fixation in the proximal humerus. The wire is passed in a figure-of-8 fashion beneath the supraspinatus tendon (*arrow*) and distally beneath the plate. The wire provides a strong purchase and acts to neutralize the deforming pull of the rotator cuff.

placement of tension band wire within the soft-tissue attachments can provide excellent anchorage. This technique was first described in the fixation of proximal humeral fractures, with better clinical results reported than those achieved with plates and screw fixation.[9,25]

A similar technique can be used to secure osteoporotic or comminuted medial malleolar fractures (Figure 4). The fracture is reduced and maintained with small Kirschner wires. The tension band wire is passed within the fibers of the deltoid ligament and proximally secured to bone by passing it around a screw placed through the tibia. The wire is placed in a figure-of-8 fashion and can be tightened by opposing twists. Tension band wires can also supplement plate and screw fixation in fractures that experience tensile loading. After securing the fracture with plate and screws, an additional tension band wire passed within adjacent tendinous attachments and then beneath the plate can help neutralize tensile forces across the construct (Figure 5).

Augmentation of Fracture Healing and Stability
Traditionally, surgeons have resorted to cancellous bone grafting to augment or help ensure rapid and complete healing of fractures. In osteoporotic bone fractures, bone grafting plays several important roles. Cancellous bone

grafts can be used to promote rapid fracture healing, improving the odds of healing in the race against eventual failure of internal fixation. Autogenous cancellous bone is osteoinductive, osteoconductive, and osteogenic and will stimulate new bone formation periosteally as well as in fracture gaps created by comminution. There is no current evidence showing that osteoporotic bone is an inferior graft material.

Bone grafting is also important in osteoporotic fractures to replace regions of skeletal loss caused by comminution or crush injury. Corticocancellous bone grafts can replace structural loss and as such can help restore skeletal stability in fracture constructs. This is especially true in metaphyseal and joint depression type fractures. Osteoporosis affects regions of cancellous bone more quickly than compact, cortical bone. Metaphyseal injury with joint depression is a typical fracture pattern associated with osteoporosis. Examples include split-depression tibial plateau fractures, intra-articular fractures of the distal radius, distal humeral fractures, and tibial plafond fractures. Surgical repair of these injuries requires elevation of the articular surface to restore joint congruity and the use of structural bone graft to fill in the crushed, metaphyseal void to provide support to the subchondral region.

The donor source for autogenous bone graft is usually the iliac crest. The morbidity associated with the harvest of autogenous bone has recently become a concern. In the elderly patient population, this is a particularly important issue. The quantity and quality of bone available at the iliac crest are often insufficient, requiring a larger exposure and increasing the risk of donor site complications. Bone graft substitutes provide an attractive alternative to autograft in osteoporotic patients. Bone graft substitutes include allograft bone, demineralized allograft bone products, and synthetic osteoconductive materials, which can be used as bone void fillers. Implants of osteoprotegerin-1, bone morphogenetic protein-2, and bone morphogenetic protein-7 are now also available. Several of these products have been shown to be useful as alternatives to autogenous graft in treating acute fractures.

In patients with severe skeletal loss, complete replacement of comminuted areas by cement may be required. Polymethylmethacrylate has been used with success, especially in supracondylar fractures of the femur. Polymethylmethacrylate has also been used to treat intertrochanteric fractures as well.[12] Although polymethylmethacrylate has proved useful, it is not an ideal material for this purpose because it becomes a permanent implant and a foreign body within bone. It also generates considerable heat with polymerization, which is harmful to bone and surrounding soft tissue. Cements made from calcium phosphate have better adhesion to bone and have the advantage of being resorbed and replaced by host bone. These cements are not used to augment screw fixation but to fill voids caused by comminution or severe osteoporosis. Calcium phosphate cements have been demonstrated to have usefulness in the treatment of intertrochanteric and distal radius fractures. It has been suggested that these new cements can provide enough support to allow earlier load bearing and decrease the dependency on internal fixation devices in fractures with metaphyseal voids.[26] However, surgeons should keep in mind that these cements offer support only in compression at loads up to 55 mPa. These materials are very weak in torsion, bending, and shear. All fractures experience loads in multiple planes, making it impossible to rely on the cement alone for support. At the present time, alterations in postoperative management from that used with traditional bone grafting cannot be supported by experience reported in the literature.

Although augmentation of the severely osteoporotic diaphysis can be accomplished using polymethylmethacrylate, another useful approach is to place an augmentation device into the medullary canal that can incorporate as bone or be resorbed. Fibular allograft struts can be used for this purpose (Figure 6). The fibular strut improves local bone stock for screw purchase and can be incorporated to provide a span across regions of diaphyseal deficiency. Creative strategies such as these can

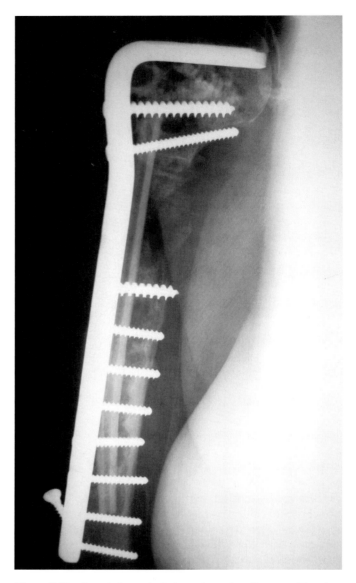

Figure 6 AP radiograph of a repair of a humeral nonunion with segmental bone loss. A fibular strut allograft was fashioned into an intramedullary peg. It spanned the defect and improved the screw purchase proximal and distal to the fracture site. The loose distal screw was hidden within soft tissues remaining from a previous attempt at reconstruction.

be extremely useful in the treatment of osteoporotic diaphyseal fractures and nonunions.

Prosthetic Replacement

Prosthetic replacement in many patients can provide superior results compared with open reduction and internal fixation of displaced femoral neck fractures, four-part fractures of the proximal humerus, extremely comminuted fractures of the distal humerus,[27,28] and unsalvageable fractures about the knee. In general, prosthetic replacement should be reserved for patients who are old enough to expect that the prosthesis will not fail during their life spans and for those whose activity expectations are limited. This is especially true when contemplating total elbow replacement for a patient with a distal humerus fracture. It is now clear that prosthetic replacement provides a more predictably successful and cost-effective outcome compared with reduction and pinning in elderly patients with displaced femoral neck fractures.[29] Findings from several studies suggest that total hip replacement may provide the best results in fit, active elderly patients with hip fractures.[30-33] Prosthetic replacement of the proximal humerus should be used only when reconstruction of the humeral head is unlikely to be successful or when the risk of osteonecrosis is high. This implies that the displaced four-part fracture with dislocation of the head and head-splitting fractures are best treated with replacement. A successful hemiarthroplasty of the shoulder requires repair of the rotator cuff via secure fixation of the greater and lesser tuberosities to the prosthesis and shaft.

Acetabular fractures in elderly patients can also be successfully managed with total hip replacement.[34] A common fracture pattern in elderly, osteoporotic patients is fracture of the anterior column and medial wall with central dislocation of the femoral head. Posterior exposure of the hip joint with resection of the femoral head provides direct exposure of the acetabulum and ready access to the posterior column and the supra-acetabular area. Major column disruptions should be stabilized. The femoral head can be useful in replacing columnar defects or defects in the medial wall. Multi-holed acetabular components can be used as internal fixation devices to improve stability. In severely osteoporotic patients, acetabular rings can be used to span defects and provide support to cemented acetabular components.

Severe fractures about the knee, especially very distal periprosthetic fractures, can be treated with revision type total knee replacements. For patients with extreme loss of the distal femur, a rotating-hinge prosthesis (tumor) megaprostheses may be needed.

Postoperative Care

It should be assumed that any patient older than middle age with a fracture in a metaphyseal region from a low-energy mechanism has osteoporosis. These patients therefore require treatment to combat further bone loss. All elderly patients with fractures should be encouraged to take calcium supplementation of approximately 1,000 to 1,500 mg per day along with a multivitamin that ensures adequate vitamin D intake. Elderly patients with fractures should also be encouraged to start bisphosphonate therapy regardless of their reported bone mineral density measurements. To date, alendronate and risedronate are the only agents proven to reduce the risk of additional fracture after a fracture of the hip.[35] Risedronate, an alternative bisphosphonate, has been shown to reduce the risk of vertebral fracture and can also be prescribed for this patient population.[36] For patients who

may be lost to follow-up in the early postoperative period, administration of a long-acting bisphosphonate such as pamidronate or zoledronic acid may be given intravenously with similar benefit. All orthopaedic surgeons who treat fractures in the elderly must accept it as their responsibility to assess and treat osteoporosis in their patients.

Pathologic Long Bone Fractures

Introduction

A pathologic fracture is a fracture that occurs through bone that has been weakened by a pathologic process. Although many processes (such as osteoporosis) can weaken bone and increase the risk of fracture, the term pathologic fracture generally refers to fractures that occur in the region of a neoplasm.

Impending pathologic fractures are neoplastic bone lesions that are destructive enough to significantly weaken the bone and place the patient at risk for fracture. Provided the patient is healthy enough to tolerate surgery, impending pathologic fractures should be treated with surgical stabilization to improve patient comfort, mobility, and independence.[37,38]

In patients younger than 40 years, most pathologic fractures are caused by primary bone tumors or infection. In patients older than 40 years, most pathologic fractures result from metastases to bone. Bone is the third most common site for tumor metastases. Cancers of the breast, lung, and prostate have a proclivity for spreading to bone. Additionally, renal and thyroid tumors may spread to bone.

Thus, because most of these bony lesions occur in adults with metastatic cancer, the underlying prognosis for these patients may be grim, and the impact of the pathologic fracture on a patient's quality of life can be devastating. This underscores the necessity for detecting these areas of bony involvement early, treating the tumor aggressively, avoiding any chance of spreading tumor cells to healthy tissue during procedures, properly controlling pain, preventing fracture, and providing the skeletal stability necessary for patients to maintain maximum independence and mobility.

Diagnostic Evaluation

The goals of evaluation of a patient with a pathologic or impending pathologic fracture include identifying tumor type, evaluating the extent of the lesion(s), and minimizing the systemic effects of the neoplastic process. All evaluations start with a thorough patient history, especially with regard to a history of malignancy, weight loss, pain, or fracture. Physical examination should be thorough but considerate of the patient's overall state. In particular, examination of the lung, thyroid, breast, and prostate should be performed to evaluate for primary malignancy in these sites.

Laboratory tests should include a complete blood cell count with differential to evaluate the oxygen-carrying capacity of the blood, rule out hematologic origin of the tumor, and identify potential clotting abnormalities. Likewise, a prothrombin time and partial thromboplastin time should be obtained. Liver function tests should be performed because the results may indicate primary or metastatic involvement of the liver. Abnormal thyroid function tests assessing T3, T4, and thyrotropin levels may indicate involvement of the thyroid gland. Serum urea nitrogen and creatinine levels should be assessed because elevation of either may be a sign of renal involvement. Serum electrolytes, calcium, magnesium, and phosphate levels may be abnormal because of bone turnover. Assessment of prostate-specific antigen and parathyroid hormone levels and erythrocyte sedimentation rate may provide additional information about the type of primary cancer. Serum and urine protein electrophoresis levels should be assessed to rule out multiple myeloma. Urinary N-telopeptides serve as an indicator for bone collagen breakdown (which parallels tumor burden) and should be assessed as a baseline by which to compare treatment progress.

Radiographic studies should include AP and lateral radiographs of the entire bone involved. Occasionally, oblique radiographs will improve the ability to measure the size of the lesion. CT scans of the chest, abdomen, and pelvis can help to identify primary tumors and to rule out metastases.

Metastatic renal and thyroid tumors can be highly vascularized and result in significant hemorrhage, even with seemingly minor surgical procedures. Patients with these bony metastases should be evaluated with arteriogram and may benefit from embolization before surgery.

CT scans of the pathologic lesion will give a more accurate assessment of the degree of bony destruction. MRI provides excellent information about the extent of the lesion in the bone and soft tissue.

A technetium bone scan may depict the site of the primary tumor and often reveals other sites of bony involvement. Multiple myeloma may not be associated with increased uptake on a bone scan, so patients with this malignancy should have a radiographic skeletal survey to identify other areas of metastasis.

Despite fairly extensive noninvasive diagnostic studies directed at identification of primary tumors, a primary tumor may not be identified in approximately 15% of patients with pathologic fractures.[39] Differentiation between a primary bone tumor and a bony metastasis is essential because proper treatment of primary bone tumors is more likely to involve surgical excision of the tumor and improved survival.[40] Therefore, a needle or open biopsy should be performed of bony lesions of unclear origin before any surgical stabilization is undertaken. If a primary bone tumor is mistaken for a metastatic lesion and treated with surgical stabilization, the patient's prognosis for limb salvage or survival may be adversely affected. For instance, if a patient had a primary malignant fibrous histiocytoma that was mistaken for a metastasis and was treated with an intramedullary rod, the radioresistance of the tumor and the intraoperative dissemination of tumor cells throughout the intramedullary canal would have a negative impact on the treatment. Thus, the diagnosis must be established before stabilization in order to avoid such a situation.

Intramedullary biopsy of a diaphyseal lesion, performed with long pituitary rongeurs or bronchial forceps, is a minimally invasive means by which reliable tissue samples can be obtained for diagnosis. Femoral reamings have been used for pathologic analysis, but they typically provide lower quality tissue samples.

Treatment Considerations

Patients with pathologic fractures usually have a poor prognosis. Most of these fractures are caused by metastatic disease, and these patients have limited survival. For instance, few patients with pathologic fractures from lung cancer survive longer than 6 months. Thus, the risks of surgical stabilization may be greater than the short-term benefit of pain relief and mobility. It is generally accepted that if survival is expected to be 2 months or less, then surgical treatment of the pathologic fracture is not indicated.

Similarly, functional status will guide the surgeon toward the best treatment. Inactive but comfortable patients can have their pathologic fractures treated without surgery.

Surgical stabilization of pathologic long bone fractures is appropriate in most patients. A stable long bone allows improved mobility and independence, better comfort, and as a consequence, fewer complications from prolonged immobility. Because many patients with this type of injury have limited life expectancy, the goal of surgery should be to achieve solid fixation that will allow immediate use of the extremity.

Surgical stabilization of impending pathologic fractures is prudent because it is generally believed that after a pathologic fracture occurs, surgical stabilization is more difficult, the surgical risks are higher, and the fracture is less likely to heal.[41]

Postoperative radiotherapy of a metastatic lesion will slow disease progression and will make fixation failure less likely. Although metastatic lung adenocarcinoma and renal adenocarcinoma tend to respond less favorably to radiotherapy and have been referred to as radioresistant, they nevertheless demonstrate a response; thus, it is in the patient's best interest to have postoperative radiotherapy to slow disease progression as much as possible. Therefore, every patient with a pathologic fracture or impending pathologic fracture should undergo postoperative radiotherapy or chemotherapy.[42]

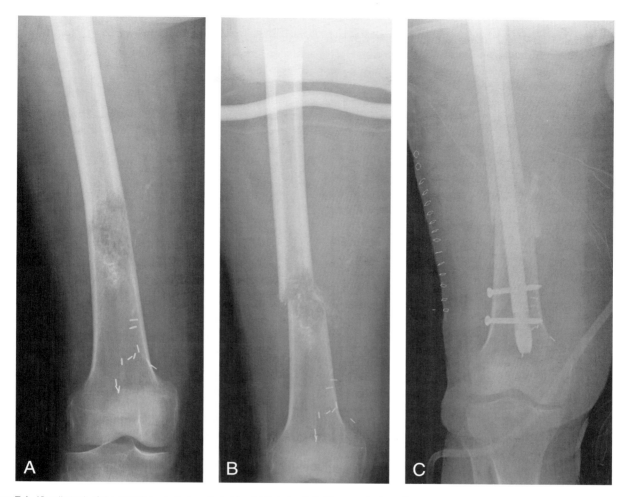

Figure 7 A, AP radiograph of the distal femur indicates a large (4-cm) lytic lesion that did not receive immediate treatment. **B,** AP radiograph of the distal femur 4 days later demonstrates pathologic fracture that occurred while the patient was sitting. Orthopaedic consultation was obtained at this time. **C,** AP radiograph of the femur demonstrates intramedullary stabilization of a pathologic distal femur fracture that occurred after needle biopsy revealed this to be metastatic adenocarcinoma of the lung. (*Courtesy of R. Rosier, MD, PhD.*)

Indications for Surgery

Surgical stabilization of a pathologic fracture is indicated when the discomfort or instability of the fracture results in a functional impairment that exceeds the surgical risk. Thus, almost every pathologic fracture of the femur, tibia, and humerus would benefit from surgical stabilization if the patient were healthy enough to tolerate the surgery. After surgical stabilization, the pathologic fracture is less painful, allows some use of the extremity, and has a greater chance of healing.

The generally accepted indications for surgical intervention for impending pathologic fractures are lesions larger than 2.5 cm, lesions involving greater than 50% of the bone diameter, and painful lesions that do not respond to radiotherapy or chemotherapy. Some authors have considered destruction of 50% of the cortical diameter or increasing bone pain (presumably caused by microfractures) as a sign of impending fracture and therefore an indication for surgical stabilization.[42,43] The rationale for surgical intervention in patients with im-

pending pathologic fractures is that because a fracture is likely and will be more difficult to treat after it occurs, the bone should be stabilized before it fractures (Figure 7).

Data suggest that the radiographic appearance of the lesion and the location of the lesion will also affect the risk of fracture.[44] Osteolytic lesions (typically metastatic thyroid and renal carcinoma) are more likely to cause fracture than mixed osteolytic/osteoblastic (breast) lesions, which are more likely to cause fracture than osteoblastic (prostate) lesions. Additionally, lesions in the intertrochanteric and subtrochanteric region of the femur are more likely to fracture because of the high concentration of forces in these areas with weight bearing.

Implant Considerations

Experience has shown that it is prudent to assume that even after proper surgical stabilization, a pathologic fracture may not heal and that the implant chosen will loosen with time. If the surgeon accepts this assumption as valid, then the chosen treatment should address these two problems before they occur. This partly explains the widespread use of intramedullary stabilization techniques for patients with pathologic fractures; complete loss of fixation is much less likely with intramedullary fixation than with extramedullary fixation.[42,45]

Periarticular lesions and fractures often leave insufficient bone for stable fixation of the articular surface. A good alternative for many of these pathologic fractures is cemented arthroplasty.[42,46] Specifically, lesions involving the femoral head, femoral neck, intercondylar femur, tibial plateau, proximal humerus, and distal humerus are indications for excision of the pathologic bone and hemiarthroplasty or total arthroplasty. Arthroplasty improves patient comfort and often allows unrestricted weight bearing. Long-stemmed arthroplasty is often necessary to bypass and stabilize lesions in the diaphyseal region. Press-fit/ingrowth implants should not be used because they are less likely to achieve ingrowth in this patient population and are more likely to be loose and/or painful.

In some patients, lesions in the metadiaphyseal or metaphyseal regions of long bones can be treated with open reduction and internal fixation after débridement of the lesion and insertion of methylmethacrylate into the void.[47]

Intertrochanteric lesions can be treated successfully with either cephalomedullary nailing or arthroplasty. Before deciding which treatment is most appropriate, surgeons must consider the likelihood that the tumor will enlarge and result in fixation failure; the needs of the patient, particularly whether the patient has the strength and balance to perform protected weight bearing after cephalomedullary nailing; and the surgeon's own skills.

Cement Use

Attempts at surgical stabilization of pathologic fractures may yield marginal fixation strength that will only weaken further with time. Augmentation of intramedullary or extramedullary fixation with methylmethacrylate cement can achieve better fixation. Typical uses for cement include filling a cavitary defect, filling an intramedullary void to achieve tighter intramedullary fixation, and insertion into screw holes to improve pullout strength of the subsequently inserted screw.[47]

Tobramycin or gentamicin are heat stable and can be added to cement to decrease the risk of early postoperative infection. This should be considered especially in patients who are immunocompromised because of their malignancy or chemotherapy. Antibiotic concentrations of 3% do not have a significant weakening effect on the cement and will cause elution of antibiotic for 1 to 3 months.[48,49]

Several precautions are necessary when using cement. First, timing is critical because the cement can harden quickly and make screw or rod insertion impossible without fragmenting and removing the cement. Second, the cement will generate a significant amount of heat during the hardening process and can cause thermal damage to nerves and other tissues nearby. It is essential to contain the cement inside the bone and to cool it with irrigation fluid while it hardens. Third, no matter how good the cement fixation is, it will only weaken with time. Thus, practical activity restrictions should be considered to preserve the fixation construct.

Lower Extremity Versus Upper Extremity Pathologic Fractures

Important differences exist between upper and lower extremity pathologic fractures. The lower extremities are used for locomotion and consequently must withstand greater forces. Thus, bony lesions in the lower extremities are more likely to cause pain and are more likely to fracture.[50] A patient with a metastatic lesion of the upper extremity can predictably protect the extremity from undue force during the course of radiation therapy and thus is less likely to experience a pathologic fracture. Because it is much more difficult to protect the lower extremity from undue forces, surgery is usually a safer option than nonsurgical treatment. Furthermore, after surgical stabilization, a lower extremity pathologic fracture is more likely to be painful during normal activity. Fixation of a lower extremity fracture is more likely to fail under applied loads.

It therefore becomes imperative to recognize and treat impending pathologic fractures of the lower extremity before the bone fractures. Intramedullary nailing or arthroplasty are the mainstay of treatment for lower extremity pathology because extramedullary fixation is likely to fail with time.

Occasionally, an upper extremity pathologic fracture will not cause much pain and can be treated with a fracture brace. This may provide good function when treating pathologic fractures of one of the forearm bones. Pathologic fractures of the humerus, however, are more likely to cause significant pain when treated in a fracture brace and are usually best treated surgically. Closed intramedullary nailing is ideal for pathologic humeral shaft fractures because it offers the benefits of intramedullary stabilization. If stable fixation does not seem likely with closed intramedullary nailing, then open nailing with cement augmentation or dual plating will provide improved fixation strength.[42,51-53]

Roles for Radiotherapy and Chemotherapy

Malignant bony lesions should be treated with radiotherapy or chemotherapy to slow or stop the neoplastic growth. It is prudent to wait 3 to 7 days after surgery to allow the incision some time for unimpeded healing. Although the specifics of radiotherapy and chemotherapy are complex, in general 800 cGy to 3,000 cGy of radiotherapy are used to treat one to several metastases, whereas chemotherapy is reserved for the treatment of multiple or widespread metastases or for painful or enlarging metastases that have already been treated with the maximum level of radiotherapy.

Bony metastatic disease can also be treated with bisphosphonates, hormone therapy, systemic radioisotopes, and immunotherapy. Bisphosphonates (such as pamidronate) inhibit osteoclasts, thereby slowing bone resorption. Although they do not have tumor-killing properties, they can decrease the pain and fracture risk of breast and prostate cancer metastases to bone.[54] Estrogen receptor blockers can have a beneficial effect on some types of metastatic breast cancer. There is widespread optimism that additional technologies to inhibit tumor growth in bone and prevent pathologic fractures will soon be developed.

Annotated References

1. World Health Organization: *The Burden of Musculoskeletal Conditions at the Start of the New Millennium.* WHO Technical Report Series Number 919, 2003. Available at: http://www.ota.org/downloads/bjdFact.doc. Accessed June 1, 2005.

2. Adachi JD, Ioannidis G, Pickard L, et al: The association between osteoporotic fractures and health-related quality of life as measured by the Health Utilities Index in the Canadian Multicentre Osteoporosis Study (CaMos). *Osteoporos Int* 2003;14:895-904.
   This multicenter study used the Health Utilities Index to document the adverse outcomes associated with lower extremity fractures resulting from osteoporosis.

3. Silver JJ, Einhorn TA: Osteoporosis and aging. *Clin Orthop* 1995;316:10-20.

4. Ekeland A, Engesaeter LB, Langeland NB: Influence of age on mechanical properties of healing fractures and intact bones in rats. *Acta Orthop Scand* 1982;53:527-534.

5. Lill CA, Fluegel AK, Schneider E: Sheep model for fracture treatment in osteoporotic bone: A pilot study about different induction mechanisms. *J Orthop Trauma* 2000;14:559-566.

6. Lill H, Hepp P, Korner J, et al: Proximal humeral fractures: How stiff should an implant be? *Arch Orthop Trauma Surg* 2003;123:74-81.
   The authors of this article assessed several different types of implants used for fixation of proximal humeral fractures. They discuss the design of osteoporosis-friendly implants and stress the importance of using flexible, load-sharing implants as opposed to traditional plates and screws.

7. Kristiansen B, Christensen S: Plate fixation of proximal humerus fractures. *Acta Orthop Scand* 1986;57:320-323.

8. Baumgaertner MR, Curtin SL, Lindskog DM, Keggi JM: The value of the tip-apex distance in predicting failure of fixation of peritrochanteric fractures of the hip. *J Bone Joint Surg Am* 1995;77:1058-1064.

9. Cornell CN: Internal fracture fixation in patients with osteoporosis. *J Am Acad Orthop Surg* 2003;11:109-119.
   This article provides a review of the principles of internal fixation in osteoporotic bone as well as an exhaustive review of the management of the most common osteoporotic fractures.

10. Einhorn TA: The structural properties of normal and osteoporotic bone. *Instr Course Lect* 2003;52:533-539.
    The author of this article reviews the basic anatomic and structural properties of normal and osteoporotic bone and discusses the consequences for the load carrying capacity of the skeleton. The clinical risk factors for fracture are also reviewed and the effect that the deficient skeleton creates for the fracture surgeon is illustrated.

11. An YH, Young FA, Fang Q, Williams KR: Effects of cancellous bone structure on screw pullout strength. *MUSC Orthop J* 2000;3:22-26.
    The authors of this article provide an analysis of the relation between screw pullout strength and the structural properties of cancellous bone.

12. Augat P, Rapp S, Claes L: A modified hip screw incorporating injected cement for the fixation of osteoporotic trochanteric fractures. *J Orthop Trauma* 2002;16:311-316.
    This article documents improved fixation in patients with unstable intertrochanteric fractures when the construct is enhanced with calcium phosphate cement that is injected through the lag screw. Increased initial stability and decreased slide were noted in patients with augmented fractures compared with control subjects.

13. Ellis T, Bourgeault CA, Kyle RF: Screw position affects dynamic compression plate strain in an in vitro fracture model. *J Orthop Trauma* 2001;15:333-337.
    This study assessed the biomechanical affects of various screw placements in experimental fractures that were stabilized with a dynamic compression plate.

14. Egol KA, Kubiak EN, Fulkerson E, Kummer FJ, Koval KJ: Biomechanics of locked plates and screws. *J Orthop Trauma* 2004;18:488-493.

The authors of this article present a review of conventional and locking plate fixation. The biomechanical problems associated with osteoporotic bone are analytically reviewed.

15. Schandelmaier P, Partenheimer A, Koenemann B, Grun OA, Krettek C: Distal femoral fractures and LISS stabilization. *Injury* 2001;329(suppl 3):SC55-SC63.

The authors of this article provide a review of the biomechanics of less invasive surgical stabilization fixation and discuss early clinical results.

16. Schutz M, Sudkamp NP: Revolution in plate osteosynthesis: A new internal fixator. *J Orthop Sci* 2003;8:252-258.

17. Stover M: Distal femoral fractures: Current results and treatment. *Injury* 2001;32(suppl 3):SC3-SC13.

This article compares and contrasts fixation with the less invasive surgical stabilization system and more conventional locking buttress plates.

18. Fankhauser F, Boldin C, Schippinger G, Haunschmid C, Szyszkowitz R: A new locking plate for unstable fractures of the proximal humerus. *Clin Orthop Relat Res* 2005;430:176-181.

This is the first clinical report of a series of patients treated with a locking proximal humeral plate.

19. Court-Brown C: Isolated tibial shaft fracture. *J Orthop Trauma* 2000;14:306-308.

20. Schultz M, Kolbeck S, Hoffman R, et al: Intramedullary nailing of femoral shaft fractures: Current status and clinical results. *Injury* 2000;30:5-20.

21. Dunlop DG, Brenkel IJ: The supracondylar intramedullary nail in elderly patients with distal femoral shaft fractures. *Injury* 1999;30:475-484.

22. Gynning JB, Hansen D: Treatment of distal femoral fractures with intramedullary nails in elderly patients. *Injury* 1999;30:43-46.

23. Kumar A, Jasani V, Butt MS: Management of distal femoral fractures in elderly patients using a titanium retrograde supracondylar nail. *Injury* 2000;31:169-173.

24. Ingman AM: Retrograde intramedullary nailing of supracondylar femoral fractures: Design and development of a new implant. *Injury* 2002;33:707-712.

The author of this article illustrates design modifications that are helpful for achieving improved stability of an intramedullary nail in osteoporotic bone.

25. Cornell CN: Proximal humerus fractures: Open reduction internal fixation, in Thompson RC (ed): *Master Techniques in Orthopedic Surgery: Fractures.* Philadelphia, PA, Lippincott-Raven, 1998.

26. Larsson S, Bauer TW: Use of injectable calcium phosphate cement for fracture fixation: A review. *Clin Orthop Relat Res* 2002;395:23-32.

The authors present a comprehensive review of current experience using injectable calcium phosphate cements as bone graft substitutes.

27. Gambirasio R, Riand N, Stern R, Hoffmeyer P: Total elbow replacement for complex fractures of the distal humerus. *J Bone Joint Surg Br* 2001;83:974-978.

28. Garcia JA, Mykula R, Stanley D: Complex fractures of the distal humerus in the elderly: The role of total elbow replacement as primary treatment. *J Bone Joint Surg Br* 2002;84:812-816.

These two articles report on the use of total elbow replacement in small series of elderly patients with complex distal humeral fractures. Both reports suggest that total elbow replacement is a useful treatment option for this patient population.

29. Bhandari M, Devereaux PJ, Swiontkowski MF, et al: Internal fixation compared with arthroplasty for displaced fractures of the femoral neck: A meta-analysis. *J Bone Joint Surg Am* 2003;85-A:1673-1681.

In this meta-analysis of the recent literature regarding the treatment of fractures of the femoral neck, the authors report that hemiarthroplasty significantly reduced the risk for reoperation but was associated with a higher risk of complications and death.

30. Rodriguez-Merchan EC: Displaced intracapsular hip fractures: Hemiarthroplasty or total arthroplasty? *Clin Orthop* 2002;399:72-77.

31. Rogmark C, Carlsson A, Johnell O, Sernbo I: A prospective randomized trial of internal fixation versus arthroplasty for displaced fractures of the femoral neck: Functional outcome of 450 patients at two years. *J Bone Joint Surg Br* 2002;84:183-188.

32. Squires B, Bannister G: Displaced intracapsular neck of femur fractures in mobile independent patients: Total hip or hemiarthroplasty. *Injury* 1999;30:345-348.

33. Tidermark J, Ponzer S, Svensson O, Soderquist A, Tornkvist H: Internal fixation compared with total hip replacement for displaced femoral neck fractures in the elderly. *J Bone Joint Surg Br* 2003;85:380-388.

The preceding four articles address the issue of whether to use arthroplasty and total hip arthroplasty to treat femoral neck fractures in fit elderly patients. These studies provide substantial support for prosthetic replacement and encourage serious consideration for adopting total replacement for this type of fracture.

34. Mears DC, Velyvis JH: Acute total hip arthroplasty for selected displaced acetabular fractures. *J Bone Joint Surg Am* 2002;84:1-9.

35. Levis S, Quandt SA, Thompson D, et al: Alendronate reduces the risk of multiple symptomatic fractures: Results of the fracture intervention trial. *J Am Geriatr Soc* 2002;50:409-415.

This landmark study demonstrates that treatment with alendronate prospectively reduces fracture risk in an elderly population by 50% at most skeletal sites.

36. Sorensen OH, Crawford GM, Mulder H, et al: Long-term efficacy of risedronate: A 5-year placebo-controlled clinical experience. *Bone* 2003;32:120-126.

The authors of this article present evidence of the effectiveness of risedronate in fracture prevention.

37. Parrish FF, Murray JA: Surgical treatment for secondary neoplastic fractures. *J Bone Joint Surg Am* 1970;52:665.

38. Zickel RE, Mouradian WH: Intramedullary fixation of pathologic fractures and lesions of the subtrochanteric region of the femur. *J Bone Joint Surg Am* 1976;58:1061-1066.

39. Rougraff BT, Kneisl JS, Simon MA: Skeletal metastases of unknown origin: A prospective study of a diagnostic strategy. *J Bone Joint Surg Am* 1993;75:1276-1281.

40. Harrington KD: The role of surgery in the management of pathologic fractures. *Orthop Clin North Am* 1977;8:841-859.

41. Ward WG, Holsenbeck S, Dorey FJ, Spang J, Howe D: Metastatic disease of the femur: Surgical treatment. *Clin Orthop* 2003;(suppl 415):S230-S244.

42. Frassica FJ, Frassica DA: Metastatic bone disease of the humerus. *J Am Acad Orthop Surg* 2003;11:282-288.

Metastatic bone disease is the most common cause of destructive bone lesions in adults, and involvement of the humerus is common. Patients with destructive humeral metastases involving < 50% of the cortex are treated nonsurgically with radiotherapy. Patients with diaphyseal lesions involving ≥ 50% of the cortex or those with pain after irradiation can be treated with intramedullary nailing. Open nailing with methylmethacrylate is appropriate for destructive lesions in which rigid fixation cannot be achieved with closed nailing. Postoperative external beam irradiation can help prevent disease progression and subsequent loss of fixation.

43. Fidler M: The incidence of fracture through metastases in long bones. *Acta Orthop Scand* 1981;52:623-627.

44. Mirels H: Metastatic disease in long bones: A proposed scoring system for diagnosing impending pathologic fractures. *Clin Orthop* 1989;249:256-264.

45. Giannoudis PV, Bastawrous SS, Bunola JA, MacDonald DA, Smith RM: Unreamed intramedullary nailing for pathological femoral fractures: Good results in 30 cases. *Acta Orthop Scand* 1999;70:29-32.

46. Lane JM, Sculco TP, Zolan S: Treatment of pathological fractures of the hip by endoprosthetic replacement. *J Bone Joint Surg Am* 1980;62:954-959.

47. Harrington KD, Sim FH, Enis JE, Johnston JO, Diok HM, Gristina JG: Methylmethacrylate as an adjunct in internal fixation of pathologic fractures: Experience with three hundred and seventy-five cases. *J Bone Joint Surg Am* 1976;58:1047-1055.

48. Kirkpatrick DK, Trachtenberg LS, Mangino PD, Von Fraunhofer JA, Seligson D: In vitro characteristics of tobramycin-PMMA beads: Compressive strength and leaching. *Orthopedics* 1985;8(9):1130-1133.

49. Klekamp J, Dawson JM, Haas DW, DeBoer D, Christie M: The use of vancomycin and tobramycin in acrylic bone cement: Biomechanical effects and elution kinetics for use in joint arthroplasty. *J Arthroplasty* 1999;14(3):339-346.

50. Swanson KC, Pritchard DJ, Sim FH: Surgical treatment of metastatic disease of the femur. *J Am Acad Orthop Surg* 2000;8:56-65.

Because the femur is the most common site of large, impending, and complete pathologic fractures, the authors of this article recommend complete preoperative evaluation of each patient with metastatic disease of the femur;

evaluation of tumor type, location, size, and extent; stable and strong fixation to allow immediate full weight bearing; that all areas of weakened bone be addressed at the time of surgery; and that postoperative radiotherapy be considered in all patients.

51. Flemming JE, Beals RK: Pathologic fractures of the humerus. *Clin Orthop* 1986;203:258-260.

52. Frassica FJ, Frassica DA: Evaluation and treatment of metastases to the humerus. *Clin Orthop Relat Res* 2003;(suppl 415):S212-S218.
    This article emphasizes the importance of radiotherapy in treating metastases to humerus and the use of hemiarthroplasty or custom arthroplasty for treating increasingly severe periarticular humerus lesions.

53. Redmond BJ, Biermann JS, Blasier RB: Interlocking intramedullary nailing of pathological fractures of the shaft of the humerus. *J Bone Joint Surg Am* 1996;78:891-896.

54. Theriault RL, Lipton A, Hortobagyi GN, et al: Pamidronate reduces skeletal morbidity in women with advanced breast cancer and lytic bone lesions: A randomized, placebo-controlled trial. Protocol 18 Aredia Breast Cancer Study Group. *J Clin Oncol* 1999;17:846-854.

Chapter 43

Periprosthetic Fractures

Ross K. Leighton, MD, FRCSC, FACS

Introduction

Periprosthetic fractures are occurring at an increasing rate, with fractures affecting primarily the femur and hip comprising the largest group. More than 200,000 arthroplasties are performed in the United States annually. With a predicted 5% annual increase in total hip replacements and an 8% increase in total knee replacements, an expanding pool of patients is at risk for this type of fracture.[1] Periprosthetic fractures occur around implants that are cemented and cementless. The treatment of fractures in patients with these implants would not be the same and should be based on the assessed stability and wear of the components.[2]

Periprosthetic Fractures of the Hip

The principles of treatment for periprosthetic fractures of the hip are based on stability of the implant, fracture location, bone quality, and medical condition of the patient.

Implant Stability

If the implant was cemented, it is essential to determine whether the cement mantle is intact. If the implant was cementless, it is important to determine whether the bone ingrowth has been damaged or disturbed.[3] If the component is stable, fracture reduction should be done to provide stability. This can be accomplished using stable internal fixation. Axial and rotational stability should be achieved with the selected implant.[4,5] The goal of rehabilitation is early mobilization, with progressive weight bearing allowed depending on the healing parameters of the involved limb. Postoperative treatment does not usually include a brace. Progressive weight bearing should be the goal over the first 3 months.

If the component is unstable, it is necessary to remove it and any cement that is present. The new revision implant should be designed and planned to achieve bone-component stability. Stability, by definition, implies that the extremity is stable under an axial or a rotational force.

If a revision implant is necessary, it should allow early mobilization, brace-free motion, and early weight bearing, with 50% weight bearing being the early goal. This is increased gradually based on healing of the fracture. In an older, confused patient or a patient with dementia who requires implant revision, captured cups or large femoral heads ($\geq$ 36 mm) should be considered as an option to reduce the dislocation rate and avoid the need for postoperative bracing.

The Vancouver classification of periprosthetic fractures includes stability of the implant, integrity of the cement mantle, and fracture location, relative to the femoral stem (Figure 1). This classification system has been very helpful in assessing stability of the implant and, therefore, determining the need for revision versus internal fixation.[6]

Patients with unstable implants and significant comorbidities typically are not candidates for implant revision. If the comorbidities are too severe, the segments of the femur should be stabilized to allow fixation with the awareness that this leaves the femoral component unstable.

Femoral Shaft Fracture

Reports in the literature regarding the prevalence of periprosthetic fracture of the hip are widespread. Postoperative periprosthetic implant fractures have been reported to occur intraoperatively, perioperatively, and postoperatively (usually as a complication of a loose implant).[6-9] Although intraoperative and perioperative femoral shaft fractures are a rare complication, they are a consistent risk for patients with implants. Patients with cemented stems average approximately a 1% prevalence of intraoperative and perioperative fractures, with one study reporting an intraoperative fracture rate of only 0.4% in more than 5,000 cemented arthroplasties.[1] Prevalence rates for intraoperative fractures in cementless arthroplasties range from 2.6% to 4.0%. Intraoperative fracture rates were reported to be highest in patients with taper design components and lowest in those with fully porous-coated press-fit collared components.[1] Post-

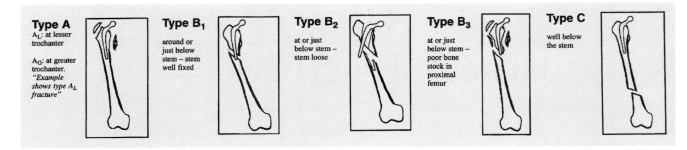

Figure 1 Vancouver classification of postoperative periprosthetic fractures of the femur. Type A fractures are located in the trochanteric region; the type A fracture shown is located at the lesser trochanter. Type B fractures are located around or just distal to the stem; type B1 is prosthesis stable; type B2 is prosthesis unstable; type B3 is bone stock inadequate. Type C fractures are located well below the stem. *(Reproduced from Duncan CP, Masri BA: Fractures of the femur after hip replacement.* Instr Course Lect *1995;44:293-304.)*

operative femoral fractures typically occur late (> 3 months after implantation) and may be caused by a loose femoral implant. Osteopenia secondary to age or stress shielding is an associated cause in many patients. Two separate, large population studies noted a 0.1% fracture rate in patients with implants.[2,3]

Classification

The American Academy of Orthopaedic Surgeons (AAOS) Committee on the Hip proposed a fracture classification system in 1990 that divided the femur into three separate regions. Level I was defined by the proximal femur and distally by the lower extent of the lesser trochanter. Level II included 10 cm of the femur distal to level I. Level III included the remainder of the femur distal to level II. These were further subdivided into six types of fractures (Table 1). Type I fractures occur proximal to the intertrochanteric line and often occur intraoperatively. Type I fractures typically require only revision of the neck resection, but a prophylactic cerclage wire is recommended to avoid problems with prostheses. Type II fractures are vertically or spirally split and do not extend past the lower extent of the lesser trochanter. Type III fractures typically extend past the lesser trochanter, but not beyond level II. Type IV fractures are typically located in the region of the femoral stem at the level III area. Type IVA fractures are spiral fractures around the tip, whereas type IVB fractures are simple transverse or short oblique fractures. Type V fractures are severely comminuted fractures around the stem in the level III area. Type VI fractures are distal to the femoral stem tip, also in level III.

A classification system is useful because it accounts for a wide variety of fracture etiologies during and after surgery. In patients with a cemented implant, the functional concerns for each type of fracture include whether it makes the femoral stem unstable and whether it compromises the integrity of the cement mantle. In patients with a cementless implant, the functional concerns are slightly different and include whether the cementless

TABLE 1 | Anatomic Level and AAOS Classification of Periprosthetic Fractures*

Anatomic Level	AAOS Classification	Description
Level I	Type I	Proximal to the intertrochanteric line
	Type II	Vertical split not extending past the lower portion of the lesser trochanter
Level II	Type III	Vertical or split extending past the lower portion of the lesser trochanter
Level III	Type IV	Fracture in the region of the tip of the femoral stem (type IVA, spiral; type IVB, transverse or short oblique)
	Type V	Severely comminuted type III or IV
	Type VI	Fracture distal to prosthesis

*Treatment is suggested by both classification schemes. This compares favorably with the new Vancouver classification.
(Reproduced with permission from Rockwood CA, Bucholz RW, Heckman JD, Green DP (eds): Rockwood and Green's Fractures in Adults, ed 4. Philadelphia, PA, Lippincott Williams & Wilkins, 2001, p 577.)

fixation is compromised by the fracture and whether the implant remains well fixed to the bone.

The stability of the implant determines the pathway or solution to the clinical presentation. The options available for fixation of these types of fractures or revision of the components includes locking plates, dynamic compression plates, cerclage wires, cerclage wire and plate combination, plate and screw combinations, retrograde nails, and revision implants.[6-14]

Intraoperative Periprosthetic Femur Fractures

The best treatment for intraoperative periprosthetic femur fractures is prevention, which requires extensive preoperative clinical and radiographic assessment of the patient. The proper equipment needed to accomplish stable fracture fixation or revision implantation must also be obtained. Additionally, the equipment that may be required should problems occur intraoperatively should also be available.

The assessment of existing screw holes and osteolytic lesions, the potential use of cortical windows, and the identification of osteopenia or osteoporosis are essential in preoperative planning to determine the surgical equipment that is required, such as cerclage wires, vertical strut allograft, cancellous autograft, and specialized revision stems and cups.

If the intraoperative fracture has not made the primary implant unstable, then the fracture should be stabilized. Internal fixation of the fracture with cerclage wires (with or without a cortical strut allograft) is the treatment of choice.

If the fracture has resulted in instability of the primary implant, a revision implant is recommended to provide a stable femoral implant and fracture stability. This usually requires the use of a longer femoral implant as well as cerclage wires and a plate and/or strut allograft.

Principles of Treatment of a Cemented Femoral Implant

A fracture that creates instability of the cement mantle or instability of the implant requires a revision to a stable implant. This includes removal of the primary implant and cement. Bone graft of the defect and stabilization of the cortical fracture with cerclage wires, plates and cerclage wires, and/or cortical struts should be performed. A strut graft is usually added to provide axial stability and improve rotational stability of the construct.[15] It has been reported, however, that strut grafts are not an absolute requirement for the treatment of all periprosthetic femoral fractures.[16] The longer the fracture (the more oblique the fracture), the less the need there is for a strut allograft. The more transverse the fracture (the more rotationally unstable), the greater the need there is for a strut graft. If the length (oblique or spiral) of the fracture extends over two or more cortical diameters, cortical struts may not be required for stability.[16]

Principles of Treatment of a Cementless Implant

Patients with a cementless component complicated by a fracture that results in instability require removal of the primary implant and fixation of the fracture with either cerclage wires and a plate or a strut allograft.[17,18] Once this is accomplished, an appropriate length implant should be inserted. The implant should pass distal to the fracture by at least two cortical diameters. If good distal fixation is achieved, axial and rotational stability should be realized.[19,20]

If the fracture does not cause instability of the stem, then stabilization of the fracture without implant revision

is recommended. This situation occurs much more commonly in patients with cementless prostheses and is not always predictable using the current classification systems. For example, a type III fracture in level II could be compatible with a stable femoral cementless implant and would not require revision. The integrity of the implant determines the treatment protocol.

The Vancouver periprosthetic hip fracture classification system is helpful in the selection of cemented components. Fracture type A can be treated with small intraoperative corrections; fracture types B1, B2, and B3 require revision; and fracture type C requires open reduction with internal fixation.[21] Cementless implants require careful evaluation to establish the integrity of the bone-component interface. This is particularly true in patients with type B1 or type B3 fractures. The treatment therefore depends on the implant design and bone-cement or bone-implant fixation (cemented versus cementless) as well as the fracture classification[22] (Figure 1).

Acetabular Fractures

Acetabular fractures can occur either intraoperatively or postoperatively. If an intraoperative fracture occurs, the first step in treatment is recognition of the problem. The second step is to select the correct fixation or implant to stabilize the acetabular component.

If a late fracture (> 3 months postoperatively) occurs, patients typically present with superior or central migration of the cup. In most instances, late fracture occurs in association with or as the result of periprosthetic osteolysis. Severe osteopenia in combination with trauma or a loose implant is another common cause of periprosthetic acetabular fracture. Initial treatment includes mobilization of the patient with progressive weight bearing when possible, allowing the fracture to unite, and planning surgical intervention at a later date. If pain prevents early patient mobilization, surgical fixation and reconstruction should be performed. Based on radiographic assessment and physical examination, a preoperative plan is designed to treat the fracture and replace the prosthesis. If the cup is unstable, removal of the loose cup and replacement with a slightly larger cementless cup with additional screw fixation should be performed. Care should be taken to avoid underreaming and thereby reduce the stress on the fractured acetabulum. A line-to-line fit with screw supplementation is ideal. In patients with osteopenic bone or more unstable fractures, an alternative technique involves using a roof ring or a cage with a cemented polyethylene liner.[23]

All of the above treatment methods may require augmentation with reconstruction plates and screws and/or bone graft, particularly in patients with anterior or posterior column fractures, central quadrilateral plate bone loss, or acetabular discontinuity. A large cementless cup with screw fixation, or a roof ring or a cage with a cemented all-polyethylene cup would complete the reconstruction. The successful use of a quadrilateral plate wire to stabilize the acetabulum and allow fixation of the cup acutely has been reported[24] (Figure 2).

In delayed reconstruction of the acetabulum after early healing of the fracture, treatment options include use of a large cementless cup with added fixation, impaction graft technique with a cemented polyethylene cup, and a roof ring or acetabular cage in association with a cemented polyethylene cup.

Bone graft is required to fill in the osseous defects secondary to the fracture. Late reconstruction allows more predictable fixation with less extensile exposure. Additional support is required to reconstruct the deformed posterior column in most patients.

To prevent dislocation, adequate tensioning of the abductors and hip girdle muscles should be achieved. If the hip appears unstable during the trial phase, steps taken to improve hip stability include increasing the femoral offset if the femoral side has been revised, increasing the head size as tolerated by the diameter of the acetabulum (32 or 36 mm or greater), or using an eccentric or lipped liner. In older patients with lower physical demands, a captured cup should be considered as a part of the armamentarium.

The use of a cemented cup alone for patients with a fractured acetabulum does not result in fracture stability.[25] The acetabulum must be supported or stabilized with a revision cup or cage to obtain predictable long-term survival.

Special Considerations

As with any loose implant, infection should be considered as a possible cause of the event. The usual workup includes a complete blood cell count and assessment of the erythrocyte sedimentation rate and C-reactive protein level. These tests should be done early and are excellent preliminary screening tools. If the results are normal, then the presence of infection is usually unlikely. If the test results show elevated levels, then a staged revision may have to be performed.

Host factors that increase the risk of infection include previous surgery, chronic remote sepsis, prolonged hospitalization, and immunosuppression (caused by diabetes, steroid use, renal failure, ethanol, and/or poor nutrition). In patients with a suspected hip infection, aspiration may or may not be used. There has been controversy in the literature as to whether hip aspiration is helpful in these patients. If the culture results are positive, treatment may be altered (for example, a two-stage procedure would be considered); if the culture results are negative, no real assumptions can be made

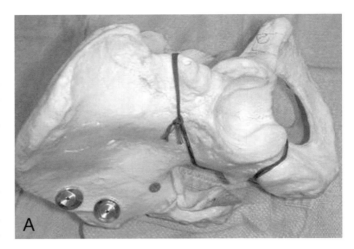

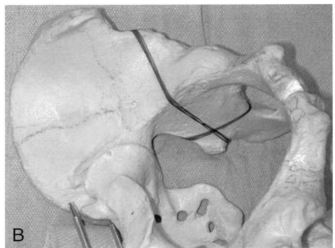

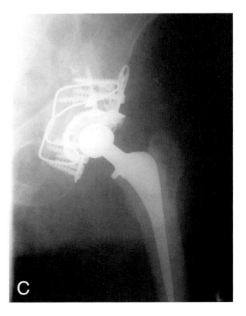

Figure 2 **A,** Outside view photograph indicating where the tie or twist of the wire or cable is created. **B,** Inside view photograph of the cables or wires used to support the quadrilateral plate. **C,** Postoperative radiograph of a periacetabular fracture repaired with the cable technique.

regarding treatment based on the reports to date. Therefore, hip aspiration would be helpful in some patients, but it should still be considered in patients with periprosthetic fractures and complex presentations.

Nuclear scanning is rarely used to assess patients with acute periprosthetic fractures because results of such diagnostic imaging would not be helpful in most instances. Its use, therefore, is discouraged.

If infection is suspected, physicians must be prepared to treat it. An infection is determined to be present at the time of revision if the erythrocyte sedimentation rate and C-reactive protein level are elevated or if the frozen section indicates more than 10 polymorphonuclear leukocytes per high-powered field. If the frozen section indicates 5 to 10 polymorphonuclear leukocytes per high-powered field, an infection is probable. However, clinical correlation is necessary in the interpretation of these results. If infection is present, removal of all the implant components is recommended in most patients. This can be combined with either a Girdlestone (excisional arthroplasty) procedure of the hip with or without an antibiotic-impregnated cement spacer or a Prostalac type of acetabular and femoral component. This type of temporary implant has a small core of metal that is completely coated with antibiotic cement and a thin polyethylene acetabulum placed in a thick cement.

If early revision is done, the fracture segment must be stabilized to the point at which the patient can be mobilized with the use of a walker or crutches. This is possible with either a Girdlestone arthroplasty, a Prostalac procedure, or a molded cement spacer. Intravenous antibiotic treatment is initiated for 6 weeks based on culture sensitivities. If the elevated complete blood cell count, erythrocyte sedimentation rate, and C-reactive protein level decrease to normal within 6 to 12 weeks and the patient is otherwise healthy, then a second-stage procedure should be performed with the appropriate revision components.

Periprosthetic Fractures of the Knee

Periprosthetic fractures about the knee have been reported to occur during surgery as well as up to 10 years after surgery.[1,26,27] Risk factors include knee manipulation with the patient under spinal or general anesthetic, rheumatoid arthritis, anterior notching of the femur, steroid use, and osteopenia. Fractures of the patella after total knee arthroplasty have been reported to be slightly more common after resurfacing the patella when compared with a nonresurfaced patella.[28] The prevalence of patellar fractures had been reported to be from 0.1% to 8.5% of patients.[29]

Classification

A modified Neer classification system has been used to classify periprosthetic fractures about the knee (Figure

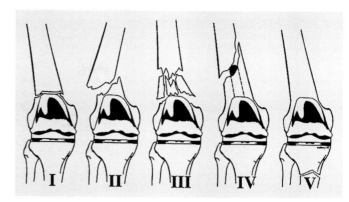

Figure 3 Classification of periprosthetic knee fractures (modified Neer classification). *(Reproduced with permission from Neer CS 2nd, Grantham SA, Shelton ML: Supracondylar fracture of the adult femur: A study of one hundred and ten cases. J Bone Joint Surg Am 1967;49:591-613.)*

3). Fracture types include type I (extra-articular and nondisplaced fractures with < 5 mm of translation and < 5° of angulation on any plane), type II (extra-articular fractures with displacement of > 5 mm or 5° of angulation), type III (fractures that are severely comminuted, with a loss of cortical contact and often significant angulation), type IV (supracondylar fractures of the femur at the tip of the revision stem, which are similar to Vancouver type C proximal fractures of the hip); also included in the Neer type 4 category are fractures of the femoral diaphysis that do not involve the prosthesis.

Fractures of the patella have been classified as type I fractures (no involvement of the implant), type II fractures (involvement of the implant, which is usually loose), type III fractures (involvement of the inferior pole, with subtype IIIA having associated patellar fracture and ligament rupture and subtype IIIB not associated with ligament rupture), and type IV fractures (fracture-dislocations of the patella).

Periprosthetic Supracondylar Femoral Fractures

The goals of treatment include returning a patient to the preinjury level of function, using a minimally invasive approach whenever possible to protect the soft tissues, avoiding the use of a brace, allowing early range of motion of the knee, and reducing the risk of infection and/or the subsequent loss of fixation. The need for a bone graft, cancellous, or strut allograft should be assessed for every fracture and is fracture- and patient-dependent.[27]

The principles of treatment are based on fracture type and implant stability. For completely nondisplaced fractures (those with stable implants), closed treatment and/or brace treatment is the treatment of choice. For displaced fractures with a stable implant, open reduction and internal fixation is recommended, with bone graft as needed. For displaced fractures with unstable implants, revision of the loose implant and fixation of the fracture is recommended.

The choice of fixation should be made in accordance with the goals of the intended outcome, which typically include providing axial and rotational stability to allow early range of motion of the knee and early patient mobility. The principal fixation options include retrograde intramedullary nail, nonlocked plate and screw systems, fixed-angle plate devices, and locked screw and plate systems. Whichever device is chosen, early range of knee motion should be allowed, but it should not be initiated with the intention of using a brace after the surgery. Preoperative planning is required to ensure that the implant is compatible with the stable component (for example, an intramedullary nail would require preoperative measurement of the intercondylar notch of the femoral implant).

Retrograde Intramedullary Nail

A retrograde intramedullary nail can be chosen when a load sharing device and percutaneous approach is required.[27] Although the length of the intramedullary nail depends on the fracture type, a longer nail is usually better. Care should be taken not to stop intramedullary nail insertion at the isthmus of the diaphysis because nail insertions that stop at the isthmus level have been linked to stress fractures. Relative indications for an intramedullary nail include obese patients with a fracture around a primary nonstemmed implant, bilateral supracondylar fractures of the femur (periprosthetic), and floating knee associated with a periprosthetic fracture. The insertion of retrograde intramedullary nails has been associated with the presence of intra-articular reaming debris and the biomechanical compatibility of the intramedullary nail and the femoral component. This construct has also been reported to result in varus and/or valgus malalignment, particularly in patients with osteoporotic bone.

Nonlocked Devices

The concerns with the use of a condylar buttress plate to treat periprosthetic fractures include the requirement for an extensile approach and the reported incidence of fracture shortening and progressive varus deformity (5% to 20%), which typically occurs secondary to angulation of the screw at the screw-plate interface.[27] These concerns have led to an increased use of fixed-angle plates and locked plates. The locked plate devices were specifically designed to address this issue.

Fixed-angle plate options can include a dynamic condylar screw, a condylar blade plate, and locked screw plates.

Concerns with the distal fixation achieved by these devices in patients with periprosthetic fractures with sta-

ble implants but minimal bone attached to the component, combined with concerns regarding the extensile approach have led to changes in the approach and the increased use of the locked plate systems. Although a new minimally invasive surgical approach addressed some of these concerns, it is not always possible to use this technique. The surgical approach is determined by the fracture pattern and the limitations imposed by instrumentation for these devices.

Locked Plate Devices

The locked screw and plate devices were designed to accommodate a minimally invasive approach and result in better distal fixation and less bone sacrifice than dynamic condylar screw devices. The instrumentation was specifically designed for a percutaneous approach. Less invasive surgical stabilization was developed to specifically minimize soft-tissue damage and reduce the risk of late deformity. The less invasive surgical approach allows for a limited approach surgically while achieving stable fixation, even for patients with severely comminuted fractures.

Fractures of the Tibia

The fractures around the proximal tibial component are typically either stress fractures of the tibial plateau at the time of insertion or fractures at the tip of the tibial cement mantle. The indications for early revision of a late fracture include uncontrollable pain, instability that cannot be corrected or controlled with open reduction and internal fixation, and inability to achieve early mobilization of the knee and the patient with internal fixation of the fracture. Implants to treat these periprosthetic fractures include the locked tibial buttress plate, regular tibial buttress plate, less invasive surgical stabilization periarticular plates (locked and unlocked), and an intramedullary nail (a very rare indication).[30,31] If the component is unstable, then it should be replaced with a new cemented component. Most revisions require stemmed implants to stabilize the fracture and reduce the stress at the fracture site. If the fracture occurs at the tip of the implant and the integrity of the cement is intact, then open reduction and internal fixation with or without bone graft is the treatment of choice.

A challenge in treating plateau fractures was providing adequate and accurate contouring of the plate while maintaining a low profile. Despite many improvements in periarticular plating systems, hardware problems are common because of the relatively thin soft-tissue coverage in this area. Several precontoured proximal tibial plates (with locked and unlocked designs in titanium as well as surgical stainless steel) have been designed, both for the medial and lateral side. Most of the advantages of

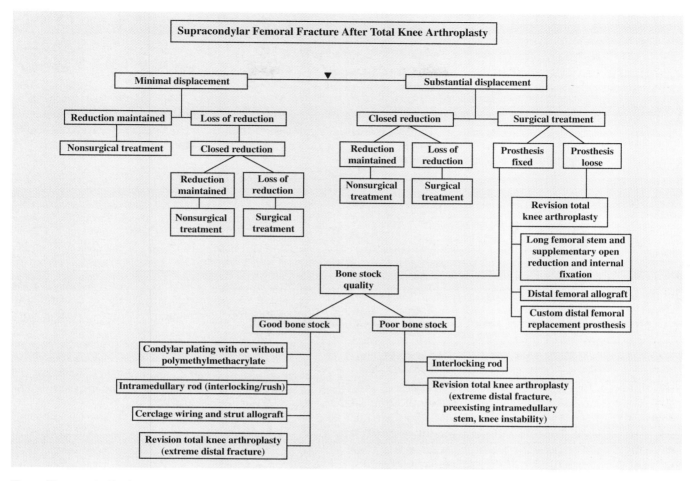

Figure 4 Treatment algorithm for supracondylar femoral fractures in patients with total knee arthroplasty. This algorithm indicates the relatively rare but absolute indications to perform a revision total knee arthroplasty in this population of patients.

the locking screws in this anatomic location appeared to occur in the proximal metaphyseal holes. The lateral locking screws allow metaphyseal support for the lateral as well as the medial tibial plateau without requiring a separate medial approach with the inherent soft-tissue damage. The locking screws prevent screw-to-plate motion, which has been associated with use of reduction in the postoperative healing phase.

Indications for Revision Total Knee Implants in Periprosthetic Fractures

There are relatively few indications for using revision total knee implants in periprosthetic fractures about the knee. Figure 4 illustrates where revision total knee arthroplasty fits into the treatment protocol for these types of injuries. When planning the surgical procedure, in addition to identifying the fracture pattern and location, it must be determined whether the implant is stable or loose and what bone stock remains on the femoral and tibial components.

If the prosthesis is considered stable and the fracture is relatively nondisplaced, then a closed treatment with a brace or a splint is the treatment of choice. If the prosthesis is stable and the fracture is displaced, then open reduction and internal fixation is usually indicated. If the prosthesis is unstable and the fracture is either nondisplaced or displaced, then a stemmed revision with fixation to achieve fracture stability is indicated to permit mobility while achieving fracture union.

Implant revision is indicated in patients with a loose, unstable, or failed component; those with very distal comminuted fractures for whom stable fixation (open or closed) is not possible; and those requiring salvage for a failed open reduction and internal fixation or a failed nonsurgical treatment. Stemmed implants with posterior stabilized or varus-valgus stabilized constrained polyethylene components are usually adequate. However, in rare instances, a hinged knee implant or treatment with major structural allograft bone may be necessary. Although there are scant data in the literature on the long-term results of this relatively rare indication for revision arthroplasty, the use of structural allografts for the treatment of periprosthetic fractures about the knee has been reported.[32]

Fractures of the Patella

Patellar fractures are rare and only occasionally have associated periprosthetic fractures of the femur and tibia. Closed treatment of patellar fractures has been recommended for those fractures that are not associated with loosening and have an intact quadriceps mechanism and an intact patellar tendon mechanism. If the patella is dislocated, loose, or disrupted, then open reduction and internal fixation is indicated to achieve continuity of the extensor mechanism.

Summary

Nondisplaced periprosthetic fractures about the knee can be treated with closed reduction with or without a hinged brace. Fixation using retrograde intramedullary nailing, fixed-angle plates, precontoured plates, or locked plates is the treatment of choice for most patients with displaced fractures and stable implants. Revision surgery for this type of injury is rarely indicated acutely; however, if the integrity of the components are compromised, early revision with stemmed implants is indicated. More commonly, revision implants are used in a delayed fashion as a salvage procedure. Although periprosthetic fractures have also been reported to occur around proximal humeral implants, elbow implants, and total ankle implants,[33-37] these are quite rare and should be treated with the same general principles used for other periprosthetic fractures. Many specialty plates are commercially available for each anatomic area. The personality of each periprosthetic fracture should be evaluated before open reduction and internal fixation or revision is attempted.

Annotated References

1. Berry DJ: Epidemiology: Hip and knee. *Orthop Clin North Am* 1999;30:183-190.

2. Dunbar MJ, Blackley HR, Bourne RB: Osteolysis of the femur: Principles of management. *Instr Course Lect* 2001;50:197-209.

    Femoral osteolysis is and will remain an important cause of total hip arthroplasty failures. The presentation is initially radiographic and patients may or may not become symptomatic. Revision of femoral components in these patients can be fraught with complications and poor results; hence, the importance of preoperative planning cannot be overemphasized.

3. Berry DJ: Periprosthetic fractures associated with osteolysis: A problem on the rise. *J Arthroplasty* 2003;18(3, suppl 1)107-111.

    Some stable, minimally displaced fractures of the pelvis and greater trochanter can be allowed to heal before revision is considered, which simplifies the operation. Unsta-

ble fractures, especially those of the femoral diaphysis, are usually treated with early repeated surgery following the established principles of periprosthetic fracture management.

4. Peters CL, Bachus KN, Davitt JS: Fixation of periprosthetic femur fractures: A biomechanical analysis comparing cortical strut allograft plates and conventional metal plates. *Orthopedics* 2003;26:695-699.

    The authors of this study compared the stability of periprosthetic femur fractures fixed using cortical allograft struts with a metal plate and report that allograft cortical struts are a biomechanically sound alternative to metal plates fixed with screws and cables for femur fracture fixation below a well-fixed femoral component.

5. Barden B, Ding Y, Fitzek JG, Loer F: Strut allografts for failed treatment of periprosthetic femoral fractures: Good outcome in 13 patients. *Acta Orthop Scand* 2003;74:146-153.

    In this series of 13 patients, strut allografts provided reliable healing with augmentation of the host bone stock despite previous femoral exposure, severe bone loss, adverse type of fracture, and persistent instability at the index operation.

6. Greidanus NV, Mitchell PA, Masri BA, Garbuz DS, Duncan CP: Principles of management and results of treating the fractured femur during and after total hip arthroplasty. *Instr Course Lect* 2003;52:309-322.

    Because the management of fractures of the femur during and after total hip arthroplasty can be difficult, treatment can be fraught with complications, and periprosthetic fractures range from the very simple (requiring no surgical intervention) to the complex (requiring major revision), a classification system of these fractures aids in understanding the principles of management and results of treatment.

7. Schmidt AH, Kyle RF: Periprosthetic fractures of the femur. *Orthop Clin North Am* 2002;33:143-152.

    The authors of this article report that periprosthetic fractures of the femur represent a heterogeneous and challenging problem for the orthopaedic surgeon. The incidence of these fractures is dramatically increasing because there are more patients with aging total joint arthroplasties.

8. Dennis MG, Simon JA, Kummer FJ, Koval KJ, Di Cesare PE: Fixation of periprosthetic femoral shaft fractures: A biomechanical comparison of two techniques. *J Orthop Trauma* 2001;15:177-180.

    The authors report that the Ogden construct provided a more rigid and stronger initial fixation of a periprosthetic fracture than the allograft construct.

9. Cook SD, Barrack RL, Santman M, Patron LP, Salkeld SL, Whitecloud TS III: Strut allograft healing to the femur with recombinant human osteogenic protein-1. *Clin Orthop* 2000;381:47-57.

Strut healing with the osteogenic protein-1 device at 4 weeks postoperatively was found to be superior to the healing in control sites at 8 weeks. The authors conclude that improving and accelerating the course of cortical strut graft healing can provide a substantial clinical benefit in lowering the risk of graft nonunion and fracture and shorten the time of protected weight bearing and functional disability.

10. Schutz M, Muller M, Krettek C, et al: Minimally invasive fracture stabilization of distal femoral fractures with the LISS: A prospective multicenter study. Results of a clinical study with special emphasis on difficult cases. *Injury* 2001;32(suppl 3):SC48-SC54.

The results of this study show that with a sound knowledge of the surgical technique and careful preoperative planning this system represents an excellent, safe procedure for the treatment of almost all distal femoral fracture types, including periprosthetic fractures of the distal femur. The authors report that there is generally no need for primary cancellous bone grafting in this patient population.

11. Venu KM, Koka R, Garikipati R, Shenava Y, Madhu TS: Dall-Miles cable and plate fixation for the treatment of peri-prosthetic femoral fractures: Analysis of results in 13 cases. *Injury* 2001;32:395-400.

The authors of this study found that the Dall-Miles cable and plate system is a useful method of internal fixation for most patients with periprosthetic femoral fractures. This method may not be suitable, however, if the femoral component is loose or if it is in varus angulation of more than 6° to the shaft of the femur.

12. Dennis MG, Simon JA, Kummer FJ, Koval KJ, DiCesare PE: Fixation of periprosthetic femoral shaft fractures occurring at the tip of the stem: A biomechanical study of 5 techniques. *J Arthroplasty* 2000;15:523-528.

The authors of this biomechanical study found that plate constructs with proximal unicortical screws and distal bicortical screws or proximal unicortical screws, proximal cables, and distal bicortical screws were significantly more stable in axial compression, lateral bending, and torsional loading than the other fixation constructs assessed.

13. Banim RH, Fletcher M, Warren P: Use of a Dall-Miles plate and cables for the fixation of a periprosthetic tibial fracture. *J Arthroplasty* 2000;15:131-133.

Although tibial periprosthetic fractures are uncommon, they are likely to be encountered more frequently with the increased use of total knee arthroplasty, and they present a challenging management problem. The authors of this article present their solution to this problem, which provided a safe, effective means of fracture management while maintaining the prosthesis.

14. Brady OH, Garbuz DS, Masri BA, Duncan CP: The treatment of periprosthetic fractures of the femur using cortical onlay allograft struts. *Orthop Clin North Am* 1999;30:249-257.

15. Haddad FS, Duncan CP: Cortical onlay allograft struts in the treatment of periprosthetic femoral fractures. *Instr Course Lect* 2003;52:291-300.

The authors of this article report that cortical struts can also be used in combination with other modalities of periprosthetic fracture treatment and they can be useful when combined with plate fixation or with revision to a long stemmed prosthesis and as adjunctive stabilizers at the junction between the host and a proximal femoral structural allograft.

16. Ricci WM, Borrelli J: Allograft struts are not required for the treatment of periprosthetic femoral shaft fractures. *Proceedings of the Orthopedic Trauma Association Meeting.* October 9-11, 2003, Salt Lake City, Utah. Available at: http://www.hwbf.org/ota/am/ota03/otapa/OTA03313.htm. Accessed August 2, 2004.

The authors report that indirect fracture reduction techniques maximize the biologic potential for fracture repair and therefore may obviate the need for strut allograft during treatment of some periprosthetic fractures around stable intramedullary implants.

17. Tsiridis E, Haddad FS, Gie GA: Dall-Miles plates for periprosthetic femoral fractures: A critical review of 16 cases. *Injury* 2003;34:107-110.

In this review of 16 patients, the authors report that the Dall-Mile plate and cable system alone is insufficient for the treatment of periprosthetic femoral fractures. It must be supplemented with additional intramedullary or extramedullary fixation.

18. Tsiridis E, Haddad FS, Gie GA: The management of periprosthetic femoral fractures around hip replacements. *Injury* 2003;34:95-105.

The authors of this article report that augmentation of intramedullary fixation with an external cortical strut to improve rotational stability and/or internally with impaction allografting to compensate for bone defects is advisable to treat patients with periprosthetic femoral fractures around hip replacement implants. Vigilant postoperative clinical and radiographic assessment following total hip replacement can identify patients with recurrent dislocation, loosening, subsidence, and osteolysis. These patients are at greatest risk of developing femoral periprosthetic fractures.

19. Haddad FS, Duncan CP, Berry DJ, Lewallen DG, Gross AE, Chandler HP: Periprosthetic femoral fractures around well-fixed implants: Use of cortical onlay allografts with or without a plate. *J Bone Joint Surg Am* 2002;84-A:945-950.

   Cortical onlay strut allografts act as biologic bone plates, serving both mechanical and biologic functions. The authors of this study found that cortical struts, either alone or in conjunction with a plate, led to a very high rate of fracture union, satisfactory alignment, and an increase in femoral bone stock at the time of short-term follow-up. These findings suggest that cortical strut grafts can be used routinely to augment fixation and healing of a periprosthetic femoral fracture.

20. Nelson CL: Periprosthetic fractures of the femur following hip arthroplasty. *Am J Orthop* 2002;31:221-223.

   The author of this article discusses the prevention, evaluation, and management of periprosthetic fractures of the femur after hip arthroplasty as well as surgical treatment techniques. The author also discusses a preferred treatment based on an algorithm developed by Duncan and Masri.

21. Berry DJ: Management of periprosthetic fractures: The hip. *J Arthroplasty* 2002; 17(suppl 1)11-13.

   Major intraoperative fractures require more complex reconstruction. Postoperative fractures associated with well-fixed implants typically are treated with open reduction and internal fixation. Postoperative fractures associated with loose implants are treated with revision and fracture stabilization, usually with specialized revision implants.

22. Macdonald SJ, Paprosky WG, Jablonsky WS, Magnus RG: Periprosthetic femoral fractures treated with a long-stem cementless component. *J Arthroplasty* 2001;16:379-383.

   The authors of this study report that because periprosthetic femoral fractures can be challenging to manage proximal femoral fractures with a loose component are best treated with revision arthroplasty.

23. Della Valle CJ, Momberger NG, Paprosky WG: Periprosthetic fractures of the acetabulum associated with a total hip arthroplasty. *Instr Course Lect* 2003; 52:281-290.

   The authors present a comprehensive classification system for guiding the management of these complex injuries.

24. Mears DC, Shirahama M: Stabilization of an acetabular fracture with cables for acute total hip arthroplasty. *J Arthroplasty* 1998;13:104-107.

25. Callaghan JJ, Kim YS, Pederson DR, Brown TD: Periprosthetic fractures of the acetabulum. *Orthop Clin North Am* 1999;30:221-234.

26. Rorabeck CH, Taylor JW: Classification of periprosthetic fractures complicating total knee arthroplasty. *Orthop Clin North Am* 1999;30:209-214.

27. Schutz M, Muller M, Krettek C, et al: Minimally invasive fracture stabilization of distal femoral fractures with the LISS: A prospective multicenter study. Results of a clinical study with special emphasis on difficult cases. *Injury* 2001;32(suppl 3):SC48-SC54.

   The results of this study show that with a sound knowledge of the surgical technique and careful preoperative planning less invasive surgical stabilization is an excellent, safe option for the treatment of almost all types of distal femoral fractures, including periprosthetic fractures of the distal femur. The authors also report that there is generally no need for primary cancellous bone grafting in this patient population.

28. Rorabeck CH, Taylor JW: Periprosthetic fractures of the femur complicating total knee arthroplasty. *Orthop Clin North Am* 1999;30:265-277.

29. Sharkey PF, Hozack WJ, Rothman RH, Shastri S, Jacoby SM: Why are total knee arthroplasties failing today? *Clin Orthop Relat Res* 2002;404:7-13.

30. Hanssen AD, Stuart MJ: Treatment of periprosthetic tibial fractures. *Clin Orthop* 2000;380:91-98.

   The authors of this article present a classification system that accounts for the anatomic location of the fracture, status of prosthesis fixation, and timing of the fracture, all of which are important in determining the appropriate treatment approach.

31. Stuart MJ, Hanssen AD: Total knee arthroplasty: Periprosthetic tibial fractures. *Orthop Clin North Am* 1999;30:279-286.

32. Wong P, Gross AE: The use of structural allografts for treating periprosthetic fractures about the hip and knee. *Orthop Clin North Am* 1999;30:259-264.

33. Worland RL, Kim DY, Arredondo J: Periprosthetic humeral fractures: Management and classification. *J Shoulder Elbow Surg* 1999;8:590-594.

34. Campbell JT, Moore RS, Iannotti JP, Norris TR, Williams GR: Periprosthetic humeral fractures: Mechanisms of fracture and treatment options. *J Shoulder Elbow Surg* 1998;7:406-413.

35. Williams GR Jr, Iannotti JP: Management of periprosthetic fractures: The shoulder. *J Arthroplasty* 2002; 17(suppl 1)14-16.

   The authors of this study report that the incidence of periprosthetic fracture during or after shoulder arthroplasty is 1% to 3% of all patients undergoing shoulder arthroplasties and speculate that this incidence may be increasing.

36. Sanchez-Sotelo J, O'Driscoll S, Morrey BF: Periprosthetic humeral fractures after total elbow arthroplasty: Treatment with implant revision and strut allograft augmentation. *J Bone Joint Surg Am* 2002;84-A:1642-1650.
    The authors of this study report that periprosthetic humeral fractures associated with a loose humeral component can be effectively treated with revision elbow arthroplasty and strut allograft augmentation. The technique is associated with a high rate of fracture union, implant survival, and satisfactory clinical results; however, the complication rate is substantial.

37. O'Driscoll SW, Morrey BF: Periprosthetic fractures about the elbow. *Orthop Clin North Am* 1999;30:319-325.

Chapter 44

Problematic Pediatric Fractures

Susan A. Scherl, MD

David S. Weisman, MD

David M. Scher, MD

Femoral Shaft Fractures in Children

There are many options available to the orthopaedist for the treatment of femoral shaft fractures in children; however, there is no "one-size-fits-all" or "cookbook" treatment algorithm. Treatment guidelines are based on the patient's age and size, fracture location and pattern, and associated injuries or illnesses. The practicing orthopaedist should have a working knowledge of the various treatment modalities and how and when to use them. There should be a high index of suspicion for the possibility of child abuse when a femoral fracture occurs in a nonambulatory child. It has been estimated that up to 70% of femoral fractures in children younger than 1 year of age are the result of abuse.[1]

Treatment options for pediatric femoral shaft fractures include traction (followed by spica casting), immediate spica casting, external fixation, fixation with flexible intramedullary nails (FIMNs) or rigid intramedullary nails, and open reduction and internal fixation (ORIF) with plates and screws. In retrospective studies, all the treatment options have demonstrated good outcomes in terms of fracture union.[2-6] Rates and types of complications vary depending on the treatment used. To date, there has been only one published prospective randomized trial comparing treatment options for femoral shaft fractures in children. This study compared fixation with FIMNs with external fixation and showed superior results in the nailing group.[7] For children between the ages of 2 to 10 years, a bayonet reduction with a 1- to 2-cm overlap at the fracture site traditionally has been recommended to counteract the effects of postfracture bony overgrowth. This treatment choice is still acceptable; however, overgrowth is generally not a complication of flexible intramedullary nailing in which a bayonet reduction is not possible.

Numerous studies have attempted to compare outcomes and costs of the various treatment methods.[8-10] Such studies are difficult to interpret and compare because of their retrospective design and differing definitions of results and costs. Overall results suggest that immediate spica casting is the most cost-effective option, that the various surgical treatments have costs that are comparable to each other and to skeletal traction, and that skeletal traction results in the longest hospital stay and thus has the greatest potential psychologic and social costs.

The Pediatric Orthopaedic Society of North America conducted a survey to determine the preferences of pediatric orthopaedists for various options for treating pediatric femoral fractures.[11] No specific consensus was found; however, there was a trend toward immediate spica casting in children younger than 6 years and for the increasing use of surgical treatment as the patient got older. General treatment guidelines for pediatric femoral fractures are shown in Table 1.

Skeletal Traction

Skeletal traction remains the gold standard in terms of reliability, outcome, and breadth of indication, but its use has decreased with the advent of newer ambulatory treatment options. A distal femoral pin inserted at the condylar flare, proximal to the physes, from medial to lateral is typically used. The use of a proximal tibial pin (as is standard in adults) can lead to physeal damage, ligamentous injury, or knee dislocation in children. The traction position is 90° of flexion at both the hip and knee. The lower leg can be supported on a sling or placed in a short leg cast and suspended by an attached ring. Initial traction weight is 10% of body weight, but no more than 10 lb. Skeletal traction is surprisingly well tolerated in children. Initially, radiographs must be taken every few days to adjust the reduction. Often, a spica cast is applied after initial callus formation. Skeletal traction has wide applicability and is minimally invasive; however, its use can result in prolonged hospitalization, pin site and skin complications, and malalignment (correct positioning requires close attention and follow-up).

Immediate Spica Casting

Immediate spica casting is generally applied with the patient in the human position (90° to 110° flexion, 45° abduction, and 20° external rotation at the hip). The use of a slight valgus mold at the fracture site is often helpful

TABLE 1 | General Treatment Guidelines for Pediatric Femoral Fractures in Children

Age	Treatment
Children younger than 6 years	Immediate spica casting
Children age 6 to 9 years	Surgical treatment with FIMNs should be considered. External fixation is usually reserved for comminuted or open fractures. ORIF can be used in comminuted or very distal or proximal fractures that are not amenable to FIMNs. Traction is always an option.
Children age 10 years and older	Surgical treatment with FIMNs, external fixation, or ORIF. Rigid intramedullary nailing should be reserved for adolescents with closed physes. If rigid nailing must be used in skeletally immature patients, the piriformis fossa entry site should be avoided (entry should be made via the greater trochanter) to decrease the incidence of osteonecrosis of the femoral head. Traction is always an option.

to prevent varus angulation. The application of a long leg cast on the affected side before incorporation into the spica cast can avoid excessive pressure on the popliteal fossa during reduction. One recent retrospective study of immediate spica casting in children younger than 10 years of age found that children older than 7 years were more likely to exhibit unacceptable limb shortening (> 1.5 cm) at 7 to 10 days after casting, which required a change in treatment plan.[12] However, with close attention to detail it is possible to manage older children with this treatment option. Immediate spica casting results in a short hospitalization and is noninvasive. Possible complications of this treatment are loss of reduction or malunion, the development of leg compartment syndrome, skin problems, and the difficulty for both the child and parents to manage the cast.

External Fixation

External fixation is especially useful for the treatment of open fractures. This treatment choice may have a somewhat higher complication rate and lower patient and family acceptance rate than other surgical treatments. The refracture rate after removal of the fixator has been reported to be as high as 22%,[13] although it averages 5% to 10%. Bilateral fractures treated with external fixation may be at particular risk for refracture. Strategies for reducing the refracture rate include early dynamization of the fixator, casting or bracing of the limb after removal, and staged removal of the fixator bar and pins. External fixation is easy to apply and adjust, can overlap reduction, and requires no general anesthetic for removal. Possible complications include refracture, pin site complication (especially infection), scarring, and knee stiffness.

Flexible Intramedullary Nails

FIMNs are indicated primarily for midshaft, transverse, or short oblique fractures without comminution because they confer minimal rotational stability; however, their use is being expanded to more distal and proximal fractures. FIMNs are usually inserted retrograde distally,

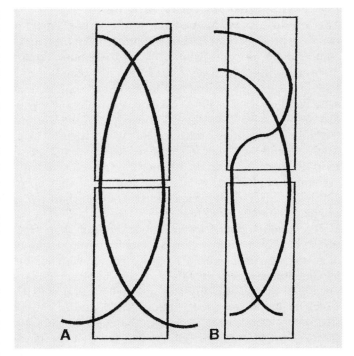

Figure 1 Schematic drawing of a midshaft diaphyseal fracture stabilized with two C-shaped nails **(A)** and one C-shaped and one S-shaped nail **(B)**. *(Reproduced with permission from Kiely N: Mechanical properties of different combinations of flexible nails in a model of a pediatric femoral fracture. J Pediatr Orthop 2002;22:424-427.)*

medially, and laterally at the flare of the femur just proximal to the physis. Antegrade insertion is useful in proximal fractures. When inserted anterograde through the greater trochanter, the lateral nail should be bent into a C shape, and the medial nail into a reverse S shape (Figure 1). One biomechanical study found no difference in the strength between two C-shaped nails inserted distally and one C-shaped and one S-shaped nail inserted proximally, for the treatment of middiaphyseal fractures.[14]

Because the nails function by three-point fixation and tensioning, it is critical to always use two nails of the same diameter, to bend them carefully to ensure tensioning (the apex of the curve should be at the level of the fracture), and to avoid crossing the nails at the fracture site. The use of FIMNs is advantageous because of their ease of insertion and the patient and family acceptance of this treatment. Negative considerations include the need for surgical removal, discomfort at insertion sites, lack of rotational stability, and the possibility of infection. There is a recent report of two patients who had intra-articular nail penetration, which caused synovitis that necessitated nail removal.[15] Results of one study of 43 fractures showed a 49% complication rate, including septic arthritis and a hypertrophic nonunion.[16]

Rigid Intramedullary Nails

Reports of femoral head osteonecrosis with the use of rigid nails inserted through a piriformis fossa entry site has led to the recommendation that rigid nails be avoided in skeletally immature patients.[17] If rigid intramedullary nails must be used, insertion through the greater trochanter is preferable.[18,19] However, there have been reports of both osteonecrosis and premature apophyseal closure with the use of the trochanteric insertion site.[20] Because the angle of insertion through the trochanter is different than through the fossa, some surgeons recommend the use of a humeral nail with its proximal bend to facilitate insertion. Pediatric rigid intramedullary nails, specifically designed for insertion through the trochanter and incorporating a bend, have recently become available. However, rigid intramedullary nailing remains a secondary treatment option in pediatric patients.

Open Reduction and Internal Fixation

Although numerous retrospective studies have shown excellent union and low complication rates with the use of plates and screws,[21,22] this treatment option has historically been used most commonly for femoral fractures in children with head injuries or with multiple injuries in whom casting or prolonged immobilization in traction were undesirable. Large incisions and the need for surgical removal are the disadvantages of this treatment choice; however, newer, minimally invasive plating techniques are being evaluated in children and may increase the use of plate and screw fixation in the future.[23]

Proximal Tibial Fractures in Children

Tibial Intercondylar Eminence Fractures

Tibial intercondylar eminence fractures typically occur as the result of a fall from a bicycle in children between 8 to 14 years of age. The mechanism of injury is forced hyperextension of the knee or a direct blow to the distal femur while the knee is flexed. This scenario produces excess tension on the anterior cruciate ligament, which then causes avulsion of the anterior tibial spine. These injuries are both intra-articular fractures and a childhood analog of an anterior cruciate ligament rupture. Meyers

and McKeever classified tibial intercondylar eminence fractures into three types: type I, nondisplaced; type II, anterior displacement with an intact posterior hinge; and type III, completely displaced. Some authors subdivide type III fractures into IIIA, with displacement only; and IIIB, with rotation in addition to complete displacement.

Type I fractures can be treated with a long leg cast with the knee in 10° to 20° of flexion. Type II fractures generally can be reduced by full extension of the knee and can then be treated in a long leg cast in the same manner as used for type I fractures. Aspiration of the knee hemarthrosis may help in reduction. Most authors agree that type III fractures require surgical reduction and fixation,[24] which historically was achieved through an open arthrotomy. More recently, good results have been shown using arthroscopic techniques.[25-28] Fixation can be achieved with sutures or hardware. Postoperatively, a long leg cast is applied with the knee in slight flexion, and a regimen of quadriceps strengthening is initiated after cast removal. Late, asymptomatic anterior knee laxity often occurs after a tibial eminence fracture, regardless of the method of treatment or quality of reduction.[29,30]

The irreducibility of type III fractures often has been attributed to soft-tissue interposition at the fracture site; however, one arthroscopic study found no soft-tissue or bony interposition in 12 irreducible type III fractures. Attachment of the anterior horn of the lateral meniscus to the fracture fragment was found. Traction on the meniscus aided in fracture reduction.[31]

Apophyseal and Epiphyseal Fractures

Fractures of the proximal tibial apophysis and epiphysis are relatively rare and generally have a good prognosis.[32,33] Tibial tubercle avulsion fractures were classified by Watson-Jones into three types. The classification was later refined by Ogden. Type I fractures occur across the secondary ossification center, at the region of the patellar tendon insertion. Type II fractures occur across the secondary ossification center at the level of the epiphysis, and type III fractures propagate proximally and posteriorly to cross the primary ossification center, and are essentially a Salter-Harris type III fracture of the epiphysis.[34]

These injuries typically occur in adolescent boys near the end of their growth period, and are often associated with jumping sports such as basketball. The mechanism of injury is thought to be forced flexion of the knee during active quadriceps contraction. Associated injuries may include patellar and quadriceps tendon avulsions, collateral and cruciate ligament tears, and meniscal tears. Recently, a patient with a tibial tubercle avulsion with associated lateral plateau rim fracture has been reported.[35]

Treatment of patients with type I tibial tubercle avulsions can be nonsurgical if there is minimal displacement. Most type II and III fractures require ORIF.

Proximal tibial epiphyseal fractures are classified using the Salter-Harris system. As with physeal fractures that occur elsewhere in the skeleton, most type I and II fractures can be treated nonsurgically, whereas most type III and IV fractures (which are intra-articular) require anatomic reduction and fixation. MRI may be useful in the diagnosis and evaluation of these fractures.[36]

Metaphyseal Fractures

Nondisplaced fractures of the proximal tibial metaphysis are prone to late valgus deformity. The mechanism of this occurrence is unknown. The deformity tends to progress for approximately 20 months after injury. Most authors recommend observation rather than surgical intervention for patients who have not reached skeletal maturity because osteotomy before the cessation of growth can result in recurrence of the deformity. Data on the occurrence of spontaneous resolution of deformity are contradictory. Two recent studies (one with 15 and the other with 7 children) reported significant improvement in angular alignment with growth,[37,38] whereas another study with 7 children reported resolution of deformity in only 2 children, both younger than 2 years.[39]

Ankle Fractures in Children

Ankle fractures in children differ somewhat from those in adults because of the presence of the open distal tibial and fibular physes. These fractures account for 5% of pediatric fractures and 15% of physeal injuries in children. Certain physeal injury patterns, such as the triplane and juvenile Tillaux fractures, occur in adolescents as the distal tibial physis is closing. They are therefore sometimes referred to as transitional fractures.

Distal Tibial and Fibular Epiphyseal Fractures

Ankle fractures in children can usually be classified according to the Salter-Harris system. As is typical in physeal injuries, most Salter-Harris type I and II fractures can be treated with closed reduction and casting, whereas most type III and IV fractures require surgical reduction and fixation. Occasionally, periosteal or soft-tissue interposition prevents closed reduction of a distal tibial Salter-Harris type II fracture. When this situation occurs, open reduction is performed with or without internal fixation. If fixation is needed, screws or Kirschner wires across the metaphyseal portion of the distal fracture fragment parallel to the physis can be used. If the physis must be crossed, smooth Kirschner wires should be used to minimize the risk of premature physeal closure.

For Salter-Harris type III and IV ankle fractures, including the transitional fractures, displacement of greater than 2 mm is the accepted criterion for open reduction. CT or MRI can be useful in assessing reduction. If not transitional, these fractures usually involve the medial malleolus. The preferred method of fixation is screws or wires in the epiphysis, distal and parallel to the physis. The risk of growth arrest, although increased in the higher Salter-Harris classification groups, can be significantly decreased with accurate open reduction.[40] Interposed periosteum should be removed from the fracture site, but the periosteum typically does not need to be repaired. One recent study of 24 patients with distal tibial growth disturbance after fracture found that patients with significant deformity were more likely to present late for treatment, have high-energy injuries, be male, and have Salter-Harris type IV or V fractures. Treatment was considered successful in 83% of the patients.[41]

Juvenile Tillaux Fractures

Juvenile Tillaux fractures occur in older adolescents during the time frame in which the anterolateral portion of the physis remains open after closure of the rest of the physis. These are Salter-Harris type III fractures of the anterolateral portion of the distal tibial physis, and occur via a mechanism of avulsion, secondary to the pull of the anteroinferior tibiotalar ligament in external rotation. They require open reduction and fixation (through an anterolateral approach to the ankle) if displaced. CT is helpful in assessing reduction. One cadaveric study found that although both plain films and CT are accurate in showing displacement of Tillaux fractures to within 1 mm, CT is more sensitive for fractures with more than 2 mm of displacement.[42] Because Tillaux fractures occur toward the end of the growth period, significant growth disturbance is uncommon. Articular congruity is the goal of open reduction.

Triplane Fractures

Triplane fractures are complicated three-dimensional fractures that occur in adolescents during the period of distal tibial physeal closure. There are two major triplane patterns: the two-part and three-part fracture (Figure 2). The two-part triplane fracture is a Salter-Harris type IV fracture and the three-part triplane fracture is a combination of Salter-Harris type II and III fractures. The Salter-Harris type III component is essentially a Tillaux fragment. CT scans are very helpful in delineating the fracture patterns and displacement and in preoperative planning for a triplane injury. However, one recent study in England found that only 38% of surgeons typically obtain a CT scan before surgical treatment of a triplane fracture.[43]

As is the case with Tillaux fractures, the growth plate is almost fused, so major growth disturbance is unlikely. The goal of reduction is articular congruity. Attempts at a closed reduction can be made by internally rotating the

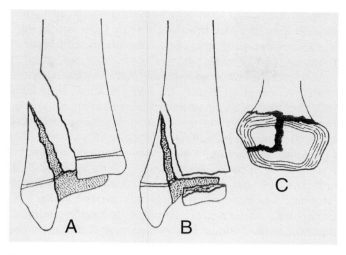

Figure 2 A, A two-part triplane fracture (Salter-Harris type IV). **B** and **C,** A three-part triplane fracture (Salter-Harris types II and III). *(Reproduced from permission from Rockwood CA Jr, Wilkins KE, King RE (eds): Fractures in Children. Philadelphia, PA, JB Lippincott, 1984, pp 1021-1027.)*

foot. This technique often is best done with the patient under general anesthesia. A long leg cast is applied and the reduction is checked by CT. Open reduction proceeds stepwise, initially using an anterolateral approach to the ankle, and adding a posteromedial incision if adequate reduction cannot be achieved from the front. A prospective study of 21 triplane fractures found most (57%) were two-part fractures. In this study, 67% of patients were treated nonsurgically; 95% of patients were pleased with the outcome. By objective measures, 67% of the patients achieved an excellent result.[44]

Proximal Femoral Fractures in Children

Hip fractures in children account for only a small number of pediatric fractures. They are usually associated with high-energy trauma or child abuse.

The proximal femur begins as one physeal anlage that divides into the greater trochanteric apophysis and the capital femoral epiphysis. The blood supply to the femoral head begins through metaphyseal vessels from the neck originating from the medial and lateral circumflex arteries. By the time a child is 4 years of age these metaphyseal vessels contribute little to circulation to the femoral head because the major blood supply now comes from the medial circumflex vessels through the postero-superior and posteroinferior retinacular vessels. The anatomy of the circulation dictates the risk of osteone-crosis because the more proximal the fracture occurs on the femoral neck the greater the likelihood of osteonecrosis.

The Delbet classification system remains the standard system for evaluating proximal femoral fractures. This system divides the fracture patterns into four types: type I, transphyseal (type IA–if the femoral head is dislo-

cated, type IB–if it is not); type II, transcervical; type III, cervicotrochanteric; and type IV, intertrochanteric.

Treatment for proximal femoral fractures involves anatomic reduction and stable internal fixation, usually accompanied by spica casting. In children younger than 2 years of age with a stable reduction of a type I fracture, casting alone is sufficient; however, close radiographic follow-up is mandatory. In the younger child, the fixation method of choice is smooth pins that cross the growth plate. If screws are necessary for fracture fixation in the older adolescent (older than 10 years), the physis may also be crossed as the overall contribution to growth of the proximal femur is 15%, and this growth plate closes earlier than others in the lower extremity. If there is a question of fracture stability, the physis may be crossed when treating children of any age. Even in the most compliant of patients, especially in a younger child, a spica cast should be used to augment the fixation.

Controversy surrounds the need to decompress the capsular hematoma in addition to providing stable fixation.[45,46] It is theorized that the tamponade effect of the hematoma contributes to the incidence of osteonecrosis, which correlates with the level of the fracture and the degree of displacement. It is reasonable to recommend that a simple aspiration could be performed in a child who is anesthetized for fracture reduction. If an open reduction is necessary, the hematoma would also be decompressed. When an open reduction is required, it should be done through an anterolateral approach.

Stress fractures of the proximal femur are rare in pediatric patients. Bone and/or MRI scans may be necessary to identify a stress fracture. Activity modification and protection of the hip are indicated. Fractures that occur before the femoral head ossifies can cause a diagnostic dilemma. These injuries may occur as a result of child abuse or a difficult delivery at birth. The hip will be positioned flexed, internally rotated, and possibly shortened. Ultrasound is an effective tool for identifying these injuries. The differential diagnosis includes infection and hip dysplasia. Patients are treated with closed reduction without hardware if the fracture is stable, and with spica casting.[47] If these fractures are discovered after healing has begun, casting should be continued until healing is complete. Unless the physis closes, there is a tremendous potential for remodeling.

Osteonecrosis is the most serious complication of proximal femoral fractures and occurs in 30% of patients overall. The highest risk for this complication occurs in type I fractures (> 90%), type II fractures (50%), and type III fractures (25%). Type IV fractures are rarely associated with osteonecrosis. Radiographic changes that show osteonecrosis may be present as early as 6 weeks after injury; however, these changes can appear as late as 2 years. MRI can be used for early identification of osteonecrosis. If osteonecrosis is unseen at 6 weeks after injury, it is unlikely to occur. Most children with posttraumatic osteonecrosis have poor results and there is no current treatment that improves their outcome.

Coxa vara is another complication that occurs more commonly with fractures that are not treated with internal fixation. The causes of this complication are malunion or asymmetric physeal closure. Total physeal closure also can occur and is more common when hardware crosses the physis. Depending on the age of the patient, total physeal closure may not contribute to a significant limb-length discrepancy. Nonunion can also occur, but as in adults, it is correlated with the adequacy of the reduction. Chondrolysis is another possible complication and is associated with persistent penetration of hardware.

Pelvic Fractures in Children

Pelvic fractures in children account for only 3% of all fractures and are associated with high-energy injuries except for the isolated avulsion fractures.[48] Most importantly, pelvic fractures can represent a significant soft-tissue trauma. Careful examination of the patient's gastrointestinal, genitourinary, and nervous systems is mandatory. A significant retroperitoneal hematoma caused by a tear to the superior and/or inferior gluteal arteries is the most common life-threatening injury directly related to an unstable pelvic fracture.

The original classification of pediatric pelvic fractures by Torode and Zieg divides these fractures into four types: type I, avulsion fractures; type II, iliac wing fractures; type III, stable ring fractures; and type IV, unstable ring fractures.[49] The Orthopaedic Trauma Association classification system can also be applied: type A, stable; type B, rotationally unstable and vertically stable; and type C, rotationally and vertically unstable.

The three primary ossification centers of the pelvis are the ilium, ischium, and pubis, which all fuse at the triradiate cartilage. The area at which the ischium and pubis fuse (the ischiopubic synchondrosis) can occasionally be mistaken for a fracture. There are multiple secondary ossification centers or apophyses including the iliac crest, ischial tuberosity, and the anterior superior and inferior iliac spine. Avulsion fractures of the secondary ossification centers occur in the following order of frequency: ischial tuberosity (38%), anterior superior iliac spine (32%), anterior inferior iliac spine (18%), lesser trochanter (9%), and iliac apophysis (3%). Symptomatic care is the only treatment that is needed. Crutches are used until comfortable ambulation without assistance is indicated.

Most pediatric pelvic ring fractures are stable and require symptomatic treatment only. Unstable fracture patterns include double vertical rami fractures, double fractures in the pelvic ring (anterior and posterior), and crush injuries producing two fractures in the pelvic ring.[50] These fractures may require traction or external or internal fixation. When external fixation is used to treat a young child, it may be necessary to place the pins anteriorly in line with the anterior iliac spine rather than in the iliac crest because of the potentially thin table of the crest relative to the anterior portion of the ilium.

Characteristics of acetabular fractures based on the Watts classification system are: type 1, small fragments resulting from a dislocation; type 2, linear fracture lines that are nondisplaced; type 3, linear fractures with joint instability; and type 4, central fracture-dislocation. The Orthopaedic Trauma Association classifies acetabular fractures as: type A, single wall/column; type B, both columns with dome attached; and type C, both columns with no dome attachment. As is the case with adults, it is important to obtain a congruous reduction in children; however, in a child it is also necessary to realign the triradiate cartilage to prevent growth arrest. This consideration would apply in any growth plate fracture.

Multiple Trauma

The treatment of a patient with multiple trauma, regardless of age, is based on the priorities of basic life support—airway, breathing, and circulation. After these critical factors have been stabilized, the evaluation of possible injury to other systems is required. Because a fracture is rarely a life-threatening injury, the examination of other systems takes priority in the emergency department.

Transporting a child with a potential head and/or neck injury requires a specialized backboard that allows the patient's neck to extend. Standard backboards, when used for children, will flex the neck because of a child's relatively large head to body ratio when compared with that of an adult. Head injury accounts for most of the morbidity and mortality after trauma.[51] A modified Glasgow Coma Scale is used for the evaluation of children. CT is preferred over MRI to evaluate head trauma because it is almost universally available and provides prompt examination results. The use of CT is indicated if the patient is unconsciousness, has neurologic findings, skull fracture, or cerebrospinal fluid leakage. MRI is effective in evaluating the cervical spine in the unconscious child and is especially useful in the diagnosis of spinal cord injury without radiographic abnormality. If the CT scan shows intracranial swelling, intracranial pressure monitoring is indicated. Cerebral perfusion pressure (mean arterial pressure minus intracranial pressure) is also monitored to maintain a level of at least 60 mm Hg. If surgical intervention is required, the intracranial pressure needs to be monitored to maintain perfusion. Any child with a head injury needs aggressive orthopaedic treatment because the probability for recovery is often good. These children are best treated with fracture fixation, which will allow for mobility and will minimize the risk of late fracture displacement from spasticity.

Abdominal trauma is best evaluated by physical examination of the responsive patient, and by CT in the unconscious patient. The CT scan can show intra-abdominal bleeding from all sources. Peritoneal lavage is not routinely used in children; however, the decision for emergent laparotomy is made based on results of the CT scan.

Thoracic trauma that causes pneumothorax greater than 15% of the lung field on radiographs and/or a hemothorax is treated with a chest tube. If the amount of blood loss exceeds 2 mL/kg/h, a thoracotomy is indicated to control bleeding. Fat embolism resulting from long bone fractures rarely occurs in children, but may be seen in adolescents. If this condition occurs, treatment with respiratory support, as is used for adults, is indicated.

Elbow Fractures in Children

Elbow fractures in children can be challenging to diagnose and treat partly because of the difficulty in visualizing the elbow with conventional radiography. The multiple bony landmark structures around the elbow become visible at different stages of development, beginning with the capitellum at approximately 2 years of age, and followed at approximately 2-year intervals by the radial head, the medial epicondyle, the trochlea, and the lateral epicondyle. To aid in the recognition of subtle injuries and to understand the exact fracture pattern and the nature of the deformity, comparison views of the uninvolved contralateral elbow should be obtained.

Supracondylar Humeral Fractures

Children are prone to supracondylar humeral fractures because the thin area of bone at the level of the olecranon and coronoid fossa is structurally weak. These injuries are divided into extension-type and flexion-type fractures. Extension-type fractures are the most common elbow fractures in children comprising 98% of supracondylar humeral fractures. The generalized ligamentous laxity of children contributes to their vulnerability to extension-type supracondylar fractures. The modified Gartland classification system divides these fractures into type I, nondisplaced fractures; type II, displaced fractures with an angulated but intact posterior cortex and a variable degree of rotation or coronal angulation; and type III, fractures with complete displacement.

Treatment of supracondylar humeral fractures depends primarily on the type of fracture. Type I fractures are routinely treated nonsurgically with splinting or casting for approximately 3 weeks. Because these fractures are nondisplaced or minimally displaced, no reduction is necessary.

There is some controversy surrounding the timing of treatment of type II and III supracondylar humeral fractures. Traditionally type III fractures have been considered orthopaedic emergencies because of the risks associated with treatment delay, such as neurovascular compromise and the need to perform open rather than closed reductions. Several recent studies have challenged the need for emergent treatment of type III fractures. In one study involving treatment delays of more than 8 hours, and in another study in which the mean delay was more than 20 hours, there was no significant increase in the number of complications or need for open reduction.[52,53] It should be noted that in these studies none of the patients had any signs of neurovascular compromise and that some patients with severe displacement underwent a provisional reduction in the emergency department.[54] The authors cautioned that their findings should serve only as guidelines to assist in the triage of patients and in timing surgery to ensure optimal equipment and staff, and not as a reason to delay prompt treatment when needed. Another recent study reported the substantial swelling and high risk for compartment syndrome when supracondylar and ipsilateral forearm fractures coexist, and recommended prompt treatment and a high degree of vigilance when these injuries occur.

Reduction of type II fractures is recommended for patients with angulation greater than 30°. When a line drawn down the anterior humerus (the anterior humeral line) falls in front of the capitellum, reduction is typically indicated. Also, the presence of varus, valgus, and rotation should be noted on the radiographs, which must be true AP and lateral views. Mild malrotation can be compensated for at the shoulder and mild valgus may be cosmetically unnoticeable. Any degree of varus, however, will be cosmetically unsatisfactory and warrants reduction.

Any reduction should be done in a controlled setting, using fluoroscopy, and should then be held with pins. The patient should be under general anesthesia during the surgery. The use of a hyperflexion cast to maintain a closed reduction can lead to severe swelling, compartment syndrome, and neurovascular compromise. Reduction and pinning allows the use of splints or casts in less than 90° of flexion, thereby reducing the risks of complications. Pins are typically placed percutaneously following a closed reduction. For most children, the use of smooth 0.062-inch Kirschner wires is optimal, except in very young children for whom 0.045-inch wires can be used.

Several recent studies have addressed the options for pin configurations, which include crossed medial and lateral pins, two parallel lateral pins, two divergent lateral pins, or one medial and two lateral pins[55-59] (Figure 3). The most stable two-pin configuration in biomechanical testing was medial and lateral pins, followed by divergent lateral pins. Two lateral pins placed with sufficient spread between them (determined to be approximately 1 cm), can usually provide sufficient stability and was not associated with a loss of reduction. The use of medial pins places the ulnar nerve at risk for injury during insertion. The optimal pin configuration should be based

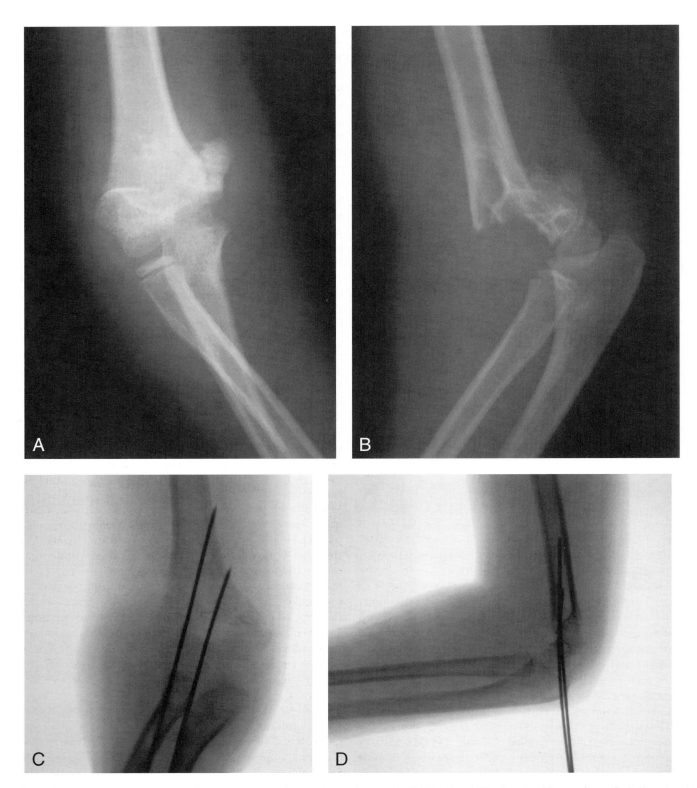

Figure 3 AP **(A)** and lateral **(B)** radiographs of a type III supracondylar humerus fracture. Postoperative AP **(C)** and lateral **(D)** radiographs of the same fracture fixed with two lateral entry pins. Note that the pins are parallel, widely spread, and the more medial pin engages the medial column of the distal humerus.

on the stability of the fracture, the degree of swelling, the fracture pattern, and the prominence of bony landmarks such as the medial epicondyle. Smooth pins should be spread as widely as possible, may be placed through any portion of the distal humeral physis, and may traverse the olecranon fossa if necessary to obtain adequate fixation because the child's arm will be continuously immobilized during the time that the pins are in place. When using a medial pin, making a small incision to place it under direct visualization is recommended.[55,60] Splint or cast immobilization is used for 3 weeks at which point the pins are removed. If the pins are placed percutaneously and remain outside the skin, they can usually be removed in an outpatient setting without the need for anesthesia or sedation.

Lateral Condyle Fractures

Lateral condyle fractures comprise the second most common pediatric elbow fracture. They often occur from a fall on an outstretched hand, which imparts either a varus force pulling the fragment off, or a valgus force pushing the fragment off. These fractures also have been associated with prior supracondylar fractures that healed in varus, thereby increasing the moment of the valgus force.

In addition to standard AP and lateral radiographs, oblique views are useful in making the diagnosis and assessing the displacement. Classifications that are typically used include the system described by Milch, based on the location of the fracture line relative to the trochlea, or by Jakob, which categorizes fractures according to the integrity of the articular surface: intact articular hinge, intra-articular fracture with disruption of the articular hinge, or intra-articular fracture with complete displacement and rotation. More recent studies, however, have divided fractures into stable or unstable based on the amount of displacement or integrity of the cartilaginous epiphysis at the level of the joint.[61,62] Fractures with 2 mm or less of displacement and no translation on any radiographic view are generally considered to be stable. Recent studies have used MRI and ultrasound to visualize the fracture line as it enters the cartilaginous epiphysis[61,62] (Figure 4). If the lateral condyle has an intact cartilaginous hinge and the fracture does not enter the joint, these fractures are deemed stable, less likely to displace, and can usually be treated nonsurgically.

Stable, nondisplaced lateral condyle fractures can be treated in a long arm cast with repeat radiographs taken every 5 to 7 days for the first 1 to 2 weeks to ensure that there is no displacement. Unstable, displaced lateral condyle fractures should be treated with an open reduction through a lateral approach, avoiding posterior dissection, and stabilized with percutaneous pins that are removed in 3 to 4 weeks. This treatment approach should be applied to any fracture with displacement at the articular surface. When there is uncertainty regarding the articu-

lar displacement, adjuvant studies such as MRI or arthrography can be useful. Nondisplaced fractures that are deemed to be unstable, either by MRI, ultrasound, intraoperative arthrography, or clinical judgment, can be managed by percutaneous pinning to prevent displacement or nonunion. Complications and consequences of lateral condyle fractures include lateral spur formation, delayed union or nonunion, cubitus varus or valgus deformity, and osteonecrosis with development of a "fishtail" deformity.

Radial Head and Neck Fractures

Fractures of the proximal radius in children are typically Salter-Harris type II fractures involving the physis and the radial neck. Displaced fractures are evident on routine radiographs, but subtle fractures may be appreciated on radiocapitellar views or inferred based on a posterior fat pad sign along with the appropriate history, signs, and symptoms.[63] Fractures are usually characterized by the Salter-Harris classification system and the degree of displacement and angulation.

Radial neck fractures with 30° or less of angulation and little or no translation can be treated nonsurgically. Fractures with more than 30° of angulation and any fractures with significant translation require manipulation with the patient either sedated or under general anesthesia. Several techniques have been described for fracture reduction in severely displaced fractures. These include the use of a percutaneous Steinmann pin to push the displaced piece up or over, the use of a percutaneous pin to "joystick" the fragment, the use of an intramedullary nail to capture the piece and rotate it onto the radial shaft, or closed manipulation which includes placing a laterally directed force on the proximal radial shaft while concurrently applying a medial force to the radial head.[64-66] After reduction, unstable fractures can be secured with percutaneous pins. Open reduction is reserved for patients with severely displaced fractures that cannot be reduced by closed or percutaneous methods. The consequences of this injury include loss of motion, osteonecrosis, and growth disturbance of the radial head. Displaced intra-articular radial head fractures (Salter-Harris types III and IV) have a poor prognosis and should be reduced anatomically.

Radial and Ulnar Fractures in Children

Fractures of both the radius and ulna in children can occur at any level along the forearm and are generally characterized according to their anatomic location — proximal, midshaft, or distal. Further classification of the fracture is based on the characteristics of the fracture itself including displacement, angulation, translation, rotation, and whether the fracture is open or closed. There is wide variation in the acceptable limits for angulation and rotation; however, angulation becomes less accept-

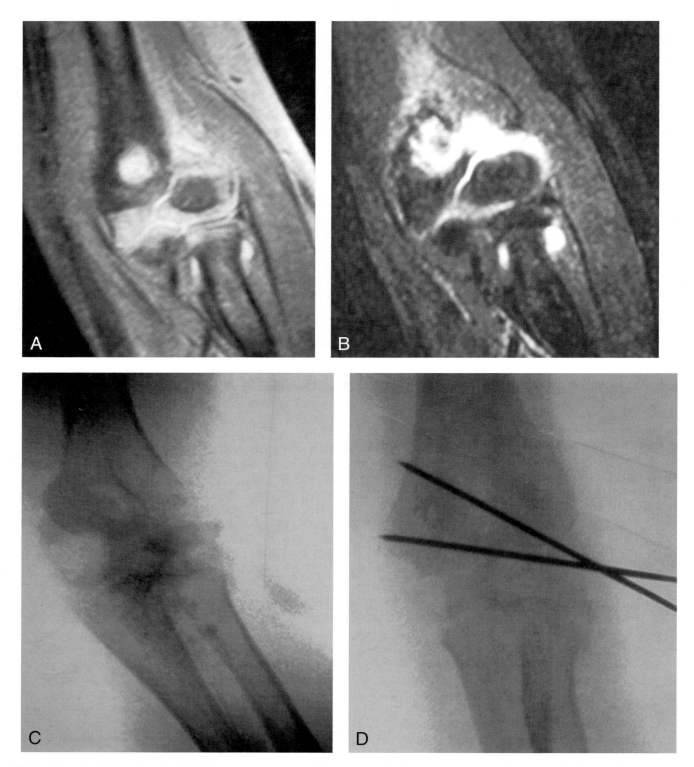

Figure 4 T1-weighted **(A)** and T2-weighted **(B)** MRI scans and an arthrogram **(C)** of a patient with a lateral condyle fracture. **D,** Postoperative AP radiograph of the same patient showing Kirschner wire fixation of the fragment.

able with the increasing age of patients, and most authors consider children older than 10 years to have limited remodeling potential.[67] Because a child's chronologic age might not reflect physiologic maturity, the radio-

graphic presence of the thumb sesamoid can be used to indicate whether the child has limited remodeling potential. Ossification of the thumb sesamoid on an AP radiograph of the hand corresponds with a bone age older than 11 years in girls and 13 years in boys. A closed reduction under adequate analgesia should be attempted. If the fracture is reduced to less then 10° to 20° of angulation, depending on the age of the child, a well-molded long arm cast can be applied and is often split to allow for swelling. An unacceptable reduction warrants a repeat reduction under general anesthesia. An open reduction may be necessary if there is a soft-tissue block to reduction.

The role for fixation of radial and ulnar fractures remains somewhat controversial, but with the frequent application of intramedullary techniques, has recently become more widespread. Indications for internal fixation include failure to maintain a reduction with a cast and a fracture for which there was extensive periosteal stripping (either from the injury or as a result of an open reduction), which consequently destabilizes the fracture. The choices for internal fixation include plates and screws or intramedullary nailing. There have been many recent reports on the successful use of intramedullary fixation with titanium elastic nails, flexible stainless steel wires, or rigid stainless steel rods (for example, Rush pins).[68,69] The advantages of intramedullary fixation include limited dissection, ease of removal, and the theoretical avoidance of complications associated with plate removal, such as refracture and restrictions on athletic participation. A disadvantage is the lack of rotational control, which will often necessitate the use of a cast. It is generally recommended that both bones be stabilized and that the wires or nails be buried beneath the skin. Although the patient must be placed under anesthesia for wire or nail removal, this technique allows the nails or wires to be left in place until there is complete healing without the risk of infection. Reangulation of forearm fractures has been described following early removal of wires.

Annotated References

1. Gross RH, Stranger M: Causative factors responsible for femoral fractures in infants and young children. *J Pediatr Orthop* 1983;3:341-343.

2. Blasier RD, Aronson J, Tursky EA: External fixation of pediatric femur fractures. *J Pediatr Orthop* 1997;17:342-346.

3. Ligier JN, Metaizeau JP, Prevot J, Lascombes P: Elastic stable intramedullary nailing of femoral shaft fractures in children. *J Bone Joint Surg Br* 1988;70:74-77.

4. Sugi M, Cole WG: Early plaster treatment for fractures of the femoral shaft in childhood. *J Bone Joint Surg Br* 1987;69:743-745.

5. Ward WT, Levy J, Kaye A: Compression plating for child and adolescent femur fractures. *J Pediatr Orthop* 1992;12:626-632.

6. Ziv I, Blackburn N, Rang M: Femoral intramedullary nailing in the growing child. *J Trauma* 1984;24:432-434.

7. Bar-On E, Sagiv S, Porat S: External fixation or flexible intramedullary nailing for femoral shaft fractures in children: A prospective, randomised study. *J Bone Joint Surg Br* 1997;79:975-978.

8. Newton PO, Mubarak SJ: Financial aspects of femoral shaft fracture treatment in children and adolescents. *J Pediatr Orthop* 1994;14:508-512.

9. Yandow SM, Archibeck MJ, Stevens PM, Shultz R: Femoral-shaft fractures in children: A comparison of immediate casting and traction. *J Pediatr Orthop* 1999;19:55-59.

10. Stans AA, Morrissy RT, Renwick SE: Femoral shaft fracture treatment in patients age 6 to 16 years. *J Pediatr Orthop* 1999;19:222-228.

11. Sanders JO, Browne RH, Mooney JF, et al: Treatment of femoral fractures in children by pediatric orthopedists: Results of a 1998 survey. *J Pediatr Orthop* 2001;21:436-441.

    In September 1998, members of the Pediatric Orthopedic Society of North America were surveyed to determine their current preferences in treating each of four middle one third femoral fracture patterns in children of four age groups. There was a statistically significant trend by pediatric orthopaedists to surgically treat femoral fractures in older children and to treat younger children nonsurgically. The consensus treatment is age dependent. The development of osteonecrosis in numerous patients after rigid rodding is a concern.

12. Ferguson J, Nicol RO: Early spica treatment of pediatric femoral shaft fractures. *J Pediatr Orthop* 2000;20:189-192.

    This prospective study examined the results of early spica casting in children 10 years or younger who presented with a femoral shaft fracture. The outcome results of 101 femoral shaft fractures treated with early spica casting showed excellent results with few complications.

13. Miner T, Carroll KL: Outcomes of external fixation of pediatric femoral shaft fractures. *J Pediatr Orthop* 2000;20:405-410.

    In this retrospective study, 37 femoral shaft fractures in 33 patients who were treated with unilateral external fixation were reviewed. The rate of refracture (21.6%) after removal of the external fixator was significantly higher than previously reported in literature.

14. Kiely N: Mechanical properties of different combinations of flexible nails in a model of a pediatric femoral fracture. *J Pediatr Orthop* 2002;22:424-427.
    This study compared the mechanical properties of different nail combinations by testing them in a model of a child's midshaft fractured femur. It was concluded that any of the tested nail combinations can be used to treat a midshaft fracture of the femur in a child.

15. Rohde RS, Mendelson SA, Grudziak JS: Acute synovitis of the knee resulting from intra-articular knee penetration as a complication of flexible intramedullary nailing of pediatric femur fractures: Report of two cases. *J Pediatr Orthop* 2003;23:635-638.
    The authors present two cases of acute synovitis of the knee (a previously unreported complication) after intra-articular penetration of the knee joint by migration of a flexible nail.

16. Luhmann SJ, Schootman M, Schoenecker PL, Dobbs MB, Gordeon JE: Complications of titanium elastic nails for pediatric femoral shaft fractures. *J Pediatr Orthop* 2003;23:443-447.
    This retrospective study reviewed 39 patients with femoral shaft fractures whose average age was 6 years. There were 21 complications (1 intraoperative, 20 postoperative) in 43 femoral fractures (49%).

17. Letts M, Jarvis J, Lawton L, Davidson D: Complications of rigid intramedullary rodding of femoral shaft fractures in children. *J Trauma* 2002;52:504-516.
    Results of this retrospective study of 54 patients showed intramedullary rodding to be an effective treatment modality for femoral fractures in skeletally mature children. In children with open femoral physes, rigid rodding should be avoided because of the rare but serious complication of osteonecrosis of the femoral head. Intramedullary rodding is not recommended for children initially treated with external fixation because of the increased risk of infection.

18. Townsend DR, Hoffinger S: Intramedullary nailing of femoral shaft fractures in children via the trochanter tip. *Clin Orthop* 2000;376:113-118.
    No patient developed osteonecrosis of the femoral head in this retrospective review of 34 patients. The trochanteric tip entry point is recommended for closed rigid intramedullary nailing of femoral shaft fractures in children and adolescents.

19. Momberger N, Stevens P, Smith J, Santora S, Scott S, Anderson J: Intramedullary nailing of femoral fractures in adolescents. *J Pediatr Orthop* 2000;20:482-484.
    In this retrospective review, 50 femoral shaft fractures were treated with reamed, interlocking intramedullary nails using a greater trochanteric starting point.

20. Green N, Letts M, Stanitski CL: Debate: A healthy 12-year-old boy with an isolated mid-diaphyseal femur fracture should be treated with an antegrade, locked, intramedullary rod. *J Pediatr Orthop* 2002; 22:821-826.
    The advantages and disadvantages of treatment with an antegrade, locked intramedullary rod are presented.

21. Eren OT, Kucukkaya M, Kockesen C: Kabukcuoglu, Kuzgun U: Open reduction and plate fixation of femoral shaft fractures in children aged 4 to 10. *J Pediatr Orthop* 2003;23:190-193.
    A retrospective review of 40 children aged 4 to 10 years with 46 femoral fractures treated with open reduction and plate fixation is presented.

22. Caird MS, Mueller KA, Puryear A, Farley FA: Compression plating of pediatric femoral shaft fractures. *J Pediatr Orthop* 2003;23:448-452.
    A retrospective review of 60 children younger than 16 years of age with femoral shaft fractures treated with compression plate fixation is presented. Outcomes of compression plate fixation of pediatric femoral fractures compared favorably to results presented in the literature for other treatment options.

23. Agus H, Kalenderer O, Eryanilmaz G, Omeroglu H: Biological internal fixation of comminuted femur shaft fractures by bridge plating in children. *J Pediatr Orthop* 2003;23:184-189.
    Fourteen children (mean age, 11.3 years) with a closed comminuted femoral shaft fracture were surgically treated by biologic internal fixation using a bridging plate. It was concluded that biologic internal fixation by bridge plating was an effective surgical treatment method for closed comminuted fractures of the proximal and distal thirds of the femoral shaft in children.

24. Fehnel DJ, Johnson R: Anterior cruciate injuries in the skeletally immature athlete: A review of treatment outcomes. *Sports Med* 2000;29:51-63.
    The authors recommend arthroscopic or arthroscopically-assisted ORIF with nonabsorbable sutures for the treatment of all displaced tibial eminence fractures.

25. Jung YB, Yum JK, Koo BH: A new method for arthroscopic treatment of tibial eminence fractures with eyed Steinmann pins. *Arthroscopy* 1999;15:672-675.

26. Osti L, Merlo F, Liu SH, Bocchi L: A simple modified arthroscopic procedure for fixation of displaced

tibial eminence fractures. *Arthroscopy* 2000;16:379-382.

A simple modified arthroscopic technique for the fixation of displaced tibial eminence fractures was used in a study of 10 consecutive patients treated for avulsion fractures of the tibial spine since 1991. Results showed a high rate of excellent and good results; no patient had fracture nonunion or related complications.

27. Reynders P, Reynders K, Broos P: Pediatric and adolescent tibial eminence fractures: Arthroscopic cannulated screw fixation. *J Trauma* 2002;53:49-54.

The authors analyzed 26 patients with displaced fractures of the intercondylar eminence of the tibia who were treated with an arthroscopically placed, intrafocal screw with spiked washer. Intrafocal screw fixation for displaced fractures of the intercondylar eminence was found to be a reliable and safe technique, although complete restoration of anteroposterior knee stability was seldom seen.

28. Yip DK, Wong JW, Chien EP, Chan CF: Modified arthroscopic suture fixation of displaced tibial eminence fractures using a suture loop transporter. *Arthroscopy* 2001;17:101-106.

The authors describe a modification of an arthroscopic technique that reduces the reliance on conventional rigid instruments and instead uses a loop transporter made from readily available suture material.

29. Wiley JJ, Baxter MP: Tibial spine fractures in children. *Clin Orthop* 1990;255:54-60.

30. Willis RB, Blokker C, Stoll TM, Patterson DC, Galpin RD: Long-term follow-up of anterior tibial eminence fractures. *J Pediatr Orthop* 1993;13:361-364.

31. Lowe J, Chaimsky G, Freedman A, Zion I, Howard C: The anatomy of tibial eminence fractures: Arthroscopic observations following failed closed reduction. *J Bone Joint Surg Am* 2002;84-A:1933-1938.

Twelve patients who had a failed manipulative reduction of a type III tibial eminence fracture underwent arthroscopic reduction and fixation of the avulsed fragment. The observation that the displaced osseous fragment was attached simultaneously to the anterior cruciate ligament and to the anterior horn of the lateral meniscus, both pulling in different directions, may explain why type III tibial eminence fractures are irreducible by manipulation.

32. Rhemrev SJ, Sleeboom C, Ekkelkamp S: Epiphyseal fractures of the proximal tibia. *Injury* 2000;31:131-134.

Data from 10 patients seen in the past 17 years with an epiphyseal (6) or apophyseal (4) fracture of the proximal tibia were reviewed. The final outcomes for all patients were good.

33. McKoy BE, Stanitski CL: Acute tibial tubercle avulsion fractures. *Orthop Clin North Am* 2003;34:397-403.

This review article examines the treatment of acute tibial tubercle avulsion fractures based on the amount of displacement and associated injuries. Nondisplaced fractures are treated nonsurgically with cast immobilization. Displaced fractures require ORIF. The outcome is usually excellent, even in type III injuries.

34. Ogden JA, Tross RB, Murphy MJ: Fractures of the tibial tuberosity in adolescents. *J Bone Joint Surg Am* 1980;62:205-215.

35. Ozer H, Turanli S, Baltaci G, Tekdemir I: Avulsion of the tibial tuberosity with a lateral plateau rim fracture: Case report. *Knee Surg Sports Traumatol Arthrosc* 2002;10:310-312.

The authors report a case of tibial tuberosity fracture with lateral plateau rim fracture in an adolescent boy, which had not been published previously in the literature. The fracture was treated with ORIF.

36. Close BJ, Strouse PJ: MR of physeal fractures of the adolescent knee. *Pediatr Radiol* 2000;30:756-762.

The authors reviewed 315 consecutive MRI examinations of pediatric knees done to assess traumatic injury. The MRI scans were reviewed for evidence of physeal fracture. Fractures were classified by the Salter-Harris system; associated findings and injuries were noted.

37. McCarthy JJ, Kim DH, Eilert RE: Posttraumatic genu valgum: Operative versus nonoperative treatment. *J Pediatr Orthop* 1998;18:518-521.

38. Tuten HR, Keeler KA, Gabos PG, Zionts LE, MacKenzie WG: Posttraumatic tibia valga in children: A long-term follow-up note. *J Bone Joint Surg Am* 1999;81:799-810.

39. Muller I, Muschol M, Mann M, Hassenplug J: Results of proximal metaphyseal fractures in children. *Arch Orthop Trauma Surg* 2002;122:331-333.

Seven children were retrospectively reexamined by review of their medical records and radiographs. Valgus deformity occurred in all patients after nonsurgical treatment, with partial remodelling was seen only in children up to the age of 5 years.

40. Kay RM, Matthys GA: Pediatric ankle fractures: Evaluation and treatment. *J Am Acad Orthop Surg* 2001;9:268-278.

The authors of this review article concluded that knowledge of common pediatric ankle fracture patterns and the pitfalls associated with their evaluation and treatment will aid the clinician in the effective management of these injuries.

41. Berson L, Davidson RS, Dormans JP, Drummond DS, Gregg JR: Growth disturbances after distal tibial physeal fractures. *Foot Ankle Int* 2000;21:54-58.

Twenty-four patients with distal tibial growth disturbance were reviewed. Patients with angular or linear deformities were more likely to be male, present late for treatment, have high-energy injuries, and have Salter-Harris types IV and V fractures. Early diagnosis and treatment of growth disturbance can prevent severe deformity.

42. Horn BD, Crisci K, Krug M, Pizzutillo PD, MacEwen GD: Radiologic evaluation of juvenile Tillaux fractures of the distal tibia. *J Pediatr Orthop* 2001; 21:162-164.

This study evaluated the accuracy of plain radiographs and CT in assessing juvenile Tillaux fractures of the distal tibia. Because of its sensitivity in detecting fractures displaced more than 2 mm, CT is the preferred imaging modality in the assessment of juvenile Tillaux fractures.

43. Jones S, Phillips N, Ali F, Fernandez JA, Flowers MJ, Smith TW: Triplane fractures of the distal tibia requiring open reduction and internal fixation: Preoperative planning using computed tomography. *Injury* 2003;34:293-298.

CT of triplane fractures provides useful information not available on conventional radiographs. A postal survey of surgeons showed that only 38% always requested CT scans before performing ORIF of displaced triplane fractures.

44. El-Karef E, Sadek HI, Nairn DS, Aldam CH, Allen PW: Triplane fracture of the distal tibia. *Injury* 2000; 31:729-736.

A prospective study of 21 triplane fractures of the distal tibia is presented. Objectively, 14 patients (67%) achieved excellent results.

45. Cheng JC, Tang N: Decompression and stable internal fixation of femoral neck fractures in children can affect the outcome. *J Pediatr Orthop* 1999;19:338-343.

46. Ng GP, Cole WG: Effect of early hip decompression on the frequency of avascular necrosis in children with fractures of the neck of the femur. *Injury* 1996; 27:419-421.

47. Hughes LO, Beaty JH: Fractures of the head and neck of the femur in children. *J Bone Joint Surg Am* 1994;76:283-292.

48. Silber JS, Flynn JM, Koffler KM, Dormans JP, Drummond DS: Analysis of the cause, classification and associated injuries of 166 consecutive pediatric pelvic fractures. *J Pediatr Orthop* 2001;21:446-450.

The authors reviewed 166 patients with pelvic fractures; 60% had multisystem injury, 50% had additional skeletal injury, and 3.6% sustained fatal injuries caused by head or visceral trauma. Anterior ring fractures were the most common. Urethral injuries were not commonly seen.

49. Blasier RD, McAtee J, White R, Mitchell DT: Disruption of the pelvic ring in pediatric patients. *Clin Orthop* 2000;376:87-95.

This article presents a retrospective review of 189 patients with pelvic fractures; 57 of the fractures were unstable. Of those available for evaluation of their treatment, 13 had been treated surgically and 30 nonsurgically. Good to excellent outcomes reported by the surgically treated patients compared to the nonsurgically treated patients were 92% versus 80%, respectively.

50. Torode I, Zeig D: Pelvic fractures in children. *J Pediatr Orthop* 1985;5:76-84.

51. Yian EH, Gullaorn LJ, Loder RT: Scoring of pediatric orthopaedic polytrauma: Correlations of different injury scoring systems and prognosis for hospital course. *J Pediatr Orthop* 2000;20:203-209.

This study compared the Trauma Score, Revised Trauma Score, Injury Severity Score, Modified Abbreviated Injury Severity Score, Pediatric Trauma Score, and TRISS-b survival statistic in 91 patients. The Trauma Score and TRISS-b were useful in predicting the prolonged need for a ventilator and complications of immobilization. The authors recommend surgical fracture treatment if prolonged days in the intensive care unit or using a ventilator are predicted.

52. Cramer KE: The pediatric polytrauma patient. *Clin Orthop* 1995;318:125-135.

53. Leet AI, Frisancho J, Ebramzadeh E: Delayed treatment of type 3 supracondylar humerus fractures in children. *J Pediatr Orthop* 2002;22:203-207.

This study is a retrospective review of 158 patients with type III supracondylar humeral fractures who presented to a tertiary care medical center with an average of 9.8 hours from injury to presentation and 21.3 hours from injury to surgical treatment. All extremities had closed injuries and were well-perfused at initial assessment. The authors found no correlation between increasing time to surgical intervention and poor outcome. Factors evaluated included longer surgical time, increased length of hospital stay, need to open the fracture, pin infection, greater than 15° of loss of motion, loss of carry angle, neurapraxia, and retained hardware.

54. Mehlman CT, Strub WM, Roy DR, Wall EJ, Crawford AH: The effect of surgical timing on the perioperative complications of treatment of supracondylar humeral fractures in children. *J Bone Joint Surg Am* 2001;83-A:323-327.

This article presents a retrospective comparison of two groups of patients with displaced supracondylar humerus fractures. One group was treated early (8 hours or less from the time of injury) and one group was treated late (more than 8 hours from the time of injury). There was no difference in the rate of perioperative complications between the two groups.

55. Gordon JE, Patton CM, Luhmann SJ, Bassett GS, Schoenecker PL: Fracture stability after pinning of displaced supracondylar distal humerus fractures in children. *J Pediatr Orthop* 2001;21:313-318.

The authors of this retrospective study of 138 patients evaluated the ability of three different pin configurations to maintain a reduction until healing. The pin configurations used were (1) two lateral pins, (2) one medial and one lateral pin, and (3) one medial and two lateral pins. The authors recommended using two lateral pins for all type II and type III fractures and adding a medial pin when rotational instability is detected after placing two lateral pins. The authors also described a radiographic technique to help make this assessment.

56. Lee SS, Mahar AT, Miesen D, Newton PO: Displaced pediatric supracondylar humerus fractures: Biomechanical analysis of percutaneous pinning techniques. *J Pediatr Orthop* 2002;22:440-443.

The authors of this study conducted biomechanical testing of three different pin configurations for a simulated supracondylar humeral fracture using a synthetic bone model. Divergent lateral pins were found to be comparable or superior to parallel lateral pins and crossed pins for all modes of testing (except axial rotation, for which crossed pins were superior).

57. Skaggs DL, Hale JM, Bassett J, Kaminsky C, Kay RM, Tolo VT: Operative treatment of supracondylar fractures of the humerus in children: The consequences of pin placement. *J Bone Joint Surg Am* 2001;83:735-740.

This retrospective review of 345 extension-type supracondylar humeral fractures was conducted to evaluate the maintenance of reduction using either lateral pins alone or crossed pins. The authors reported no loss of reduction with either pin configuration, but the use of crossed pins was associated with ulnar nerve injury. The risk of ulnar nerve injury was increased when the medial pin was inserted with the elbow hyperflexed. The authors did not recommend routine use of a medial pin and cautioned that when one is used the elbow should not be hyperflexed during insertion.

58. Skaggs DL, Cluck MW, Mostofi A, Flynn JM, Kay RM: Lateral entry pin fixation in the management of supracondular fractures in children. *J Bone Joint Surg Am* 2004;86:702-707.

The authors of this study investigated the adequacy of a lateral pin configuration in maintaining fracture reduction by evaluating a consecutive series of patients treated exclusively with lateral pins, thereby removing selection bias. There was no significant loss of reduction in this series and no nerve injury. The authors emphasized the use of the term "lateral-entry pin" rather than "lateral pin" because these pins begin laterally but should engage the medial column of the distal humerus just proximal to the fracture. They also made the following recommendations for optimal pin placement: pin separation at the fracture site, engagement of the medial and lateral columns of the distal humerus in the region just proximal to the fracture, engagement of sufficient bone in the proximal-medial and distal-lateral portions of the fragments, and use of a third lateral pin when necessary to ensure sufficient fixation.

59. Zionts LE, McKellop HA, Hathaway R: Torsional strength of pin configurations used to fix supracondylar fractures of the humerus in children. *J Bone Joint Surg Am* 1994;76:253-256.

60. Green DW, Widmann RF, Frank JS, Gardner MJ: Low incidence of ulnar nerve injury with crossed pin placement for pediatric supracondylar humerus fractures using a mini-open technique. *J Orthop Trauma* 2005;19:158-163.

The authors describe a mini-open technique for medial pin placement that involves direct visualization of the medial epicondyle during pin insertion. In this series, no permanent ulnar nerve injuries occurred, and one patient had transient sensory neuropathy that resolved in 1 week. The authors recommend the use of a crossed pin configuration for rotationally unstable fracture and suggest that this technique be used for insertion of the medial pin.

61. Horn BD, Herman MJ, Crisci K, Pizzutillo PD, MacEwen GD: Fractures of the lateral humeral condyle: Role of the cartilage hinge in fracture stability. *J Pediatr Orthop* 2002;22:8-11.

In this study, MRI was used to determine fracture stability of lateral condyle fractures based on the integrity of the articular cartilage. The authors found that MRI accurately demonstrated the extent of the fracture within the chondroepiphysis and the presence of intra-articular extension of the fracture, allowing categorization of fractures as stable or unstable. In the one instance in which a fracture had been presumed stable based on radiographic evidence and then subsequently displaced, the MRI scan demonstrated that the articular hinge was in fact disrupted. The authors concluded that MRI can be useful to clarify the stability of some fractures in the absence of clear evidence on conventional radiographs.

62. Vocke-Hell AK, Schmid A: Sonographic differentiation of stable and unstable lateral condyle fractures of the humerus in children. *J Pediatr Orthop B* 2001; 10:138-141.

High-resolution ultrasound was used to successfully visualize the extension of lateral condyle fractures into the chondroepiphysis in six children. The authors report that this method is a rapid and inexpensive method of characterizing the stability of a lateral condyle fracture without the need for sedation.

63. Skaggs DL, Mirzayan R: The posterior fat pad sign in association with occult fracture of the elbow in children. *J Bone Joint Surg Am* 1999;81:1429-1433.

64. Metaizeau JP, Lascombes P, Lemelle JL, Finlayson D, Prevot J: Reduction and fixation of displaced radial neck fractures by closed intramedullary pinning. *J Pediatr Orthop* 1993;13:355-360.

65. Neher CG, Torch MA: New reduction technique for severely displaced pediatric radial neck fractures. *J Pediatr Orthop* 2003;23:626-628.

    The authors describe a technique for closed reduction of radial neck fractures that emphasizes placing a laterally (radially) directed force on the radial shaft.

66. Schmittenbecher PP, Haevernick B, Herold A, Knorr P, Schmid E: Treatment decision, method of osteosynthesis, and outcome in radial neck fractures in children: A multicenter study. *J Pediatr Orthop* 2005;25:45-50.

    This study assessed a case series of patients from several different institutions who underwent internal fixation for the treatment of displaced radial neck fractures after both closed and open reductions. Most of the patients who required a reduction underwent elastic stable intramedullary nailing (23 patients), and three patients had Kirschner wire fixation. Seventy-eight percent of the patients who underwent elastic stable intramedullary nailing had good or excellent results, but 22% had fair or poor results because of restriction of forearm rotation. The results of open reduction were worse independent of the method of fixation.

67. Wyrsch B, Mencio GA, Green NE: Open reduction and internal fixation of pediatric forearm fractures. *J Pediatr Orthop* 1996;16:644-650.

68. Shoemaker SD, Comstock CP, Mubarak SJ, Wenger DR, Chambers HG: Intramedullary Kirschner wire fixation of open or unstable forearm fractures in children. *J Pediatr Orthop* 1999;19:329-337.

69. Lee S, Nicol RO, Stott NS: Intramedullary fixation for pediatric unstable forearm fractures. *Clin Orthop Relat Res* 2002;402:245-250.

    The authors of this study conducted a retrospective review of 49 patients with radial and ulnar fractures that were treated surgically using intramedullary fixation of one or both bones. Approximately one third of the patients who had intramedullary fixation of the ulna alone had a loss of reduction in the first several weeks after surgery. The authors also reported that two patients had progressive angulation of fractures after early removal of wires that had been placed percutaneously. They concluded that surgical management of radial and ulnar fractures in children using intramedullary fixation should consist of fixation of both bones and the tips of the wires or nails should be buried to prevent the need for early removal.

Index

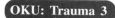